NON-NEOPLASTIC ADVANCED LUNG DISEASE

LUNG BIOLOGY IN HEALTH AND DISEASE

Executive Editor

Claude Lenfant
Director, National Heart, Lung, and Blood Institute
National Institutes of Health
Bethesda, Maryland

ADDITIONAL VOLUMES IN PREPARATION

The opinions expressed in these volumes do not necessarily represent the views of the National Institutes of Health.

NON-NEOPLASTIC ADVANCED LUNG DISEASE

Edited by

Janet R. Maurer
Hartford, Connecticut, U.S.A.

MARCEL DEKKER, INC.   NEW YORK · BASEL

Library of Congress Cataloging-in-Publication Data
A catalog record for this book is available from the Library of Congress.

ISBN: 0-8247-4077-7

This book is printed on acid-free paper.

Headquarters
Marcel Dekker, Inc.
270 Madison Avenue, New York, NY 10016
tel: 212-696-9000; fax: 212-685-4540

Eastern Hemisphere Distribution
Marcel Dekker AG
Hutgasse 4, Postfach 812, CH-4001 Basel, Switzerland
tel: 41-61 260-6300; fax: 41-61-260-6333

World Wide Web
http://www.dekker.com

The publisher offers discounts on this book when ordered in bulk quantities. For more information, write to Special Sales/Professional Marketing at the headquarters address above.

Current printing (last digit):
10 9 8 7 6 5 4 3 2 1

PRINTED IN THE UNITED STATES OF AMERICA

INTRODUCTION

Both today's medicine and our hope for medicine in the future are dominated by genetic research and the expectation that the discovery of genes, and the understanding of their function and regulation, will improve public health considerably. Many lung diseases are candidates for such benefits.

Although genomic research and gene discovery are progressing swiftly, the application of this new knowledge to the practice of medicine remains sparse, spotty, and slow. Meanwhile, for a variety of reasons, the prevalence of lung diseases has increased and their treatment remains largely palliative. Many lung diseases are chronic conditions that progress over long periods of time and often culminate unavoidably in a fatal outcome. Fortunately, there are many approaches that are available to care quite effectively for these patients. They include medical and surgical interventions as well as pharmacological, rehabilitative, and behavioral regimens.

Because this volume presents all of these approaches, and describes how they can be applied depending on the specific pathology, this is truly a book for the physician clinician. The editor, Janet Maurer, and the contributors are themselves individuals who care for patients. The readership will be reminded of the many options from which the patients can, and will, benefit.

As the Executive Editor of the Lung Biology in Health and Disease series, I welcome the opportunity to introduce this volume.

Claude Lenfant, M.D.
Bethesda, Maryland

PREFACE

In the late 1980s, the emergence of lung transplantation as a therapeutic option for patients with a variety of end-stage lung diseases focused attention on this disparate group of suffering but often minimally managed patients. Transplant teams working with potential lung-transplant candidates discovered that much could be done to improve the lives of these patients, even though their diseases were advanced and irreversible. It became clear that certain simple interventions—e.g., pulmonary rehabilitation and oxygen—could greatly improve a patient's life. It also became clear that the disparate physiologies of different end-stage diseases made it necessary to tailor interventions to each specific disease. Thus this text contains sections on the pathologies and physiologies of different end-stage processes as well as the state-of-the-art medical management of these processes.

The other aspect of managing chronically ill patients that is nearly always a factor in their function and survival is their social and mental health. It is not possible to optimally treat a patient with advanced disease without bringing these issues into focus and addressing them directly; thus the section on quality of life. Part of this, of course, involves assisting patients and their families in preparing for a patient's death and the disruption that this will cause for everyone.

An aging population in the setting of high-technology health care means that an increasing number of patients will live long lives with severe chronic illness. This text is designed to assist those who care for these patients in treating their lung disease, their age- and risk-factor-related comorbidities, and their quality of life.

Janet R. Maurer

CONTRIBUTORS

Susan E. Abbey, M.D., F.R.C.P.C. Associate Professor, Department of Psychiatry, University of Toronto, and Director, Program in Medical Psychiatry, University Health Network, Toronto, Ontario, Canada

Loutfi Sami Aboussouan, M.D., F.C.C.P. Associate Professor, Division of Pulmonary, Critical Care, and Sleep Medicine, Department of Medicine, Wayne State University School of Medicine, Detroit, Michigan, U.S.A.

Vivek N. Ahya, M.D. Assistant Professor, Pulmonary, Allergy, and Critical Care Division, Department of Medicine, University of Pennsylvania School of Medicine, and University of Pennsylvania Medical Center, Philadelphia, Pennsylvania, U.S.A.

Fortune O. Alabi, M.D. Senior Staff, Division of Pulmonary and Critical Care Medicine, Department of Medicine, Henry Ford Hospital, Detroit, Michigan, U.S.A.

Robert M. Aris, M.D. Associate Professor, Division of Pulmonary Medicine, Department of Medicine, University of North Carolina at Chapel Hill, Chapel Hill, North Carolina, U.S.A.

William R. Auger, M.D. Professor, Department of Internal Medicine, University of California, San Diego, San Diego Medical Center, San Diego, California, U.S.A.

Robyn J. Barst, M.D. Department of Pediatric Cardiology, Columbia University College of Physicians and Surgeons, New York, New York, U.S.A.

Sue. A Brown, M.D. Assistant Professor, Division of Endocrinology, Department of Medicine, University of North Carolina at Chapel Hill, Chapel Hill, North Carolina, U.S.A.

Francis C. Cordova, M.D. Assistant Professor, Division of Pulmonary and Critical Care Medicine, Department of Medicine, Temple University School of Medicine, and Temple Lung Center, Philadelphia, Pennsylvania, U.S.A.

Eva C. Creutzberg, Ph.D. Department of Pulmonology, University Hospital Maastricht, Maastricht, The Netherlands

Gerard J. Criner, M.D. Professor and Director, Division of Pulmonary and Critical Care Medicine, Department of Medicine, Temple University School of Medicine, and Temple Lung Center, Philadelphia, Pennsylvania, U.S.A.

Jim J. Egan, M.D., F.R.C.P.I., F.R.C.P. Medical Director, Advanced Lung Disease, and Irish National Lung Transplant Program, Mater Misericordiae Hospital and St. Vincent s University Hospitals, Dublin, Ireland

Carol F. Farver, M.D. Staff Pathologist, Department of Anatomic Pathology, Cleveland Clinic Foundation, Cleveland, Ohio, U.S.A.

Peter F. Fedullo, M.D. Professor, Division of Pulmonary and Critical Care Medicine, Department of Medicine, University of California, San Diego, and Director, Medical Intensive Care Unit, San Diego Medical Center, San Diego, California, U.S.A.

Stanley B. Fiel, M.D. Professor and Chief, Division of Pulmonary and Critical Care Medicine, Department of Medicine, Drexel University College of Medicine, Philadelphia, Pennsylvania, U.S.A.

Kevin R. Flaherty, M.D., M.S. Assistant Professor, Division of Pulmonary and Critical Care Medicine, Department of Medicine, University of Michigan, Ann Arbor, Michigan, U.S.A.

Adaani E. Frost, M.D., F.R.C.P.(C) Professor, Division of Pulmonary and Critical Care Medicine, Department of Medicine, Baylor College of Medicine, Houston, Texas, U.S.A.

Sean P. Gaine, M.D., Ph.D., F.R.C.P.I. Consultant Respiratory Physician, Department of Respiratory Medicine, University College Dublin, and Mater Misericordiae Hospital, Dublin, Ireland

Steven E. Gay, M.D. Clinical Assistant Professor, Division of Pulmonary and Critical Care Medicine, Department of Medicine, University of Michigan, Ann Arbor, Michigan, U.S.A.

John Hansen-Flaschen, M.D. Professor and Chief, Pulmonary, Allergy and Critical Care Division, Department of Medicine, University of Pennsylvania School of Medicine, Philadelphia, Pennsylvania, U.S.A.

Stuart W. Jamieson, M.B., F.R.C.S. Professor and Head, Division of Cardiothoracic Surgery, Department of Surgery, University of California, San Diego, San Diego Medical Center, San Diego, California, U.S.A.

Paul W. Jones, Ph.D., F.R.C.P. (Lond) Professor of Respiratory Medicine, Department of Physiological Medicine, St. George's Hospital Medical School, London, England

David P. Kapelanski, M.D., F.A.C.S. Clinical Professor, Division of Cardiothoracic Surgery, Department of Surgery, University of California, San Diego, San Diego Medical Center, San Diego, California, U.S.A.

J. Michael Kay, M.D., F.R.C.P.C., F.R.C.Path. Professor Emeritus, Department of Pathology and Molecular Medicine, McMaster University, Hamilton, Ontario, Canada

Kim M. Kerr, M.D. Assistant Professor, Division of Pulmonary and Critical Care Medicine, Department of Medicine, University of California, San Diego, San Diego Medical Center, San Diego, California, U.S.A.

Joseph P. Lynch III, M.D. Professor, Division of Pulmonary and Critical Care Medicine, Department of Medicine, University of Michigan, Ann Arbor, Michigan, U.S.A.

Donald A. Mahler, M.D. Professor, Department of Medicine, Dartmouth Medical School, Lebanon, New Hampshire, U.S.A.

Fernando J. Martinez, M.D., M.S. Professor, Division of Pulmonary and Critical Care Medicine, Department of Medicine, University of Michigan, Ann Arbor, Michigan, U.S.A.

Janet R. Maurer, M.D., M.B.A., A.B.I.M., F.R.C.P.(C), F.C.C.P. Senior Medical Director, Lifesource, CIGNA HealthCare, Hartford, Connecticut, U.S.A.

Francis X. McCormack, M.D. Associate Professor, Division of Pulmonary and Critical Care Medicine, Department of Internal Medicine, University of Cincinnati School of Medicine, Cincinnati, Ohio, U.S.A.

Edward Moloney, M.D. Adult Intensive Care Unit, Imperial College School of Medicine, National Heart and Lung Institute, and Royal Brompton Hospital, London, England

Denis E. O'Donnell, M.D., F.R.C.P.(I), F.R.C.P.(C) Professor and Head, Division of Respiratory and Critical Care Medicine, Department of Medicine, Queen's University, Kingston, Ontario, Canada

David A. Ontjes, M.D. Professor, Division of Endocrinology, Department of Medicine, University of North Carolina at Chapel Hill, Chapel Hill, North Carolina, U.S.A.

Annemie M. W. J. Schols, Ph.D. Department of Pulmonology, University Hospital Maastricht, Maastricht, The Netherlands

James K. Stoller, M.D., M.S. Vice Chairman, Division of Medicine; Associate Chief of Staff and Head, Section of Respiratory Therapy; and Professor, Department of Pulmonary and Critical Care Medicine, Cleveland Clinic Foundation, Cleveland, Ohio, U.S.A.

Gregory Tino, M.D. Associate Professor, Pulmonary, Allergy, and Critical Care Division, Department of Medicine, and Director, Pulmonary Outpatient Practices, University of Pennsylvania School of Medicine, and University of Pennsylvania Medical Center, Philadelphia, Pennsylvania, U.S.A.

Joseph F. Tomashefski, Jr., M.D. Professor, Department of Pathology, Case Western Reserve University School of Medicine, and Chair, Department of Pathology, MetroHealth Medical Center, Cleveland, Ohio, U.S.A.

Nha Voduc, M.D., F.R.C.P. Clinical Fellow, Division of Respirology and Critical Care Medicine, Department of Medicine, Queen's University, Kingston, Ontario, Canada

Idelle M. Weisman, M.D. Chief, Department of Clinical Investigation, Pulmonary Critical Care Service, William Beaumont Army Medical Center, El Paso, and Clinical Professor, Division of Pulmonary and Critical Care

Medicine, University of Texas Health Science Center at San Antonio, San Antonio, Texas, U.S.A.

Allison C. Widlitz, M.S., P.A. Department of Pediatric Cardiology, Columbia University College of Physicians and Surgeons, New York, New York, U.S.A.

Emiel F. M. Wouters, Ph.D. Department of Pulmonology, University Hospital Maastricht, Maastricht, The Netherlands.

CONTENTS

NON-NEOPLASTIC
ADVANCED
LUNG DISEASE

1

Pathology of Advanced Obstructive Lung Disease
Emphysema, Chronic Bronchitis, Bronchiolitis Obliterans, and Bronchiectasis

JOSEPH F. TOMASHEFSKI, JR.

Case Western Reserve University School of Medicine
and MetroHealth Medical Center
Cleveland, Ohio, U.S.A.

I. Introduction

Diseases of chronic airflow obstruction (CAO) can be separated into two major categories: (1) emphysema, a destructive process of lung parenchyma, and (2) diseases of large and small airways. CAO is one of the most important causes of chronic respiratory failure and a leading indication for lung transplantation. In this chapter the pathological anatomy of four major pathways of CAO are considered: emphysema, chronic bronchitis, bronchiolitis obliterans, and bronchiectasis. In each condition, morphological features are correlated with the pathogenesis and physiological parameters of deranged lung function.

II. Emphysema

Pulmonary emphysema is a process in which expansion of distal airspaces is the result of alveolar septal destruction without obvious fibrosis (1). The consequence of this slowly evolving remodeling of lung architecture is a hyperinflated, overly compliant organ having a markedly diminished number of greatly dilated and simplified gas exchanging units. There are two important and distinctive anatomical variants of emphysema, suggesting unique

1

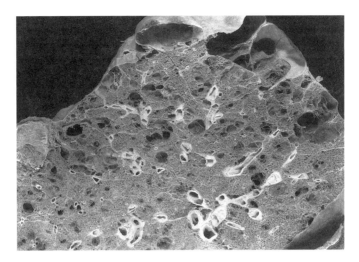

Figure 3 Moderate centriacinar emphysema with apical bulla (Reid type II). (Barium sulfate impregnation.)

Panacinar emphysema, in contrast, denotes uniform destruction of the entire acinus and lobule, tends to be more diffusely distributed, and is the variant of emphysema most common in homozygous alpha$_1$-antitrypsin deficiency (3,9). Grossly, panacinar emphysema imparts a marked loss of consistency to the lung parenchyma, which is replaced by uniformly dilated

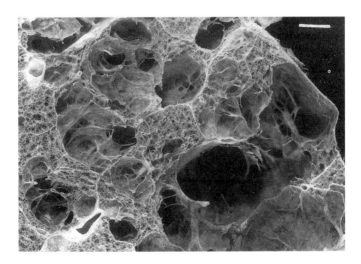

Figure 4 Confluent centriacinar emphysema. Emphysematous lesions are interspersed with islands of relatively preserved parenchyma. (Barium sulfate impregnation; scale equals 0.5 cm.)

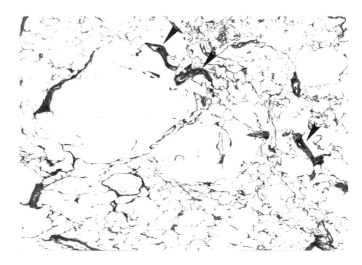

Figure 5 Centriacinar emphysema. Respiratory bronchiole is destroyed. Note sclerotic pulmonary artery branches (arrowheads) and apparently detached alveolar septa.

airspaces with enlarged interalveolar fenestrae (Fig. 6) (10). In advanced emphysema of alpha$_1$-antitrypsin deficiency, the lower lobe tends to be more severely involved, but all lobes are significantly affected (9). Panacinar emphysema can also be regional and confined to part of a lobe. Histologically

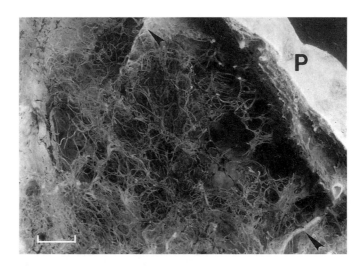

Figure 6 End-stage panacinar emphysema. Emphysematous airspaces completely efface secondary lobules. Remnants of interlobular septa (arrowheads) extend from visceral pleura (p). (Barium sulfate impregnation; scale equals 1 cm.)

panacinar emphysema exhibits diffuse, extreme loss of alveolar tissue, with negligible fibrosis. In both panacinar and centriacinar emphysema, alveolar septal attachments to small airways are reduced (Fig. 7) (11). Panacinar emphysema is also caused by cigarette smoke; frequently, mixtures of panacinar and centriacinar emphysema are seen in the same lung, with one form predominating (12). Morphometric assessment of the internal surface area (ISA) of the lung and the surface area per unit volume correlates inversely with the anatomical extent of emphysema, regardless of the histological subtype (13).

A unique form of panacinar emphysema afflicts intravenous drug abusers who chronically inject aqueous suspensions of talc-containing pharmaceutical tablets (14,15). Histologically, numerous brightly birefringent interstitial talc particles are associated with mild perivascular fibrosis and panacinar emphysema (15) (Figs. 8 and 9). Individuals with talc-induced emphysema progress from predominantly restrictive to severe obstructive lung disease, with increased residual volume, decreased FEV_1/FVC ratio, and decreased DL_{CO} (14). The mechanism by which foreign-body microemboli induce emphysema may relate to repeated episodes of intracapillary neutrophil sequestration and release of inflammatory mediators and proteases (16).

The small pulmonary artery branches in severe emphysema usually exhibit morphological signs of pulmonary hypertension. Vascular remodeling includes arterial and venous medial muscle hypertrophy and intimal fibrosis, with longitudinally oriented arterial subintimal smooth muscle cells (Fig. 5) (17). Smooth muscle is also seen to extend into normally nonmuscularized

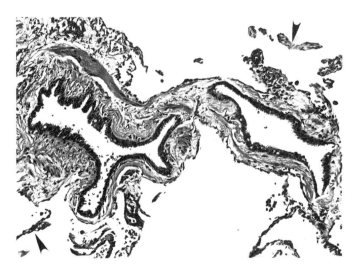

Figure 7 Panacinar emphysema. Two membranous bronchioles, nearly devoid of alveolar septal attachments, reside in emphysematous airspaces. "Apparently detached" septa (arrowheads) are a histological marker of emphysema.

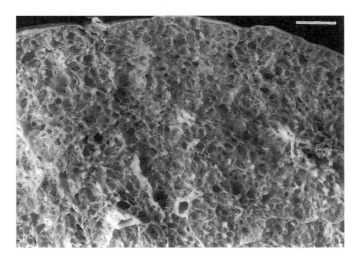

Figure 8 Intravenous drug abuse with diffuse, uniform, fine panacinar emphysema. (Barium sulfate impregnation; scale equals 0.5 cm.)

arteries (17). The cause of these vascular changes is thought to be chronic hypoxia and sustained vasoconstriction (18). Because of its large reserve, loss of the pulmonary capillary bed in emphysema makes only a minor contribution to pulmonary hypertension and right ventricular hypertrophy.

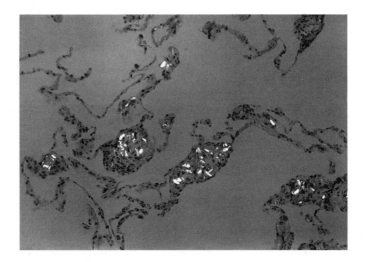

Figure 9 Diffusely emphysematous airspaces associated with interstitial perivascular deposits of birefringent talc particles, accompanied by mild fibrosis (partially polarized light).

A. Emphysematous Bullae

A *bulla* is a ballon-like emphysematous airspace, at least 1 cm in diameter, usually located in close proximity to the visceral pleura. In contrast, a *bleb* represents loculated air that has dissected into the interstitial compartment of the visceral pleura (19). Reid has defined three morphological types of emphysematous bullae: a narrow-necked bulla that protrudes above the pleural surface of the excised lung (type I); a broad-based bulla that extends superficially into the underlying lung parenchyma (type II) (Fig. 3); and the giant bulla, which reaches deeply into the underlying lung, replacing a major portion of the lobe (type III) (Fig. 10) (19). Type III bullae are frequently associated with respiratory compromise due to compression of adjacent lung tissue. Bullae may be seen in any of the morphological variants of emphysema. The term *bullous emphysema* generically refers to any anatomical subtype of emphysema in which bullae are prominent.

B. Clinicopathological Correlations

Panacinar and centriacinar emphysema usually cannot be distinguished on the basis of symptoms, pulmonary function tests or conventional chest x-rays (20). Physiological parameters of airflow obstruction and increased lung volumes are seen in both variants. The correlation between lung function tests and anatomical severity of emphysema is variable and tends to be nonlinear (20). Using excised lungs, Pratt and colleagues demonstrated marked air trapping and diminished expiratory flow in symptomatic patients with panacinar emphysema and, in nonsymptomatic patients, increased total lung capacity (TLC) with only mildly decreased flow rates and air trapping (21,22). In lungs with centriacinar emphysema, increasing TLC was observed with increasing extent of emphysema. Elevated residual volume and decreased FEV_1 were seen in all lungs with more than 30% destruction by centriacinar emphysema (23).

The radiological diagnosis of emphysema is correlated with increasing anatomical severity of disease; however, even mild grades of anatomical emphysema may be detected on chest x-ray (20,24). Although many criteria have been proposed for the radiological diagnosis of emphysema, the most consistent abnormalities are depressed and flattened diaphragms and irregular radiolucencies of lung fields on the posteroanterior roentgenogram, an abnormal retrosternal airspace, and flattening or even concavity of the diaphragmatic contour on the lateral roentgenogram (24).

Computed tomography (CT) has been shown to be a useful adjunct in assessing the presence and severity of emphysema (25). Using high-resolution CT (HRCT), emphysema can be detected by the presence of areas of abnormally low attenuation, and centriacinar and panacinar emphysema can often be discriminated. On HRCT, lesions of centriacinar emphysema are characterized as multiple small, spotty, or centrilobular lucencies with an upper

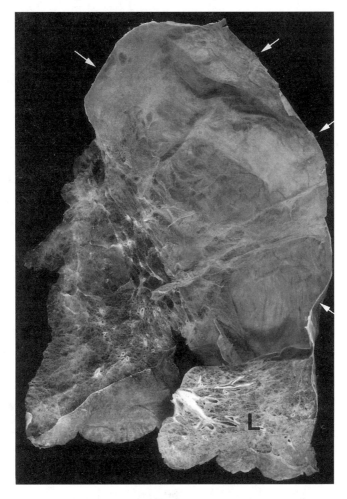

Figure 10 Giant bulla (Reid type III) (arrows) which replaces nearly the entire upper lobe and compresses the lower lobe (L). There is also diffuse panacinar emphysema. (Barium sulfate impregnation.)

lobe predominance, whereas panacinar emphysema presents as lucent lung containing small pulmonary vessels with a diffuse or lower lobe accentuation (26).

C. Pathogenesis

The overriding concept of the pathogenesis of emphysema, which has evolved from the initial observation by Eriksson of severe emphysema in patients with congenital deficiency of alpha$_1$-antitrypsin, is that of a protease-antiprotease imbalance, followed by enzymatic degradation of the structural protein elastin (6,27,28). Cigarette smoke functions in several ways as a mediator of tissue destruction. Smoking stimulates pulmonary inflammatory cells (neutrophils and macrophages) to accumulate and activate. Both neutrophil and macrophage elastase may be important in the dissolution of lung elastin (29,30). Respiratory bronchiolitis, the earliest anatomical lesion seen in young cigarette smokers, channels the centriacinar accumulation of macrophages and sets the stage for ensuing centriacinar emphysema (31). The morphological degree of lung parenchymal destruction has been correlated with increased cellularity (presumably inflammatory cells) in the alveolar walls (32).

Concomitantly, oxidants present in cigarette smoke inhibit the activity of alpha$_1$-antitrypsin, the most important serum protease inhibitor (33). Recent observations by Hogg and colleagues further suggest that latent adenoviral infection predisposes to more frequent and more severe chronic obstructive pulmonary disease (COPD), possibly explaining the sporadic occurrence of emphysema in persons with similar smoking histories (34). As alveolar septa are destroyed, lung elastic recoil is diminished. The reduced number of alveolar septa tethered to small airways leads to closure of these airways at higher lung volumes, resulting in air trapping.

III. Chronic Bronchitis

Chronic bronchitis is defined clinically as chronic cough and sputum production for three successive months in at least two successive years (3). The causes of chronic bronchitis are many, including industrial irritants and fumes, repeated infections, and—most importantly—tobacco smoke. Chronic bronchitis frequently accompanies and contributes to airflow obstruction due to emphysema; however, chronic bronchitis is rarely a sole cause of end-stage CAO (20,35).

The morphological hallmark of chronic bronchitis is a thickened bronchial wall due to mural edema, chronic inflammation, and mucous gland hyperplasia (Figs. 11 and 12) (3,36). The inflammatory cell population in the central airways of cigarette smokers consists largely of macrophages and T lymphocytes (mainly CD8 + lymphocytes), which infiltrate the submucosa and bronchial glands (37,38). The number of CD8 + T cells has been shown to correlate with the degree of airflow limitation (37,38).

Enlargement of the submucosal mucous glands includes an increase of mucus-secreting acini with an elevated proportion of mucous to serous cells. Mucous gland hyperplasia is morphologically assessed using the gland-to-wall ratio (Reid index), which is calculated by dividing the thickness of the glandular layer by the distance between the bronchial perichondrium and the mucosal basement membrane in a well-oriented bronchial cross section (39). In general, a Reid Index greater than 0.5 is associated with chronic bronchitis (3). The surface epithelial changes seen in chronic bronchitis include squamous

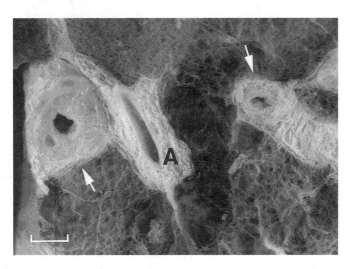

Figure 11 Chronic bronchitis. Bronchial cross sections (arrows) demonstrate severe mural thickening and luminal narrowing. Adjacent lung parenchyma is involved by fine panacinar emphysema. (A, pulmonary artery.) (Barium sulfate impregnation; scale equals 0.5 cm.)

metaplasia and goblet cell hyperplasia, although mucus secretion from surface goblet cells is a minor contribution to overall mucus production. In contrast to bronchial asthma, the smooth muscle layer of the bronchial wall tends to be less hypertrophic in chronic bronchitis (40). Mucous stasis and luminal

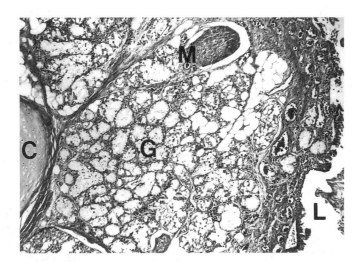

Figure 12 Chronic bronchitis. Mucous gland layer (G) is markedly hypertrophied (Reid index, 0.8). (C, cartilage; L, lumen; M, smooth muscle.)

narrowing due to a thickened airway wall each potentially contribute to airflow obstruction.

A. Changes in Small Airways

A constant finding in the lungs of patients with chronic bronchitis is inflammation and structural remodeling of small airways (less than 2 mm in diameter). The histological features in the small airways include chronic inflammation, fibrosis, smooth muscle hyperplasia, squamous metaplasia, goblet cell hyperplasia, mucous stasis, and luminal narrowing (41). In patients with emphysema, inflammation of small airways is most common in centriacinar emphysema; it tends to be less intense in panacinar emphysema, including that associated with alpha$_1$-antitrypsin deficiency (9,29). Compared to nonsmokers, smokers with or without chronic bronchitis exhibit increased goblet cells and inflammatory cells, including neutrophils, macrophages, and CD8 + T lymphocytes in their peripheral airways (42,43). Most likely, small airways disease is not directly caused by chronic bronchitis or emphysema but is due to a common initiating insult, such as cigarette smoke.

Hogg and colleagues have identified the small airways as the most important site of increased airflow resistance in patients with CAO. They found that airways less than 3 mm in internal diameter contribute approximately 80% of the total lung resistance in patients with emphysema (44). Smokers have fewer alveolar attachments to the bronchiolar perimeter than do nonsmokers (11,45). A correlation between the number of alveolar attachments and a decline in FEV_1 has also been shown, but the relative contribution to airway resistance caused by inflammation and fibrosis versus the loss of airway stability and early collapse due to decreased alveolar tethering is uncertain (11).

IV. Bronchiolitis Obliterans

Another important disease of small airways which is both an indication for lung transplantation and a complication of it, is bronchiolitis obliterans (46,47). Bronchiolitis obliterans occurs as a result of an inflammatory process in which the lumens of respiratory and membranous bronchioles are narrowed or completely obstructed by fibrous tissue. Clinically, patients exhibit dyspnea and often severe obstructive physiology. The radiographic features include nodular densities, alveolar opacities, and hyperinflation. The long-term complications of bronchiolitis obliterans are those attributable to unilateral hypertransradiency (McLeod's syndrome), atelectasis, or bronchiectasis (48,49). Most cases of bronchiolitis obliterans are idiopathic; however, a large number of specific entities either directly cause bronchiolitis obliterans or are associated with it (Table 1).

Histologically, bronchiolitis obliterans represents the severe end of the spectrum of bronchiolar inflammation and is preceded by acute bronchiolitis, followed by chronic mural inflammation and mucosal ulceration (50,51). Two

Table 1 Causes of Constrictive and Proliferative Bronchiolitis Obliterans

Constrictive or proliferative	Primarily constrictive
Viral and mycoplasmal infections	Inflammatory bowel disease
Organ transplantation	Mineral dust
Rheumatoid arthritis	Asthma, chronic bronchitis
Toxic fumes	*Sauropus androgynus*
Diffuse alveolar damage	Diffuse panbronchiolitis
Extrinsic allergic alveolitis	Cryptogenic constrictive bronchiolitis
Cystic fibrosis	obliterans
Drug reactions	
Idiopathic	
	Primarily proliferative
	Bacterial and fungal infections
	Aspiration
	Postobstruction
	Eosinophilic pneumonia
	Idiopathic BOOP[a]

[a] Bronchiolitis obliterans organizing pneumonia.
Source: Ref. 47.

distinctive histological forms of bronchiolitis obliterans are recognized: proliferative (polypoidal) and constrictive (47). Both variants may be associated with the same underlying causes (Table 1).

A. Proliferative Bronchiolitis Obliterans

Proliferative bronchiolitis obliterans is characterized by polyps of fibromyxoid tissue that occlude terminal and respiratory bronchioles and frequently extend into alveolar ducts. Associated chronic bronchiolar and peribronchiolar inflammation, intra-alveolar foamy (lipid-laden) macrophages, and varying degrees of organizing pneumonia complete the histological picture (Fig. 13). When organizing pneumonia is prominent, the process is designated as bronchiolitis obliterans organizing pneumonia (BOOP) or cryptogenic organizing pneumonia (52,53). BOOP may have the same underlying causes as proliferative bronchiolitis in general, although it usually presents as restrictive lung disease and radiographically exhibits peripheral alveolar infiltrates. In contrast to other forms of bronchiolitis obliterans or usual interstitial pneumonia, BOOP tends to be responsive to corticosteroids. However, when interstitial fibrosis is also prominent or diffusely present, the clinical course of BOOP evolves more rapidly and is likely to progress toward end-stage respiratory failure (Fig. 14) (54,55).

The histological features of proliferative bronchiolitis are fairly stereotypic; however, subtle features may indicate specific etiologies. Small

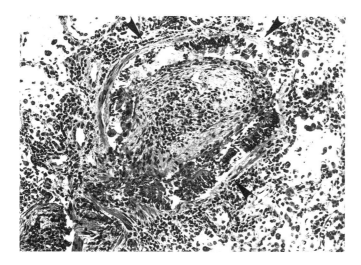

Figure 13 Proliferative bronchiolitis obliterans. Lumen of terminal bronchiole (arrowheads) is occluded by polypoid tuft of organizing fibroblastic tissue. There is chronic peribronchiolar inflammation.

epithelioid granulomas and nonspecific interstitial pneumonia suggest hypersensitivity pneumonitis, whereas food particles, including birefringent cellulose fibers, entrapped in the organizing luminal fibrous tissue indicate chronic

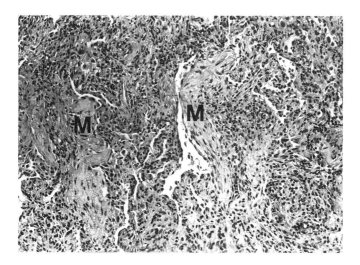

Figure 14 Bronchiolitis obliterans organizing pneumonia (BOOP), aggressive variant. Tongues of fibroblastic tissue [Masson bodies (M)] occlude alveolar ducts. The intervening lung parenchyma is fibrotic and chronically inflamed.

aspiration. Bronchiolitis obliterans with chronic eosinophilic pneumonia has been associated with rheumatoid arthritis (56,57). As proliferative bronchiolitis matures, the bronchiole is effaced by scar tissue. The localization of the scar adjacent to a muscular pulmonary artery or the demonstration of bronchiolar elastic fibers or smooth muscle by elastic tissue stains are useful morphological features indicative of end-stage bronchiolitis obliterans (Figs. 15 and 16) (47,51).

B. Constrictive Bronchiolitis

Constrictive bronchiolitis is characterized by concentric or eccentric mural or peribronchiolar fibrous tissue producing a rigid bronchiole with a narrow lumen (Fig. 16) (47). Constrictive bronchiolitis is probably synonymous with other clinically similar entities such as *adult bronchiolitis*, *small airways disease*, and *cryptogenic obliterative bronchiolitis* (58–60). In constrictive bronchiolitis, the presenting symptom is cough followed by dyspnea. Chest x-ray usually shows hyperinflation. Pulmonary function tests are consistent with severe airflow obstruction. A minority of patients appear to respond to steroid therapy.

The major causes of constrictive bronchiolitis are indicated in Table 1. Constrictive bronchiolitis in the setting of collagen vascular disease is usually associated with rheumatoid arthritis. Penicillamine therapy is an important cause of drug-induced bronchiolitis obliterans, which may confound the presentation of rheumatoid lung diseases. A recent epidemic of constrictive

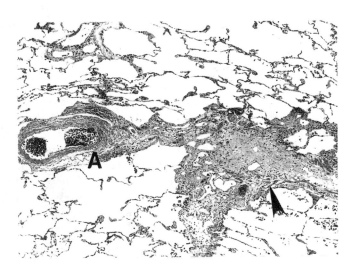

Figure 15 Juxta-arterial scar (arrowhead) consistent with completely obliterated bronchiole (lung transplant bronchiolitis obliterans). A, muscular pulmonary artery.

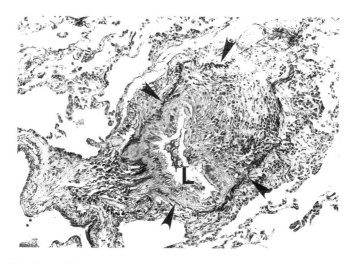

Figure 16 Constrictive bronchiolitis obliterans, idiopathic. There is eccentric submucosal fibrosis with luminal (L) narrowing and distortion. Remnant elastic lamina designates boundary of original bronchiolar lumen. (Movat pentachrome stain.)

bronchiolitis in Taiwan has been linked to ingestion of an extract from the plant *Sauropus androgynus* for the purpose of weight reduction (61). Idiopathic constrictive bronchiolitis obliterans is a rare cause of slowly progressive CAO, occurring mainly in female nonsmokers who have no other known cause of bronchiolitis. Histopathologically, very subtle inflammatory features are seen, primarily in membranous bronchioles (60). As designated in Table 1, there is significant overlap in the causes of both proliferative and constrictive bronchiolitis obliterans, suggesting that some cases of constrictive bronchiolitis may represent the chronic, fibrotic phase of proliferative bronchiolitis obliterans.

Another important variant of constrictive bronchiolitis is diffuse panbronchiolitis, which is mainly characterized as a form of sinopulmonary disease among East Asian people (62). There have been a few reports, however, of North Americans of Asian or non-Asian descent who have acquired diffuse panbronchiolitis (63,64). Clinically the disease resembles cystic fibrosis, as patients develop chronic cough, sputum production, and dyspnea on exertion. Chest x-rays typically show small nodular shadows with hyperinflation. The progression of the disease is toward worsening bronchiectasis. Histologically, diffuse panbronchiolitis causes mural thickening of respiratory bronchioles with infiltration by lymphocytes, plasma cells, and histiocytes; intraluminal neutrophils; and localization of foamy macrophages within the bronchiolar wall (63).

Regardless of the underlying cause, constrictive bronchiolitis ranges histologically from chronic inflammation with mild scarring to complete obliteration of the bronchiolar lumen. The early lesion is usually a cellular inflammatory infiltrate, mainly of lymphocytes in the mucosa, bronchiolar wall, and peribronchiolar connective tissue. Intraluminal neutrophils and mucosal necrosis may also be seen. Submucosal fibrosis narrows the bronchiolar lumen either eccentrically or concentrically (Fig. 16). Bronchiolar narrowing tends to be variably located within the lung. Histological identification of bronchiolitis obliterans may require multiple samples with serial sections.

C. Transplant Bronchiolitis Obliterans

Bronchiolitis obliterans is also a major complication of lung transplantation and an important cause of transplant failure (47). Patients present with dyspnea and progressive obstruction. The pathogenesis of transplant bronchiolitis obliterans is thought to represent chronic rejection.

The pathology of lung transplant–associated bronchiolitis obliterans is primarily that of constrictive bronchiolitis (Fig. 15). The distribution is patchy but extensive (65). In the early stages, the histological features include cellular lymphocytic bronchiolitis with ulceration and intraluminal and submucosal granulation tissue. As the connective tissue matures, the process takes on the appearance of constrictive bronchiolitis. Associated histological features include postobstructive cholesterol pneumonia, peribronchiolar fibrosis, and perivascular lymphocytic infiltrates of acute rejection (47,65,66). Bronchiectasis with mucous stasis develops in some patients (66,67).

Physiologically, posttransplant bronchiolitis obliterans initially contributes to a reduction in $FEF_{25-75\%}$ with preservation of the FEV_1/FVC ratio. As obstruction worsens, FEV_1 and FVC decline while RV increases due to air trapping. TLC may be slightly reduced due to decreased chest wall compliance related to the transplant procedure and/or mild interstitial pulmonary fibrosis, which is frequently seen in transplanted lungs (47,66).

V. Bronchiectasis

Bronchiectasis, simply defined, is dilatation of bronchi. Included in this broad definition are conditions such as traction bronchiectasis secondary to parenchymal scarring; airway dilatation accompanying atelectasis or parenchymal loss, as in emphysema; or transient airway dilatation associated with pneumonic consolidation. A more selective definition of bronchiectasis is that of fixed airway dilatation associated with inflammation and destruction of bronchial mural components. In this section *bronchiectasis* refers to this latter entity (68,69).

Bronchiectasis can be further categorized as localized or diffuse. Localized bronchiectasis due to endobronchial obstruction is most commonly the result of a neoplasm but may also evolve from events such as aspirated foreign body, extrinsic compression due to enlarged lymph nodes (e.g., right middle-lobe syndrome), or erosion and obstruction by a calcified lymph node (broncholith). Localized bronchiectasis may also have an infectious etiology, most important of which is pulmonary tuberculosis. Localized bronchiectasis is usually treated by surgical resection or elimination of the cause of bronchial obstruction.

Bronchiectasis that is most likely to be associated with end-stage respiratory failure possibly necessitating lung transplantation is nonobstructive diffuse or multifocal bronchiectasis (Table 2). The usual identified cause of this type of bronchiectasis is chronic or recurrent infection. Frequently, an underlying congenital or acquired condition will play a role by predisposing the airways to repeated infectious insults (Table 2). In approximately 50% of cases of bronchiectasis, however, a specific inciting factor is not identified—i.e., "idiopathic bronchiectasis" (70). In these patients, childhood respiratory infections, especially those likely to have produced bronchiolitis obliterans, are often presumed to have initiated the process of bronchiectasis (49,70). Congenital syndromes, such as cystic fibrosis or primary ciliary dyskinesia, by impeding bronchial clearance, promote endobronchial infection, leading to a recurrent cycle of repeated infection and escalating bronchial injury that culminates in bronchiectasis (71). *Congenital bronchiectasis* (Williams-Campbell syndrome), on the other hand, refers to isolated bronchiectasis, present from birth, which is usually due to a deficiency or abnormality of bronchial cartilage (72).

Patients with bronchiectasis typically present clinically with cough, purulent sputum production, wheezing, recurrent pneumonia, and hemoptysis (69). Frequently purulent sinusitis accompanies bronchiectasis and may

Table 2 Major Causes and/or Predisposing Conditions of Diffuse/Multifocal Bronchiectasis

Chronic infections
  Tuberculosis and nontuberculous mycobacterial infections
  Respiratory infections of childhood (presumed cause of idiopathic bronchiectasis)
    Bacterial (pertussis)
    Viral (adenovirus, respiratory syncytial virus, measles virus)
Hypogammaglobulinemia
Primary ciliary dyskinesia (immotile cilia syndrome, Kartagener's syndrome)
Cystic fibrosis
Young's syndrome
Alpha$_1$-antitrypsin deficiency (rare)
Allergic bronchopulmonary aspergillosis
Rheumatoid arthritis (rarely other collagen vascular diseases)
Ulcerative colitis
Congenital bronchiectasis (Williams-Campbell syndrome)

contribute to its development. The symptoms of bronchiectasis are readily explained by the pathological anatomical features.

The usual gross appearance of bronchiectasis is that of abnormally dilated airways, which extend almost to the visceral pleura. Reid defined three patterns of bronchiectasis based on their bronchographic appearance: cylindrical, saccular, and varicose (68). In cylindrical bronchiectasis, dilated bronchi form tube-like structures of uniform caliber. Varicose bronchiectasis appears as intermittent constriction and dilatation of the bronchial lumen. By far the most common pattern seen grossly is that of saccular bronchiectasis, wherein bronchi exhibit progressive dilatation from hilum to periphery (Figs. 17 and 18). With increasing severity of bronchiectasis, there is more pronounced simplification of the arborizing airway pattern, with loss of branch points (73). In the most advanced form—i.e., cystic bronchiectasis—lung tissue is replaced by contiguous, thin-walled cysts.

The distribution of bronchiectasis correlates incompletely with its underlying cause. For example, in cystic fibrosis, upper-lobe bronchiectasis may predominate, although all lung zones tend to be affected (74). Bronchiectasis due to allergic bronchopulmonary aspergillosis also predominates in the upper lobes, where classically it exhibits central rather than peripheral airway dilatation. In general, in idiopathic bronchiectasis, the lower lobes are more heavily involved.

Just as the macroscopic features of bronchiectasis are stereotypic, the microscopic anatomy tends to be relatively nonspecific and does not indicate the underlying cause. The bronchial wall is fibrotic and atrophic with loss of component structures such as smooth muscle, glands, and cartilage (Fig. 19) (73,75). A variable degree of chronic inflammation, mainly lymphocytes and plasma cells, infiltrates the bronchial wall and surrounding tissue. Lymphoid hyperplasia is prominent in follicular bronchiectasis, which may be the result of an underlying autoimmune or viral etiology (76). Ectatic airway branches become apposed as the intervening parenchyma is destroyed by chronic pneumonia and fibrosis (Fig. 19).

The bronchial mucosa may retain its ciliated, pseudostratified configuration, albeit distorted by irregular folds or pseudopapillary projections, or the mucosa may be replaced by metaplastic squamous epithelium. Mucosal inflammation is constant, often associated with epithelial erosion or frank ulceration, in which vascularized granulation tissue becomes a locus of left-to-right shunting and a source of hemoptysis. The bronchial lumen frequently contains mucopurulent exudate (Fig. 19). In cystic fibrosis, luminal secretions, which are extraordinarily viscid, fill and further distend the bronchial lumen. In allergic bronchopulmonary aspergillosis, on the other hand, the exudate is granular, with degenerated eosinophils and Charcot-Leyden crystals. The cavernous interior of bronchiectatic airways is suitable for fungal colonization, sometimes leading to mycetoma formation.

A striking and constant feature of bronchiectasis is hypertrophy of bronchial arteries (Fig. 20). An increased number of bronchial artery profiles,

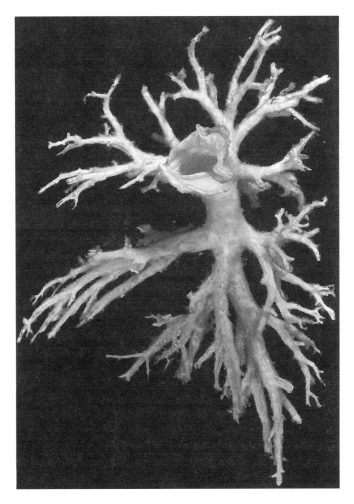

Figure 17 Normal bronchial tree of right lung dissected free of lung parenchyma. Bronchial caliber is tapered from hilum to periphery. Middle-lobe bronchi extend diagonally to the left.

many having bizarre patterns of muscular hypertrophy, extend through the bronchial wall into submucosal positions. Erosion of the exposed artery by an overlying ulcer is a cause of massive, life-threatening hemoptysis. Pulmonary artery branches also exhibit medial hypertrophy and intimal fibrosis, which may correlate with pulmonary hypertension.

The morphological features of bronchiectasis are consistent with concepts of pathogenesis. Sustained inflammation, accompanied by proteolysis and inflammatory mediators, destroys and weakens the bronchial wall, which becomes increasingly distended by traction from adjacent scarred or collapsed

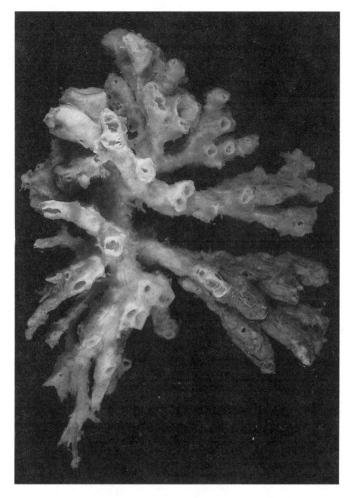

Figure 18 Saccular bronchiectasis from a patient with cystic fibrosis. Thick-walled bronchi project peripherally as dilated, blind-ended pouches. Middle-lobe bronchi course diagonally to the right.

parenchyma. The accumulation of luminal exudate provides an additional internal distending force. Sustained inflammation and structural remodeling ultimately lead to blind-ended conduits incapable of supporting ventilation.

A. Cystic Fibrosis

End-stage cystic fibrosis (CF)–associated lung disease is an important cause of respiratory failure due to bronchiectasis. In general, the pathology of bronchiectasis in CF conforms to the descriptions of bronchiectasis elaborated above. Massive dilation of bronchiectatic airways (i.e., cystic bronchiectasis) is

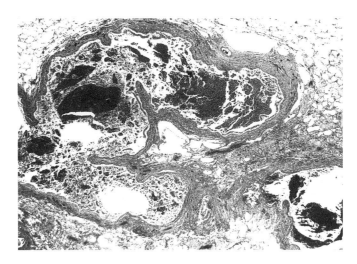

Figure 19 Bronchiectasis, cystic fibrosis. Dilated airways, with atrophic, fibrotic walls, contain mucopurulent exudate.

recognized as thin-walled cysts on chest x-ray. Rupture of peripheral bronchiectatic cysts represents a cause of spontaneous pneumothorax in CF patients (77). Other salient features of CF-associated lung disease include marked chronic bronchitis with variable hyperplasia or atrophy of bronchial

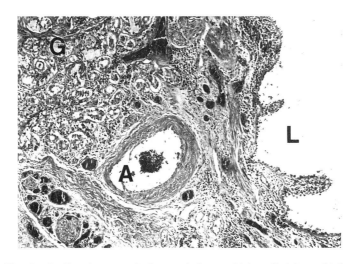

Figure 20 Cystic fibrosis, central airway. A large, thick-walled bronchial artery (A) approaches the denuded mucosal surface. There is chronic inflammation and adjacent mucous gland (G) hyperplasia. L, bronchial lumen.

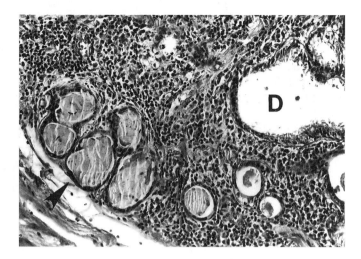

Figure 21 Cystic fibrosis, central airway. Atrophic mucous glands consist of dilated tubules containing inspissated secretion (arrowhead). There is surrounding intense chronic inflammation, and the gland duct (D) is dilated.

glands. Atrophic acini and ductules contain dense, waxy, inspissated eosinophilic secretion (Fig. 21) (71). Chronic endobronchial infection in CF, frequently by mucoid strains of *Pseudomonas aeruginosa*, leads to massive accumulation of mucopurulent exudate within bronchial lumens (Fig. 19). Small airways show typical features of purulent bronchiolitis and chronic constrictive bronchiolitis obliterans (71). Recurrent acute and chronic organizing bronchopneumonia leads to peribronchial scar formation. The pathological features of pneumonia due to *Burkholderia cepacia* resembles those attributable to *P. aeruginosa*. *B. cepacia* may also be associated with a rapidly progressive clinical course due to severe necrotizing pneumonia (78). Emphysema is usually minimal in CF, affecting less than 10% of the parenchymal lung tissue (74,79,80).

References

1. Fletcher CM, Gilson JG, Hugh-Jones P, Scadding JG. Terminology, definitions, and classification of chronic pulmonary emphysema and related conditions. A report of the conclusions of a CIBA guest symposium. Thorax 1959; 14:286–299.
2. Pratt PC, Kilburn KH. A modern concept of the emphysemas based on correlations of structure and function. Hum Pathol 1970; 1:443–463.
3. Thurlbeck WM. Chronic airflow obstruction. In: Thurlbeck WM, ed. Pathology of the Lung. New York: Thieme, 1988:519–576.

4. Sobonya RE. Normal anatomy and development of the lung. In: Baum GL, Wolinsky E, eds. Textbook of Pulmonary Diseases. Boston: Little Brown, 1989:3–21.

5. Snider GL, Kleinerman J, Thurlbeck WM, Bengali ZH. The definition of emphysema. Am Rev Respir Dis 1985; 132:182–185.

6. Wright JL. Emphysema: concepts under change—a pathologist's perspective. Mod Pathol 1995; 8:873–880.

7. Heard BE. A pathological study of emphysema of the lungs with chronic bronchitis. Thorax 1958; 13:136–149.

8. Leopold TG, Gough J. The centrilobular form of emphysema and its relation to chronic bronchitis. Thorax 1957; 12:219–235.

9. Greenberg SD, Jenkins DE, Stevens PM, Schweppe HI. The lungs in homozygous alpha-1 antitrypsin deficiency. Am J Clin Pathol 1973; 60:581–592.

10. Nagai A, Ihano H, Matsuba K, Thurlbeck WM. Scanning electronmicroscopic morphometry of emphysema in humans. Am J Crit Care Med 1994; 150:1411–1415.

11. Nagai A, Yamawaki I, Takizawa T, Thurlbeck WM. Alveolar attachments in emphysema of human lungs. Am Rev Respir Dis 1991; 144:888–891.

12. Kim WD, Eidelman DG, Izquierdo J, Ghezzo H, Saetta M, Cosio MG. Centrilobular and panlobular emphysema in smokers. Two distinct morphologic and functional entities. Am Rev Respir Dis 1991; 144:1385–1390.

13. Butler C. Lung surface area in various morphologic forms of human emphysema. Am Rev Respir Dis 1976; 114:347–352.

14. Pare JP, Cote G, Fraser RS. Long-term follow-up of drug abusers with intravenous talcosis. Am Rev Respir Dis 1989; 139:233–241.

15. Schmidt RA, Glenny RW, Godwin JD, Hampson NB, Cantino ME, Reichenbach D. Panlobular emphysema in young intravenous Ritalin abusers. Am Rev Respir Dis 1991; 143:649–656.

16. Farber HW, Fairman RP, Millan JE, Rounds S, Glauser FL. Pulmonary response to foreign body microemboli in dogs: release of neutrophil chemoattractant activity by vascular endothelial cells. Am J Respir Cell Molec Biol 1989; 1:27–35.

17. Semmens M, Reid L. Pulmonary arterial muscularity and right ventricular hypertrophy in chronic bronchitis and emphysema. Br J Dis Chest 1974; 68:253–263.

18. Shelton DM, Keal E, Reid L. The pulmonary circulation in chronic bronchitis and emphysema. Chest 1977; 715:303S–306S.

19. Reid L. The Pathology of Emphysema. London: Loyd-Luke, 1967:211–241.

20. Thurlbeck WM, Henderson JA, Fraser RG, Bates DV. Chronic obstructive lung disease. A comparison between clinical, roentgenologic, functional and morphologic criteria in chronic bronchitis, emphysema, asthma and bronchiectasis. Medicine 197; 49:81–145.

21. Pratt PC, Haque MA, Klugh GA. Correlation of postmortem function and structure in normal and emphysematous lungs. Am Rev Respir Dis 1961; 83:856–865.

22. Pratt PC, Haque MA, Klugh GA. Correlation of postmortem function and structure in panlobular pulmonary emphysema. Lab Invest 1962; 11:177–187.

23. Pratt PC, Jutabha O, Klugh GA. Quantitative relationship between structural extent of centrilobular emphysema and postmortem volume and flow characteristics of lungs. Med Thorac 1965; 22:197–208.

24. Pratt PC. Role of conventional chest radiography in diagnosis and exclusion of emphysema. Am J Med 1987; 82:998–1006.
25. Bergin C, Muller N, Nichols DM, Lillington G, Hogg JC, Mullen B, Grymaloski MR, Osborne S, Pare PD. The diagnosis of emphysema. A computer tomographic-pathologic correlation. Am Rev Respir Dis 1986; 133:541–546.
26. Webb WR, Muller NL, Naidich D. High-Resolution CT of the Lung. Philadelphia: Lippincott Williams & Wilkins, 2001:421–466.
27. Eriksson S. Studies in alpha-1-antitrypsin deficiency. Acta Med Scand (Suppl) 1965; 432:1–85.
28. Kimbel P. Proteolytic mechanisms of lung injury in the pathogenesis of emphysema. Chest 1984; 85:39S–41S.
29. Cosio MG, Guerrassimov A. Chronic obstructive pulmonary disease. Inflammation of small airways and lung parenchyma. Am J Respir Crit Care Med 1999; 160:S21–S25.
30. Shapiro ED. The macrophage in chronic obstructive pulmonary disease. Am J Respir Crit Care Med 1999; 160:S29–S32.
31. Niewoehner DE, Kleinerman J, Rice D. Pathologic changes in the peripheral airways of young cigarette smokers. N Engl J Med 1974; 291:755–758.
32. Eidelman D, Saetta MP, Ghezzo H, Wang N-S, Hordal JR, King M, Cosio, MG. Cellularity of the alveolar walls in smokers and its relation to alveolar destruction. Functional implications. Am Rev Respir Dis 1990; 141:1547–1552.
33. Repine JE, Bast A, Lankhorst I, and the Oxidative Stress Study Group. Oxidative stress in chronic obstructive pulmonary disease. Am J Respir Crit Care Med 1997; 156:341–357.
34. Hogg JC. Childhood viral infection and the pathogenesis of asthma and chronic obstructive lung disease. Am J Respir Crit Care Med 1999; 160:S26–S28.
35. Greenberg SD, Boushy SF, Jenkins DE. Chronic bronchitis and emphysema: correlation of pathologic findings. Am Rev Respir Dis 1967; 96:918–928.
36. Reid LM. Pathology of chronic bronchitis. Lancet 1954; 1:275–278.
37. Di Stefano A, Turato G, Maestrelli P, Mapp LE, Ruggieri MP, Roggeri A, Boschetto P, Fabbri LM, Saetta M. Airflow limitation in chronic bronchitis is associated with T-lymphocyte and macrophage infiltration of the bronchial mucosa. Am J Respir Crit Care Med 1996; 153:629–632.
38. O'Shaughnessy TC, Ansari TW, Barnes NC, Jeffery PK. Inflammation in bronchial biopsies of subjects with chronic bronchitis: inverse relationship of CD8+ T lymphocytes with FEV1. Am J Respir Crit Care Med 1997; 155:852–857.
39. Reid LM. Measurement of the bronchial mucous gland layer: a diagnostic yardstick in chronic bronchitis. Thorax 1960; 15:132–141.
40. Dunnill MS. Pulmonary Pathology. London: Churchill Livingstone, 1982:33–49.
41. Cosio M, Ghezzo H, Hogg JC, Corbin R, Loveland M, Dosman J, Macklem PT. The relations between structural changes in small airways and pulmonary functions tests. N Engl J Med 1977; 298:1277–1281.
42. Bosken C, Hands J, Gatter K, Hogg JC. Characterization of the inflammatory reaction in the peripheral airways of cigarette smokers using immunohistochemistry. Am Rev Respir Dis 1992; 145:911–917.
43. Saetta M, Turato G, Baraldao S, Zanin A, Braccioni F, Mapp CE, Maestrelli P, Cavallesco G, Papi A, Fabbri LM. Goblet cell hyperplasia and epithelial inflammation in peripheral airways of smokers with both symptoms of chronic

bronchitis and chronic airflow limitation. Am J Respir Crit Care Med 2000; 161:1016–1021.

44. Hogg JC, Macklem PT, Thurlbeck WM. Site and nature of airway obstruction in chronic obstructive lung disease. N Engl J Med 1968; 278:1355–1360.

45. Saetta M, Ghezzo H, Kim WD, King M, Angus GE, Wang N-S, Cosio MG. Loss of alveolar attachments in smokers. Am Rev Respir Dis 1985; 132:894–900.

46. Gosink BB, Friedman PJ, Liebow AA. Bronchiolitis obliterans. Roentgenologic-pathologic correlation. Am J Roentgenol Radiat Ther Nucl Med 1973; 97:816–832.

47. Wright JL, Cagle P, Churg A, Colby TV, Myers J. Diseases of small airways. Am Rev Respir Dis 1992; 146:240–262.

48. Reid L, Simon G, Zorab PA. The development of unilateral hypertransradiency of the lung. Br J Dis Chest 1967; 61:190–192.

49. Becroft DMO. Bronchiolitis obliterans, bronchiectasis, and other sequelae of adenovirus type 21 infection in young children. J Clin Pathol 1971; 24:72–82.

50. McLean KH. The pathology of acute bronchiolitis—a study of its evolution. Part I: The exudative phase. Aust Ann Med 1956; 5:254–267.

51. McLean KH. The pathology of acute bronchiolitis—a study of its evolution. II. The repair phase. Aust Ann Med 1957; 6:29–43.

52. Epler GR, Colby TV, McCloud TC, Carrington CB. Gaensler EA. Bronchiolitis obliterans organizing pneumonia. N Engl J Med 1985; 312:152–158.

53. Bellomo R, Finlay M, McLaughlin P, Tai E. Clinical spectrum of cryptogenic organizing pneumonitis. Thorax 1991; 46:554–558.

54. Cohen AJ, King TE Jr, Downey GP. Rapidly progressive bronchiolitis obliterans with organizing pneumonia. Am J Respir Crit Care Med 1994; 149:1670–1675.

55. Yousem SA, Lohr RH, Colby TV. Idiopathic bronchiolitis obliterans organizing pneumonia/cryptogenic organizing pneumonia with unfavorable outcome: pathologic features. Mod Pathol 1997; 10:864–871.

56. Beheshti J, Mino M, Mark EJ. Chronic eosinophilic pneumonia, bronchiolitis obliterans organizing pneumonia overlap syndrome; analysis of twelve cases. Mod Pathol (suppl) 2002; 15:315A.

57. Cooney TP. Interrelationship of chronic eosinophilic pneumonia, bronchiolitis obliterans, and rheumatoid disease: a hypothesis. J Clin Pathol 1981; 34:129–137.

58. Dorinsky PM, Davis B, Lucas JG, Weiland JE, Gadek JE. Adult bronchiolitis. Evaluation by bronchoalveolar lavage and response to prednisone therapy. Chest 1985; 88:58–63.

59. Macklem PT, Thurlbeck WM, Fraser RG. Chronic obstructive disease of small airways. Ann Intern Med 1971; 74:167–177.

60. Kraft M, Mortenson RL, Colby TV, Newman L, Waldron JA Jr, King TE Jr. Cryptogenic constrictive bronchiolitis. A clinicopathologic study. Am Rev Respir Dis 1993; 148:1093–1101.

61. Chang H, Wang J-S, Tseng H-H, Lai R-S, Su J-M. Histopathological study of *Sauropus androgynus* associated constrictive bronchiolitis obliterans: a new cause of constrictive bronchiolitis obliterans. Am J Surg Pathol 1997; 21:35–42.

62. Homma H, Yamanaka A, Tanimoto S, Tamura M, Chijimatsu Y, Sira S, Izumi T. Diffuse panbronchiolitis. A disease of the transitional zone of the lung. Chest 1983; 83:63–69.

63. Fisher MS, Rush WL, Rosado-de-Christenson ML, Goldstein ER, Tomski SM, Wempe JM, Travis WD. Diffuse panbronchiolitis. Histologic diagnosis in

unsuspected cases involving North American residents of Asian descent. Arch Pathol Lab Med 1997; 122:156–160.

64. Fitzgerald JE, King TE Jr, Lynch DA, Tader RM, Schwarz MI. Diffuse panbronchiolitis in the United States. Am J Respir Crit Care Med 1996; 154:497–503.
65. Yousem SA, Burke CM, Billingham ME. Pathologic pulmonary alterations in long-term human heart-lung transplantation. Hum Pathol 1985; 16:911–923.
66. Scott JP, Peters SG, McDougall JL, Berk KC, Midthun DE. Posttransplantation physiologic features of the lung and obliterative bronchiolitis. Mayo Clin Proc 1997; 72:170–174.
67. Husain AN, Siddiqui MT, Reddy VB, Yeldandi V, Montoya A, Garrity ER. Postmortem findings in lung transplant recipients. Mod Pathol 1996; 9:752–761.
68. deMello D, Reid L. Bronchiectasis. In: Saldana, ML, ed. Pathology of Pulmonary Disease. Philadelphia: Lippincott, 1994:295–308.
69. Baum GL, Hershko EL. Bronchiectasis. In: Baum GL, Wolinsky E, eds. Textbook of Pulmonary Diseases, 4th ed. Boston: Little Brown, 1989:567–588.
70. Pasteur MC, Helliwell SM, Houghton SJ, Webb SC, Foweraker JE, Coulden RA, Flower CD, Bilton D, Keogan MT. An investigation into causative factors in patients with bronchiectasis. Am J Respir Crit Care Med 2000; 152:1277–1284.
71. Tomashefski JF Jr, Dahms BB, Abramowsky CI. The pathology of cystic fibrosis. In: Davis PB, ed. Cystic Fibrosis. New York: Marcel Dekker, 1993:435–489.
72. Williams H, Campbell P. Generalized bronchiectasis associated with deficiency of cartilage in the bronchial tree. Arch Dis Child 1960; 35:182–191.
73. Reid LM. Reduction in bronchial subdivision in bronchiectasis. Thorax 1950; 5:233–247.
74. Tomashefski JF Jr, Bruce M, Goldberg HI, Dearborn, DG. Regional distribution of macroscopic lung disease in cystic fibrosis. Am Rev Respir Dis 1986; 133:535–540.
75. Ogrinc G, Kampalath B, Tomashefski JF Jr. Destruction and loss of bronchial cartilage in cystic fibrosis. Hum Pathol 1998; 29:65–73.
76. Whitwell F. A study of the pathology and pathogenesis of bronchiectasis. Thorax 1952; 7:213–239.
77. Tomashefski JF Jr, Bruce M, Stern RC, Dearborn DG, Dahms B. Pulmonary air cysts in cystic fibrosis: relation of pathologic features to radiologic findings and history of pneumothorax. Hum Pathol 1985; 16:253–261.
78. Tomashefski JF Jr, Thomassen MJ, Bruce MC, Goldberg HI, Konstan M, Stern, RC. *Pseudomonas cepacia* associated pneumonia in cystic fibrosis. Relation of clinical features to histopathologic patterns of pneumonia. Arch Pathol Lab Med 1988; 112:166–172.
79. Bedrossian CWM, Greenberg, SD, Singer DB, Hansen JJ, Rosenberg, HS. The lung in cystic fibrosis. A quantitative study including prevalence of pathologic findings among different age groups. Hum Pathol 1976; 7:195–204.
80. Sabonya R, Taussig, LM. Quantitative aspects of lung pathology in cystic fibrosis. Am Rev Respir Dis 1986; 134:290–295.

2

Pathology of Advanced Interstitial Diseases
Pulmonary Fibrosis, Sarcoidosis, Pulmonary Histiocytosis X, Autoimmune Pulmonary Disease, and Lymphangioleiomyomatosis

CAROL F. FARVER

Cleveland Clinic Foundation
Cleveland, Ohio, U.S.A.

I. Introduction

The pathology of advanced interstitial lung disease usually consists of extensive fibrosis, which leads to bilateral honeycomb changes within the lung. Multiple diseases can cause similar honeycomb pathology and a specific etiological diagnosis usually requires correlation of the pathological features with radiological and clinical findings. However, some diseases have characteristic morphological features that will help in defining the etiology in these end-stage lungs. The following discussion highlights the characteristic gross and microscopic features of the advanced pathology of pulmonary fibrosis, sarcoidosis, pulmonary histiocytosis X, autoimmune pulmonary disease, and lymphangioleiomyomatosis.

II. Pulmonary Fibrosis

Pulmonary fibrosis or scarring is the end stage of a number of diseases that affect the lung. These diseases include systemic diseases such as connective tissue disease, pulmonary disease secondary to occupational exposures, and pulmonary infections. However, most pulmonary fibrosis is idiopathic (1). Pulmonary fibrosis is most common in middle-aged men and women and, in its chronic stage, presents with similar clinical characteristics, including dyspnea, cough, restrictive physiology, and chest imaging studies that show disease predominantly in the lower lobes. Though early imaging studies may show a ground-glass appearance, these findings are followed by reticulonodular infiltrates, coarse linear shadows, and, finally, small lungs with honeycomb changes (2).

A. Macroscopic Features of Advanced Pulmonary Fibrosis

The gross features of lungs from patients with end-stage pulmonary fibrosis are firm and stiff with dense white fibrous tissue diffusely involving the pulmonary parenchyma, resulting in a weight of two to three times that of a normal lung. The scarring of the pulmonary parenchyma begins in the periphery and advances to eventually involve the majority of the lung. As the fibrosis advances, the obstruction of small airways leads to a remodeling of these peripheral airspaces into cystically dilated spaces of honeycombing (Fig. 1). This honeycombing and the irregular scarring of the underlying lung parenchyma leads to the characteristic nodular appearance of the pleural surface (Fig. 2). These gross features appear more marked in the lower lobes though this may be the result of the greater volume of the lower lobes (1).

B. Histopathology of Advanced Pulmonary Fibrosis

Multiple patterns of tissue injury give rise to pulmonary fibrosis (3) through a sequence of cellular events consisting of inflammation, tissue destruction, and remodeling (4). This sequence is most commonly seen in the setting of the idiopathic interstitial pneumonias, including usual interstitial pneumonia (UIP), nonspecific interstitial pneumonia/fibrosis (NSIP), and diffuse alveolar damage (DAD). In UIP, this sequence begins at different foci and different times, producing a pattern of fibrosis of varying ages throughout the lung (Fig. 3). The progression from inflammation to fibrosis includes interstitial widening and epithelial injury due to a mixed inflammatory infiltrate, followed by epithelial sloughing, fibroblastic infiltration, and organizing fibrosis (5). Deposition of collagen by these fibroblasts occurs in the latter stages of repair; therefore the histopathological picture of UIP is a continuum of inflammation at the peripheral edge of ongoing injury to irreversible, dense collagen within the older, inactive areas of the lesion. The presence of the abundant collagen produces stiff lungs that are unable to clear the airway secretions, leading to recurrent inflammation of the bronchiolar epithelium with eventual fibrosis and breakdown of the airway structure. This remodeling produces mucus-filled ectatic spaces giving rise to the honeycomb spaces of the advanced pathology (Fig. 4) and may produce a hyperplasia of smooth muscle around the alveolar ducts and respiratory bronchioles (Fig. 5). Because it occurs predominantly in the periphery of the lung, involving the subpleura and interlobular septa, the gross picture is one of more advanced peripheral disease.

In NSIP and DAD, the injury to the tissue occurs at the same time, producing a pattern of inflammation and fibrosis that is similar in age throughout the affected areas of the lung (6). In NSIP, this injury consists of a widening of the interstitium with chronic, inflammatory cells and varying amounts of collagen deposition which determines the grade (1–3) of the lesion, with grade 3 containing the most collagen (Fig. 6). Recent studies show that 73% of these lungs can go on to form honeycomb changes that arise out of a diffuse pattern of interstitial collagen deposition (7).

In those lungs involved by DAD, the organizing and irreversible fibrosis occurs within both the alveolar space and the interstitium and may also result from collapse of alveolar walls (8). The histopathological picture is one of thickened alveolar septa, intra-alveolar granulation tissue, microcyst formation, and areas of irregular alveolar scarring (Fig. 7). These microcysts may progress to large cysts, an adult equivalent of bronchopulmonary dysplasia; however, this is rare (8).

III. Sarcoidosis

Sarcoidosis is a systemic disease that involves the lung in over 90% of the cases (9). It most commonly presents in the 20- to 40-year age group; a female involvement predominates, and, in the United States, African Americans are more commonly affected than Caucasians (10). The clinical presentation of pulmonary sarcoidosis is quite variable and 30 to 60% of the patients are asymptomatic (11). The most common symptoms are cough and dyspnea with restrictive pulmonary function tests (12). Chest imaging studies are abnormal in over 90% of patients with sarcoidosis, and the most common finding is bilateral hilar lymph node enlargement. Within the lung parenchyma, reticular, reticulonodular, and focal alveolar opacities are most characteristic (13). In long-standing sarcoidosis, cysts, large bullae, cystic bronchiectasis, or enlarged pulmonary arteries secondary to pulmonary hypertension may be seen (13,14).

A. Macroscopic Features of Advanced Sarcoidosis

The gross appearance of the lungs in early sarcoidosis is a network of fine nodules following the lymphatics in the subpleura, down the interlobular septa, and around the bronchovascular bundle (Fig. 8a). As this pathology advances, nodules of fibrosis and irregular fibrous scars can be seen and honeycombing may appear, especially in the upper lobes. Involvement of bronchi and bronchioles by these granulomas can produce fibrotic narrowing and occlusion; upper-lobe bronchiectasis (Fig. 9) of either the saccular or cylindrical types is seen (15). Cicatricial emphysema may develop in the area of scarring, adding to the destruction of the adjacent lung parenchyma, and bulla may form and rupture, resulting in spontaneous pneumothoraces that can be seen in patients with end-stage sarcoidosis (16). In patients with cystic

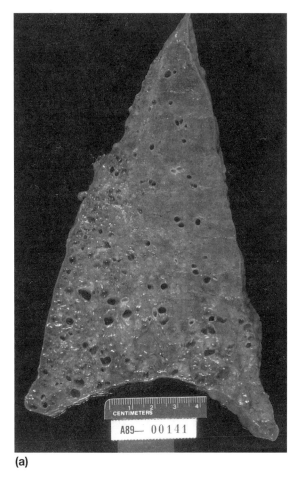

(a)

Figure 1 Sagittal section of lung with advanced idiopathic pulmonary fibrosis. Honeycomb changes are present in the basilar peripheral zones, as is typical (a). Honeycomb changes consist of ectatic airspaces with mucous plugging (b).

end-stage sarcoidosis, aspergillomas can be seen (Fig. 10) and may cause major or massive hemoptysis (17).

B. Histopathology of Advanced Sarcoidosis

Epithelioid granulomas, predominantly nonnecrotizing, are the characteristic feature of this disease. They consist of activated macrophages with scattered giant cells, usually the Langhans' type, with peripherally arranged nuclei, and a rim of lymphocytes. The granulomas may have early central necrosis but not the significant necrosis found in infectious granulomas. A variety of inclusions including Schaumann and asteroid bodies may be seen. These are not specific

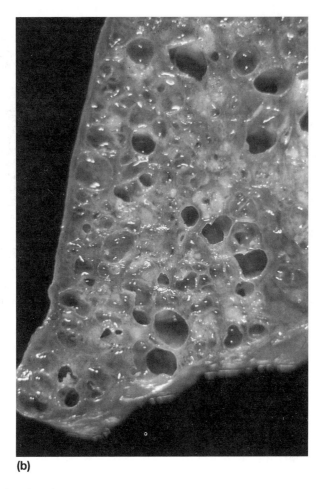

(b)

Figure 1 Continued

to sarcoidosis but can be found in a number of granulomatous diseases (18). The distribution of the granulomas in sarcoidosis tends to occur in the upper two-thirds of the lung and follows the lines of the pulmonary lymphatics (19)— in the subpleura, around the bronchovascular bundle, and within the interlobular septa (Figure 8b). Granulomas involving the mucosa and submucosa of larger airways may be seen by the bronchoscopist as small white nodules. In nodular sarcoidosis, the granulomas become confluent and present as nodular masses within the lung that may measure up to 5 cm in diameter (20). In active, early sarcoidosis, there can be an accompanying interstitial pneumonitis; however, this is not a usual feature of the pathology and if present, will decrease with chronicity (21). The pulmonary blood vessels are often involved by granulomas, given their distribution along the lymphatic

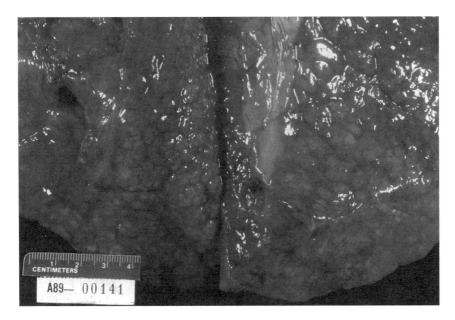

Figure 2 Pleural surface of lungs with advanced idiopathic pulmonary fibrosis. The nodular surface is typical of these lungs and is similar to that seen in cirrhotic livers.

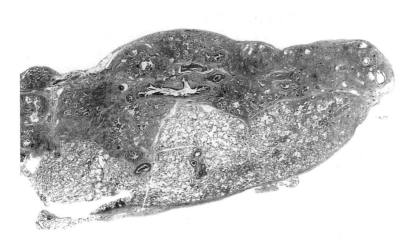

Figure 3 Open lung biopsy showing variable areas of inflammation, fibrosis and honeycomb change adjacent to areas of normal lung typical of UIP ($\times 8$).

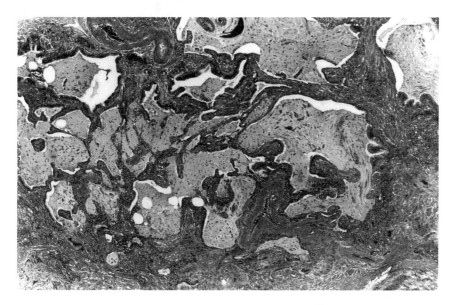

Figure 4 Honeycomb change in UIP with enlarged airspaces with mucous pooling and intervening dense fibrosis (× 16).

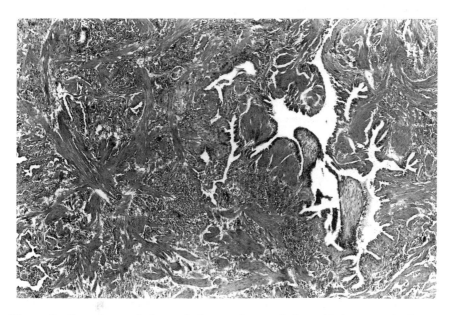

Figure 5 Smooth muscle hyperplasia seen in association with honeycomb changes (× 16).

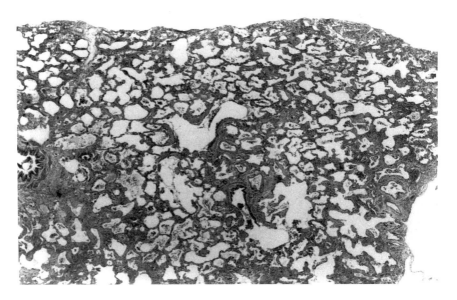

Figure 6 Nonspecific interstitial pneumonia/fibrosis, grade 3, with diffuse interstitial fibrosis (× 16).

routes (22). This granulomatous vasculitis may involve either the pulmonary arteries or veins and is characterized by granulomas within the vessel wall that may narrow or obliterate the lumina (Fig. 11) (23).

Chronic pulmonary sarcoidosis is characterized by scarring and fibrosis, with increased fibroblasts and deposition of type 1 collagen in the distribution of the granulomas along the lymphatics. This fibrosis involves the interstitium, causing alveolar wall collapse, and produces large air-filled spaces with a honeycombing appearance, predominantly in the upper lobes. In end-stage sarcoidosis, granulomas may be difficult to find, with only the lymphatic distribution of the fibrosis helpful for making the pathological diagnosis (Fig. 12). This fibrosis has a hyalinized and lamellar character and may contain giant cells and Schaumann bodies as the only remnant of the previous granulomatous inflammation (Fig. 13). Pulmonary vascular scarring secondary to granulomatous involvement is commonly seen (24); however, secondary pulmonary hypertension is unusual (25).

IV. Pulmonary Histiocytosis X (Eosinophilic Granuloma, Langerhans Cell Granulomatosis of the Lung)

Pulmonary histiocytosis X is one of three systemic diseases that are characterized by an abnormal proliferation of Langerhans cells. The clinical spectrum of diseases includes localized lesions, usually in bones or lungs, and disseminated disease with a clinically aggressive course. (26–28). Pulmonary histiocytosis X, unlike the other two systemic diseases, involves the lungs exclusively. It is found most commonly in young adults between their third and fourth decades (29), who present with cough, dyspnea, chest pain, and spontaneous pneumothorax (30). No gender predominance or occupational risk is seen; however, more than 95% of the patients are active or former smokers (27). The role of cigarette smoking in the pathogenesis of pulmonary histiocytosis X is not understood (31,32). Chest x-rays are usually abnormal in symptomatic patients (33) but may be nonspecific. The characteristic image reveals a bilateral reticulonodular infiltrate in the middle and upper lung zones with sparing of the costophrenic angles (34).

A. Macroscopic Features of Advanced Histiocytosis X

The gross features of pulmonary histiocytosis X vary with age and severity of disease. Early lesions consist of nodules up to 1 cm in diameter and may, on rare occasions, contain cavitation (28). These lesions are usually surrounded by emphysematous change and have a firm white stellate appearance (Fig. 14). As the disease progresses to more severe and, finally, end-stage pulmonary histiocytosis X, the lung develops extensive scarring and cyst formation (Fig. 15), producing the pneumothoraces that can be seen in this disease (28,33).

B. Histopathology of Advanced Pulmonary Histiocytosis X

To understand the pathological features of advanced pulmonary histiocytosis X, it is important to understand the progression of the disease from its early cellular form through its proliferative phase, where the pattern of fibrosis of its healed phase is established. Early active lesions are bronchiolocentric and composed predominantly of Langerhans cells along with scattered eosinophils, lymphocytes, plasma cells, and polymorphonuclear leukocytes (Fig. 16). Though identifiable by routine light microscopy, Langerhans cells are more readily seen using special techniques such as immunohistochemical studies for S-100 protein or CD1a (35–37) and by ultrastructural analysis, where the Langerhans cells of histiocytosis X contain distinct cytoplasmic racquet-shaped granules referred to as Birbeck granules (Fig. 17) (38).

As the lesions progress, the Langerhans histiocytes proliferate and spread to adjacent alveolar walls and vessels, while the numbers of eosinophils, lymphocytes and plasma cells increase. This extension into the lung interstitium produces a star-shaped appearance from low power (Fig. 18). The underlying bronchiole becomes obliterated by the inflammatory infiltrate and a desquamative interstitial pneumonitis reaction can be seen in adjacent alveolar spaces (39). Organizing or intraluminal fibrosis may be seen in adjacent alveoli and early interstitial fibrosis begins in the peribronchiolar area. This proliferating phase progresses to a fibrotic phase, where the lesions are characteristically acellular with collagen deposition in the areas of the infiltrate, causing obliteration and scarring of bronchioles, vessels, and adjacent alveolar

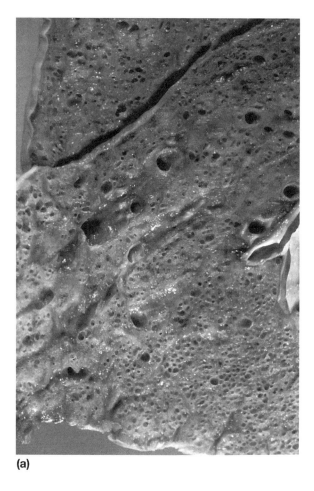

(a)

Figure 7 Autopsy lung with advanced diffuse alveolar damage with dense consolidation and microcyst formation (a). Thickened alveolar septa which give rise to microcyst formation in organizing DAD (b) (× 40).

walls in a stellate pattern (Fig. 15b). With these lesions, it may be difficult to diagnosis pulmonary histiocytosis X, given the lack of Langerhans cells present. The pathologist may need to search multiple tissue sections to find active lesions and depend on clinical information to support less definitive findings. Unlike UIP, which has large, irregular patches of scarring with intervening interstitial inflammation, the fibrosis that results from pulmonary histiocytosis X produces a symmetrical, discrete, focal scarring with minimal inflammation in the adjacent alveoli.

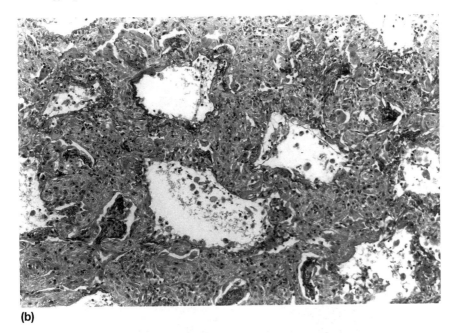

(b)

Figure 7 Continued

Though most patients recover from pulmonary histiocytosis X, approximately 10% develop progressive pulmonary disease that results in end-stage fibrosis (28,40). In this advanced form of the disease, the bronchiolar-based scarring becomes confluent causing significant distortion of the normal pulmonary architecture giving rise to thin-walled cysts, a scarred and nodular pleural surface, and irreversible fibrosis and honeycomb lung indistinguishable from UIP (27). In addition, pulmonary hypertension is commonly seen, with one series reporting a greater than 90% incidence in patients who came to transplantation (41). This hypertension may be the result of the vascular medial thickening that can be found in advanced pulmonary histiocytosis X. It may represent a sequela of a vasculitis secondary to the inflammation from the adjacent bronchocentric nodule (27).

V. Autoimmune Pulmonary Disease

Autoimmune diseases are among the most common of the systemic diseases that involve the lung (42). These represent a heterogenous group of diseases, the most common of which include systemic lupus erythematosus (SLE), rheumatoid arthritis (RA), progressive systemic sclerosis (PSS), Sjörgren's disease, mixed connective tissue disease (MCT), and dermatomyositis-polymyositis (DPM). These clinical manifestations vary depending on the

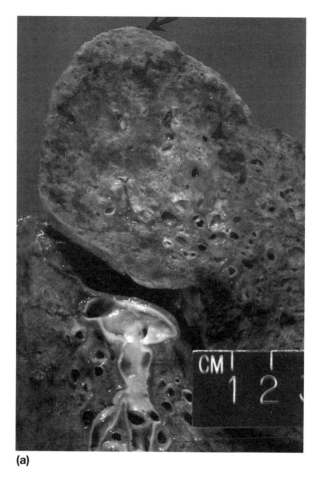

(a)

Figure 8 Apex of lung with fibrosis from sarcoid, with predominant fibrosis in subpleura (arrow) and around the bronchovascular bundles (arrowhead) (a). The distribution of the granulomas in sarcoidosis following the pulmonary lymphatics—in the subpleura, interlobular septa and around the bronchovascular bundle (b) (×8).

disease. However, the common feature that links this group is the immunologically mediated inflammatory changes within the connective tissues of the body (43), including the musculoskeletal and vascular system. Within the lung, this may include the lung parenchyma, tracheobronchial tree, pulmonary vasculature, pleura, and respiratory muscles (42).

Patients with autoimmune diseases involving the lung usually present with a myriad of pulmonary symptoms (44). Common symptoms include shortness of breath, pleuritic chest pain, and restrictive physiology with imaging studies, including interstitial and alveolar infiltrates, pleural effusions,

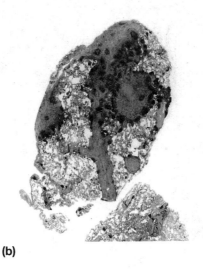

(b)

Figure 8 Continued

and, occasionally, nodules or mass-like lesions (45). As the pulmonary involvement progresses, the symptoms and imaging studies of many these patients resemble clinically those of patients with advanced pulmonary fibrosis with severe dyspnea and features of honeycomb changes (42).

A. Histopathology of Advanced Autoimmune Pulmonary Disease

The pulmonary pathology of autoimmune pulmonary disease includes a variety of patterns of injury involving the pleura, parenchyma, small airways, and vessels. However, the specific pathology for each disease is difficult to define for a number of reasons. First, the clinical diseases have considerable overlap, and, second, the pathological patterns are not specific for a particular disease. Nonetheless, some generalizations can be made regarding which pathological patterns are more likely to be found in each collagen vascular disease. These are summarized in Table 1.

Pleuritis, either acute or chronic, is the most common pathological pattern found in the collagen vascular diseases (42) and can give rise to pleural fibrosis. Advanced pleural fibrosis with dense, irreversible collagen deposition is most commonly found in patients with rheumatoid arthritis (46). In this patient population, necrobiotic (rheumatoid) nodules can also be found but are seen rarely, mostly in men with advanced seropositive rheumatoid arthritis who also have subcutaneous nodules (47). The nodules may enlarge to form cavities within the subpleural area that can result in hemoptysis and hemothorax or become secondarily infected (48).

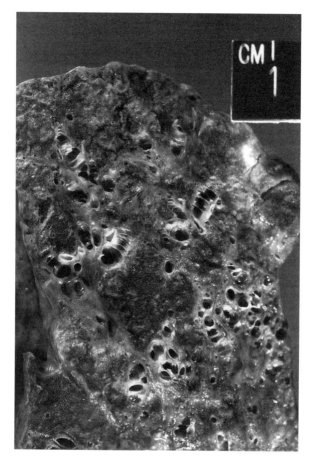

Figure 9   Upper-lobe bronchiectasis in advanced sarcoidosis.

Parenchymal diseases involving both the interstitium and the alveolar space may progress to advanced disease in many of these collagen vascular diseases. The pattern of advanced pathology of many of the interstitial diseases, such as NSIP and UIP, is indistinguishable to that previously described (see Sec. II). However, in some diseases, the pulmonary fibrosis may have distinguishing features. In progressive systemic sclerosis, it may be less active and result in a finer, more diffuse fibrosis (49). In rheumatoid arthritis, the fibrosis has a UIP-type pattern, but prominent areas of reactive bronchus-associated lymphoid tissue (BALT) and increased numbers of fibroblastic foci of young connective tissue (Fig. 19) may distinguish it from idiopathic UIP (50).

Table 1 Pathological Patterns in Collagen Vascular Diseases[a]

	SLE	RA	PSS	Sjörgren's disease	Mixed connective tissue disease	Poly-dermato-myositis
NSIP	+	+		+		+
BOOP	+	+		+		
DAD	+			+		
UIP		+	+	+		+
Pulmonary fibrosis, not UIP			+			
LIP				+		
Lymphoma				+		
Vascular intimal sclerosis	+		+		+	
Vasculitis	+	+	+		+	
Pulmonary hypertension	+	+	+		+	
Intra-alveolar hemorrhage	+				+	
Pleuritis	+	+	+		+	+
Necrobiotic nodules		+				
Constrictive bronchiolitis		+				
Follicular bronchiolitis		+				
Amyloidosis		+				

[a] + = pathologic pattern is found; rare incidence not included.
Key: SLE, systemic lupus erythematosus; RA, rheumatoid arthritis; PSS, progressive systemic sclerosis; NSIP, nonspecific interstitial pneumonia; BOOP, bronchiolitis obliterans organizing pneumonia; DAD, diffuse alveolar damage; UIP, usual interstitial pneumonia; LIP, lymphocytic interstitial pneumonia.

Advanced airway pathology in collagen vascular diseases usually takes the form of constrictive bronchiolitis (49). This irreversible scarring of the small airways arises out of a chronic lymphocytic bronchiolitis producing submucosal and eventually transmural scarring of the airway that leads to complete replacement of the lumen with collagen. Bronchiectasis, though rare, may also be found, and both pathological patterns are most commonly found in rheumatoid arthritis (51).

Chronic vascular pathology in the collagen vascular diseases usually takes the form of pulmonary hypertensive arteriopathy with fibrointimal thickening and muscular hypertrophy or more advanced changes of fibrointimal obliteration and angiomatoid lesions. These changes are most commonly seen in the setting of progressive systemic sclerosis where a concentric fibrotic narrowing of the lumen (Fig. 20) may result in pulmonary hypertension (52).

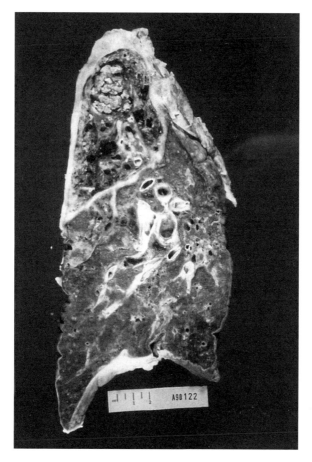

Figure 10 Cystic end-stage sarcoidosis with aspergilloma in apical cavity. (Courtesy of J. Tomashefski, Jr., MetroHealth Medical Center, Cleveland, Ohio.)

VI. Lymphangioleiomyomatosis

Lymphangioleiomyomatosis (LAM) is a rare disease characterized by the abnormal proliferation of smooth muscle cells within the parenchyma of the lung and occasionally within extrapulmonary sites such as the lymphatics and lymph nodes of the retroperitoneum and mediastinum (53). It occurs exclusively in females in their reproductive years, with an average age at diagnosis of 30 to 35 years (54), though a case in a man has been reported (55). Caucasians are most commonly affected and no familial tendency has been described. A wide variety of lesions have been associated with LAM, including tuberous sclerosis and/or renal angiomyolipomas (56–58). The most common presenting symptoms are exertional dyspnea and pneumothorax with

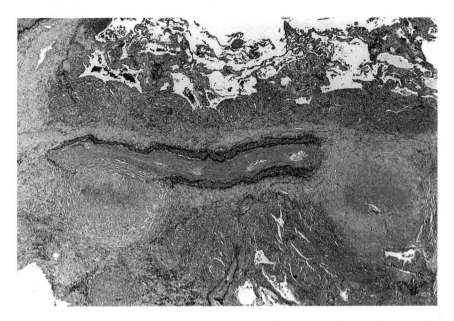

Figure 11 Obliteration of pulmonary artery by sarcoidal granulomas. The artery has some intimal fibroplasia secondary to adjacent inflammation (×20).

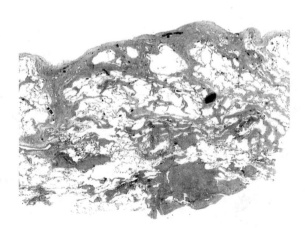

Figure 12 End-stage sarcoidosis with scarring in the distribution of the lymphatics and areas of large air-filled spaces with honeycomb-like appearance due to alveolar wall collapse (×8).

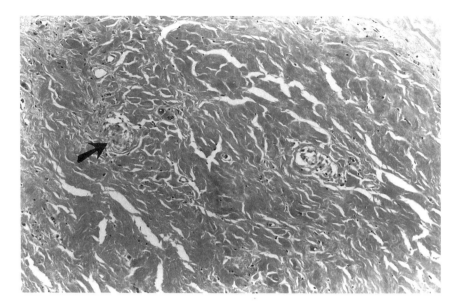

Figure 13 End-stage sarcoidosis with area of hyalinized collagen and scattered giant cells (arrow) as the only remnant of previous granulomas (×100).

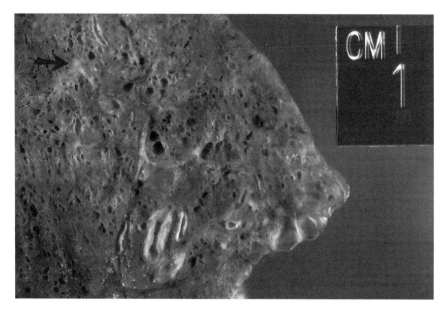

Figure 14 Pulmonary histiocytosis X with early emphysematous changes and stellate lesions (arrow).

hemoptysis, chest pain, and chylous pleural effusions commonly developing during the course of the disease (59). Chest x-rays in LAM usually show a generalized, symmetrical reticulonodular interstitial infiltrate with normal lung volumes. However, as the disease progresses, the chest x-ray may show honeycombing differing from that of end-stage interstitial fibrosis in that it appears more "delicate" (60). Computed tomography (CT) of the chest or high resolution CT will show extensive cystic degeneration (61).

A. Macroscopic Features of Advanced Lymphangioleiomyomatosis

Lungs involved by LAM have diffuse, small, thin-walled cysts that range in size from 5 to 50 mm, are round or polygon-shaped, and are scattered throughout the lung without a clear predilection (61). As the disease progresses, the cysts may become bigger and coalesce, producing a honeycomb appearance (Fig. 21). However, unlike end-stage lungs of interstitial fibrosis—which are small and dense, with thick, gray-white fibrous tissue—advanced LAM lungs have a tan/brown color from the smooth muscle and hemosiderin deposition and are of normal size (62). In between the cysts may be areas of normal lung parenchyma, though these are rare in advanced disease. The pleural surface has blebs protruding throughout and the pleural cavity may have dense fibrous adhesions because of ruptured cysts and recurrent pneumothoraces. Surgeons have described a weeping of chylous fluid from the pleural surface due to the lymphatic obstruction (63).

B. Histopathology of Advanced Lymphangioleiomyomatosis

The lesions of LAM show abnormal accumulations of smooth muscle cells in the adventitia of the terminal bronchi, in the alveolar walls, around lymphatics and venules, and in the pleura (Fig. 22). These smooth muscle cells are plump, spindle-shaped cells with round or ovoid nuclei (Fig. 23). Ultrastructurally, they contain numerous electron-dense membrane-bound granules consisting of fine crystal-like lamellae (64). Immunohistochemical studies reveal that they are immunoreactive to alpha smooth muscle–specific actin, confirming their myoid lineage (65) and to HMB-45, a monoclonal antibody for melanomas and melanocytic lesions (64). Within the alveoli are reactive type II pneumocytes and hemosiderin-laden macrophages. The hemosiderin present in these lungs is thought to be a result of microhemorrhages secondary to venous obstruction by the smooth muscle cells.

Early lesions of LAM occur mainly around lymphatics; as the disease advances, however, these smooth muscle cell proliferations increasingly involve terminal and respiratory bronchiolar walls, causing their collapse, promoting emphysema, and contributing to the parenchymal cysts and pneumothorax (66,67). The amount of smooth muscle gradually increases and—by the time the disease is at end stage—the entire lung consists of thick nodules of smooth muscle cells between large, irregular emphysematous spaces (Fig. 24). These

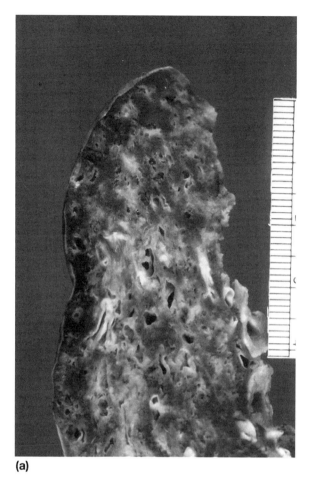

(a)

Figure 15 End-stage pulmonary histiocytosis X with advanced scarring and early cyst formation (a). (Courtesy of J. Tomashefski, Jr., MetroHealth Medical Center, Cleveland, Ohio.) Fibrotic phase of end-stage pulmonary histiocytosis X with obliteration and scarring of bronchioles and vessels, producing a stellate pattern of fibrosis with adjacent emphysema (b) ($\times$ 16).

nodules contain more collagen than those found in early-stage LAM (53). In addition, around and within the nodules of smooth muscle are slit-like spaces distended with lymph fluid due to the obstruction of lymphatics. The venules may also be obliterated, causing pulmonary venous hypertension and hemoptysis (68).

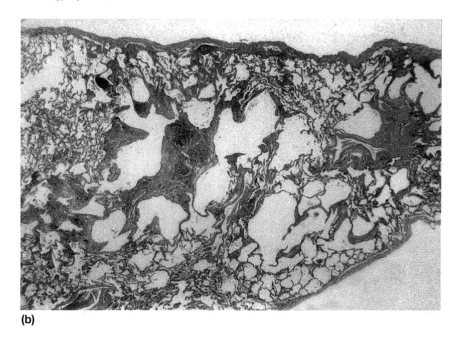

(b)

Figure 15 Continued

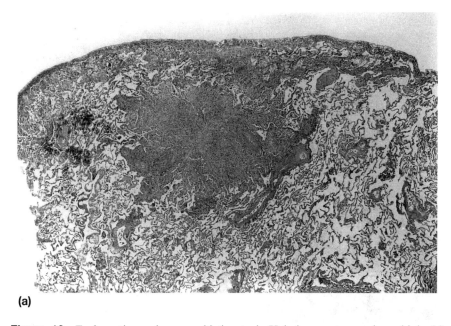

(a)

Figure 16 Early active pulmonary histiocytosis X lesion center on bronchiole (a) (×16). Inflammatory infiltrate is composed of scattered eosinophils, lymphocytes, plasma cells, and Langerhans cells (b) (×200).

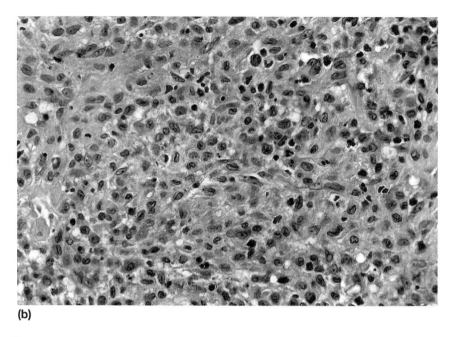

(b)

Figure 16   Continued

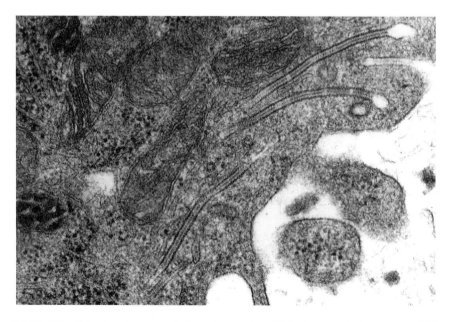

Figure 17   Cytoplasmic racquet-shaped granules (Birbeck granules) present within Langerhans cell cytoplasm.

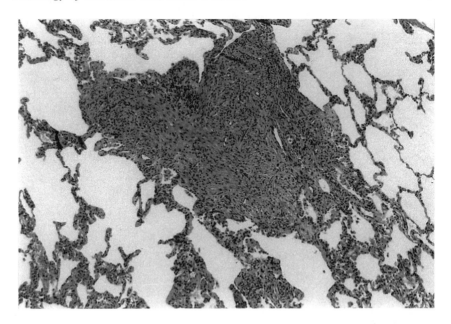

Figure 18 Active lesion of pulmonary histiocytosis X with spread of inflammatory cells into adjacent alveolar walls, producing a stellate appearance (×40).

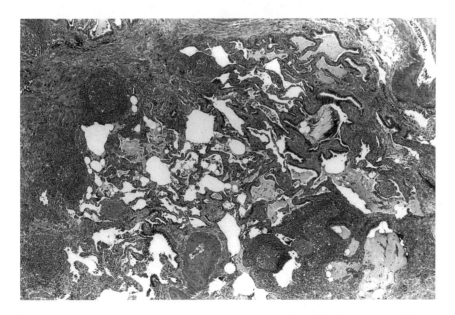

Figure 19 Lung from patient with rheumatoid arthritis and UIP pattern of fibrosis with prominent areas of reactive BALT (×16).

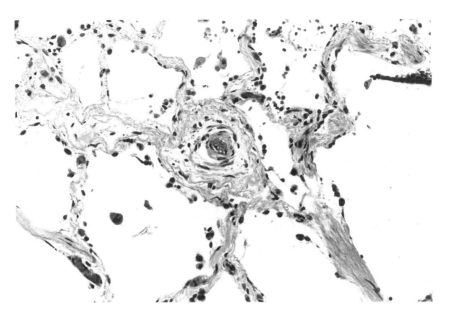

Figure 20 Small arteriole with concentic fibrotic narrowing in lung from patient with progressive systemic sclerosis (× 100).

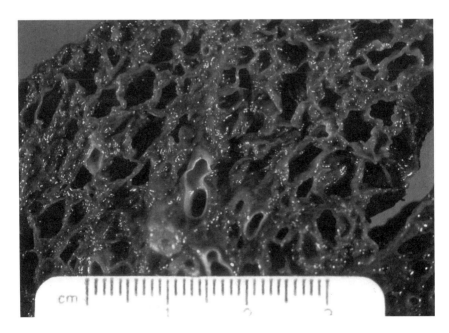

Figure 21 Cut surface of an explant lung from patient with lymphangioleiomyomatosis showing large cysts that coalesce to produce a honeycomb-like appearance.

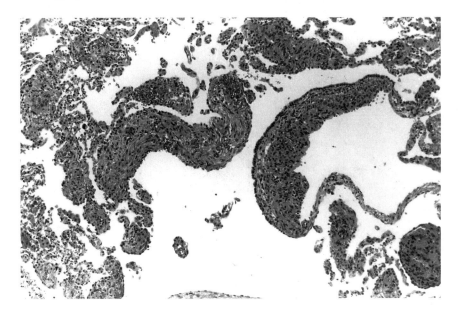

Figure 22 LAM smooth muscle cells around bronchioles and vessels in lung involved by lymphangioleiomyomatosis (× 100).

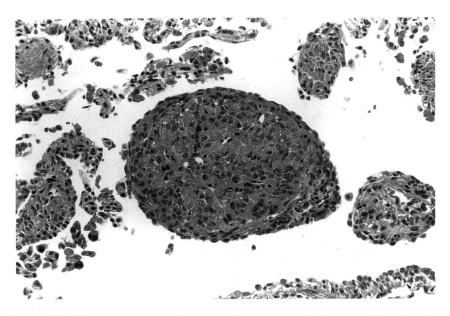

Figure 23 Plump smooth muscle cells with round or fusiform nuclei in fascicles (× 200).

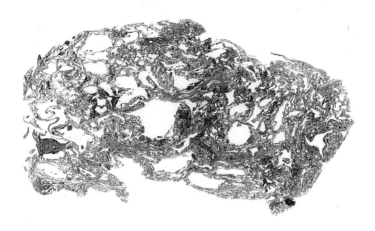

Figure 24 End-stage lymphangioleiomyomatosis with thick nodules of smooth muscle cells between large, irregular emphysematous spaces (× 8).

References

1. Hammer SP. Idiopathic interstitial fibrosis. In: Dail DH, Hammer SP, eds. Pulmonary Pathology. New York: Springer-Verlag, 1994:647–678.
2. Akira M, Sakatani M, Ueda E. Idiopathic pulmonary fibrosis: progression of honeycombing at thin-section CT. Radiology 1993; 189:687–691.
3. Colby TV, Churg AC. Patterns of pulmonary fibrosis. Pathol Annu 1986; 277–309.
4. Crystal RG, Bitterman PB, Rennard SI, Hance AJ, Keogh BA. Interstitial lung diseases of unknown cause: disorders characterized by chronic inflammation of the lower respiratory tract. N Engl J Med 1984; 310(3):154–164.
5. Wolff G, Crystal RG, Biology of pulmonary fibrosis. In: Crystal RG, West JB, Weibel ER, Barnes PJ, eds. The Lung. Philadelphia: Lippincott-Raven, 1997:2509–2524.
6. Katzenstein A-L, Fiorelli RF. Nonspecific interstitial fibrosis: histologic features and clinical significance. Am J Surg Pathol 1994; 18(2):136–147.
7. Nagai S, Kitaichi M, Itoh H, Nishimura K, Izumi T, Colby TV. Idiopathic nonspecific interstitial pneumonia/fibrosis: comparison with idiopathic pulmonary fibrosis and BOOP. Eur Respir J 1998; 12(5):1010–1019.
8. Tomashefski JF, Jr. Pulmonary pathology of the adult respiratory distress syndrome. Clin Chest Med 1990; 11(4):593–619.
9. Thomas PD, Hunninghake GW. Current concepts of the pathogenesis of sarcoidosis. Am Rev Respir Dis 1987; 135:747–760.
10. Hosoda Y, Yamaguchi M, Hiraga Y. Global epidemiology of sarcoidosis. Clin Chest Med 1997; 18(4):681–694.
11. Reich JM, Johnson RE. Course and prognosis of sarcoidosis in a nonreferral setting: analysis of 86 patients observed for 10 years. Am J Med 1985; 89:61–66.

12. DeRemee RA. Sarcoidosis. Mayo Clin Proc 1995; 70:177–184.
13. Chiles C, Putnam CE. Pulmonary sarcoidosis. Semin Respir Med 1992; 13:345–357.
14. Zak HJ, Cole RP. Bullous emphysema occuring in pulmonary sarcoidosis. Respiration 1995; 62:290–293.
15. McCann BG, Harrison BDW. Bronchiolar narrowing and occlusion in sarcoidosis—correlation of pathology with physiology. Respir Med 1991; 85:65–67.
16. Mayock RI, Bertrand P, Morisson CE, Scott JH. Manifestations of sarcoidosis. Am J Med 1963; 35:67–89.
17. Israel HL, Ostrow A. Sarcoidosis and aspergillloma. Am J Med 1969; 47:243–250.
18. Carr I, Norris P. The fine structure of human macrophage granules in sarcoidosis. J Pathol 1977; 122:29–32.
19. Katzenstein A-L. Systemic diseases involving the lung. In: Katzenstein and Askin's Surgical Pathology of Non-Neoplastic Lung Disease. Philadelphia: Saunders, 1997:168–192.
20. Romer FK. Sarcoidosis with large nodular lesions simulating pulmonary metastases: an analysis of 126 cases of intrathoracic sarcoidosis. Scand J Respir Dis 1977; 58:11–16.
21. Mitchell DM, Mitchell DN, Emerson CH. Transbronchial lung biopsy through fiberoptic bronchoscope in diagnosis of sarcoidosis. Br Med J 1980; 280:679–681.
22. Carrington CB, Gaensler EA, Mikus JP, Schachter AW, Burke GH, Goff AM. Structure and function in sarcoidosis. Ann NY Acad Sci 1976; 278:265–283.
23. Rosen Y, Moon S, Huang C, Gourin A, Lyons HA. Granulomatous pulmonary angiitis in sarcoidosis. Arch Pathol Lab Med 1977; 101:170–174.
24. Takemura T, Matsui Y, Saiki S, Mikami R. Pulmonary vascular involvement in sarcoidosis: a report of 40 autopsy cases. Hum Pathol 1992; 23:1216–1223.
25. Smith L, Lawrence J, Katzenstein A. Vascular sarcoidosis: a rare cause of pulmonary hypertension. Am J Med Sci 1983; 38:38–44.
26. Lichtestein L: Histiocytosis X: Integration of eosinophilic granuloma of bone, "Letterer-Siwe disease" and "Schuller-Christian disease" as related manifestations of a single nosologic entity. Arch Pathol 1953; 56:84–102.
27. Travis WD, Borok Z, Roum JH, Zhang J, Feuerstein I, Ferrans VJ, Crystal RG. Pulmonary Langerhans cell granulomatosis (histiocytosis X): a clinicopathologic study of 48 cases. Am J Surg Pathol 1993; 17(10):971–986.
28. Colby TV, Lombard C. Histiocytosis X in the lung. Hum Pathol 1983; 14:847–856.
29. Prophet D. Primary pulmonary histiocytosis X. Clin Chest Med 1982; 3:643–653.
30. Lewis JG. Eosinophilic granuloma and its variants with special reference to lung involvement. Q J Med 1964; 33:377 386.
31. Youkeles JS, Grizzanti JS, Liao Z, Chang CJ, Rosenstreich DL. Decreased tobacco-glycoprotein-induced lymphocyte proliferation in vitro in pulmonary eosinophilic granuloma. Am J Respir Crit Care Med 1995; 151(1):145–150.
32. Aguayo SM, King TE Jr, Waldron JA Jr, Sherritt KM, Kane MA, Miller YE. Increased pulmonary neuroendocrine cells with bombesin-like immunoreactivity in adult patients with eosinophilic granuloma. J Clin Invest 1990; 86(3):838–844.
33. Friedman PJ, Liebow AA, Sokologg J. Eosinophilic granuloma of the lung. Medicine 1983; 60:385–396.
34. Hoffman L, Cohn JE, Gaensler EA. Respiratory abnormalities in eosinophilic granuloma of the lung. N Engl J Med 1962; 267:577–589.

35. Flint A, Lloyd RV, Colby TB. Pulmonary histiocytosis X: immunoperoxidase staining for HLA-DR antigen and S-100 protein. Arch Pathol Lab Med 1986; 110(10):930–933.

36. Auerswald V, Barth J, Magnussen H. Value of CD-1 positive cells in bronchoalveolar lavage fluid for the diagnosis of pulmonary histiocytosis X. Lung 1991; 169:305–309.

37. Soler P, Chollet S, Jacque C, Fukuda Y, Ferrans JV, Basset F. Immunocytochemical characterization of pulmonary histiocytosis X cells in lung biopsies. Am J Pathol 1985; 118(3):439–451.

38. Gracey DR, Divertie MB, Brown AL Jr. Primary pulmonary histiocytosis X: electron microscopic study of eight cases. Chest 1971; 59(1):5–9.

39. Bedrossian CWM, Kuhn CIII, Luna MA, Conklin RH, Byrd RB, Kaplan PD. Desquamative interstitial pneumonia-like reaction accompanying pulmonary lesions. Chest 1977; 72:166–169.

40. Powers MA, Askin FB, Cresson DH. Pulmonary eosinophilic granuloma. 25-year follow-up. Am Rev Respir Dis 1984; 129(3):503–507.

41. Harari S, Brenot F, Barberis M, Simmoneau G. Advanced pulmonary histiocytosis X is associated with severe pulmonary hypertension. Chest 1997; 111(4):1142–1144.

42. Wiedemann HP, Matthay RA. Pulmonary manifestations of the collagen vascular diseases. Chest 1989; 10:677–722.

43. Matthay RA, Schwarz MI, Petty TL. Pleuro-pulmonary manifestations of connective tissue diseases. Clin Notes Respir Dis 1977; 16:3–9.

44. King TE Jr. Connective tissue disease. In: Interstitial Lung Disease. Hamilton, Ontario: Decker, 1998:451–506.

45. Hunninghake GW, Fauci AS. Pulmonary involvement in the collagen vascular diseases. Am Rev Respir Dis 1979; 119:471–503.

46. Shiel WC Jr, Prete PE. Pleuropulmonary manifestations of rheumatoid arthritis. Semin Arthritis Rheum 1984; 13:235–243.

47. Hull S, Mathews JA. Pulmonary necrobiotic ndules as a presenting feature of rheumatoid arthritis. Ann Rheum Dis 1982: 41:21–24.

48. Ziff M. The rheumatoid nodule. Arthritis Rheum 1990; 33:761–767.

49. Colby TV. Pulmonary pathology in patients with systemic autoimmune diseases. Clin Chest Med 1998; 19(4):587–612.

50. Travis WD, Koss MN, Feerrans VJ. The lung in connective tissue disorders. In: Haselton PS, ed. Spencer's Pathology of the Lung. New York: McGraw-Hill, 1996:803–834.

51. Shadick NA, Fanta CH, Weinblatt ME, O'Donnell W, Coblyn JS. Bronchiectasis. A late feature of severe rheumatoid arthritis. Medicine (Baltimore) 1994; 73:161–170.

52. Young RH, Mark EJ. Pulmonary vascular changes in scleroderma. Am J Med 1978; 64:998–1004.

53. Johnson S. Rare Diseases—lymphangioleiomyomatosis: clinical features, management and basic mechanism. Thorax 1999; 54(3):254–264.

54. Sullivan E. Lymphangioleiomyomatosis: a review. Chest 1998; 114(6):1689–1703.

55. Aubry MC, Myers JL, Ryu JH, Henske EP, Logginidou H, Jala SM, Tazelaar H. Pulmonary lymphangioleiomyomatosis in a man. Am J Respir Crit Care Med 2000; 162:749–752.

56. Corrin B, Liebow AA, Friedman PJ. Pulmonary lymphangiomyomatosis: a review. Am J Pathol 1975; 79:347–382.
57. Capron F, Amille J, LeClerc P, Mornet P, Barbagellata M, Reynes M, Rochemaure J. Pulmonary lymphangioleiomyomatosis and Bourneville's tuberous sclerosis with pulmonary involvement: the same disease. Cancer 1983; 52(5): 851–855.
58. Lack EE, Dolan MF, Finisio J, Grover G, Singh M, Triche TJ. Pulmonary and extrapulmonary lymphangioleiomyomatosis: report of a case with bilateral renal angiomyolipomas, multifocal lymphangioleiomyomatosis and a glial polyp of the endocervix. Am J Surg Pathol 1986; 10(9):650–657.
59. Taylor JR, Ryu J, Colby TV, Raffin TA. Lymphangioleiomyomatosis: clinical course in 32 patients. N Engl J Med 1990; 323(18):1254–1260.
60. Carrington CB, Cugell DW, Gaensler EA, Marks A, Redding RA, Schaaf JT, Tomasian A. Lymphangioleiomyomatosis: physiologic-pathologic-radiologic correlations. Am Rev Respir Dis 1977; 116(6):977–995.
61. Muller NL, Chiles C, Kullnig P. Pulmonary lymphangiomyomatosis: correlation of CT with radiographic and functional findings. Radiology 1990; 175:335–339.
62. Colby TV, Carrington CB. Interstitial Lung Disease. In: Thurlbeck WM, Churg AM, eds. Pathology of the Lung. New York: Thieme, 1995:589–737.
63. Dail D. Uncommon tumors. In: Dail DH, Hammer SP, eds. Pulmonary Pathology. New York: Springer-Verlag, 1994:1279–1461.
64. Bonetti F, Chiodera PL, Pea M, Martignoni G, Bosi F, Zamboni G, Mariuzzi GM. Transbronchial biopsy in lymphangiomyomatosis of the lung. Am J Surg Pathol 1993; 17(11):1092–1102.
65. Kalassian KG, Doyle R, Kao P, Ruoss S, Raffin TA. Lymphangioleiomyomatosis: new insights. Am J Respir Crit Care Med 1997; 155:1183–1186.
66. Sobonya RE, Quan SF, Fleishman JS. Pulmonary lymphangioleiomyomatosis: quantitative analysis of lesions producing airflow limitation. Hum Pathol 1985; 16:1122–1128.
67. Fukuda Y, Kawamoto M, Yamamoto A, Ishizaki M, Bassett F, Masugi Y. Role of elastic fiber degradation in emphysema-like lesions of pulmonary lymphangiomyomatosis. Hum Pathol 1990; 21:1252–1261.

3

Pathology of Advanced Pulmonary Vascular Disease

J. MICHAEL KAY

McMaster University
Hamilton, Ontario, Canada

I. Introduction

A. Nomenclature and Classification of Pulmonary Hypertension

Pulmonary hypertension is a common condition that has many causes and associations and has been the subject of many attempts at classification. In the majority of patients, clinical examination together with relevant investigations reveals a cause such as underlying heart or lung disease. These cases have been classified as *secondary* pulmonary hypertension. In a small minority of patients, the cause of the pulmonary hypertension remains unexplained despite exclusion of predisposing lesions by history, physical examination, chest imaging, lung function tests, and cardiac catheterization. In 1975, a committee of the World Health Organization (WHO) suggested that such cases should be designated *primary* pulmonary hypertension (1). Unfortunately, many authors have used this term to refer to the specific entity of unexplained pulmonary arteriopathy with plexiform lesions, so that in practice it has had two different meanings. The term *unexplained* pulmonary hypertension was then introduced to refer to cases of pulmonary hypertension in which clinical examination and investigation revealed no cause (2). Pulmonary hypertension has also been classified as *hyperkinetic*, *passive*, *obstructive*, and *vasoconstrictive*, according to the dominant pathophysiological mechanism involved (3,4). The plethora of classifications has confused patients, insurance carriers, and some physicians (5). In an attempt to remedy this problem, a new diagnostic classification of pulmonary hypertension was proposed at a WHO meeting in 1998 (Table 1). This classification recognizes that the tissue pathology of pulmonary hypertension caused by different agents may be similar and the treatment may be identical (6).

B. Risk Factors for Pulmonary Hypertension

A risk factor for pulmonary hypertension is any factor or condition that is suspected to play a causal or facilitating role in the development of the disease. Risk factors—which may include drugs, demographic factors, and other diseases—must be present prior to the onset of pulmonary hypertension. When it is not possible to determine whether a factor was present before the onset of the pulmonary hypertension and it is thus unclear whether it played a causal role, the term *associated condition* is used. The precise mechanisms by which some risk factors produce pulmonary hypertension have not been established. A subcommittee of the WHO has categorized risk factors according to the strength of their association with pulmonary hypertension and their probable causal role (Table 2) (6). *Definite* indicates an association based on several different observations, including a major controlled study or a clear epidemic. *Very likely* indicates several concordant observations or a general consensus among experts. *Possible* indicates an association based on case series, registries, or expert opinions. *Unlikely* indicates risk factors that have been proposed but have not been found to have any association from controlled studies. Definite risk factors are considered to play a causal role in the development of pulmonary hypertension.

Based on current available evidence and on personal experience, the present author differs from the WHO subcommittee and would classify amphetamines as unlikely and portal hypertension/liver disease, collagen vascular diseases, and congenital systemic-pulmonary cardiac shunts as definite risk factors for pulmonary hypertension.

C. Causes of Advanced Pulmonary Vascular Disease

The conditions that are commonly encountered in patients who present for medical or surgical treatment of advanced pulmonary vascular disease are as follows:

Systemic-to-pulmonary shunts
Primary pulmonary arterial hypertension
Chronic pulmonary thrombotic and/or embolic disease
Pulmonary veno-occlusive disease
Pulmonary capillary hemangiomatosis

The pathology of these conditions is reviewed in the following paragraphs.

Table 1 WHO Classification of Pulmonary Hypertension

A. **Pulmonary arterial hypertension**
   1 Primary pulmonary hypertension
      a. Sporadic
      b. Familial
   2 Related to:
      a. Collagen vascular disease
      b. Congenital systemic-to-pulmonary shunts
      c. Portal hypertension
      d. HIV infection
      e. Drugs/toxins
          i.   Anorexigens
          ii. Other
      f. Persistent pulmonary hypertension of the newborn
      g. Other
B. **Pulmonary venous hypertension**
   1 Left-sided atrial or ventricular heart disease
   2 Left-sided valvular heart disease
   3 Extrinsic compression of central pulmonary veins
      a. Fibrosing mediastinitis
      b. Adenopathy/tumors
   4 Pulmonary veno-occlusive disease
   5 Other
C. **Pulmonary hypertension associated with disorders of the respiratory system and/or hypoxemia**
   1 Chronic obstructive pulmonary disease
   2 Interstitial lung disease
   3 Sleep-disordered breathing
   4 Alveolar hypoventilation disorders
   5 Chronic exposure to high altitude
   6 Neonatal lung disease
   7 Alveolar-capillary dysplasia
   8 Other
D. **Pulmonary hypertension due to chronic thrombotic and/or embolic disease**
   1 Thromboembolic obstruction of proximal pulmonary arteries
   2 Obstruction of distal pulmonary arteries
      a. Pulmonary embolism (thrombus, tumor, ova and/or parasites, foreign material)
      b. In situ thrombosis
      c. Sickle cell disease
E. **Pulmonary hypertension due to disorders directly affecting the pulmonary vasculature**
   1 Inflammatory
      a. Schistosomiasis
      b. Sarcoidosis
      c. Other
   2 Pulmonary capillary hemangiomatosis

Key: WHO, World Health Organization; HIV, human immunodeficiency virus.

Table 2 WHO Classification of Risk Factors for Pulmonary Hypertension

A.	**Drugs and toxins**

A. **Drugs and toxins**
    1. Definite
        a. Aminorex
        b. Fenfluramine
        c. Toxic rapeseed oil
    2. Very likely
        a. Amphetamines
        b. L-tryptophan
    3. Possible
        a. Meta-amphetamines
        b. Cocaine
        c. Chemotherapeutic agents
    4. Unlikely
        a. Antidepressants
        b. Oral contraceptives
        c. Estrogen therapy
        d. Cigarette smoking
B. **Demographic and medical conditions**
    1. Definite
        a. Gender
    2. Possible
        a. Pregnancy
        b. Systemic hypertension
    3. Unlikely
        a. Obesity
C. **Diseases**
    1. Definite
        a. HIV infection
    2. Very likely
        a. Portal hypertension/liver disease
        b. Collagen vascular diseases
        c. Congenital systemic-to-pulmonary cardiac shunts
    3. Possible
        a. Thyroid disorders

Key: WHO, World Health Organization; HIV, human immunodeficiency virus.

There is considerable variation in pulmonary vascular reactivity from individual to individual. This means that the same cause of pulmonary hypertension may be present in various subjects to the same extent, but the degree of pulmonary hypertension and the severity of the hypertensive pulmonary vascular disease may vary considerably.

II. Systemic-to-Pulmonary Shunts

Shunts between the systemic and pulmonary circulations will increase pulmonary blood flow. Pulmonary hypertension may develop if the shunt is large enough and if there is no accompanying pulmonary stenosis to protect the pulmonary circulation. It is helpful to consider a shunt as being either pre- or posttricuspid because the risk to the pulmonary circulation is different in each case.

Pretricuspid shunts occur at the level of the atria and include high atrial septal defects such as those of the secundum or sinus venosus type (Table 3). The major factor influencing the magnitude of the left-to-right shunt is the distensibility of the two ventricles. At birth, the thickness of the ventricles is similar and their distensibilities do not differ significantly. Therefore there is little or no shunting of blood through the atrial septal defect. However, once the right ventricular pressure falls, the wall of the right ventricle becomes thinner relative to the left ventricle while its distensibility becomes relatively greater. As a result, a left-to-right shunt develops through the atrial septal defect, thereby increasing the pulmonary blood flow. In young people with pretricuspid shunts, the pulmonary blood flow may be three times greater than normal, but the pulmonary vascular resistance is not elevated because of the enormous distensibility of the pulmonary vasculature. However, an increase in pulmonary blood flow of this magnitude for many years eventually leads to the development of pulmonary hypertension in about 30% of subjects (3). Hypertensive pulmonary vascular disease is usually delayed until the fourth decade, only rarely occurring in childhood or early adult life (7).

Posttricuspid shunts are the result of large communications between the left ventricle or aorta on one hand and the right ventricle or pulmonary arteries

Table 3 Causes of Systemic-to-Pulmonary Shunts

Pretricuspid shunts
  Atrial septal defects
  Anomalous pulmonary venous drainage
Posttricuspid shunts
  Ventricular septal defect
  Persistent truncus arteriosus
  Single ventricle
  Eisenmenger's complex
  Patent ductus arteriosus
  Aortopulmonary septal defect
  Complete atrioventricular canal defect
  Rupture of aortic aneurysm into pulmonary artery
  Rupture of ventricular septum after myocardial infarction
  Postoperative systemic-to-pulmonary shunt procedure

on the other. Most of the diseases with posttricuspid shunts are congenital anomalies of the heart and great vessels, such as ventricular septal defect (Table 3). Rarely, a posttricuspid shunt may be acquired, as in the case of rupture of the interventricular septum following myocardial infarction (8). In posttricuspid shunts such as ventricular septal defect, the magnitude of the shunt is proportional to the area of the defect and to the difference in pressure between the two ventricles (3). Associated stenosis of the pulmonary valve increases the resistance to outflow from the right ventricle and diminishes the magnitude of the left-to-right shunt. Conversely, stenosis of the aortic valve elevates left ventricular pressure and increases the shunt of blood into the right ventricle. At birth, there is normally a rapid fall in pulmonary vascular resistance as the ductus arteriosus closes and the pulmonary arteries dilate. If a large ventricular septal defect is present, this fall in pulmonary vascular resistance and pressure may be delayed for several weeks. Only when the resistance begins to decline does the left-to-right shunt increase. Thus, affected infants do not usually develop symptoms during the first 4 weeks of life. The combination of high pressure and high flow may produce pulmonary vascular disease as early as the second year of life.

A. Pulmonary Vascular Disease in Systemic-to-Pulmonary Shunts

Hypertensive pulmonary vascular disease develops only in those cases of systemic to pulmonary shunt in which critical levels of pulmonary artery pressure and flow are reached and exceeded. The brunt of the disease falls on the muscular pulmonary arteries and pulmonary arterioles, which may show spectacular and characteristic changes. Less prominent lesions also occur in the pulmonary veins and lung parenchyma.

B. Muscular Pulmonary Arteries and Pulmonary Arterioles

Progressive changes develop in the intima and media of muscular pulmonary arteries and pulmonary arterioles in patients with systemic-to-pulmonary shunts (9). The lesions tend to follow a sequence irrespective of the precise nature of the defect causing the shunt but related to a progressive increase in pulmonary artery pressure and pulmonary vascular resistance on the one hand and a reduction in pulmonary blood flow on the other. The earliest structural change is medial hypertrophy of muscular pulmonary arteries, accompanied by muscularization of pulmonary arterioles. In more severe cases, this is complicated by a cellular intimal proliferation, which may be followed by concentric laminar intimal fibrosis. The changes encountered in patients presenting with advanced pulmonary vascular disease comprise severe concentric laminar intimal fibrosis, plexiform lesions, dilation lesions, fibrinoid necrosis, and arteritis. These lesions are associated with high, fixed levels of pulmonary vascular resistance.

A growing body of literature based on in vivo and in vitro research supports the concept of phenotypic heterogeneity within the smooth muscle cell population of the arterial media (10). Numerous functions are required of smooth muscle cells under both normal and pathological conditions. These include contraction, proliferation, and synthesis of matrix proteins. These different smooth muscle cell functions may require different phenotypes. In chronic pulmonary hypertension, some medial smooth muscle cells are likely to hypertrophy and retain contractile functions, whereas others are likely to exhibit increased proliferation and/or synthesis of collagen and elastin. These cellular responses are stimulated by hypoxia, mechanical stress, blood-borne and locally produced mitogens, and growth factors that activate a cascade of intracellular signaling mechanisms that promote smooth muscle cell growth and/or matrix protein synthesis (11).

Muscularization and Medial Hypertrophy

The earliest histological evidence of pulmonary hypertension is muscularization of pulmonary arterioles. The walls of pulmonary arterioles (less than 100 µm in diameter), which are usually devoid of histologically discernible smooth muscle, develop a thick muscular media sandwiched between distinct internal and external elastic laminae. Even arterial vessels as small as 30 µm in diameter become muscularized and resemble small muscular pulmonary arteries instead of venules, as they do in the normal lung. Ultrastructural studies in lung biopsy material from children with congenital heart defects have shown that the new media arises as a result of hypertrophy, division, and differentiation of precursor smooth muscle cells, pericytes, and intermediate cells, which are normally found in the nonmuscular and partially muscular pulmonary arterioles, respectively (12). There is also synthesis of elastic tissue with the formation of a new internal elastic lamina.

The media of muscular pulmonary arteries becomes hypertrophied and may be as thick as 25% of the external diameter of the vessel. Ultrastructural studies have shown that the increase in medial thickness is due both to hypertrophy of the smooth muscle cells and to a significant increase in collagen fibers and elastin. There is a rough correlation between medial thickness of the muscular pulmonary arteries on one hand and elevation of pulmonary arterial pressure and calculated resistance, on the other (13,14). The endothelial cells of hypertrophied muscular pulmonary arteries show increased expression of endothelin-1, which is vasoconstrictor agent and mitogen for smooth muscle cells and fibroblasts (15).

Intimal Proliferation

Ultrastructural studies of thick muscular pulmonary arteries from patients with congenital heart disease and primary pulmonary arterial hypertension have disclosed two distinct types of vascular smooth muscle cell. Most have abundant electron-lucent cytoplasm, but a minority are more elongated, with electron-dense cytoplasm—the so-called dark smooth muscle cells. There is intimate association of light and dark smooth muscle cells. Protuberances of dark cells often fit into depressions on the surfaces of light smooth muscle cells (16). Dark smooth muscle cells from the inner half of the media migrate into the intima through gaps in the internal elastic lamina (17). These gaps may be natural or may arise in pulmonary hypertension as a result of elastase activity. The lumen becomes narrowed as a result of intimal thickening caused by the accumulation of smooth muscle cells between the endothelial basement membrane and the internal elastic lamina. The intimal smooth muscle cells commonly form concentric rings with much intercellular proteoglycan. Histologically this appears as "onionskin" proliferation. The neointimal smooth muscle cells synthesize collagen and elastin so that the lumens of pulmonary arterioles and muscular pulmonary arteries are progressively narrowed by concentric laminar intimal fibroelastosis. In histological sections, concentric laminar intimal fibrosis is commonly identified in muscular pulmonary arteries 100 to 150 μm in diameter, close to their origins from parent vessels (Fig. 1). It is uncommon below the age of 2 years.

Plexiform Lesions

Plexiform lesions, which signify an advanced form of hypertensive pulmonary vascular disease, occur in pulmonary arterial branches measuring between 100 and 150 μm in diameter, shortly after their origin from larger arteries. They are slightly more common in supernumerary arteries than in symmetrical regular dichotomous branches (18). About one-third of plexiform lesions are intra-acinar and about two-thirds are preacinar (19). The typical plexiform lesion has a striking appearance and has two basic elements (Fig. 2). The first consists of a circumscribed dilatation of a pulmonary artery branch close to its origin from a parent artery. In this dilated segment, there is destruction of the arterial wall, with pronounced thinning of the media, loss of smooth muscle cells, as well as disappearance of the internal elastic lamina (Fig. 3) and sometimes also the external elastic lamina. The second element is a collection of narrow, slit-like channels within the dilated segment. These channels, which are lined by cells with hyperchromatic nuclei, resemble a vascular plexus. The distal part of the plexiform lesion drains into a dilated and thin-walled vessel, the wall of which usually consists of a single elastic lamina. This channel, or its branches, terminates in the alveolar capillaries (20). Plexiform lesions vary in structure according to their age. In the early stage of their development, they are cellular, and the vascular spaces are lined by numerous plump cells that have been identified as endothelial cells (21). The tissue separating the vascular spaces contains rounded cells and small quantities of collagen. The media of the parent artery often contains a focus of fibrinoid necrosis that may extend into the wall of the sac. The vascular spaces commonly contain thrombi. More advanced plexiform lesions contain large quantities of collagen, which is deposited between the vascular channels and may encroach on them. The regions of fibrinoid necrosis and thrombosis undergo organization to form masses of collagen. Finally, elastic fibers become deposited. These mature

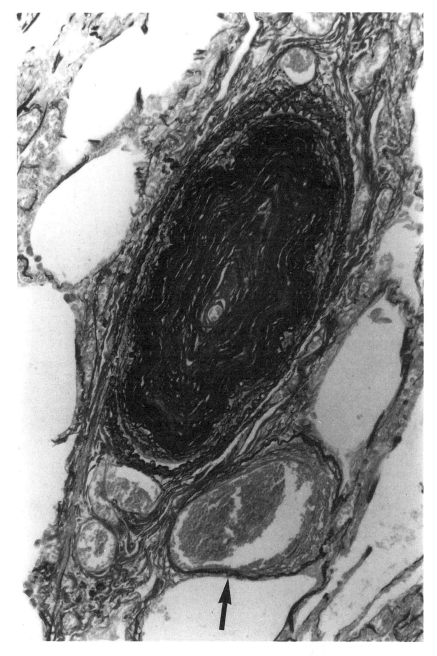

Figure 1 Muscular pulmonary artery from a 25-year-old man with severe pulmonary hypertension due to a large aortopulmonary septal defect. The lumen is narrowed due to severe concentric laminar intimal fibrosis. The media is atrophic. A dilated vein-like branch is located at the lower right side of the artery (arrow). [Miller elastic Van Gieson stain (EVG), ×200.]

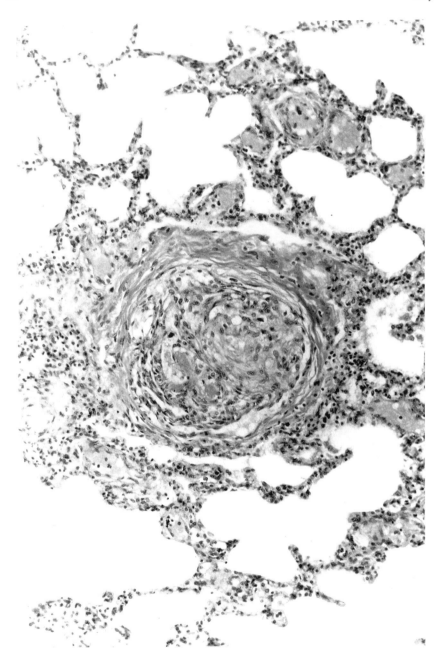

Figure 2 Transverse section of a muscular pulmonary artery showing a plexiform
lesion. There is thinning of the media and loss of smooth muscle cells. The lumen is
occupied by a plexus of slit-like vascular channels lined by proliferated endothelial cells.
From an autopsy performed on a 10-month-old female infant with a large ventricular
septal defect. [Hematoxylin and eosin stain (HE), × 200.]

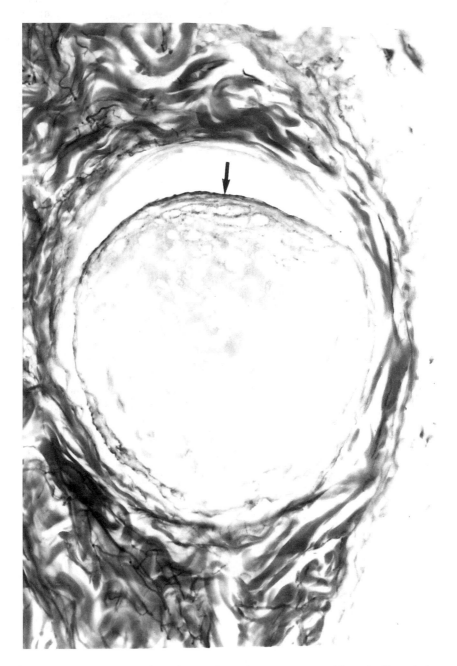

Figure 3 Transverse section of muscular pulmonary artery with a plexiform lesion. There is destruction of the internal elastic lamina and part of the external elastic lamina. An arrow indicates the remaining external elastic lamina. From the infant illustrated in Figure 2. (EVG, × 500.)

plexiform lesions may appear different from the younger ones but can still be recognized as dilated sacs containing irregular bands of fibroelastic tissue in which a plexus of vascular channels persists (Fig. 4). Such mature plexiform lesions can be mistaken for organized thrombi. Plexiform lesions are observed mainly in adolescents and adults and are uncommon below the age of 2 years, although they have been described in infants as young as 8 weeks (22). Their numbers vary greatly. In some cases, numerous plexiform lesions may be seen in a single histological section; in other cases, they are so scarce that multiple sections, sometimes from different blocks are necessary to find them.

Dilatation Lesions

Advanced pulmonary vascular disease is characterized by pronounced dilatation, often over a considerable length, of pulmonary arterial vessels, leading to thinning of the arterial wall (Fig. 5). This may decrease the average thickness of the arterial media considerably. Such an artery may mimic a normal muscular pulmonary artery. There is progressive replacement of medial smooth muscle by fibrous tissue. Eventually, virtually all the media may disappear with the formation of dilatation lesions known as *vein-like branches of hypertrophied muscular pulmonary arteries* (9) (Fig. 6). The rare *angiomatoid lesion* is a dilatation lesion in which widening of the channels associated with dilatation and tortuosity of the surrounding distal branches produces a fairly large, angioma-like mass (20). Dilatation lesions are common in severe pulmonary hypertension, particularly in adults. They are frequently found in lungs that contain plexiform lesions, but they may occur in the absence of these alterations. They seem to occur in a small muscular pulmonary artery just proximal to a fibrotic occlusion.

Fibrinoid Necrosis and Arteritis

Fibrinoid necrosis usually affects small muscular pulmonary arteries and pulmonary arterioles. The media is swollen with loss of nuclear detail. It stains intensely and homogeneously with eosin and by the picro-Mallory and Martius scarlet blue methods for fibrin. The lumen frequently contains a thrombus. Fibrinoid necrosis may be the sole lesion in a hypertensive pulmonary artery, but it is frequently complicated by arteritis. There is an infiltrate of neutrophil polymorphs that affects all layers of the wall and usually extends beyond the adventitia into the surrounding lung tissue (Fig. 7). Older lesions undergo organization with the development of granulation tissue, which involves the adventitia as well as the media. There is often fragmentation of the elastic laminae.

Other Vascular and Parenchymal Lesions

Fresh and organizing thrombi are encountered in the muscular pulmonary arteries of about 30% of patients with congenital heart disease (23). They are

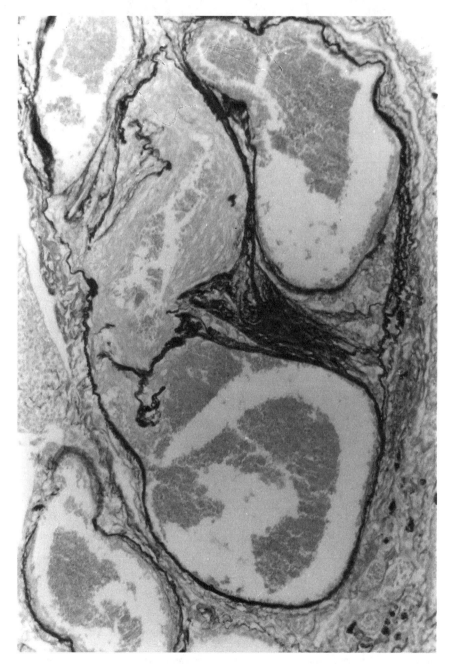

Figure 4 Muscular pulmonary artery with a mature plexiform lesion. The vessel is represented by a dilated sac containing irregular bands of fibroelastic tissue, which separate the vascular channels. From the patient illustrated in Figure 1. (EVG, × 200.)

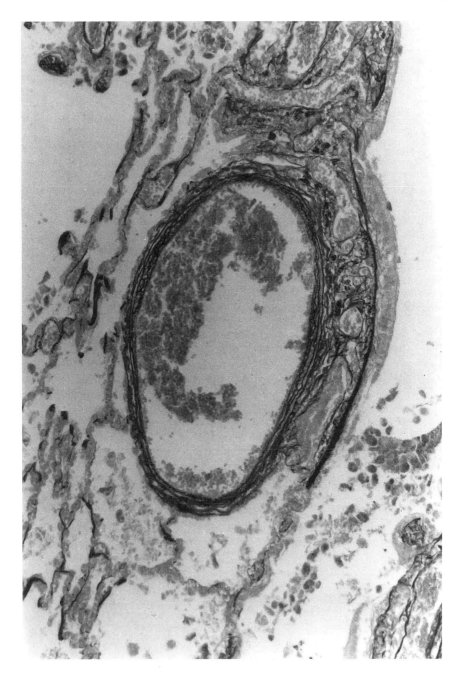

Figure 5 Transverse section of a muscular pulmonary artery from the patient with severe pulmonary hypertension illustrated in Figure 1. Dilatation of the vessel has caused thinning of the media so that it resembles a normal muscular pulmonary artery. (EVG, × 200.)

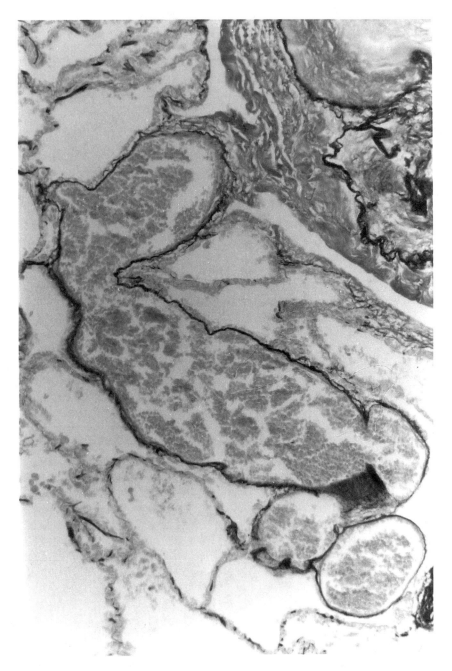

Figure 6 Dilated vein-like branch of muscular pulmonary artery. The edge of the parent artery is seen at the top right corner of the picture. From the patient with the aortopulmonary septal defect shown in Figure 1. (EVG, × 200.)

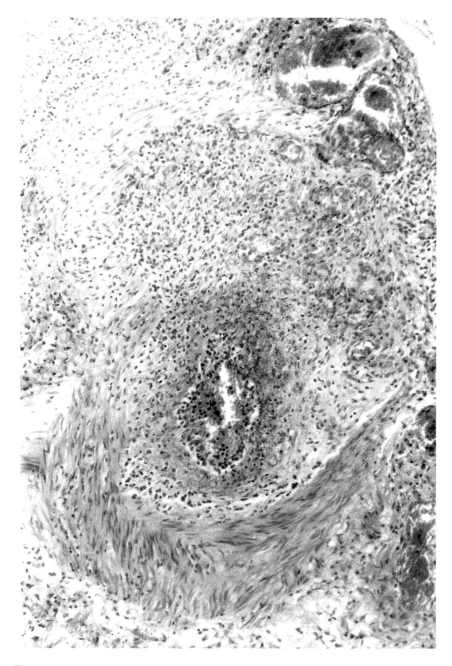

Figure 7 Muscular pulmonary artery showing acute arteritis. The media in the lower half of the picture is intact. In the upper half, it is necrotic and infiltrated by neutrophil polymorphs that extend into the adventitia. From a 12-year-old girl with cor triloculare biatriatum. (HE, × 200.)

probably secondary to endothelial injury caused by the hemodynamic disturbances (24,25). Longitudinal smooth muscle is commonly encountered in muscular pulmonary arteries in hypertensive pulmonary vascular disease of any severity (26). This is a nonspecific change that is not related to the underlying cause of the pulmonary hypertension. It is frequently seen in patients over the age of 11 years with congenital heart disease (23). The smooth muscle cells are arranged in bundles in the intima, where they are situated within a reduplication of the internal elastic lamina. Longitudinal smooth muscle may also be encountered within the media or adventitia.

In almost all patients over the age of 5 years with congenital heart disease, the pulmonary veins show a fibrous or fibrocellular intimal proliferation (23,27). Many patients show muscularization of the pulmonary veins, with the development of a medial coat of smooth muscle separated by two elastic laminae. These venous lesions are probably the consequence of increased levels of pulmonary blood flow, which may be especially high in atrial septal defect (9).

Lung parenchymal lesions that occur in patients with pulmonary hypertension due to congenital heart disease include the presence of increased numbers of alveolar macrophages, intra-alveolar hemorrhage, hemosiderin-laden macrophages, focal intra-alveolar fibrosis, cholesterol granulomas, mast cell hyperplasia, increased neuroendocrine cells in the distal bronchioles, and peribronchial lymphoid aggregates (4,23).

Reversibility of Pulmonary Hypertension and Vascular Disease

The relation between arterial lesions in open-lung biopsy specimens and the reversibility of pulmonary hypertension has been examined in patients studied immediately after the closure of the defect (28) and from 24 hr to 25 years after surgery (27,29,30). Such studies have shown that medial hypertrophy and intimal fibrosis of muscular pulmonary arteries are associated with pulmonary hypertension, which is potentially reversible, while the presence of plexiform lesions and dilatation lesions is associated with high fixed levels of pulmonary vascular resistance and irreversible pulmonary hypertension.

It has been possible to study the regression of hypertensive pulmonary vascular lesions in patients with congenital heart disease in whom banding of the pulmonary artery was performed (31,32). Two lung biopsy specimens were available in these patients, one taken at the time of banding and one several years later at the time of corrective surgery. From such investigations it appears that medial hypertrophy, cellular intimal proliferation, and mild concentric laminar intimal fibrosis (occluding less than 20% of the lumen) are largely reversible. On the other hand, severe concentric laminar intimal fibrosis, plexiform lesions, dilatation lesions, and fibrinoid processes are irreversible.

It should be understood that the presence of potentially reversible pulmonary vascular disease is not always synonymous with operability and immediate postoperative survival (33). Infants and young children with congenital heart disease and severe medial hypertrophy of the muscular pulmonary arteries are especially prone to pulmonary hypertensive crises, which may cause death during surgery or in the postoperative period. Presumably these events result from intense vasoconstriction provoked by such factors as hypoxia and hypovolemia.

III. Primary Pulmonary Arterial Hypertension

The pulmonary vascular and parenchymal lesions that occur in patients with primary pulmonary arterial hypertension are similar to those found in subjects with systemic-to-pulmonary shunts. The muscular pulmonary arteries may show medial hypertrophy, concentric laminar intimal fibrosis (Fig. 8), plexiform lesions (Figs. 9 and 10), dilatation lesions, fibrinoid necrosis, and arteritis. In 1975, an expert committee of the WHO recommended that this pattern of hypertensive pulmonary vascular disease be designated *plexogenic pulmonary arteriopathy* (1). Plexogenic pulmonary arteriopathy was envisaged as a disease with a sequence of changes that might eventually include plexiform lesions. *Plexogenic pulmonary arteriopathy* is a subtle term that implies the potential to develop plexiform lesions. According to the WHO, plexogenic pulmonary arteriopathy can be diagnosed in the absence of plexiform lesions. Using this criterion, only 70 to 89% of the cases designated plexogenic pulmonary arteriopathy actually have plexiform lesions (34–38). The remaining cases have either medial hypertrophy and intimal fibrosis or isolated medial hypertrophy (Table 4). The recommendation of the WHO has either been misunderstood or misinterpreted by many pathologists and clinicians, resulting in much confusion in the literature. Some authors have restricted the diagnosis of plexogenic pulmonary arteriopathy to cases in which plexiform lesions are actually present (35). To add to the confusion, reference has even been made to *preplexiform lesions* (38). Since it is desirable that pathologists make morphological diagnoses based on what they can see rather than speculating on what might develop later, the consultant pathologists associated with the National Heart, Lung, and Blood Institute Registry of Primary Pulmonary Pulmonary Hypertension recommended the use of the term *pulmonary arteriopathy with plexiform lesions* (37). The criterion for making this diagnosis is the identification of plexiform lesions in tissue sections.

A. Muscular Pulmonary Arteries and Pulmonary Arterioles

The frequency with which plexiform lesions, isolated medial hypertrophy, and medial hypertrophy with intimal fibrosis were found in three retrospective and two prospective studies is shown in Table 4. The pattern of pulmonary vascular disease that was most commonly encountered was pulmonary arteriopathy with plexiform lesions. Its incidence in the three retrospective studies ranged from 70 to 89%, while in the two prospective studies it ranged from 75 to 84%. The incidence of isolated medial hypertrophy ranged from 0 to 11%, while the

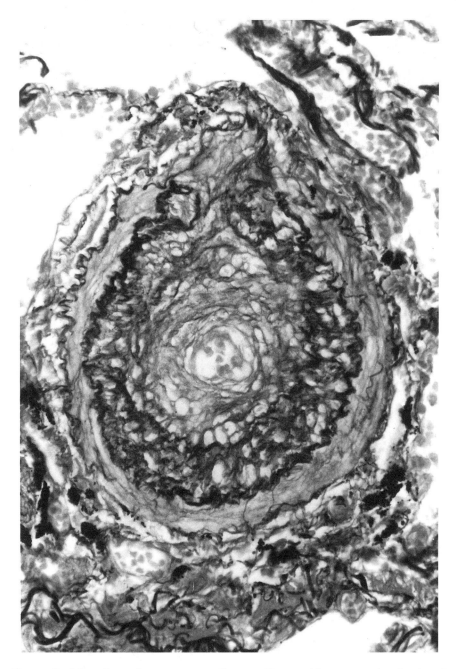

Figure 8 Muscular pulmonary artery from a 62-year-old woman who developed primary pulmonary arterial hypertension after taking aminorex. There is mild medial hypertrophy and severe concentric laminar intimal fibrosis. The edge of an emerging lateral branch is seen at the 12 o'clock position. (EVG, × 500.)

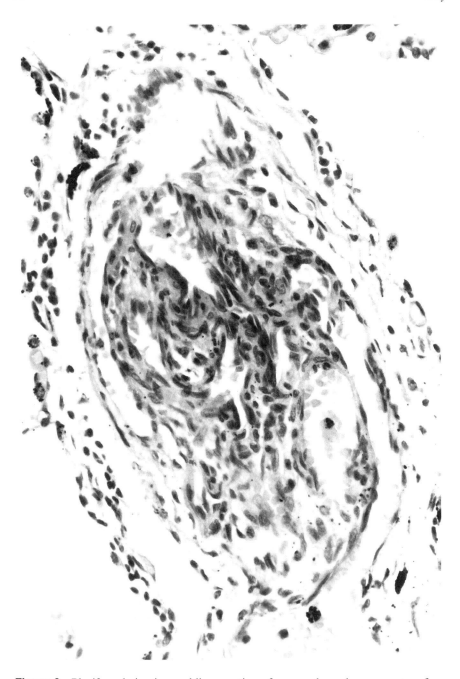

Figure 9 Plexiform lesion in an oblique section of a muscular pulmonary artery from a 42-year-old woman with primary pulmonary arterial hypertension. The lumen contains a plexus of slit-like vascular channels lined by proliferated endothelial cells. (HE, × 500.)

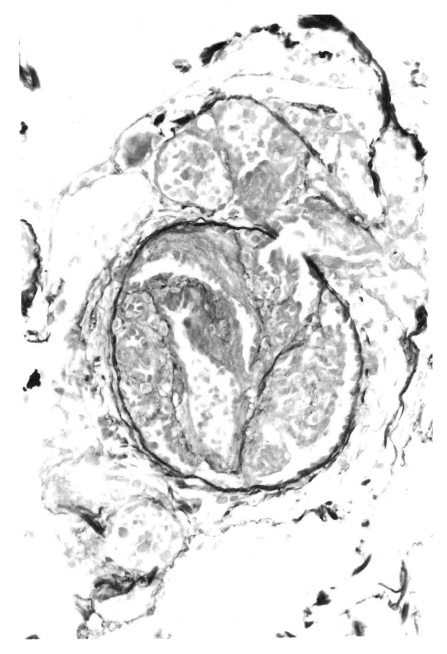

Figure 10 Transverse section of another plexiform lesion from the 42-year-old woman with primary pulmonary arterial hypertension shown in Figure 9. There is destruction of the internal elastic lamina and media. The wall is represented by the external elastic lamina. The lumen contains a plexus of slit-like vascular channels lined by proliferated endothelial cells. (EVG, × 500.)

Table 4 Relative Frequency of Lesions in Muscular Pulmonary Arteries in Three Retrospective and Two Prospective Studies of Primary Pulmonary Arterial Hypertension

Type of study	Wagenvoort and Wagenvoort (34), multicenter, retrospective		Bjornsson and Edwards (35), single center, retrospective		Burke et al. (36), multicenter, retrospective		Pietra et al. (37), multicenter, prospective		Madden et al. (38), single center, prospective	
	N	%	N	%	N	%	N	%	N	%
Plexiform lesions	77	70	22	78	56	89	25	84	15	75
Isolated medial hypertrophy	—	—	3	11	—	—	1	3	—	—
Intimal fibrosis and medial hypertrophy	33	30	—	—	7	11	4	13	5	25
Isolated arteritis	—	—	3	11	—	—	—	—	—	—
Total	110		28		63		30		20	

incidence of medial hypertrophy and intimal fibrosis ranged from 0 to 30%. One retrospective series was unusual in that it included three cases (11%) of isolated pulmonary arteritis (35). Perhaps the most accurate estimate of the relative frequency of lesions may be obtained from the National Heart, Lung, and Blood Institute Registry of Primary Pulmonary Hypertension. The purpose of the Registry was to analyze in a systematic and prospective manner the natural history, epidemiology, pathology, and treatment of unexplained pulmonary hypertension in a cohort of patients in whom the diagnosis was established by standardized clinical and laboratory criteria. In a group of 30 patients with primary pulmonary arterial hypertension, 25 had pulmonary arteriopathy with plexiform lesions (84%), 4 had medial hypertrophy and intimal fibrosis (13%), and 1 had isolated medial hypertrophy (37).

The endothelial cells of hypertrophied muscular pulmonary arteries show increased expression of endothelin-1, which is a vasoconstrictor agent and mitogen for smooth muscle cells and fibroblasts (15). There is ultrastructural evidence that the cellular intimal proliferation is derived from smooth muscle cells from the inner half of the tunica media, which migrate into the intimal through gaps in the internal elastic lamina (16,17). Immunohistochemical studies have suggested that smooth muscle cells in the media and neointima actively synthesize collagen in patients with severe primary pulmonary arterial hypertension (39) and that this process may be modulated by transforming growth factor-β (40). Fibrosis also occurs in the adventitia of the muscular pulmonary arteries (41). Muscularization of pulmonary arterioles occurs but is less common than in patients with systemic-to-pulmonary shunts (23,38). Plexiform lesions are relatively sparse; they involve 3.9% of arteries in biopsy tissues and 7% of arteries in autopsy tissues (37). In contrast to systemic-to-pulmonary shunts, the majority are associated with intra-acinar arteries (19). In 70% of cases, the plexiform lesions are scantily infiltrated by T cells, B cells, and macrophages (42). The endothelial cell proliferation in the plexiform lesions of primary pulmonary arterial hypertension has been reported to be monoclonal, in contrast to secondary pulmonary hypertension, where it is reported to be polyclonal (21,43). There is no correlation between the numbers of plexiform lesions and the pulmonary artery pressure (35,36,44). In two retrospective studies, dilatation lesions were identified in 50 and 73% of patients, respectively (35,36). However, in a prospective study, dilatation lesions were rarely seen (37). Fibrinoid necrosis and arteritis are uncommon lesions, occurring in about 11% of patients (36).

B. Other Vascular and Parenchymal Lesions

Thrombotic lesions have been reported as occurring in the pulmonary arteries in 27 to 65% of patients with primary pulmonary arterial hypertension (23,36–38). They are absent or scarce in children but common in adults (45). The number of organized and recanalized thrombi in tissue sections appears to be related to the duration of the illness but not the stage of the disease (45). The occurrence of thrombi is independent of the presence of plexiform lesions (45). Thrombotic lesions occur with equal frequency in pulmonary vascular disease secondary to systemic-to-pulmonary shunts (23). Apparently the combination of sustained pulmonary hypertension and age, possibly through endothelial injury, may elicit thrombosis and its sequelae, which in turn may aggravate the pulmonary arterial pressure (45). Long-term oral anticoagulant therapy has been shown to improve survival in patients with primary pulmonary arterial hypertension (46).

Longitudinal smooth muscle cells are commonly seen in muscular pulmonary arteries in patients with primary pulmonary arterial hypertension (23). The smooth muscle cells are arranged in bundles or layers, particularly in the intima, where they are situated within a reduplication of the internal elastic lamina. Longitudinal smooth muscle cells may also be seen in the media or adventitia.

In the majority of patients with primary pulmonary arterial hypertension, the pulmonary veins show a nonocclusive fibrocellular or fibrous intimal proliferation (23,35–38). In a few cases, this is accompanied by the development of a thick medial coat of smooth muscle separated by two elastic laminae.

The lung parenchymal lesions that occur in primary pulmonary arterial hypertension are identical to those encountered in systemic-to-pulmonary shunts (4,23).

C. Risk Factors and Associated Conditions

The hypertensive pulmonary vascular disease associated with aminorex (Fig. 8), fenfluramine, dexfenfluramine, HIV infection, portal hypertension/liver disease, and collagen vascular disease is identical to that encountered in primary pulmonary arterial hypertension (4). The plexiform lesions in two women who developed severe pulmonary hypertension after receiving fenfluramine were reported to show a monoclonal endothelial cell proliferation (47).

IV. Chronic Pulmonary Thrombotic and/or Embolic Disease

The terms *thrombotic pulmonary arteriopathy* (48) and *pulmonary arteriopathy with thrombotic lesions* (37) are preferable to the term *thromboembolic pulmonary hypertension*, since it is impossible to distinguish between embolic thrombi and in situ thrombi by microscopy alone (35). Although the embolic nature of thrombotic pulmonary arteriopathy has been emphasized (34), sources of such emboli in the systemic veins and the right side of the heart frequently cannot be demonstrated at autopsy (49–52). It has therefore been suggested that, in some cases, in situ thrombosis of the pulmonary arteries may occur (35,51,53).

Clinically apparent pulmonary embolism recurs in from 8 to 20% of patients treated for pulmonary thromboembolism (54,55). In view of these statistics, it is surprising that chronic pulmonary hypertension following pulmonary embolism is such a rare condition, with a prevalence at autopsy ranging from 0.15 to 0.38% (54,56). In one study, serial lung scans done in patients with acute pulmonary thromboemboli showed complete normalization of the perfusion defects in 86% of patients over a 1-year period, and it was estimated that less than 2% of these would develop chronic pulmonary hypertension (51). In a more recent study, 78 patients with acute pulmonary thomboembolism were subjected to a 1-year follow-up by serial echocardiography Doppler and a 5-year clinical follow-up. Four patients (5.1%) developed chronic pulmonary hypertension, and 3 underwent pulmonary thromboendarterectomy (57).

Chronic pulmonary thrombotic and/or embolic disease occurs in two forms (50,51). There may be occlusion of the proximal pulmonary arteries or there may be widespread occlusion of distal muscular pulmonary arteries. Some patients with occlusion of the proximal pulmonary arteries may complain of hemoptysis and recurrent episodes of pleuritic pain (50), but the majority present with increasing dyspnea on exertion (50,58). Patients with widespread thrombotic occlusion of the distal muscular pulmonary arteries may be clinically indistinguishable from those with primary pulmonary arterial hypertension.

A. Thrombotic Obstruction of Proximal Pulmonary Arteries

Chronic thrombotic occlusion of the proximal pulmonary arteries is a rare entity with an incidence at autopsy ranging from 0.02 to 0.2% (49,56). In most instances, it is impossible at autopsy to distinguish with certainty between organized thromboemboli and thrombi formed in situ (49). Some authors have denied the existence of primary thrombosis of the proximal pulmonary arteries and stated that the diagnosis is the result of inadequate examination for sources of emboli (59). However, there are undoubted cases of primary thrombotic occlusion of the proximal pulmonary arteries in which no source for embolism could be discovered at autopsy (50,52).

At autopsy, the affected proximal pulmonary arteries are dilated and either stenosed or completely occluded by gray or yellow firmly adherent laminated thrombus (49,52). On microscopic examination, small blood vessels and fibrous connective tissue attach the thrombus to the intimal surface and extend for a variable distance into the thrombus. The intima shows fibrous thickening and the underlying media frequently shows basophilic degeneration resembling cystic medial necrosis (49). Nonocclusive thrombi tend to organize into fibrous intimal plaques. If the vessel was occluded by the thrombus, the end result is likely to be a fibrous band (Fig. 11) stretching in a variety of somewhat bizarre patterns across the lumen of the artery (60). Such fibrous bands are relatively frequent in elastic pulmonary arteries (Fig. 12) and are a

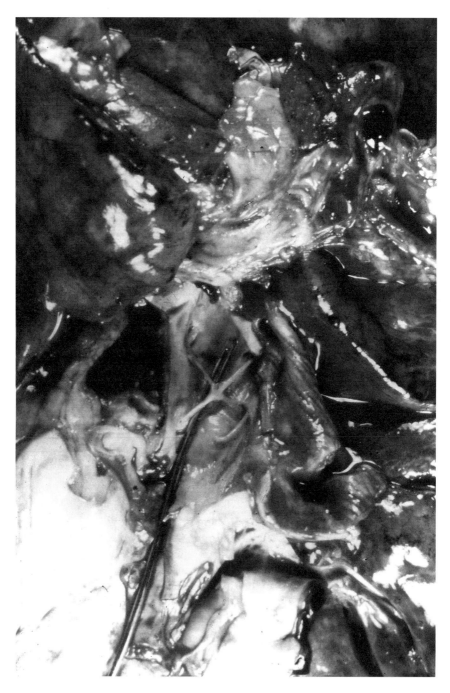

Figure 11 Intraluminal fibrous band in a lobar pulmonary artery at autopsy. This structure represents an old organized and recanalized occluding thrombus.

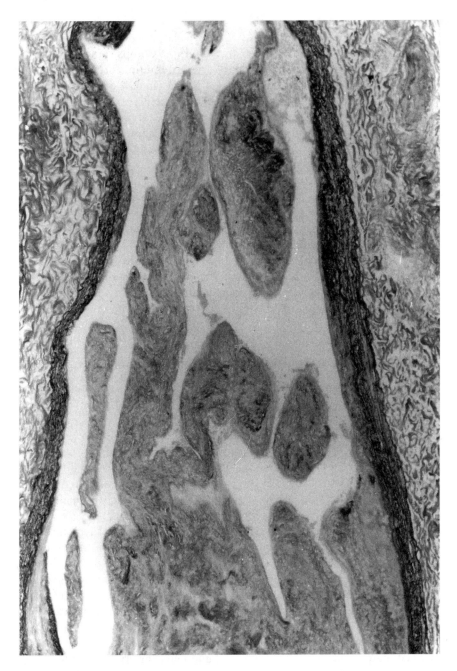

Figure 12 The lumen of this longitudinally sectioned elastic pulmonary artery contains a complex fibroelastic band representing an old organized and recanalized thrombus. From a 44-year-old man with autopsy-proven chronic thromboembolic pulmonary hypertension. (EVG, ×80.)

clear indication of previous thrombotic episodes. They may give rise to systolic murmurs over the lung fields (58) and can be visualized by pulmonary angiography and pulmonary angioscopy (61). In an autopsy study of 68 cases of thrombosis of the proximal pulmonary arteries, multiple organized thrombi were noted in the distal muscular pulmonary arteries in 65% of patients. Recent pulmonary infarcts were present in 13% of patients, and 74% had right ventricular hypertrophy. In 35% of cases, the distal muscular pulmonary arteries were microscopically normal; in 51%, they showed medial hypertrophy; in 13%, there was intimal proliferation (49). Plexiform lesions were not reported.

It is important to consider the diagnosis of thrombosis of the proximal pulmonary arteries in any patient who presents with dyspnea on exertion, since this condition can be treated surgically (58,61). There is no surgical plane of cleavage between the organized thrombus and the intima, so it is necessary to carry out thromboendarterectomy rather embolectomy. The surgical pathology specimen consists of partially organized pale red thrombus adherent to firm, resilient, gray organized thrombus that merges with the fibrotic intima (Fig. 13). The underlying media may include abnormal thick vascular channels representing bronchopulmonary arterial anastomoses.

B. Thrombotic Obstruction of Distal Pulmonary Arteries

The muscular pulmonary arteries and pulmonary arterioles show cushion-like eccentric patches of intimal fibrosis (Fig. 14). When traced in serial sections, postthrombotic intimal fibrosis, although almost completely occlusive, often extends over relatively short distances. Consequently, in random histological sections, many pulmonary arteries show no intimal thickening at all, and occluded vessels are often uncommon. When the amount of intimal fibrosis is assessed morphometrically, the average value is usually low compared to other forms of hypertensive pulmonary vascular disease, in which intimal fibrosis affects long segments of the arteries (34). Recanalization may give rise to colander-like lesions (Fig. 15) and intravascular fibrous septa. Fresh thrombus is rare (37). It has been stated that medial hypertrophy is either mild or absent (48), but it was observed in 64% of cases of thrombotic pulmonary arteriopathy in a retrospective series of cases of unexplained pulmonary hypertension (35). In a prospective study of unexplained pulmonary hypertension, there was no significant difference in the frequency of medial hypertrophy when thrombotic pulmonary arteriopathy was compared with pulmonary arteriopathy with plexiform lesions (37). Plexiform lesions and dilatation lesions have not been described in patients with thrombotic pulmonary arteriopathy (34–37,49). Pulmonary arteritis rarely occurs (35). In a paper purporting to demonstrate plexiform lesions in patients with chronic thromboembolic pulmonary hypertension (62), the illustrations depict recanalized thrombi rather than plexiform lesions (63).

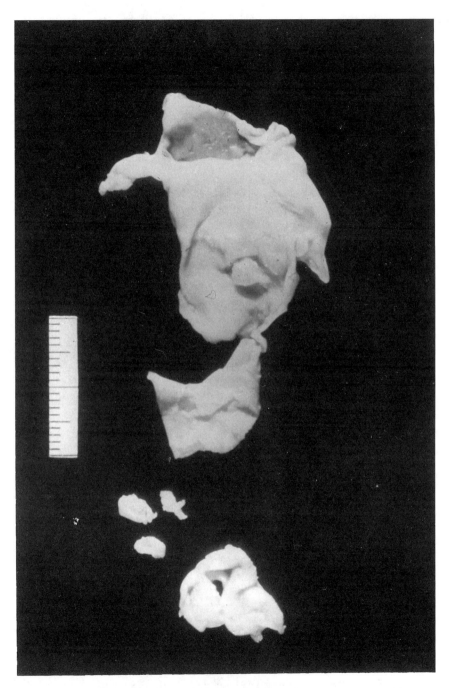

Figure 13 Pulmonary thromboendarterectomy specimen from a 21-year-old woman with chronic thromboembolic pulmonary hypertension.

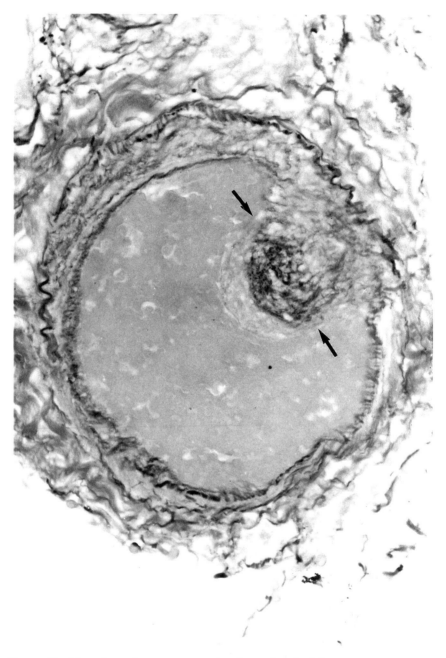

Figure 14 Muscular pulmonary artery showing a sharply defined intimal fibroelastic plaque (between two arrows) characteristic of an old organized mural thrombus. Note the absence of medial hypertrophy. From a 44-year-old man with chronic thromboembolic pulmonary hypertension. (EVG, × 500.)

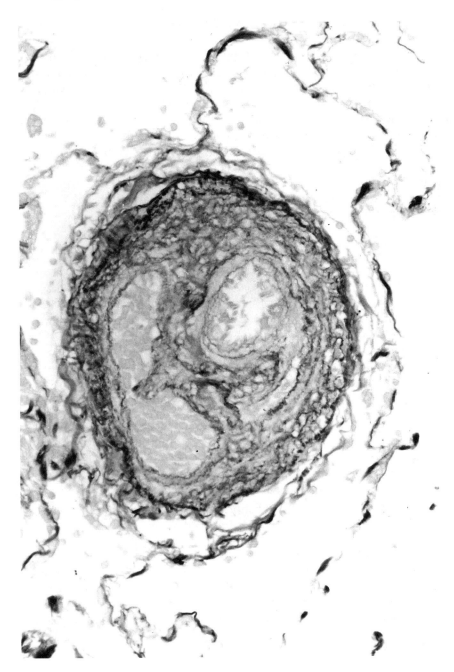

Figure 15 The lumen of this muscular pulmonary artery contains multiple fibroelastic septa (colander-like lesion) characteristic of an old organized and recanalized thrombus. From the patient with chronic thromboembolic pulmonary hypertension illustrated in Figure 14. (EVG, × 500.)

V. Pulmonary Veno-occlusive Disease

The first well-documented case of pulmonary veno-occlusive disease was published by Höra in 1934 (64). Subsequently, several cases were reported under a variety of names until *pulmonary veno-occlusive disease* became the generally accepted term in 1966 (65). Approximately 150 cases have now been reported in the literature (66). Pulmonary veno-occlusive disease affects all age groups and has been reported from all over the world. About 60% of patients are male and the age range is from 11 days to 76 years. About 40% of patients are aged 16 years or less. In pulmonary veno-occlusive disease, the predominant lesions are in the pulmonary veins, but there are also significant changes in the alveolar capillaries, muscular pulmonary arteries, lymphatics, and lung parenchyma.

A. Pulmonary Veins

The intrapulmonary veins and venules are narrowed or occluded by intimal fibrosis (Fig. 16) (65,67). This may consist of either loose, myxoid connective tissue or dense collagen and elastic tissue, sometimes including occasional smooth muscle cells (68). Colander lesions and intravascular fibrous septa indicative of recanalized thrombus are present in the pulmonary veins in most cases (Fig. 17), but recent thrombus is rarely identified (69). In most cases the pulmonary veins in the interlobular fibrous septa and the intra-acinar veins and venules are involved. However, in some cases the lesions are virtually restricted to the small intra-acinar veins and venules. This makes histological diagnosis difficult because of the problem of distinguishing small pulmonary veins and venules from pulmonary arterioles. The proportion of veins and venules affected varies between 30 and 90% (67). In most cases the venous changes are equally and evenly distributed throughout both lungs. In a few cases, however, the veins in some parts of the lungs are affected more than in others. The pulmonary veins often show medial hypertrophy. Sometimes the thickened layer of smooth muscle is located between distinct internal and external elastic laminae. This appearance is termed *arterialization*, because the affected pulmonary veins resemble muscular pulmonary arteries. In some cases, these features are probably secondary to increased pressure in the pulmonary veins resulting from obstruction in the larger distal venous trunks. In other cases, where the larger veins are widely patent, the medial hypertrophy and arterialization may result from direct injury to the vessel wall (69). The lesions in the pulmonary veins are usually bland, but occasional cases of nonspecific pulmonary phlebitis (70) and granulomatous pulmonary phlebitis (71) have been described.

B. Alveolar Capillaries

The alveolar capillaries may show dilatation and severe congestion, particularly in relation to occluded or narrowed pulmonary venules. Electron

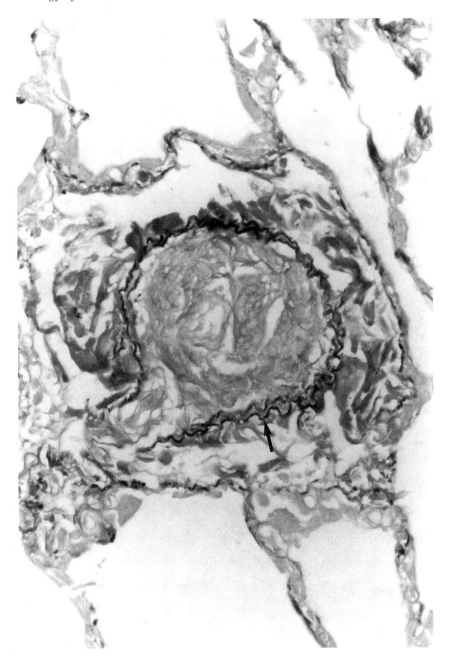

Figure 16 Pulmonary veno-occlusive disease. Transverse section of a pulmonary vein located in a fibrous interlobular septum. Note the elastic tissue in its wall (arrow). The lumen is severely narrowed by fibrous tissue. A venule joins the vein at the 7 o'clock position. Its lumen is also occluded. Open-lung biopsy from a 17-year-old boy with severe pulmonary hypertension. (EVG, × 500.)

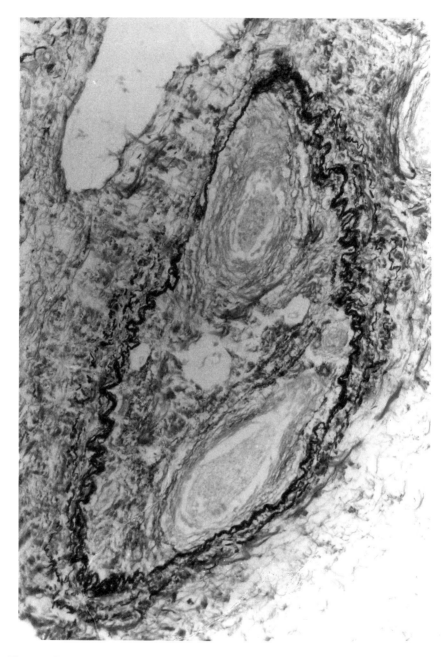

Figure 17   Pulmonary veno-occlusive disease. The lumen of this pulmonary vein is occupied by fibrous tissue perforated by two or three vascular channels (colander-like lesion) indicative of old organized and recanalized thrombus. A dilated lymphatic vessel is seen at the top left corner of the picture. From the autopsy performed on the 17-year-old boy illustrated in Figure 16. (EVG, × 200.)

microscopy has shown thickening of the endothelial cell basement membrane and electron-dense deposits representing disintegrating extravasated erythrocytes (68).

C. Muscular Pulmonary Arteries

In the majority of cases of pulmonary veno-occlusive disease, the muscular pulmonary arteries show medial hypertrophy (Fig. 18). In 75% of cases, there is eccentric intimal fibrosis that appears to be postthrombotic in origin. Intravascular fibrous septa and recent thrombi are encountered in the pulmonary arteries in 25% of cases (69). Thrombotic lesions in elastic pulmonary arteries may cause abnormal perfusion lung scans (72). Plexiform lesions and dilatation lesions have not been identified. Pulmonary arteritis has been reported but is rare (73).

D. Lymphatics

The lymphatic vessels in the interlobular fibrous septa and in the perivascular and peribronchiolar connective tissue are frequently dilated (Fig. 19). The presence of dilated lymphatic vessels within thickened and edematous interlobular fibrous septa is the morphological basis of the Kerley B lines, which are seen in the chest radiographs of 20% of cases of pulmonary veno-occlusive disease. In a patient with pulmonary hypertension, the detection of Kerley B lines in the absence of left atrial enlargement may be an important clue to the clinical diagnosis of pulmonary veno-occlusive disease (74).

E. Lung Parenchyma

Interstitial edema is common and most easily recognized in the interlobular fibrous septa, which become abnormally wide. In long-standing cases, interstitial fibrosis, which may be severe and extensive, develops in the alveolar walls (67). A proliferation of type II pneumonocytes (68) and an infiltrate of lymphocytes and plasma cells frequently accompanies the fibrosis, so that the histology mimics usual interstitial pneumonia (Fig. 20) (67). Hemosiderin, derived from extravasated erythrocytes, is present in alveolar macrophages (Fig. 21) or deposited within the interstitium. Occasionally, hemosiderin encrusts elastic fibers in the walls of pulmonary blood vessels (Fig. 22) and alveolar septa, where it may evoke a giant cell reaction. The hemosiderosis may be so prominent that a diagnosis of idiopathic pulmonary hemosiderosis is entertained. Nodules of metaplastic bone may occur within the alveolar spaces. Pulmonary infarction has been observed in a few cases.

F. Etiology of Pulmonary Veno-occlusive Disease

The cause of pulmonary veno-occlusive disease is unknown, but the character of the venous lesions indicates that thrombosis is an essential factor in the majority of cases if not all. Changes in the pulmonary arteries have attracted

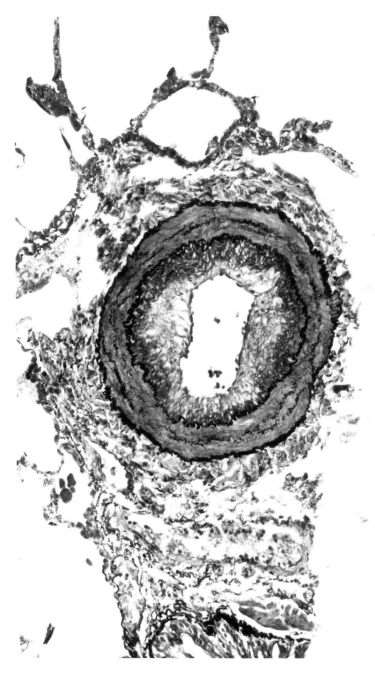

Figure 18 Muscular pulmonary artery showing moderate medial hypertrophy and severe intimal fibrosis. Open-lung biopsy from patient with pulmonary veno-occlusive disease. (EVG, ×200.)

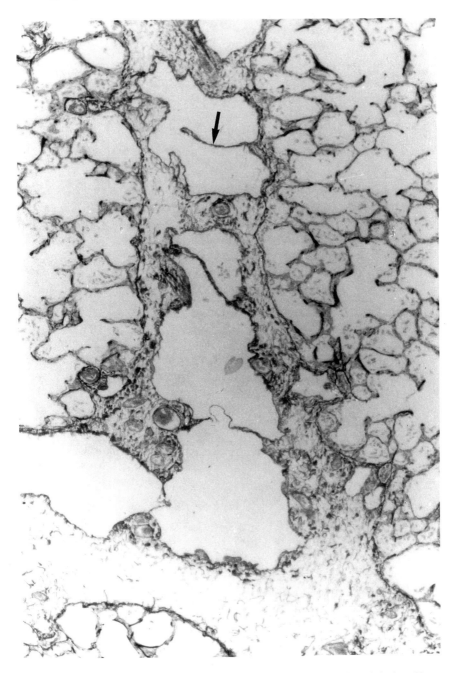

Figure 19 Dilated lymphatic vessel in widened edematous interlobular fibrous septum. Note the delicate valve leaflets in the lumen (arrow). Autopsy specimen from the 17-year-old boy with pulmonary veno-occlusive disease illustrated in Figures 16 and 17. Kerley B lines were visible in his chest radiograph. (EVG, ×80.)

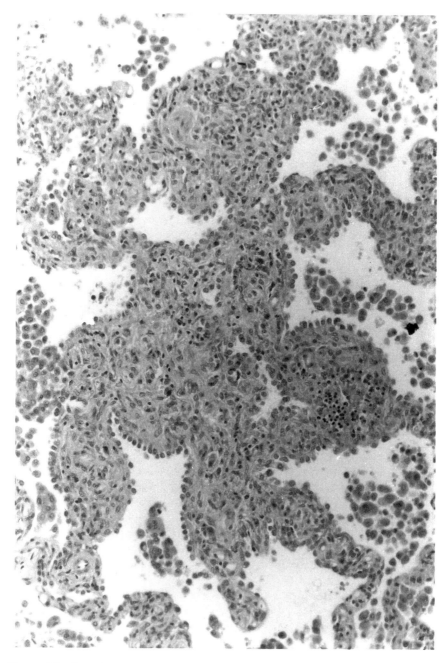

Figure 20   Open-lung biopsy from a 57-year-old man with pulmonary veno-occlusive disease. There is interstitial fibrosis accompanied by a scanty infiltrate of lymphocytes and plasma cells and a proliferation of type II pneumonocytes. The alveoli contain abundant macrophages. (HE, ×200.)

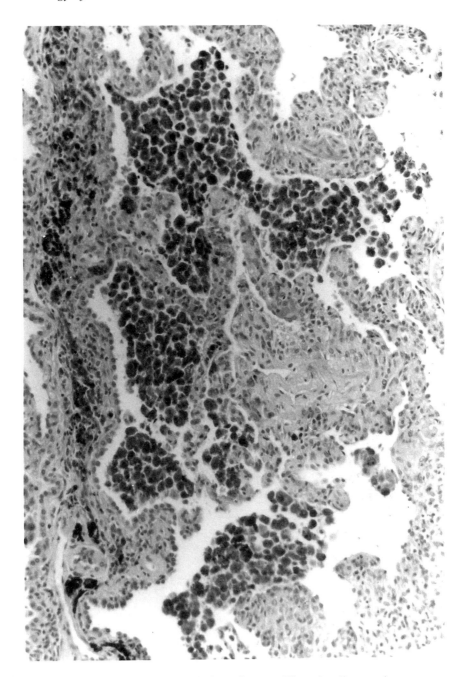

Figure 21 Pulmonary veno-occlusive disease. The alveoli contain numerous hemosiderin-laden macrophages. There are interstitial deposits of hemosiderin on the left side of the picture. Open-lung biopsy from the 57-year-old man shown in Figure 20. (HE, × 200.)

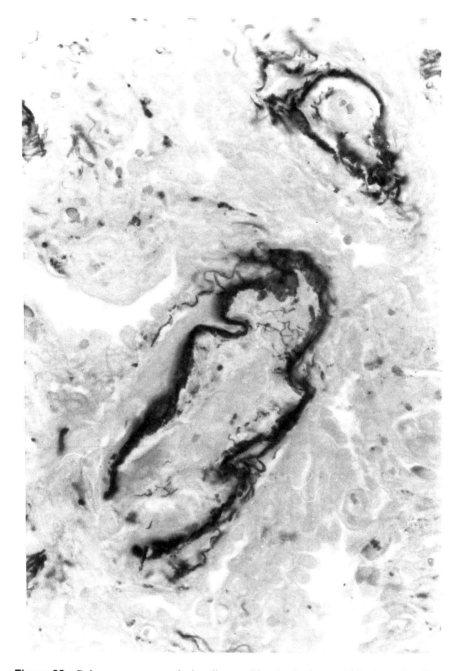

Figure 22 Pulmonary veno-occlusive disease. The elastic tissue within the walls of two pulmonary venules is heavily impregnated with hemosiderin. From the 57-year-old man illustrated in Figures 20 and 21. (Perls Prussian blue stain, × 500.)

less attention than those in the pulmonary veins despite the fact that they are sometimes as severe (69). This suggests that the process is a pulmonary vascular occlusive disease rather than a condition limited to the pulmonary veins (75,76). In some cases, the lesions in the arteries appear to be more recent than those in the veins. This suggests that the process may commence in the pulmonary veins and that the arteries are affected later. It may be that the pulmonary veins are more susceptible to injury than the pulmonary arteries. Normal pulmonary venous endothelium contains less plasminogen activator than pulmonary arterial endothelium. If an infective or toxic agent damaged pulmonary vascular endothelium, plasminogen activator might be depleted in the pulmonary veins before the pulmonary arteries, with the subsequent encouragement of thrombosis in the pulmonary veins (77).

A wide variety of risk factors and associations of pulmonary veno-occlusive disease have been described (Table 5). Most of these are based on

Table 5 Conditions Associated with Pulmonary Veno-occlusive Disease

Genetic factors
    Occurrence in siblings
    Intrauterine occurrence
Infection
    Toxoplasmosis
    Measles
    Epstein-Barr virus infection
    Cytomegalovirus infection
    Human immunodeficiency virus infection
Toxic exposures
    Household cleaning powder
    Bleomycin
    Mitomycin
    Carmustine
Transplantation
    Bone marrow
    Kidney
Autoimmune disorders
    Rheumatoid arthritis
    Systemic lupus erythematosus
    Systemic sclerosis
Hormonal factors
    Pregnancy
    Oral contraceptives
Miscellaneous
    Hypertrophic obstructive cardiomyopathy
    Myocarditis
    Sarcoidosis
    Unilateral hypertransradiant lung

reports of single cases and small series of cases. Discussion of these is outside the scope of this chapter; they are reviewed in detail elsewhere (4,78). It is unlikely that a single etiological agent is responsible for all cases of pulmonary veno-occlusive disease. It is probably best regarded as a syndrome rather than an etiological entity, although a final common pathway, probably thrombosis, is likely (78).

VI. Pulmonary Capillary Hemangiomatosis

This is a rare cause of pulmonary hypertension. It was first described in 1978 (79), and by 2000 a total of 28 cases had been reported (80). Males and females are affected in approximately equal numbers, with an age range from 12 to 71 years (mean 27 years). About 25% of patients are aged 14 years or less.

A. Pathology

The condition is characterized by an aggressive proliferation of small vessels resembling capillaries, which invade the interlobular fibrous septa, pleura, alveolar septa (Fig. 23), and walls of bronchi, pulmonary arteries, and pulmonary veins (Fig. 24) (81). Perineural and intraneural involvement has also been reported (82). In the alveolar walls, a reticulin stain reveals contiguous back-to-back masses of capillaries growing on both sides of the septa (81,83). The infiltration of the walls of pulmonary veins and venules commonly induces partial obstruction or even occlusion of the lumen (Fig. 25). There is intimal fibrosis and many veins show arterialization, with a distinct media of smooth muscle bounded by internal and external elastic laminae. Some of the capillaries that infiltrate the walls of small pulmonary veins increase in size to form thin-walled, sinusoids that protrude into the lumen (84). Other thin-walled vessels form vascular halos around small pulmonary veins and pulmonary arterioles (85). In most cases of pulmonary capillary hemangiomatosis, the endothelial cells have bland nuclei. However, in one case there was hyperchromasia and pleomorphism of endothelial nuclei (79).

The pulmonary arteries show medial hypertrophy, and there is muscularization of pulmonary arterioles. Plexiform lesions, arteritis, and organized thrombi have not been seen in the small pulmonary arteries. The alveoli show recent and old hemorrhage. They contain large aggregates of hemosiderin-laden macrophages. There may be iron encrustation of elastic tissue in the pulmonary arteries and veins and alveolar septa. Subpleural bone metaplasia has been reported, but significant interstitial fibrosis is uncommon.

B. Etiology

Pulmonary hypertension in pulmonary capillary hemangiomatosis appears to be secondary to occlusion of veins and venules by invading capillaries (81,82).

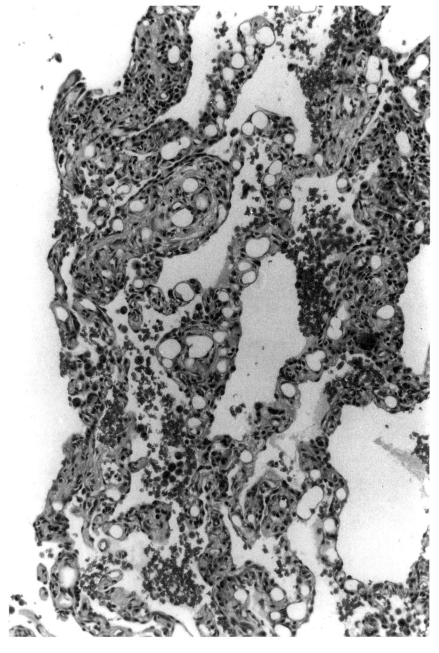

Figure 23 Pulmonary capillary hemangiomatosis. Numerous small vessels resembling capillaries infiltrate the alveolar walls; they appear as empty round or oval spaces. Open-lung biopsy from a 31-year-old man with severe pulmonary hypertension. (HE, × 200.)

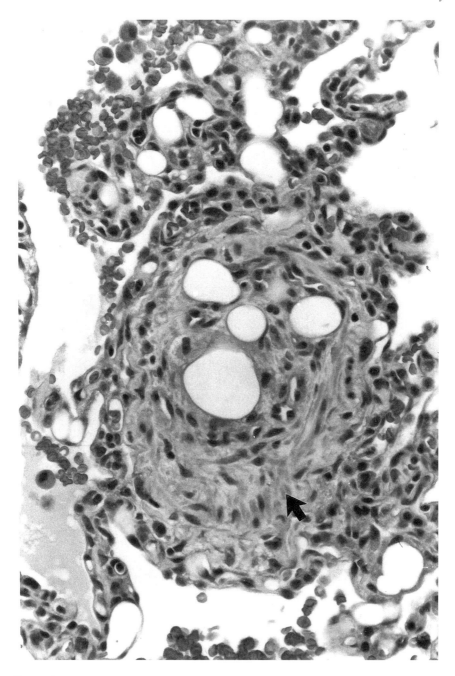

Figure 24 Pulmonary capillary hemangiomatosis. Transverse section of a pulmonary venule occluded by capillary hemangiomatosis. Note the smooth muscle in the wall of the venule (arrow) and the involvement of the adjacent alveolar walls by capillary hemangiomatosis. From the 31-year-old man shown in Figure 23. (HE, × 500.)

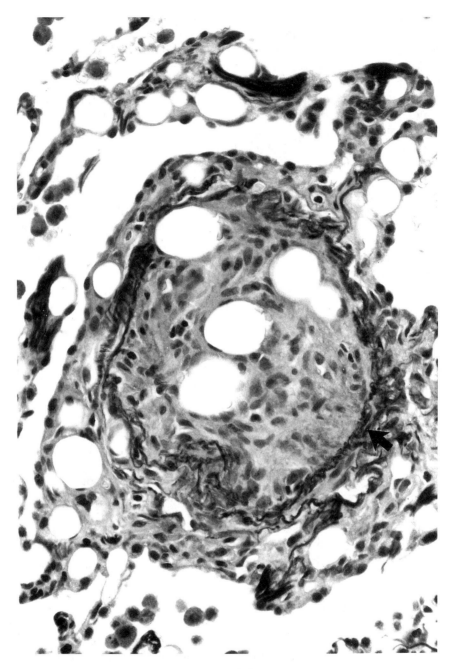

Figure 25 Pulmonary capillary hemangiomatosis. Transverse section of a pulmonary venule occluded by capillary hemangiomatosis. Note the elastic tissue in the wall of the venule (arrow) and the involvement of the adjacent alveolar walls by capillary hemangiomatosis. From the 31-year-old man shown in Figures 23 and 24. (EVG, × 500.)

About 50% of patients complain of hemoptysis, and hemothorax occurs in about 15% of cases. Hemoptysis is rare in pulmonary veno-occlusive disease. The nature of pulmonary capillary hemangiomatosis is unclear. The existence of sheets of small blood vessels in the lung is suggestive of a hamartoma (85). However, if the disease is hamartomatous, it is surprising that the mean age of the patients is 27 years and that the disease has been reported in a 71-year-old man (79). The aggressively infiltrative nature of the process, which sometimes involves nerves, and the occasional occurrence of hyperchromasia and pleomorphism of nuclei are more in keeping with a low-grade vascular neoplasm.

Pulmonary capillary hemangiomatosis must be distinguished from Kaposi's sarcoma. Capillary hemangiomatosis is characterized by fairly regular, well-formed capillaries rather than the irregular slits lined by spindle cells that occur in Kaposi's sarcoma. Most cases of pulmonary Kaposi's sarcoma show eosinophilic, hyaline, periodic acid–Schiff (PAS)-positive intracytoplasmic globules (86), which have not been described in pulmonary capillary hemangiomatosis. The condition must also be distinguished from diffuse pulmonary hemangiomatosis that occurs in children (87). The latter appears to be a true vascular malformation, often involving several organs. The vascular channels resemble cavernous hemangiomas and are much larger than than those of pulmonary capillary hemangiomatosis. Pulmonary capillary hemangiomatosis appears to be a distinct morphological entity separate from pulmonary veno-occlusive disease (81). However, some authors (36) have had difficulty in distinguishing pulmonary capillary hemangiomatosis from pulmonary veno-occlusive disease with so-called pseudoangiomatous features (88).

Pulmonary capillary hemangiomatosis has been described in association with hypertrophic cardiomyopathy, systemic lupus erythematosus, Takayasu's aortoarteritis, and scleroderma (80,89). In one study, isolated foci of pulmonary capillary hemangiomatosis were identified in 8 of 148 (5.7%) consecutive autopsies (80). The lesions ranged in diameter from 0.6 to 5 cm and were visible on gross examination in three cases. There was minimal invasion of small pulmonary arteries and veins but no vascular occlusion. The patients did not have pulmonary hypertension and there was no capillary proliferation in other organs.

VII. Lung Biopsy in Advanced Pulmonary Vascular Disease

A biopsy specimen measuring $2.5 \times 2 \times 1$ cm from an adult lung or a proportionately smaller specimen from a child will usually include blood vessels that are representative of the lungs as a whole (90). The lingula of the left upper lobe is a favorite site for biopsy because of its accessibility. It has been suggested that the lingula is inappropriate because the pulmonary arteries in this segment have thicker medial and intimal layers (91). However, other studies have failed to observe any significant differences between the pulmonary arteries in various parts of the lungs, including the lingula (92,93). Accordingly, there seems to be no good reason why the lingula should be excluded as a biopsy site.

Surgical lung biopsy specimens should be fixed in a state of distention. Otherwise, collapse of lung tissue may lead to crenation of the elastic laminae and induce a state of spurious medial hypertrophy in muscular pulmonary arteries. Lung biopsy specimens are most conveniently fixed by injecting them through multiple punctures in the pleura with a 25-gauge butterfly needle connected to a 5-mL syringe (94). This technique may induce slight edema of the interlobular fibrous septa. This does not lead to difficulties in interpretation and is a small price to pay for the excellent display of pulmonary microanatomy.

The walls of blood vessels are composed essentially of collagen, smooth muscle, and elastic tissue. Using the conventional hematoxylin and eosin staining method, all these tissues appear pink and cannot be distinguished from one another. Accordingly, it is necessary to use a connective tissue stain such as the Miller elastic–van Gieson method (95) for evaluating the pulmonary vasculature. Representative sections should also be stained by the Perls Prussian blue method for ferric iron to detect hemosiderosis, which is one of the features of chronic pulmonary venous hypertension (Figs. 21 and 22).

A. Lung Biopsy in Systemic-to-Pulmonary Shunts

In most patients with congenital heart disease, careful measurements of the pulmonary vascular resistance and calculation of the ratio between the pulmonary vascular resistance and the systemic vascular resistance give reliable indications of the state of the pulmonary vascular bed, obviating the need for routine open-lung biopsies. If a reliable assessment of the pulmonary vascular resistance cannot be made, it may be necessary to perform a lung biopsy to evaluate the state of the pulmonary arteries and decide whether the defect should be repaired. An open-lung biopsy in such patients may yield valuable information, but it should not be undertaken without careful consideration of the risks involved. Mortality and morbidity rates of 20 and 13%, respectively, have been reported when an open-lung biopsy has been used as an isolated procedure in children with congenital heart disease (33) Intraoperative frozen sections are inadequate to assess hypertensive pulmonary vascular disease because of the necessity for multiple well-stained sections (33,48).

B. Lung Biopsy in Unexplained (Primary) Pulmonary Hypertension

Histopathological classification of hypertensive pulmonary vascular disease in lung biopsy specimens can be achieved accurately and reproducibly, as shown by the 96% interobserver agreement between the pathologists and by the good correlation between premortem and postmortem diagnoses in the National

Heart, Lung and Blood Institute Registry of Primary Pulmonary Hypertension (37).

In patients with clinically unexplained pulmonary hypertension, plexiform lesions are pathognomic for primary pulmonary arterial hypertension, but it is important to realize that 27 to 63% of patients with plexiform lesions may also show recanalized thrombi. Thrombotic obstruction of distal pulmonary arteries is diagnosed by seeing evidence of organized thrombi in the absence of plexiform lesions. Fresh thrombus is rarely seen in open-lung biopsies from patients with thrombotic pulmonary arteriopathy. Occasionally, difficulty may be encountered in distinguishing between an organized recanalized thrombus with a florid endothelial cell proliferation (Fig. 26) and a plexiform lesion. Pulmonary arteries containing organized and recanalized thrombi usually have intact internal and external elastic laminae (Fig. 27), whereas these structures are destroyed at the site of plexiform lesions (Fig. 10).

Chronic pulmonary venous hypertension, such as occurs in pulmonary veno-occlusive disease and pulmonary capillary hemangiomatosis, produces profound changes in the lung parenchyma. Mistaken diagnoses of usual interstitial pneumonia and idiopathic pulmonary hemosiderosis are not uncommon in lung biopsy specimens from patients with pulmonary veno-occlusive disease. If a lung biopsy shows interstitial fibrosis or hemosiderosis, it is important to pay particular attention to the pulmonary veins and venules to avoid an erroneous diagnosis. In most cases of pulmonary veno-occlusive disease, the muscular pulmonary arteries show medial hypertrophy and eccentric intimal fibrosis. Sometimes the arterial lesions may be more prominent than those in the pulmonary veins, so it is important to examine the pulmonary veins in detail to avoid missing occlusive lesions. The diagnosis of pulmonary veno-occlusive disease may be particularly difficult when the occlusive lesions are restricted to the intra-acinar veins and venules because of the difficulty in distinguishing them from pulmonary arterioles. Some cases of pulmonary capillary hemangiomatosis may be misdiagnosed as pulmonary veno-occlusive disease. A reticulin stain and immunohistochemistry for factor 8 and CD 31 (Fig. 28) are very helpful in identifying the invasive capillary proliferation. Plexiform lesions do not occur in either pulmonary veno-occlusive disease or pulmonary capillary hemangiomatosis.

VIII.   Risks and Benefits of Lung Biopsy

Open-lung biopsy is potentially hazardous, and it may be questioned whether it is worthwhile subjecting the patient to the risk of the procedure. In individual patients, the value of the information to be gained must be carefully weighed against the risks of the procedure. In a prospective study of unexplained pulmonary hypertension, 1 of 23 patients submitted to open-lung biopsy died as a result of the procedure (37).

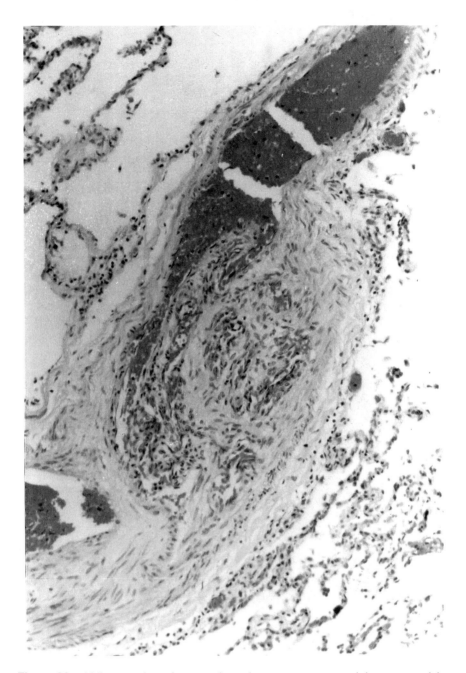

Figure 26 Oblique section of a muscular pulmonary artery containing an organizing thrombus with a florid endothelial cell proliferation that might be misinterpreted as a plexiform lesion. From the patient with chronic thromboembolic pulmonary hypertension illustrated in Figures 14 and 15. (HE, × 200.)

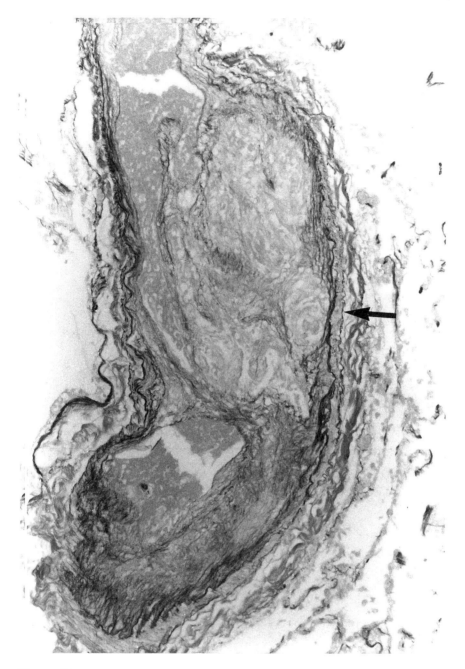

Figure 27 Oblique section of the same muscular pulmonary artery, as shown in Figure 26, containing an organizing thrombus with a florid endothelial cell proliferation. Note the intact internal and external elastic laminae (arrow), which distinguish a thrombus from a plexiform lesion. Compare with Figure 10. (EVG, ×200.)

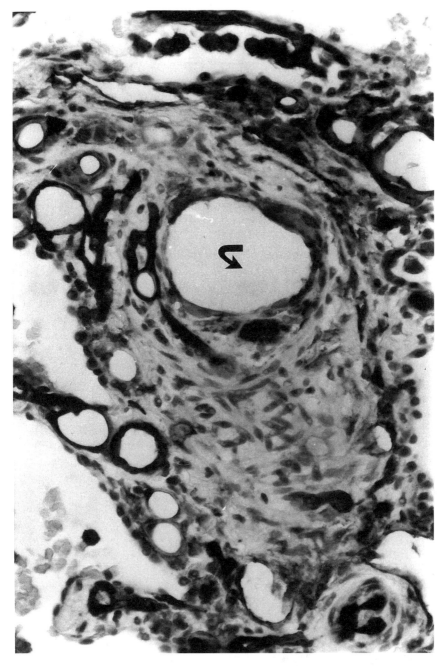

Figure 28 Pulmonary capillary hemangiomatosis. The cells lining the infiltrating capillary-like structures express CD 31 and appear as black circles and ovals. The large oval space (curved arrow) just above the center of the picture is the narrow lumen of a pulmonary venule. (Immunohistochemistry for CD 31, × 500.)

The therapies currently available for treating patients with unexplained pulmonary hypertension are vasodilators, anticoagulants, and lung or heart-lung transplantation. Qualitative histological examination of lung tissue does not provide a basis for predicting how individual patients will respond to vasodilator agents (96). However, quantitative morphological analysis of the initial open-lung biopsy specimen did prove helpful in predicting acute responsiveness to vasodilator agents and the subsequent clinical course of patients with primary pulmonary arterial hypertension and thrombotic obstruction of distal pulmonary arteries. An intimal area of more than 18% of the vascular cross-sectional area had an 85% predictive value for identifying the patients who did poorly during the first 36 months of follow-up (96).

At the World Symposium on Primary Pulmonary Hypertension in 1998, it was stated that there is little evidence that lung biopsy provides clinically useful information in most patients and that it was not recommended as a part of the routine evaluation of patients with suspected primary pulmonary hypertension (6). A disadvantage of not performing lung biopsy is that a definitive diagnosis will not be established, because primary pulmonary arterial hypertension, thrombotic obstruction of distal pulmonary arteries, pulmonary veno-occlusive disease, and pulmonary capillary hemangiomatosis are often indistinguishable clinically (37). These four conditions are distinct pathological entities with diverse etiologies. Unless a biopsy is performed, the clinician will not know which disease is being treated. Pulmonary vasodilators have an established role in the treatment of primary pulmonary arterial hypertension, but there are theoretical reasons why vasodilators may not be effective in pulmonary veno-occlusive disease and pulmonary capillary hemangiomatosis and may, in fact, worsen the cardiopulmonary status. If the muscular pulmonary arteries dilate but the resistance of the pulmonary veins remains fixed, an increase in transcapillary hydrostatic pressure may ensue and produce florid pulmonary edema (78). Fatal pulmonary edema has been reported in patients with pulmonary veno-occlusive disease (66) and pulmonary capillary hemangiomatosis (89) treated with vasodilator agents.

References

1. Hatano S, Strasser T. Primary Pulmonary Hypertension. Report of Committee. Geneva: World Health Organization, 1975.
2. Fishman AP. Unexplained pulmonary hypertension. Circulation 1982; 65:651–652.
3. Dexter L. Pulmonary vascular disease in acquired and congenital heart disease. Arch Intern Med 1979; 139:922–928.
4. Kay JM. Vascular disease. In: Thurlbeck WM, Churg AM, eds. Pathology of the Lung, 2nd ed. New York: Thieme, 1995:931–1066.
5. Voelkel NF, Tuder RM. Severe pulmonary hypertensive diseases: a perspective. Eur Respir J 1999; 14:1246–1250.

6. Rich S. Executive Summary from the World Symposium on Primary Pulmonary Hypertension. Geneva: World Health Organization, 1998.
7. Haworth SG. Pulmonary vascular disease in secundum atrial septal defect in childhood. Am J Cardiol 1983; 51:265–272.
8. Shillingford JP, Kay JM, Heath D. Perforation of interventricular septum following myocardial infarction. Am Heart J 1970; 80:562–569.
9. Heath D, Edwards JE. The pathology of hypertensive pulmonary vascular disease. A description of six grades of structural changes in the pulmonary arteries with special reference to congenital cardiac septal defects. Circulation 1958; 18:533–547.
10. Stenmark KR, Mecham RP. Cellular and molecular mechanisms of pulmonary vascular remodeling. Annu Rev Physiol 1997; 59:89–144.
11. Voelkel NF, Tuder RM. Cellular and molecular mechanisms in the pathogenesis of severe pulmonary hypertension. Eur Respir J 1995; 8:2129–2138.
12. Meyrick B, Reid L. Ultrastructural findings in lung biopsy material from children with congenital heart defects. Am J Pathol 1980; 101:527–542.
13. Yamaki S, Wagenvoort CA. Plexogenic pulmonary arteriopathy. Significance of medial thickness with respect to advanced pulmonary vascular lesions. Am J Pathol 1981; 105:70–75.
14. Wagenvoort CA, Nauta J, Van der Schaar PJ, Weeda HWH, Wagenvoort N. Effect of flow and pressure on pulmonary vessels. A semiquantitative study based on lung biopsies. Circulation 1967; 35:1028–1037.
15. Giaid A, Yanagisawa M, Langleben D, Michel RP, Levy R, Shennib H, Kimura S, Masaki T, Duguid WP, Stewart DJ. Expression of endothelin-1 in the lungs of patients with pulmonary hypertension. N Engl J Med 1993; 328:1732–1739.
16. Heath D, Smith P, Gosney J. Ultrastructure of early plexogenic pulmonary arteriopathy. Histopathology 1988; 12:41–52.
17. Smith P, Heath D, Yacoub M, Madden B, Caslin A, Gosney J. The ultrastructure of plexogenic pulmonary arteriopathy. J Pathol 1990; 160:111–121.
18. Yaginuma G, Mohri H, Takahashi T. Distribution of arterial lesions and collateral pathways in the pulmonary hypertension of congenital heart disease: a computer aided reconstruction study. Thorax 1990; 45:586–590.
19. Jamison BM, Michel RP. Different distribution of plexiform lesions in primary and secondary pulmonary hypertension. Hum Pathol 1995; 26:987–993.
20. Wagenvoort CA. The morphology of certain vascular lesions in pulmonary hypertension. J Pathol Bacteriol 1959; 78:503–511.
21. Tuder RM, Lee S-D, Cool CC. Histopathology of pulmonary hypertension. Chest 1998; 114:1S–6S.
22. Wagenvoort CA. The pulmonary arteries in infants with ventricular septal defect. Med Thorac 1962; 19:354–361.
23. Caslin AW, Heath D, Madden B, Yacoub M, Gosney JR, Heath D. The histopathology of 36 cases of plexogenic pulmonary arteriopathy. Histopathology 1990; 16:9–16.
24. Hall SM, Haworth SG. Onset and evolution of pulmonary vascular disease in young children: abnormal postnatal remodelling studied in lung biopsies. J Pathol 1992; 166:183–186.
25. Hoffman JIE, Rudolph AM, Heymann MA. Pulmonary vascular disease with congenital heart lesions: pathologic features and causes. Circulation 1981; 64:873–877.

26. Heath D. Longitudinal muscle in pulmonary arteries. J Pathol Bacteriol 1963; 85:407–412.

27. Haworth SG. Pulmonary vascular disease in ventricular septal defect: structural and functional correlations in lung biopsies from 85 patients, with outcome of intracardiac repair. J Pathol 1987; 152:157–168.

28. Heath D, Helmholz HF, Burchell HB, DuShane JW, Kirklin JW, Edwards JE. Relation between structural changes in the small pulmonary arteries and immediate reversibility of pulmonary hypertension following closure of ventricular and atrial septal defects. Circulation 1958; 18:1167–1174.

29. Rabinovitch M, Keane JF, Norwood WI, Castaneda AR, Reid L. Vascular structure in lung tissue obtained at biopsy correlated with pulmonary hemodynamic findings after repair of congenital heart defects. Circulation 1984; 69:655–667.

30. Braunlin EA, Moller JH, Patton C, Lucas RV, Lillehei CW, Edwards JE. Predictive value of lung biopsy in ventricular septal defect: long-term follow-up. J Am Coll Cardiol 1986; 8:1113–1118.

31. Dammann JF, McEachen JA, Thompson WM, Smith R, Muller WH. The regression of pulmonary vascular disease after the creation of pulmonary stenosis. J Thorac Cardiovasc Surg 1961; 42:722–734.

32. Wagenvoort CA, Wagenvoort N, Draulans-Noe Y. Reversibility of plexogenic pulmonary arteriopathy following banding of the pulmonary artery. J Thorac Cardiovasc Surg 1984; 87:876–886.

33. Wilson NJ, Seear MD, Taylor GP, LeBlanc J, Sandor GGS. The clinical value and risks of lung biopsy in children with congenital heart disease. J Thorac Cardiovasc Surg 1990; 9:460–468.

34. Wagenvoort CA, Wagenvoort N. Primary pulmonary hypertension. A pathologic study of the lung vessels in 156 clinically diagnosed cases. Circulation 1970; 42:1163–1184.

35. Bjornsson J, Edwards WD. Primary pulmonary hypertension: a histopathologic study of 80 cases. Mayo Clin Proc 1985; 60:16–25.

36. Burke AP, Farb A, Virmani R. The pathology of primary pulmonary hypertension. Mod Pathol 1991; 4:269–282.

37. Pietra GG, Edwards WD, Kay JM, Rich S, Kernis J, Schloo B, Ayres SM, Bergofsky EH, Brundage BH, Detre KM, Fishman AP, Goldring RM, Groves BM, Levy PS, Reid LM, Vreim CE, Williams GW. Histopathology of primary pulmonary hypertension. A qualitative and quantitative study of pulmonary blood vessels from 58 patients in the National Heart, Lung, Blood Institute, Primary Pulmonary Hypertension Registry. Circulation 1989; 80:1198–1206.

38. Madden BP, Gosney J, Coghlan JG, Kamalvand K, Caslin AW, Smith P, Yacoub M, Heath D. Pretransplant clinicopathological correlation in end-stage primary pulmonary hypertension. Eur Respir J 1994; 7:672–678.

39. Botney MD, Liptay MJ, Kaiser LR, Cooper JD, Parks WC, Mecham RP. Active collagen synthesis by pulmonary arteries in human primary pulmonary hypertension. Am J Pathol 1993; 143:121–129.

40. Botney MD, Bahadori L, Gold LI. Vascular remodeling in primary pulmonary hypertension. Potential role for transforming growth factor-β. Am J Pathol 1994; 144:286–295.

41. Chazova I, Loyd JE, Zhdanov VS, Newman JH, Belenkov Y, Meyrick B. Pulmonary artery adventitial changes and venous involvement in primary pulmonary hypertension. Am J Pathol 1995; 146:389–397.
42. Tuder RM, Groves BM, Badesch DB, Voelkel NF. Exuberant endothelial cell growth and elements of inflammation are present in plexiform lesions of pulmonary hypertension. Am J Pathol 1994; 144:275–285.
43. Lee SD, Shroyer KR, Markham NE, Cool CD, Voelkel NF, Tuder RM. Monoclonal endothelial cell proliferation is present in primary but not secondary pulmonary hypertension. J Clin Invest 1998; 101:927–934.
44. Yamaki S, Wagenvoort CA. Comparison of primary plexogenic pulmonary arteriopathy in adults and children. A morphometric study in 40 patients. Br Heart J 1985; 54:428–434.
45. Wagenvoort CA, Mulder PGH. Thrombotic lesions in primary plexogenic pulmonary arteriopathy. Similar pathogenesis or complications? Chest 1993; 103:844–849.
46. Chaouat A, Weitzenblum E, Higenbottam T. The role of thrombosis in severe pulmonary hypertension. Eur Respir J 1996; 9:356–363.
47. Rubin RM, Radisavljevic Z, Shroyer KR, Polak JM, Voelkel NF. Monoclonal endothelial cells in appetite suppressant-associated pulmonary hypertension. Am J Respir Crit Care Med 1998; 158:1999–2001.
48. Wagenwoort CA, Mooi WJ. Biopsy Pathology of the Pulmonary Vasculature. London: Chapman & Hall, 1989.
49. Presti B, Berthrong M, Sherwin RM. Chronic thrombosis of major pulmonary arteries. Hum Pathol 1990; 21:601–606.
50. Goodwin JF, Harrison CV, Wilcken DEL. Obliterative pulmonary hypertension and thrombo-embolism. Br Med J 1963; 1:701–711, 777–783.
51. Rich S, Levitsky S, Brundage BH. Pulmonary hypertension from chronic pulmonary thrombo-embolism. Ann Intern Med 1988; 108:425–434.
52. Case Records of the Massachusetts General Hospital (Case 38–1981). N Engl J Med 1981; 305:685–693.
53. Egermayer P, Peacock AJ. Is pulmonary embolism a common cause of chronic pulmonary hypertension? Limitations of the embolic hypothesis. Eur Respir J 2000; 15:440–448.
54. Widimsky J. Acute pulmonary embolism and chronic thromboembolic pulmonary hypertension: is there a relationship? Eur Respir J 1991; 4:137–140.
55. Carson JL, Kelley MA, Duff A, Weg JG, Fulkerson WJ, Palevsky HI, Schwartz JS, Thompson BT, Popovich J Jr, Hobbins TE, Spera MA, Alavi A, Terrin ML. The clinical course of pulmonary embolism. N Engl J Med 1992; 326:1240–1245.
56. Owen WR, Thomas WA, Castleman B, Bland EF. Unrecognized emboli to the lungs with subsequent cor pulmonale. N Engl J Med 1953; 249:919–926.
57. Ribeiro A, Lindmarker P, Johnsson H, Juhlin-Dannfelt A, Jorfeldt L. Pulmonary embolism: one-year follow-up with echocardiography Doppler and five year survival analysis. Circulation 1999; 99:1325–1330.
58. Moser KM, Auger WR, Fedullo PF, Jamieson SW. Chronic thrombo-embolic pulmonary hypertension: clinical picture and surgical treatment. Eur Respir J 1992; 5:334–342.
59. McLachlin J, Paterson JC. Some basic observations on venous thrombosis and pulmonary embolism. Surg Gynecol Obstet 1951; 93:1–8.

60. Perez MT, Alexis JB, Ferreira T, Garcia H. Pulmonary artery fibrous bands. Report of a case with extensive lung infarction andsuperinfection with *Coccidioides immitis, Pseudomonas*, and acid fast bacilli. Arch Pathol Lab Med 1999; 123:170–172.

61. Peterson KL. Acute pulmonary thromboembolism. Has its evolution been rededfined? Circulation 1999; 99:1280–1283.

62. Moser KM, Bloor CM. Pulmonary vascular lesions occurring in patients with chronic major vessel thromboembolic pulmonary hypertension. Chest 1993; 103:685–692.

63. Kay JM. Pulmonary vascular lesions in chronic thromboembolic pulmonary hypertension (correspondence). Chest 1994; 105:1619–1620.

64. Höra J. Zur Histologie der klinischen "primaren Pulmonalsklerose." Frankf Z Pathol 1934; 47:100–108.

65. Heath D, Segel N, Bishop J. Pulmonary veno-occlusive disease. Circulation 1966; 34:242–248.

66. Holcomb BW Jr, Loyd JE, Ely EW, Johnson J, Robbins IM. Pulmonary veno-occlusive disease. A case series and new observations. Chest 2000; 118:1671–1679.

67. Wagenvoort CA, Wagenvoort N. The pathology of pulmonary veno-occlusive disease. Virchows Arch (A) 1974; 364:69–79.

68. Kay JM, deSa DJ, Mancer JFK. Ultrastructure of lung in pulmonary veno-oclcusive disease. Hum Pathol 1983; 14:451–456.

69. Wagenvoort CA, Wagenvoort N, Takahashi T. Pulmonary veno-occlusive disease. Involvement of pulmonary arteries and review of the literature. Hum Pathol 1985; 16:1033–1041.

70. McDonnell PJ, Summer WR, Hutchins GM. Pulmonary veno-occlusive disease. Morphological changes suggesting a viral cause. JAMA 1981; 246:667–671.

71. Crissman JD, Koss M, Carson RP. Pulmonary veno-occlusive disease secondary to granulomatous venulitis. Am J Surg Pathol 1980; 4:93–99.

72. Thadani U, Burrow C, Whitaker W, Heath D. Pulmonary veno-occlusive disease. Q J Med 1975; 44:133–159.

73. Heath D, Scott O, Lynch J. Pulmonary veno-occlusive disease. Thorax 1971; 26:663–674.

74. Rambihar VS, Fallen EL, Cairns JA. Pulmonary veno-occlusive disease: antemortem diagnosis from roentgenographic and hemodynamic findings. Can Med Assoc J 1979; 120:1519–1522.

75. Pääkko P, Sutinen S, Remes M, Paavilainen T, Wagenvoort CA. A case of pulmonary vascular occlusive disease: comparison of postmortem radiography and histology. Histopathology 1985; 9:253–262.

76. Hasleton PS, Ironside JW, Whittaker JS, Kelly W, Ward C, Thompson GS. Pulmonary veno-occlusive disease. A report of four cases. Histopathology 1986; 10:933–944.

77. Annotation: Pulmonary veno-occlusive disease. Br Med J 1972; 3:369.

78. Mandel J, Mark EJ, Hales CA. Pulmonary veno-occlusive disease. Am J Respir Crit Care Med 2000; 164:1964–1973.

79. Wagenvoort CA, Beetstra A, Spijker J. Capillary haemangiomatosis of the lungs. Histopathology 1978; 2:401–406.

80. Havlik DM, Massie LW, Williams WL, Crooks LA. Pulmonary capillary hemangiomatosis-like foci. An autopsy study of 8 cases. Am J Clin Pathol 2000; 113:655–662.

81. Tron V. Magee, F. Wright JL, Colby T, Churg A. Pulmonary capillary hemangiomatosis. Hum Pathol 1986; 17:1144–1150.
82. Faber CN, Yousem SA, Dauber JH, Griffith BP, Hardesty RL, Paradis IL. Pulmonary capillary hemangiomatosis. A report of three cases and a review of the literature. Am Rev Respir Dis 1989; 140:808–813.
83. Magee F, Wright JL, Kay JM, Peretz D, Donevan R, Churg A. Pulmonary capillary hemangiomatosis. Am Rev Respir Dis 1985; 132:922–925.
84. Heath D, Reid R. Invasive pulmonary haemangiomatosis. Br J Dis Chest 1985; 79:284–294.
85. Whittaker JS, Pickering CAC, Heath D, Smith P. Pulmonary capillary haemangiomatosis. Diag Histopathol 1983; 6:77–84.
86. Purdy LJ, Colby TV, Yousem SA, Battifora H. Pulmonary Kaposi's sarcoma. Premortem histologic diagnosis. Am J Surg Pathol 1986; 10:301–311.
87. Rowen M, Thompson JR, Williamson RA. Diffuse pulmonary hemangiomatosis. Radiology 1978; 127:445–451.
88. Daroca PJ, Mansfield RE, Ishinose H. Pulmonary veno-occlusive disease: report of a case with pseudoangiomatous features. Am J Surg Pathol 1977; 1:349–355.
89. Gugnani MK, Pierson C, Vanderheide R, Girgis RE. Pulmonary edema complicating prostacyclin therapy in pulmonary hypertension associated with scleroderma. A case of pulmonary capillary hemangiomatosis. Arthritis Rheum 2000; 43:699–703.
90. Wagenvoort CA. Open lung biopsies in congenital heart disease for evaluation of pulmonary vascular disease. Predictive value with regard to corrective operability. Histopathology 1985; 9:417–436.
91. Heath D, Best PV. The tunica media of the arteries of the lung in pulmonary hypertension. J Pathol Bacteriol 1958; 76:165–174.
92. Haworth SG, Reid L. A morphometric study of regional variation in lung structure in infants with pulmonary hypertension. A justification of open lung biopsy. Br Heart J 1978; 40:825–831.
93. Gianoulis M, Wright JL. An autopsy study of the small vessels in biopsies from the lingula and upper and lower lobes: implications for vascular assessment. Mod Pathol 1990; 3:567–569.
94. Churg AM. An inflation procedure for open lung biopsies. Am J Surg Pathol 1983; 7:69–71.
95. Miller PJ. An elastic stain. Med Lab Technol 1971; 28:148–149.
96. Palevsky HI, Schloo BL, Pietra GG, Weber KT, Janicki JS, Rubin E, Fishman AP. Primary pulmonary hypertension. Vascular structure, morphometry, and responsiveness to vasodilator agents. Circulation 1989; 80:1207–1221.

4

Management of Advanced Chronic Obstructive Pulmonary Disease

DENIS E. O'DONNELL and NHA VODUC

Queen's University
Kingston, Ontario, Canada

I. Introduction

Chronic obstructive pulmonary disease (COPD) is a common cause of morbidity and mortality worldwide. It is currently the fourth leading cause of death in North America and the only major cause of death and disability that continues to rise (1–4). Over the next 20 years it is projected that unprecedented numbers of patients with advanced symptomatic COPD will require expert medical assistance (5). This review discusses a comprehensive management approach for patients with severe COPD. Such an approach is primarily based on our current understanding of the pathophysiological underpinnings of this diverse group of obstructive disorders. Particular emphasis is placed on how best to achieve effective symptom control, since this is the most challenging goal for the management of patients with more advanced disease. The rationale for the various current pharmacological and nonpharmacological interventions and their relative clinical efficacy in achieving improvements in dyspnea, exercise capacity, and health status are reviewed.

In the recent GOLD consensus statement (5), COPD is defined as "a disease state characterized by airflow limitation that is not fully reversible." This airflow limitation is generally progressive and is the result of an abnormal inflammatory response of the airways and lung parenchyma to tobacco smoke and other noxious exposures. Clearly, COPD is a complex group of disorders with diverse pathophysiological and clinical manifestations. Given this diversity, an individualized approach to management that is based on a rigorous evaluation of the patient's impairment and disability is likely to yield best results.

In this review, advanced COPD is defined as severe airway obstruction (i.e., forced expiratory volume in one second $(FEV)_{1.0} < 50\%$ predicted) with persistent incapacitating dyspnea and exercise intolerance. In such patients, troublesome symptoms may persist despite escalating bronchodilator therapy. To manage these patients effectively, considerable health care resources are required: the components of a comprehensive management plan are outlined in Figure 1. The goals of management are presented in Table 1 (5).

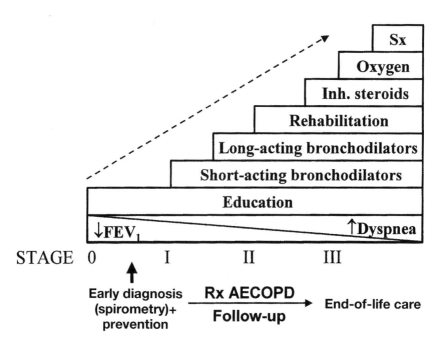

Figure 1 Stepwise approach to management of COPD. Therapy is escalated as the disease progresses. Sx = surgery; Inh = inhaled.

Table 1 Goals of COPD Management

Prevent disease progression
Relieve symptoms
Improve exercise tolerance
Improve health status
Prevent and treat complications
Prevent and treat exacerbations
Reduce mortality

Source: Ref. 5.

II. Pathophysiology of Exercise Intolerance in COPD

A. Exercise Limitation in COPD

In order to develop a rationale for the management of the disabled COPD patient, we must first consider the pathophysiology of exercise intolerance and dyspnea.

Exercise limitation is multifactorial in COPD. Recognized contributing factors include (1) ventilatory limitation due to impaired respiratory system mechanics and ventilatory muscle dysfunction, (2) metabolic and gas exchange abnormalities, (3) peripheral muscle dysfunction, (4) cardiac impairment, (5) intolerable exertional symptoms, and (6) any combination of these interdependent factors. The predominant contributing factors to exercise limitation vary among patients with COPD or, indeed, in a given patient over time. The more advanced the disease, the more of these factors come into play in a complex integrative manner.

B. Ventilatory Mechanics in COPD

COPD is a heterogeneous disorder characterized by dysfunction of the small and large airways and by parenchymal and vascular destruction, in highly variable combinations. Although the most obvious physiological defect in COPD is expiratory flow limitation, due to reduced lung recoil (and airway tethering effects) as well as intrinsic airway narrowing, the most important mechanical consequence of this is a "restrictive" ventilatory deficit due to dynamic lung overdistention or hyperinflation (DH) (6,7). When expiratory flow limitation reaches a critical level, lung emptying becomes incomplete during resting tidal breathing and lung volume fails to decline to its natural equilibrium point (i.e., the relaxation volume of the respiratory system). End-expiratory lung volume (EELV), therefore, becomes dynamically and not statically determined and represents a higher resting lung volume than in health (6,8). In flow-limited patients, EELV is, therefore, a continuous variable that fluctuates widely with rest and activity. When ventilation ($\dot{V}_E$) increases in flow-limited patients, as, for example, during exercise, increases in EELV (or DH) are inevitable (Figs. 2 and

3). Minor DH can occur in the healthy elderly, but at much higher $\dot{V}_E$ and oxygen consumption ($\dot{V}_{O_2}$) than in COPD (6). For practical purposes, the extent of DH during exercise depends on the extent of expiratory flow limitation, the level of baseline lung hyperinflation, the prevailing ventilatory demand, and the breathing pattern for a given ventilation (6).

The extent and pattern of DH development in COPD patients during exercise is highly variable. Clearly, some patients do not increase EELV during exercise, whereas others show dramatic increases (i.e., > 1 L) (6,9,10). We recently studied the pattern and magnitude of DH during incremental cycle exercise in 105 patients with COPD ($FEV_{1.0} = 37 \pm 13\%$ predicted; mean $\pm$ SD) (6) (Figs. 2 and 3). In contrast to age-matched healthy control subjects, the majority of this sample (80%) demonstrated significant increases in EELV above resting values: dynamic inspiratory capacity (IC) decreased significantly by 0.37 ± 0.39 L (or $14 \pm 15\%$ predicted) from rest (6). Similar

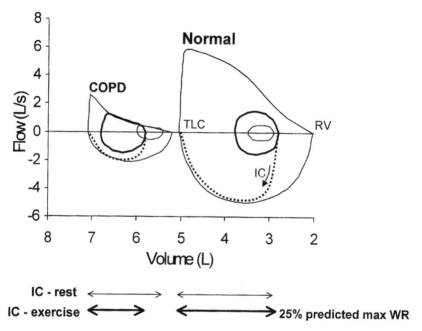

Figure 2 Flow-volume loops showing the effects of exercise on tidal volume in COPD and in health. The outer loops represent the maximal limits of flow and volume. The smallest loops represent the resting tidal volumes. The thicker loops represent the increased tidal volumes and flows seen with exercise. The dotted lines represent the IC maneuver to TLC, which is used to anchor tidal flow-volume loops within the respective maximal loops. Healthy subjects are able to increase both their tidal volumes and inspiratory and expiratory flows. In COPD, expiratory flow is already maximal during resting ventilation. In order to increase expiratory flow further, these patients must hyperinflate.

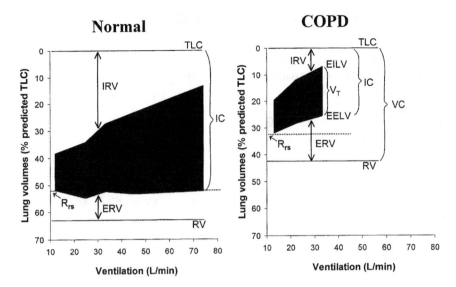

Figure 3 Changes in operational lung volumes are shown as ventilation increases with exercise in COPD and in age-matched healthy subjects. End-expiratory lung volume (EELV) increases above the relaxation volume of the respiratory system (Rrs) in COPD, as reflected by a decrease in inspiratory capacity (IC), while EELV in health either remains unchanged or decreases. "Restrictive" constraints on tidal volume (V_T, solid area) expansion during exercise are significantly greater in the COPD group from both below (increased EELV) and above (reduced IRV as EILV approaches TLC). IRV = inspiratory reserve volume; ERV = expiratory reserve volume; EILV = end-inspiratory lung volume; TLC = total lung capacity. (From Ref. 6.)

levels of DH have recently been reported in COPD patients after completing a 6-min walking test while breathing without an imposed mouthpiece (11). For the same $FEV_{1.0}$, patients with lower diffusion capacity ($DL_{CO} < 50\%$ predicted), and presumably more emphysema, had faster rates of DH at lower exercise levels, earlier attainment of critical volume constraints (peak V_T), greater exertional dyspnea, and lower peak $\dot{V}_E$ and $\dot{V}_{O_2}$ when compared with patients with a relatively preserved DL_{CO} (6). In the latter group, the magnitude of change in EELV from rest to peak exercise was similar to that of the group with low DL_{CO}, but air trapping occurred predominantly at a higher $\dot{V}_{O_2}$ and $\dot{V}_E$ at the end of exercise. Patients with predominant emphysema likely had faster rates of DH because of reduced elastic lung recoil (and airway tethering) and an increased propensity to expiratory flow limitation. In this group, DH is often further compounded by a greater ventilatory demand as a result of higher physiological dead space, reflecting greater ventilation perfusion abnormalities (12). The extent of DH during exercise is inversely correlated with the level of resting lung hyperinflation: patients who were severely hyperinflated at rest showed minimal further DH during exercise (6).

Tidal Volume Restriction and Exercise Intolerance

The resting inspiratory capacity (IC) and, in particular, the dynamic IC during exercise [and not the resting vital capacity (VC)] represent the true operating limits for V_T expansion in any given patient. Therefore, when V_T approximates the peak dynamic IC during exercise, or the dynamic end-inspiratory lung volume (EILV) encroaches on the total lung capacity (TLC) envelope, further volume expansion is impossible, even in the face of increased central drive and electrical activation of the diaphragm (13) (Figs. 2 and 3).

In our study, using multiple regression analysis with symptom-limited peak $\dot{V}_{O_2}$ as the dependent variable and several relevant physiological measurements as independent variables [including $FEV_{1.0}$ and $\dot{V}_E$ expressed as a percent of maximal ventilatory capacity] peak V_T (standardized as percent predicted VC) emerged as the strongest contributory variable, explaining 47% of the variance (6). Peak V_T, in turn, correlated strongly with both the resting and peak dynamic IC. It is noteworthy that this correlation was particularly strong ($r = 0.9$) in approximately 80% of the sample, who had a diminished resting and peak dynamic IC (i.e., <70% predicted). Studies by Tantucci et al. (14) have provided evidence that such patients with a diminished resting IC have demonstrable resting expiratory flow limitation by the negative expiratory pressure (NEP) technique. Recent studies have confirmed that patients with a reduced resting IC and evidence of resting expiratory flow limitation have poorer exercise performance when compared with those with a better preserved resting IC with no evidence of expiratory flow limitation at rest (6,15,16).

DH and Inspiratory Muscle Dysfunction

DH results in increased elastic loading of the inspiratory muscles and compromises their ability to generate pressure. The net effect of DH during exercise in COPD is, therefore, that the V_T response to increasing exercise is progressively constrained despite near maximal inspiratory efforts (17). The ratio of tidal esophageal pressure swings relative to maximum (P_{es}/PI_{max}) to tidal volume (expressed as V_T/VC or V_T/predicted IC) is significantly higher at any given work rate or ventilation in COPD as compared with health (17). The negative effects of DH are listed in Table 2.

C. Dynamic Hyperinflation and Dyspnea

Dyspnea intensity during exercise has been shown to correlate well with concomitant measures of dynamic lung hyperinflation (17,18). In a multiple regression analysis with Borg ratings of dyspnea intensity as the dependent variable versus a number of independent physiological variables, the change in EILV (expressed as percent of TLC) during exercise emerged as the strongest independent correlate ($r^2 = 0.63$, $p = 0.001$) in 23 patients with advanced COPD (average $FEV_{1.0}$, 36% predicted) (18). The change in EELV and change in V_T

Table 2 Negative Effects of Dynamic Hyperinflation During Exercise

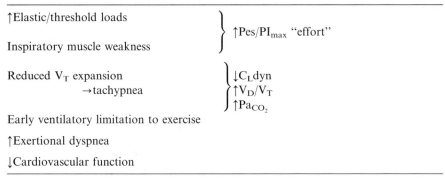

↑Elastic/threshold loads

Inspiratory muscle weakness
} ↑Pes/PI_{max} "effort"

Reduced V_T expansion
        →tachypnea
} ↓C_Ldyn
↑V_D/V_T
↑Pa_{CO_2}

Early ventilatory limitation to exercise

↑Exertional dyspnea

↓Cardiovascular function

(components of EILV) emerged as significant contributors to exertional breathlessness and, together with increased breathing frequency, accounted for 61% of the variance in exercise Borg ratings (18). A second study showed equally strong correlations between the intensity of perceived inspiratory difficulty during exercise and EILV/TLC ($r^2 = 0.69$, $p < 0.01$) (17). Dyspnea intensity also correlates well with the ratio of effort (P_{es}/PI_{max}) to tidal volume response (V_T/VC) (17). This increased effort-displacement ratio in COPD ultimately reflects neuromechanical dissociation (or uncoupling) of the ventilatory pump (Fig. 4).

Current evidence suggests that breathlessness is not only a function of the amplitude of central motor output but is also importantly modulated by peripheral feedback from a host of respiratory mechanoreceptors (for comprehensive reviews, see Refs. 19–22). Thus, the psychophysical basis of neuromechanical dissociation likely resides in the complex central processing and integration of signals that mediate (1) central motor command output (23–25) and (2) sensory feedback from various mechanoreceptors that provide precise instantaneous proprioceptive information about muscle displacement (muscle spindles and joint receptors), tension development (Golgi tendon organs), and change in respired volume or flow (lung and airway mechanoreceptors) (26–35). Awareness of the disparity between effort and ventilatory output may elicit patterned psychological and neurohumoral responses that culminate in respiratory distress, which is an important affective dimension of perceived inspiratory difficulty.

Further indirect evidence of the importance of DH in contributing to exertional dyspnea in COPD has come from a number of studies showing that dyspnea was effectively ameliorated by interventions that reduced operational lung volumes (either pharmacologically or surgically) or that counterbalanced the negative effects of DH on the inspiratory muscles (continuous positive airway pressure) (36–43). Consistently strong correlations have been reported between reduced Borg ratings of dyspnea and reduced DH during exercise in a

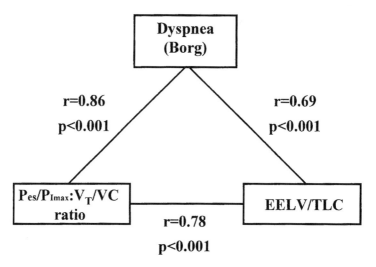

Figure 4 Statistical correlations between Borg dyspnea ratings, end-expiratory lung volume (EELV), and the ratio of inspiratory effort (esophageal pressure relative to maximum, Pes/PI_{max}) to the tidal volume response (V_T standardized for vital capacity) at a standardized level of exercise in COPD. (Data from Ref. 17.)

number of studies following various bronchodilators and lung volume reduction surgery (36–43).

It must be emphasized that dyspnea is a complex, multidimensional symptom in COPD and that the mechanical factors outlined above and/or alterations in ventilatory demand, although instrumental, may not explain dyspnea causation in all patients with COPD. In some patients, other factors may be predominant (e.g., inspiratory muscle weakness, arterial oxygen desaturation or hypercapnia (28) independent of increased ventilation, or cardiac factors that are currently poorly understood). It follows, therefore, that each patient should be assessed on an individual basis so that identifiable and potentially reversible factors can be recognized.

D. Ventilatory Limitation and Gas Exchange Abnormalities in COPD

Arterial hypoxemia during exercise commonly occurs in patients with severe COPD as a result of the effect of a fall in mixed venous oxygen tension on low ventilation/perfusion lung units and shunting (44). In severe COPD, both the ability to increase lung perfusion and distribute inspired ventilation throughout the lungs during exercise is compromised (44). Resting physiological dead space is often increased, reflecting ventilation/perfusion inequalities, and fails to decline further during exercise as is the case in health (12,44,45). To maintain appropriate alveolar ventilation and blood gas homeostasis in the face of increased physiological dead space (V_D/V_T), minute ventilation must increase. In this regard, several studies have confirmed high levels of submaximal ventilation during exercise in COPD compared with health (12,46,47).

In more advanced COPD, arterial hypoxemia during exercise occurs as a result of alveolar hypoventilation (48,49). The reduced exercise ventilation relative to metabolic demand may reflect reduced output of the central controller or a preserved or amplified central respiratory drive in the presence of an impaired mechanical/ventilatory muscle response. The evidence that CO_2 retention during exercise is the result of reduced central or peripheral chemosensitivity or inspiratory muscle fatigue is inconclusive. We recently concluded that CO_2 retention during exercise occurred in part because of greater dynamic restrictive constraints on tidal volume (secondary to DH) in the setting of a fixed high physiological dead space during exercise (50).

Increased Ventilatory Demand During Exercise in COPD

The effects of the mechanical derangements in COPD outlined above are often amplified by concomitantly increased ventilatory demand (Fig. 5). A high V_D/V_T that fails to decline with exercise is the primary stimulus for increased submaximal ventilation in this population. Other factors contributing to increased submaximal ventilation include early lactic acidosis, hypoxemia, high metabolic demands of breathing, low arterial CO_2 set points, and other nonmetabolic sources of ventilatory stimulation (i.e., anxiety). As we have seen, the extent of DH and its consequent negative sensory consequences in flow-limited patients will vary with ventilatory demand (6). There is abundant evidence that increased ventilatory demand contributes to the causation of dyspnea in COPD: intensity of dyspnea during exercise has been shown to correlate strongly with the change in $\dot{V}_E$ or with $\dot{V}_E$ expressed as a fraction of maximal ventilatory capacity (18). Flow-limited patients with the highest ventilation will develop limiting ventilatory constraints on flow and volume generation and greater dyspnea early in exercise (6). For a given $FEV_{1.0}$, patients who have greater ventilatory demands have been shown, in one study, to have more severe chronic activity-related dyspnea (12). Moreover, relief of exertional dyspnea and improved exercise endurance following interventions such as exercise training (51), oxygen therapy (52), and opiates (53) have been shown to result in part from the attendant reduction in submaximal ventilation (see below).

E. Peripheral Muscle Dysfunction and Exercise Intolerance in COPD

Recently, there has been heightened interest in the role of abnormalities of peripheral muscle structure and function in exercise limitation in COPD (for excellent comprehensive reviews, see Refs. 54 and 55). The importance of

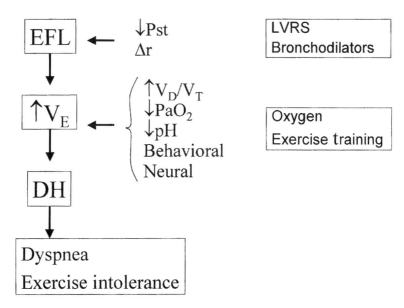

Figure 5 The combination of expiratory flow limitation (EFL) and accelerated ventilation ($\dot{V}_E$) during exercise contributes to dynamic lung hyperinflation (DH) and exercise intolerance. V_D/V_T = physiological dead space; Pst = static lung recoil; Δr = airway resistance; LVRS = lung volume reduction surgery.

increased leg effort as an exercise-limiting symptom in COPD was first highlighted by Killian et al. (56).

Peripheral muscle dysfunction is a potentially reversible cause of exercise curtailment in COPD and is currently the focus of intense study (57–66). Abnormalities of peripheral muscle structure and function have now been extensively documented in COPD (54,55). Many of these abnormalities ultimately represent the effects of reduced activity levels or immobility because of overwhelming dyspnea. These abnormalities include loss of muscle mass and mitochrondrial (aerobic) potential and compromised oxidative phosphorylation, which results in an exaggerated dependence on high-energy phosphate transfer and anaerobic glycolysis (57,62). Severe peripheral muscle weakness, due in part to disuse atrophy, has been reported in several studies (57,59). In a number of studies, lactate thresholds (i.e., the $\dot{V}_{O_2}$ at which lactate begins to increase) have been shown to be lower in COPD than in health (63,64). Thus, in exercising COPD patients, there is excessive accumulation of metabolic byproducts that impair contractility and increase the propensity to fatigue. Early metabolic acidosis (and increased CO_2 production through acid buffering effects) may stimulate increased ventilation and hasten the onset of critical ventilatory limitation. Moreover, an acidic milieu, with an altered ionic status (e.g., increased potassium) of the active peripheral muscle, may also stimulate resident metaboreceptors, which may have important effects on ventilatory and sympathetic stimulation, as has been demonstrated in patients with congestive heart failure (54,67,68).

Muscle biopsies in COPD have shown reduced capillarization with preserved or decreased capillary to fiber ratios (60–62). These muscles show consistent reductions in type I slow-twitch, high-oxidative, low-tension, fatigue-resistant muscle fibers (60–62). There is an increased preponderance of type II fibers, which would be expected to be associated with an increased velocity of contraction, a reduced mechanical efficiency, and increased fatigability (68). General muscle wasting (cachexia) in COPD has been associated with low circulating levels of anabolic steroids, growth hormone, and altered circadian rhythms of leptin production in COPD (69–72). It has recently been shown that exercise in COPD patients accelerated free radical formation (73). If these free radicals are not scavenged by antioxidants, they can result in extensive damage to membranes and the cation cycling proteins (74). Other well-recognized factors that contribute to peripheral muscle weakness in COPD under certain circumstances include chronic oral steroid therapy, malnutrition, and the effects of hypoxia, hypercapnia, and acidosis (54).

III. Assessment of the Dyspneic Patient

Current stratification of COPD severity is primarily based on the measurement of $FEV_{1.0}$. However, the $FEV_{1.0}$ correlates poorly with disability and health status. A more rigorous evaluation of patients can be undertaken by quantification of impairment, disability, and handicap (Table 3). This more comprehensive approach is likely to be more valuable in optimizing management and evaluating therapeutic responses.

A. The Patient Interview

The first step in evaluating dyspnea intensity and the resultant functional disability in a given patient is a comprehensive history and physical examination. Generally, dyspnea is first experienced during activity and progresses insidiously over time, so that the patient is rarely certain about the precise onset of his or her symptoms. Avoidance of activity is an effective dyspnea-relieving strategy in symptomatic COPD patients. Patients are often unaware that they have made significant lifestyle modifications so as to avoid provoking dyspnea. Thus, they may learn to accomplish a given physical task at a considerably reduced pace or to avoid certain activities that they know will precipitate dyspnea. Because of this long-term behavioral adaptation, the caregiver may have to question the patient extensively to uncover the specific circumstances where dyspnea is experienced during common daily activities. A number of simple questions have traditionally been used to elicit the magnitude of the task required to induce dyspnea in a given individual. These include the

Table 3 Patient Evaluation/Stratification

Symptoms (BDI, MRC)	
Body mass index (BMI)	
Spirometry	impairment
Hyperinflation (IC, FRC)	
DL_{CO} and CT scan	
Exercise performance:	disability
Peak $\dot{V}_{O_2}$	
Ventilatory reserve	
Gas exchange	
Peripheral muscle strength	
Health status	handicap

following: "How far can you walk on a level surface before experiencing shortness of breath?" "How many flights of stairs can you climb before getting short of breath?" "While walking, can you keep pace with someone who does not have breathing problems?" "Can you talk and walk at the same time?" The intensity of dyspnea and the resultant functional disability can be assessed by "self-rated" magnitude-of-task questionnaires, such as the Medical Research Council (MRC) scale, or by an interview using the more comprehensive Baseline Dyspnea Index (BDI) (75–80). Cardiopulmonary exercise testing (CPET) can also be used to accurately evaluate exertional dyspnea intensity and functional disability (see below).

B. Physical Examination

Physical examination is notoriously unreliable in assessing the presence or severity of COPD. The relationship between specific physical findings and dyspnea intensity is poorly defined. Simply observing the patient during the minor activity of undressing or moving to the examination couch may confirm historical information related to the level and intensity of the patient's activity-related dyspnea. Respiratory distress may be evident in an inability to complete sentences. Patients may be seen to spontaneously adopt pursed-lip breathing or to favor the leaning forward position in their efforts to ameliorate dyspnea. Physical findings may give clues to the underlying pathophysiology and source of dyspnea in some patients. Severe thoracic hyperinflation is readily identified in patients with more advanced disease. However, the physical evaluation of lesser levels of hyperinflation is insensitive. Physical features that are suggestive of lung hyperinflation include an overexpanded chest, accessory muscle use at rest, reduced thoracic motion despite maximal inspiratory efforts, tracheal tug, supraclavicular and intercostal recession during inspiration, indrawing of the lateral aspects of the lower ribs during tidal or deep inspiration (originally described by William Stokes in 1837) (81), and a tympanic percussion note over the thorax with diminished cardiac and liver dullness. Auscultation of the chest may be insufficiently sensitive to detect airway obstruction in patients with COPD, but markedly reduced breath sounds bilaterally in the face of maximal inspiratory effort are suggestive of emphysema. Prolonged forced expiratory time (measured by stethoscope at the trachea) may be the only auscultatory abnormality in some patients with COPD (82). Wheeze and crackles are nonspecific but may cause the clinician to suspect additional cardiopulmonary pathology, which may contribute to dyspnea in a particular patient.

C. Investigations

A chest radiograph may reveal features of lung overinflation or highlight possible comorbid conditions. Simple spirometry ($FEV_{1.0}$), forced vital capacity (FVC) and the $FEV_{1.0}$/FVC ratio are useful for diagnostic purposes and to assess the severity of airway obstruction. Spirometric inspiratory capacity (IC) and slow (or timed) vital capacity (VC) provide indirect information about the level of resting lung hyperinflation (i.e., functional residual capacity and residual volume, respectively). Patients with a resting IC of <70% predicted generally have resting expiratory flow limitation (6,15,16). The $FEV_{1.0}$/FVC ratio may suggest a concomitant restrictive ventilatory problem. Maximal and tidal flow–volume loops give qualitative, imprecise information about the extent of expiratory flow limitation present at rest. If possible, the rate of decline of the various pulmonary function parameters over time should be evaluated in order to assess the time course of disease progression in that individual.

Single-breath diffusion capacity for carbon monoxide (DL_{CO}) is also measured and is characteristically reduced in emphysema or other conditions where the pulmonary vasculature is attenuated. For a given $FEV_{1.0}$, those with a reduced diffusion capacity (i.e., <50%) have greater chronic activity-related dyspnea, greater exertional dyspnea, and poorer exercise tolerance than those with a better preserved DL_{CO} (6,12). Plethysmographic lung volumes quantify the level of lung hyperinflation and identify coexistent restriction. Bronchodilator reversibility testing with a short acting $beta_2$ agonist may identify patients with acute reversible bronchoconstriction. However, a single negative test in the laboratory is an insensitive measure of potential long-term clinical responses and should not, therefore, influence pharmacological choices. Bronchodilator responsiveness testing using bronchodilator combinations, while measuring changes in lung volume as well as expiratory flow rates may predict sustained clinical benefits of bronchodilators better than the traditional approach (83). In patients with severe resting hyperinflation, substantial reductions in air trapping (i.e., >0.5 L reduction in residual volume) can occur in the absence of change in the $FEV_{1.0}$ (84).

A high-resolution computed tomography (CT) scan may be indicated to demonstrate the extent and pattern of emphysema and the presence of bullae, usually suspected from the plain radiograph. Newer high-resolution CT scanning techniques are likely to provide more precise quantification of emphysema and airway abnormalities than currently available technologies. In dyspneic patients for whom volume reduction surgery is being considered, CT imaging together with radioisotope ventilation perfusion scanning can provide information about the pattern and heterogeneity of disease and can help identify discrete areas of emphysema that can be targeted for removal. Maximal inspiratory pressures (MIPs) measured at functional residual capacity (FRC) and residual volume (RV) by a manometer using a mouth occlusion technique, as well as maximal expiratory pressures (MEPs) measured at TLC, may identify ventilatory muscle weakness as a potential contributor to dyspnea. These tests are highly motivation-dependent and imprecise but may identify patients with persistent critical inspiratory muscle weakness who will require more formal neuromuscular evaluation. The patient's weight and nutritional status should also be recorded: patients with progressive weight loss may need additional nutritional and diagnostic assessment. Weight has been shown to be an important prognostic indicator in COPD.

D. Cardiopulmonary Exercise Testing (CPET) in COPD

CPET, using an incremental cycle ergometry protocol, has traditionally been used to evaluate exercise performance in COPD. Standard CPET measures the following physiological responses: metabolic load [oxygen uptake ($\dot{V}_{O_2}$) and carbon dioxide output ($\dot{V}_{CO_2}$)], peak power output, ventilation ($\dot{V}_E$), breathing pattern, arterial oxygen saturation, heart rate, electrocardiogram, oxygen pulse, and blood pressure. Increasingly, exertional symptom assessment using validated scales (i.e., Borg and visual analogue scales) is being used during CPET, and this constitutes an important advance (85,86). Common physiological responses to incremental cycle exercise in COPD are now well established (Table 4). Conventional CPET has the potential to yield important clinical information on an individual patient basis: (1) it provides an accurate assessment of the patient's exercise capacity that cannot be predicted from resting physiological measurements; (2) it measures the perceptual responses to quantifiable physiological stimuli (i.e., $\dot{V}_{O_2}$, ventilation, and power output); (3) it can provide insight into the pathophysiological mechanisms of exercise intolerance and dyspnea in a given patient (e.g., excessive ventilatory demand, arterial oxygen desaturation); and (4) it can identify other coexistent conditions that contribute to exercise limitation (i.e., cardiac disorders, intermittent claudication, musculoskeletal problems, etc.). The results of CPET can also assist in developing individualized exercise training protocols, and sequential CPET can be used to evaluate the impact of therapeutic interventions in patients with COPD.

Exercise Flow-Volume-Loop Analysis

One shortcoming of traditional CPET is that it gives little or no information about the prevailing dynamic ventilatory mechanics during exercise. This

concentrations and increased capillary density after supervised training (148). $\dot{V}_{O_2}$ kinetics are faster after training and blood lactate levels are lower at a standardized work (149). Perceived leg discomfort is significantly less at any given work rate following exercise training and contributes to improved exercise endurance, particularly in patients where leg discomfort was the primary locus of sensory limitation prior to program entry (47,51).

Upper Limb Training

Many patients with advanced COPD may experience severe breathlessness during upper extremity activity (e.g., combing hair, showering, lifting objects, etc.) (150–153). In some instances, dyspnea during this type of activity may exceed that experienced during lower limb weight bearing tasks. Dyspnea during arm exercise may result from the associated high ventilatory demands for a given $\dot{V}_{O_2}$, which potentially could aggravate dynamic hyperinflation in flow-limited patients (150–152). Additionally, the upper limb muscles are anchored to the thorax and can serve as accessory muscles of inspiration. It follows that if these muscles are used for their peripheral locomotor function in patients who depend on their supportive role in ventilation, dyspnea may arise when other inspiratory muscles such as the diaphragm are suddenly burdened with a greater share of the work of breathing. In several studies, weight training of upper extremities resulted in greater improvement in endurance and reduced dyspnea during upper limb exercise compared with control in patients with advanced COPD (152–155). Upper limb training should, therefore, be incorporated into multimodality exercise training protocols and may be particularly beneficial in those patients whose dyspnea is regularly provoked by upper extremity exercise.

E. Breathing Retraining

Various breathing retraining techniques have been advocated for the improvement of dyspnea in symptomatic patients with COPD (155–160). Attempts to retrain patients to adopt a slower, deeper breathing pattern are variably successful. The rationale behind retraining is that the adoption of a more efficient breathing pattern, with reduced relative physiological dead space and improved efficiency of CO_2 elimination, will cause $\dot{V}_E$ reduction, which should, in turn, reduce perceived dyspnea. Many patients trained in this technique adopt a slower, deeper pattern when supervised but generally quickly resort to their spontaneous faster breathing pattern when they believe they are unobserved. This is not surprising, since the rapid, shallow breathing pattern characteristically adopted by patients with more advanced disease, particularly during activity, likely represents the optimal compensatory strategy for intrinsic mechanical loading (i.e., elastic loading). A rapid, shallow breathing pattern would act to minimize the intrathoracic pressure perturbations and the associated respiratory discomfort. Moreover, a slower, deeper pattern may actually accentuate mechanical loading and breathing discomfort in some patients, and this is clearly not desirable.

Diaphragmatic breathing (159,160) has been advocated for many years as a dyspnea-relieving strategy in advanced COPD. The patient is instructed to allow the abdominal wall to move outward during slow inspiration, usually in conjunction with slow expiration through pursed lips (159,160). Some studies have provided evidence that this technique provides some alleviation of dyspnea, while others have not. The potential mechanisms of dyspnea relief during diaphragmatic breathing are also unclear. Putative mechanisms include altered pattern of ventilatory muscle recruitment or avoidance of excessive increases in breathing frequency during or following activity, with resultant avoidance of dynamic hyperinflation. Diaphragmatic breathing may serve to distract patients from distressing dyspnea and may serve as an anxiety-relieving strategy or relaxation technique that hastens recovery from acute dyspneic episodes.

Alterations in breathing pattern (i.e., increased tidal volume, reduced frequency) as a result of interventions that increase resting IC, such as pharmacological volume reduction, are likely to be more successful than breathing retraining in contributing to dyspnea relief (146). Under these circumstances, a slower, deeper breathing pattern has been shown to contribute to improved Borg ratings of dyspnea during exercise (146).

Pursed-Lip Breathing

Pursed lip breathing (PLB) is a breathing technique adopted spontaneously by many patients with COPD as a dyspnea-relieving strategy, usually during acute episodes provoked by activity, anxiety, or intercurrent respiratory tract infections. Traditionally, patients are taught this technique as a component of pulmonary rehabilitation programs. PLB involves active expiration through a resistance created by constricting or pursing the lips (155,156). The nasopharynx has been shown to be occluded during PLB (161). Expiration is prolonged, and tidal volume generally increases, with modest transient improvements in gas exchange. PLB is thought to be more common in patients with advanced COPD, particularly those with emphysema. While patients who spontaneously adopt PLB clearly derive symptomatic relief, symptomatic responses in those who are instructed in the technique are highly variable and unpredictable. The mechanisms of dyspnea relief during PLB are conjectural, and current mechanistic theories are mainly based on clinical observation. Attempts have been made to study the possible physiological mechanisms of dyspnea relief during PLB by applying external resistive loads, but these loads imperfectly simulate actual PLB. Possible dyspnea-relieving factors during PLB include altered breathing pattern (i.e., slower and deeper) with improved ventilation/perfusion ($\dot{V}/\dot{Q}$) relationships, improved arterial oxygen desaturation (156,162) and CO_2 elimination, altered pattern of ventilatory muscle recruitment (i.e., more expiratory muscle recruitment, which can optimize diaphragmatic length and assist inspiration), attenuation of dynamic airway compression (163) and reduced lung hyperinflation as a result of reduced breathing frequency and prolongation of expiratory time. Like diaphragmatic breathing, PLB may serve as a useful relaxation technique that relieves anxiety and helps patients avoid regression to respiratory panic during acute episodes of dyspnea. While no consensus exists about the precise neurophysiological mechanisms of dyspnea relief during PLB, clinical experience has shown that the technique is undoubtedly beneficial in some patients. Thus, instruction in PLB should be provided by skilled instructors as part of the rehabilitation program. Those who derive symptomatic benefit will habitually resort to this technique during episodes of dyspnea.

F. Inspiratory Muscle Training

When inspiratory muscles are functionally weakened, greater motor command output or effort is required to maintain a given ventilation during rest and exercise (21,26). Intensity of dyspnea has been shown to increase when the inspiratory force required during tidal breathing increases as a fraction of maximal force-generating capacity (21). Theoretically, therefore, interventions that increase inspiratory muscle strength should reduce the level of neural activation and inspiratory effort required during tidal breathing, with resultant reduction in dyspnea. In practice, the effectiveness of specific inspiratory muscle training using a variety of techniques (voluntary isocapneic hypercapnia, inspiratory resistive loading, and inspiratory threshold loading) has been inconsistent (164). One metanalysis of 17 clinical studies concluded that there is insufficient evidence to recommend specific inspiratory muscle training for routine clinical purposes (165). Earlier studies, which employed resistive loading, have been criticized because of the uncertainty of the training stimulus, since breathing pattern was not controlled. Similarly, breathing frequency was not targeted in a number of studies employing inspiratory muscle threshold loading. Definitive conclusions from the literature are, therefore, difficult to draw and the prevalence of true inspiratory muscle weakness among patients with COPD remains unknown. One drawback is that the current measurements of inspiratory muscle strength, such as maximal occlusion pressures, are highly effort-dependent and are also dependent on the lung volume at which they are measured (166). Thus, the validity and reproducibility of these measurements are uncertain. More accurate assessments of muscle function, using techniques such as phrenic electromagnetic stimulation or sniff esophageal pressure recording, have limited availability (167,168). Patients deemed to have inspiratory muscle weakness based on MIPs may not have actual functional weakness. In fact, a recent study has provided evidence that inspiratory muscle strength is preserved or even relatively increased in severe COPD (169). Patients with advanced COPD may not respond to inspiratory muscle training if weakness is due to severe nutritional depletion, chronic hypoxia and hypercapnea, steroid myopathy, or electrolyte imbalance. Notwithstanding the general lack of evidence that specific inspiratory muscle training is a useful dyspnea-relieving measure, a few important controlled studies have shown that inspiratory muscle training, using targeted resistive or inspiratory threshold training, improves dyspnea and exercise endurance in patients with COPD and that these improvements correlate with physiological data (i.e., increased MIP) (170,171).

Further studies are required to identify the subgroup of patients with COPD who are more likely to benefit from specific inspiratory muscle training. Studies are also needed to define the optimal mode of training, including training threshold and duration. While we await definitive information on the value of inspiratory muscle training, it seems reasonable to identify patients with severe inspiratory muscle weakness and to institute specific measures to improve function aimed at reversing the underlying problem (i.e., nutritional supplementation, correction of electrolytes, withdrawal of high-dose steroid therapy, etc.). These measures, in conjunction with an exercise training program where the training stimulus is targeted to high and sustained ventilation levels, should conjointly improve inspiratory muscle function to a level comparable to that achieved by inspiratory muscle training (146). Studies are currently under way to assess the effects of treatment with anabolic steroids or a growth hormone analogue, in conjunction with exercise training, on ventilatory muscle function, dyspnea, and exercise duration in patients with advanced COPD.

Follow-Up

Most controlled studies to date, have focused on the short-term benefits of pulmonary rehabilitation. One recent study by Griffiths et al. (172) has shown that over a period of 1 year, many of the subjective and objective benefits of exercise training are lost. Careful follow-up to ensure adherence to home-based exercise programs together with a vigorous proactive approach to the management of COPD exacerbations would likely yield better long-term results, but this remains to be established in clinical studies.

V. Oxygen Therapy

While large, controlled studies have provided convincing evidence of the beneficial effects of continuous oxygen therapy on survival in severely hypoxemic patients with COPD, the effects of such therapy on chronic symptoms is unknown (174–177). The effect of oxygen on dyspnea in a given individual with symptomatic COPD is entirely unpredictable, and the mechanism(s) of dyspnea relief in those who do respond are not fully understood. Potential mechanisms include reduced ventilatory drive and hypoventilation as a result of diminished hypoxic drive from peripheral chemoreceptors (175,176) or from reduced activity generated metabolic acidosis (177).

Interpretation of the available literature on this subject is compounded by considerable interstudy variability in (1) baseline dyspnea severity and degree of resting and exercise hypoxemia in study patients, (2) the concentration of added oxygen, (3) the exercise protocols used (i.e., endurance versus incremental), and (4) the mode of oxygen delivery (high flow versus demand reservoir). Therefore it is not surprising that studies which have specifically addressed mechanisms of dyspnea relief during added oxygen have yielded conflicting results. In particular, the question of whether the relief of dyspnea is solely a function of the attendant reduction of ventilation or is independent of this effect has not been conclusively answered. Some studies in normals and in patients with COPD, during rest and exercise, have shown that dyspnea relief is independent of ventilation (175,176), while others have not (177,178). Reduced peripheral chemoreceptor activity in response to oxygen, and the attendant reduced ventilation, has long been thought to be a primary mechanism of dyspnea relief in COPD (175,176). However, one recent study has shown that other mechanisms are equally plausible. In patients with advanced disease but with mild hypoxemia, reduction of standardized Borg ratings during added oxygen compared with room air was shown to be directly related to reduced submaximal ventilation, which, in turn, correlated strongly with reduced metabolic acidosis (i.e., reduced blood lactate concentrations) (52,177). Reduced blood lactate concentrations likely reflect improved oxygen delivery and/or utilization at the peripheral muscle level during supraphysiological levels of oxygen (i.e., oxygen 60%).

Several other studies have shown that dyspnea decreases at a given ventilation during added oxygen or that the reduction in dyspnea during oxygen seemed disproportionate to the small reductions in ventilation that were induced (175–180). Possible explanations for this phenomenon include a variety of oxygen-induced physiological effects: (1) reduced respiratory muscle impedance as a result of reduced airways resistance (181) or reduced dynamic hyperinflation (secondary to altered breathing pattern for a given $\dot{V}_E$), (2) delay in inspiratory muscle fatigue because of increased oxygen enriched blood perfusion to the muscles, (3) altered central perception of dyspneogenic stimuli, and (4) decreased afferent inputs from pulmonary vasculature or right heart chambers secondary to acute or chronic decreases in pulmonary artery pressure (175–182). The relative importance of these various factors are difficult if not impossible to quantify and likely vary between individuals. Moreover, several of these factors in combination (i.e., reduced $\dot{V}_E$ and factors that reduce dyspnea for a given $\dot{V}_E$) may have additive effects on dyspnea relief.

Three recent studies have provided evidence that patients with moderate to severe COPD but with only mild exercise hypoxemia benefit from supplemental oxygen therapy during exercise in terms of reduced exertional dyspnea and improved exercise endurance (52,177,183,184). Improvement in exercise endurance during oxygen was related to reduced ventilation, with an attendant decrease in the rate of DH and a concomitant increase in submaximal inspiratory reserve volumes (Fig. 9). Reduced operating lung

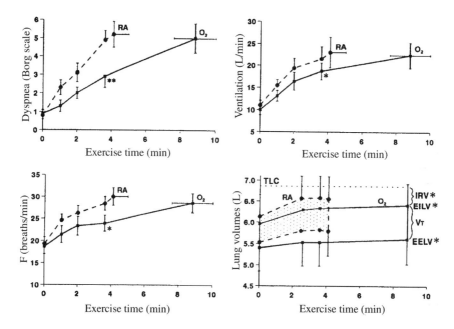

Figure 9 Exercise responses during hyperoxia (breathing 60% O_2) and room air (RA) are shown in patients with advanced COPD. During hyperoxia, dyspnea and exercise endurance are significantly improved during constant-load exercise. Ventilation, breathing frequency (F) and operating lung volumes are significantly reduced (*$p < 0.05$, difference at isotime exercise). See text for abbreviations. (Adapted from Ref. 247.)

volumes delayed critical mechanical limitation of ventilation, with corresponding improvements in dyspnea and exercise endurance (177). In normoxic COPD patients, improvements in operating lung volumes and endurance time increase in a dose-dependent manner with the fractional concentration of oxygen (FI_{O_2}) until reaching a plateau at the 50% level ($FI_{O_2} = 0.5$) (184).

Ambulatory oxygen may serve as a useful adjunct to exercise reconditioning, promoting increased mobility and activity levels in symptomatic COPD patients. Ambulatory oxygen therapy may be used as an adjunct to formal exercise training, allowing patients to achieve and sustain higher training levels, and theoretically helping them to achieve greater physiological training effects.

There is no consensus on what level of arterial oxygen desaturation should warrant consideration for ambulatory oxygen in patients who are not hypoxemic at rest. Reimbursement criteria for ambulatory oxygen from various government agencies and insurance companies vary greatly, and general recommendations cannot be made at this time in the absence of evidence for long-term beneficial effects. One approach suggested by the ATS is that ambulatory oxygen should be recommended for patients whose resting arterial oxygen is less than 55 mmHg or between 55 and 60 mmHg with significant desaturation during activity (174). Currently, there is no agreement as to what constitutes significant arterial oxygen desaturation during exercise. Since a positive symptomatic response to oxygen therapy is unpredictable in a given patient, a single-blind, case-controlled study should be conducted to identify responders. We employ a treadmill constant-load endurance test at approximately 70% of the patients predetermined maximum work rate or $\dot{V}_{O_2}$, the patient is randomized to room air or oxygen, and endurance times and Borg ratings of dyspnea are recorded. The added oxygen should be sufficient to maintain oxygen saturations greater than 90% during exercise. We recommend ambulatory oxygen for those patients whose endurance times on oxygen are prolonged by greater than 25% of the control value or whose Borg ratings are diminished by greater than one unit at a standardized exercise time (highest equivalent work rate) (52,177). Alternative protocols involve stair climbing or walking (including 6 MWD) with a reliable pulse oximeter, with measurement of endurance time and dyspnea at the end of exercise.

Further studies are required to examine the long-term effects of oxygen (continuous or ambulatory) on chronic activity related dyspnea, functional status, and quality of life. Studies are under way to assess the value of adjunct ambulatory oxygen therapy during exercise training in COPD. Given the cost of long-term ambulatory oxygen, evidence-based criteria need to be developed for patient selection, oxygen prescription, and optimal mode of delivery.

For patients with COPD in the terminal phases of their illness, who are dyspneic at rest, oxygen therapy may provide some relief regardless of their level of resting hypoxemia (185,186). Therefore a trial of oxygen is justified in these patients for palliative purposes and treatment should be offered to those who are shown to derive benefit.

VI. Case Summary

To illustrate the effectiveness of a combined-modality approach in the management of a patient with severe COPD, changes in resting and exercise physiological data are provided in response to treatment with bronchodilators, ambulatory oxygen, and exercise training. It is clear that a myriad of small changes of physiological parameters (that are not normally measured) culminate in clinically meaningful improvements in the patient's symptoms and exercise capacity (Fig. 10) (Table 7).

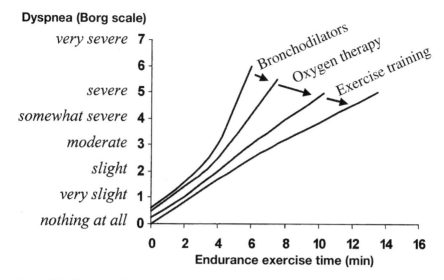

Figure 10   Sequential plots of dyspnea intensity (Borg scale ratings) over time during constant-load submaximal cycle exercise testing in a breathless patient with advanced COPD. Note the cumulative effects of various interventions on dyspnea and exercise endurance. (From Ref. 248.)

Table 7   Management of Dyspnea in COPD: Postintervention Changes (Δ) from Baseline

Transition Dyspnea Index	~3
$\Delta FEV_{1.0}$	↑ 6% predicted
ΔFRC	↓ 400 mL
$\Delta EELV_{dyn}$ (standard exercise)	↓ 420 mL
ΔIRV_{dyn} (standard exercise)	↑ 350 mL
ΔVentilation (standard exercise)	↓ 5 L/min
ΔBreathing frequency (standard exercise)	↓ 6 breaths per minute
ΔMIP	↑ 30% (~22 cmH$_2$O)
ΔMEP	↑ 25% (~23 cmH$_2$O)
ΔInspiratory muscle endurance	↑ ~3 ×
ΔQuadricep strength	↑ 25%
ΔQuadricep endurance	↑ 40%

VII. Adjunctive Therapies

A. Narcotic and Sedative Drugs
Opiates

Opiate therapy has been used for centuries in the treatment of respiratory distress. Over time, the knowledge that these drugs are powerful respiratory depressants has led to their more restricted use as dyspnea-relieving medications. A number of controlled, crossover, randomized studies have shown that oral opiates (morphine, dihydrocodeine, hydrocodone) in small numbers of patients with COPD have shown modest but significant acute improvements in exertional dyspnea and in exercise capacity compared with placebo (183–194). However, side effects during acute opiate administration are commonly reported and include drowsiness, hypercapnia, hypotension, confusion, and constipation (188–198).

The mechanisms of acute dyspnea alleviation during opiate therapy in COPD are multifactorial. Opiates have been shown to depress respiratory drive, both at rest and during exercise. Reductions in submaximal exercise ventilation and hypercapnia have been reported in a number of acute studies (187,188). As is the case during oxygen therapy, reduced ventilation or a reduced rate of rise of submaximal ventilation may result in improved dynamic mechanics in flow-limited patients and a delay of the point of ventilatory limitation, with attendant improvement in dyspnea and exercise capacity. Additionally, reduced central motor command output may, of itself, modulate dyspnea independent of the changes in mechanics and inspiratory muscle function that may accompany reduced ventilation. The study of Light et al. (187) demonstrated that relief of dyspnea at a standardized submaximal exercise work rate was related to reduced ventilation. However, these authors also noted that dyspnea ratings were diminished at any given submaximal ventilation. This latter observation suggests that other factors are instrumental in dyspnea relief, such as altered central processing of neural signals that would otherwise mediate dyspnea. These mechanisms have been postulated to explain opiate-induced increases in breath-holding time (199) and increased tolerance to hypoxia and hypercapnia (189). Additionally, opiates may alter mood, cause euphoria, or address the affective dimension of breathlessness in some individuals, thus allaying anxiety and respiratory panic.

Despite the favorable results of acute opiate administration in the laboratory setting (187,194), the results of studies examining the long-term effects of opiate therapy have yielded inconsistent results (192). Woodcock et al. (195) demonstrated that higher-dose hydrocodeine (30 mg three times daily) provided symptom alleviation but resulted in intolerable side effects, whereas lower dosages (15 mg three times a day), provided significant dyspnea relief and improved exercise tolerance, with minimal side effects (196). In the study of Rice et al. (200), COPD patients were randomized to codeine (30 mg four times a day) or promethazine (25 mg four times a day) for a 1-month period and showed no improvement in either dyspnea or exercise tolerance, while significant side effects developed in some patients. Small but significant increases in Pa_{CO_2} in the group as a whole were noted during codeine administration. Eiser and coworkers (197) conducted a placebo-controlled study of oral diamorphine (2.5 or 5 mg for 2 weeks each) in 8 patients with severe COPD and noted no improvement in dyspnea or exercise intolerance but also no increased drowsiness or hypercapnia.

Opiates delivered by nebulizers have not been shown to be superior to any mode of opiate delivery in symptomatic COPD patients. Earlier theories that topical opiates may exert their dyspnea-relieving effects via pulmonary opiate receptors have not been substantiated (193,201,202). The efficacy of inhaled opiates appears to depend on the degree to which the drug is absorbed into the bloodstream and the consequent reduction in central ventilatory drive (202).

While the role of long-term opiates in advanced symptomatic COPD remains controversial, it is generally accepted that these drugs are very useful as a palliative measure for some patients in the terminal phases of their illness (203–206). Dosages must be carefully individualized to obtain maximum symptomatic benefit while minimizing adverse effects to the patient. From a perusal of the available literature, the routine use of opiates cannot be recommended for symptomatic COPD patients, given the propensity of these drugs to cause serious side effects. Further studies are required to develop more precise guidelines for their use. Studies are also required to determine if the earlier introduction of lower dosages of opiates in a subpopulation of severely dyspneic COPD patients can diminish the respiratory depressant effects of the drugs that occur when higher dosages are administered acutely to patients with ventilatory compromise. Tolerance to the respiratory depressant effects have been reported in patients in whom long-term low-dose opiates are prescribed primarily for pain relief (207); it is not known whether similar tolerance could develop in COPD patients when opiates are prescribed for dyspnea relief.

B. Anxiolytics

Anxiolytics have the potential to relieve dyspnea by depressing respiratory drive in response to hypoxemia or hypercapnia or by altering the affective response to perceived respiratory discomfort. Despite the earlier demonstration of a beneficial effect of diazepam in a small, single-blinded study in "pink and puffing" COPD patients (208), several subsequent controlled studies have failed to show consistent improvements in dyspnea and exercise tolerance over placebo (205,206). Moreover, these drugs were often poorly tolerated and caused excessive drowsiness. Studies using diazepam, alprazolam, and promethazine in symptomatic COPD patients did not demonstrate improvements in dyspnea or exercise capacity, at least when examining group responses. However, negative group responses obscured impressive improvements in some individuals (192,199,208–210). Buspirone, a newer anxiolytic agent, has been tested in dyspneic COPD patients on the basis of this drug's theoretical advantage of not causing respiratory depression. In a randomized controlled study by Singh et al. (211), 6-week therapy with buspirone (10 to 20 mg PO), in 11 COPD patients with mild to moderate anxiety did not result in significant improvements over placebo in dyspnea, exercise tolerance, or anxiety scores. By contrast, Argyrapoulous et al. (212) showed significant improvements in mood, dyspnea, and exercise endurance using buspirone (20 mg daily) in patients with moderately severe COPD. In this study, the drug was well tolerated and there was no depression in respiratory drive or deterioration in arterial blood gases.

The limitations of the available studies on sedatives and anxiolytics include small sample sizes and uncertainty as to whether study subjects actually suffered from morbid anxiety in addition to dyspnea. There is currently insufficient evidence to recommend the routine use of anxiolytics in breathless COPD patients. However, a trial of anxiolytic therapy is reasonable on an individual basis in dyspneic patients, particularly those with severe anxiety or frequent respiratory panic attacks. Pharmacological treatment should ideally be provided in conjunction with psychological counseling and instruction in relaxation techniques. Simple measures such as avoidance of excessive beta$_2$-agonist medication, instruction in breathing relaxation techniques, and short-acting anxiolytics such as lorazepam may successfully abort spiraling respiratory panic attacks in those predisposed to them.

C. Lung Volume Reduction Surgery

Bullectomy has been advocated for many years for patients with COPD who have disabling breathlessness and localized bullous disease (213). There is evidence that this procedure can provide impressive and often sustained symptomatic relief in selected patients with giant, well-demarcated bullae (greater than one-third of the hemithorax) that are judged to be compressing or collapsing more normally functioning adjacent lung tissue (212–219). Patients with smaller bullae and more diffuse background emphysema are less likely to attain significant long-term benefits (289–293). The overall success rate of bullectomy in a given individual is dictated by the balance between the functional gains achieved by surgery and the rate of decline of pulmonary function with time. Although bullectomy has been performed for more than 50 years, the mechanisms of symptom benefit have only recently been systematically explored. The objective outcome measure of interest in previous studies has traditionally been the $FEV_{1.0}$, which may only indirectly reflect alterations in the ventilatory mechanics relevant for dyspnea relief; parameters such as reduced thoracic gas volume are likely more important (218).

Another type of surgical procedure for volume reduction was proposed by Brantigan in the late 1950s and has recently been reevaluated by Cooper and others (219,100), who have brought significant technical advancements to the original procedure. Volume reduction surgery (VRS) for patients with severe thoracic hyperinflation is currently being investigated in large, randomized controlled trials. The original concept behind Brantigan's procedure was that the removal of peripheral, nonfunctioning, space-occupying emphysematous lung tissue should enhance static recoil of the surgically reduced lung (219). This should result in an associated increase in radial tethering of hitherto collapsed airways in expiration and should promote lung emptying. Brantigan did not emphasize the additional potential benefits of this surgery with respect to ventilatory mechanics and inspiratory muscle function (219).

There are many parallels between the mechanical effects of giant bullectomy and modern volume reduction procedures with respect to the potential underlying mechanisms of their common benefits in patients with advanced COPD (i.e., reduced dyspnea and improved exercise tolerance). Both procedures result in reduction of plethysmographically determined thoracic gas volumes with reduced end-expiratory volume of the lung and chest wall (213,215,220,221). In both procedures, total lung capacity and residual volume have been shown to contract (213,215,220,221). Both procedures lead to volume recruitment (to a variable degree) of previously compressed or collapsed lung (283).

Dynamic expiratory flow rates have been shown to increase with both procedures, likely as a result of a combination of volume recruitment (i.e., increased VC) and enhanced static recoil of the lung in expiration (222,233). Following removal of space-occupying destroyed alveolar units, transpulmonary pressures can more effectively expand the adjacent, presumably more normally compliant alveolar units. VC recruitment after VRS usually occurs in association with reduced residual volume, due to more effective lung emptying on expiration. The shift of the static recoil curve downward and to the right has been demonstrated with both procedures (223–225). Part of the improvement in dynamic flow rates undoubtedly relates to this mechanism; however, it must be remembered that the effects of enhanced recoil would be expected to be less marked in patients in whom irreversible intrinsic airways disease contributes importantly to baseline (preoperative) flow limitation. Following removal of noncommunicating bullae or peripheral alveolar units, $FEV_{1.0}/FVC$ ratios show little change (i.e., $FEV_{1.0}$ increase commensurate with FVC) (225,226). The effects of both procedures on expiratory flow limitation are variable, and significant flow limitation may still be present after surgery, albeit at lower operational lung volumes (226).

Bullectomy has been shown to improve inspiratory muscle function (227,228). In one study, MIPs measured at FRC increased significantly by 40% ($p < 0.01$) 3 months postsurgery in 8 patients with severe COPD and unilateral bullectomy (226). The MIPs improve in the short term, presumably because of enhanced length-tension relationships of the diaphragm and other inspiratory muscles. Volume reduction surgery also has been shown to improve geometric configuration of the diaphragm (reduced radius of curvature), to reduce elastic loading, and to enhance ventilatory muscle coordination.

Improvements in arterial oxygenation are also common to both procedures, likely a result of enhanced $\dot{V}/\dot{Q}$ relationships in the newly recruited and previously compressed alveolar units (215,220,221). As expected, a reduction in the resting physiological dead-space ratio is rarely seen following bullectomy, as the majority of bullae are believed to be noncommunicating (215). Similarly, physiological dead space would not be expected to change after VRS, since the peripheral emphysematous tissue targeted for resection is believed to be largely redundant and nonfunctioning. However, relative dead space may be reduced because of increased tidal volume.

Effects of Volume Reduction Surgery on Exertional Dyspnea

Both bullectomy and VRS have been shown to reduce activity-related dyspnea and improve exercise endurance. Following unilateral bullectomy and VRS in 8 patients with advanced COPD, 99% of the variance in improved Borg ratings was explained by a combination of reduced end-expiratory lung volume, reduced breathing frequency, and increased VC (226). The mechanisms of dyspnea relief following VRS have been investigated in two recent studies. Martinez et al. (40) showed that reduced Borg ratings of exertional dyspnea following VRS correlated well with reduced EELV and reduced autoPEEP. Thus, VRS reduces the threshold and elastic loads on the inspiratory muscles. Laghi et al. (41) found a close association between improved exertional dyspnea and exercise endurance as well as enhanced neuromechanical coupling of the diaphragm as a result of reduced lung volumes following volume reduction surgery.

Other beneficial effects of VRS that could contribute to alleviation of dyspnea include (1) reduced mechanical constraints on tidal volume expansion and reduced breathing frequency for a given ventilation, (2) increased efficiency of CO_2 elimination because of reduced relative physiological dead space, (3) improved $\dot{V}/\dot{Q}$ relations and increased arterial oxygen saturation, (4) reduced ventilatory demand in some patients, and (5) favorable hemodynamic effects (218). The net effect of VRS is to improve the relationship between inspiratory muscle effort, which diminishes relative to maximum, and the tidal volume response to exercise. Therefore, as is the case with bullectomy, less effort is required for a given tidal volume after VRS (228,229).

VRS and exercise training likely have important synergistic effects; improved mechanics, reduced ventilatory demand, and improved peripheral and ventilatory muscle function all combine to achieve greater symptom control and activity levels. In most centers offering VRS, the procedure is bracketed by supervised exercise retraining programs (100). VRS, therefore, would appear to have a sound physiological rationale and should be considered as an option for greatly debilitated patients who remain severely breathless despite optimal pharmacotherapy, oxygen therapy, and pulmonary rehabilitation. While early results are promising, it would appear that only a minority of selected patients with localized heterogeneous emphysema who do not have any comorbid conditions are suitable (222). Because of an unacceptable mortality risk, VRS is contraindicated in patients with homogeneous emphysema who have a DL_{CO} of less than 25% predicted (228). It must be remembered that the magnitude of symptom alleviation achieved with this costly surgery, which carries a significant morbidity, is in some instances comparable to that achieved by supervised exercise training. A great deal of additional information is required to determine the ultimate role of VRS as a dyspnea-relieving procedure in patients with disabling COPD. In particular, controlled studies must determine whether the beneficial effects seen in acute studies are sustained in the long term.

VIII. Management of Acute Exacerbation of COPD

There is no current consensus with respect to the definition of acute exacerbation of COPD (AECOPD). In 1999, the Aspen Lung Conference attempted to formulate a working definition of AECOPD as "a sustained worsening of the patients' condition from the stable state, and beyond day-to-day variations, necessitating a change in regular medications in patients with underlying COPD" (229). Dyspnea is usually the most prominent symptom of exacerbations. Acute COPD exacerbations that require hospitalization carry a 10% mortality (230–233). Mortality rates are even higher (40–59%) in older patients with comorbid illnesses (233). Exacerbations result from tracheobronchial infections and air pollution, in variable combinations. Viral infections with the rhinovirus and influenza A and B are now believed to be more common in causing AECOPD than previously thought. Health-related quality of life has been shown to be negatively influenced by AECOPD (234,235). Symptoms of severe dyspnea and exercise intolerance may persist for months following AECOPD, with little change in the $FEV_{1.0}$ (234,235). AECOPD can quickly neutralize the subjective and objective benefits of exercise training programs in advanced COPD. Several recent studies have shown that therapeutic interventions such as inhaled steroids, ipratropium, salmeterol, and tiotropium can reduce the frequency and/or severity of AECOPD (98,99,113,114,236). The effects likely reflect the more sustained and effective symptom control with these agents, leading to diagnostic "downgrading" of AECOPD to common colds or upper respiratory tract infections.

The pathophysiology of AECOPD is complex. Small airway dysfunction and increased expiratory flow limitation in the setting of increased ventilatory demand (secondary to $\dot{V}/\dot{Q}$ inequalities or fever), causes severe dynamic lung hyperinflation (DH) (Fig. 11). The attendant reduced exercise capacity results in rapid deconditioning and skeletal muscle weakness, which may be aggravated by high-dose oral steroids and possibly by the release of systemic inflammatory mediators. Management should be directed toward suppressing inflammation, treating bacterial infection if present, improving small airway

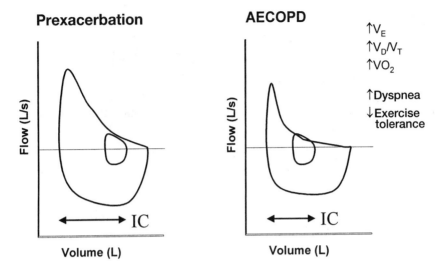

Figure 11 An example showing the impact of acute exacerbations of COPD (AECOPD) on lung function. Expiratory airflow limitation (EFL) is increased and the tidal flow-volume loop shifts toward TLC, indicating a reduced inspiratory capacity (IC) and dynamic lung hyperinflation (DH). The combination of increased ventilatory demand and EFL amplifies DH. $\dot{V}_E$ = ventilation; V_D/V_T = physiological dead space; $\dot{V}_{O_2}$ = oxygen uptake.

function, reducing lung hyperinflation, and active mobilization (low-level exercise training) to avoid rapid deconditioning.

The management of AECOPD in patients presenting to the physician's office is briefly outlined below. Management of AECOPD requiring hospitalization is comprehensively reviewed elsewhere.

Bronchodilators

The principal goal of management is the optimization of pulmonary function. Bronchodilators play a key role in this regard. A combination of short-acting inhaled beta$_2$ agonists (salbutamol) and anticholinergics (ipratroprium) is recommended; although, strictly speaking, this has not been demonstrated to be superior to either agent alone in the setting of COPD *exacerbations* (237). These inhaled medications may be administered by metered-dose inhaler (MDI, with spacer) or nebulizer. Despite evidence suggesting that MDI is equal to a nebulizer (238) or possibly even superior to one (239), many clinicians will opt for the latter during severe exacerbations, recognizing that patients with severe exacerbations may not be sufficiently cooperative to use the MDI. There is no evidence suggesting that long-acting beta$_2$ agonists improve pulmonary function above that provided by regular dosing with short-acting medications in the setting of COPD exacerbation. In the rare situation where inhaled bronchodilators are not available, intravenous beta$_2$ agonists may be used, although studies involving exacerbations of *asthma* have failed to demonstrate any benefit with the addition of intravenous beta$_2$ agonists to regular dosing with inhaled bronchodilators (240). Previously, methylxanthines (theophylline) were routinely used in the treatment of exacerbations. However, two randomized clinical trials (RCTs) specifically examining the effect of methylxanthines on COPD exacerbations failed to demonstrate any additive benefit above standard inhaled bronchodilator therapy (241,242,244).

Steroids

Steroids are frequently used during exacerbations of COPD. Prior to 1999, the evidence supporting this practice was very limited. A double-blind, RCT by Albert et al., involving 44 patients, suggested an improvement in $FEV_{1.0}$ compared to placebo 24 hr after the initiation of therapy (243). However the clinical significance of this finding is unknown. Other studies had failed to demonstrate that steroids consistently reduce hospitalization, intubation, or mortality.

Two RCTs on this topic were published during the summer of 1999. The larger of the two (in fact, the largest RCT up to date on this subject) was the Veterans Affairs Cooperative Study (SCCOPE) (244). This trial included 271 patients with COPD exacerbations randomized to one of three arms: placebo, 2 weeks of systemic steroids, and 8 weeks of steroids. Despite no difference in mortality and intubation rates, the authors reported a significant reduction in "treatment failures." The clinical relevance of this finding is questionable when one considers that commencement of steroids by the treating physician outside of study protocol was included in the definition of "treatment failure." The only clear clinical benefit was a marginally shorter duration of hospitalization (9.7 versus 8.5 days, $p=0.03$) in patients treated with steroids.

The smaller RCT (56 patients) by Davies et al. (245) was able to demonstrate a 60-mL improvement in $FEV_{1.0}$ at 5 days using only 30 mg prednisolone for 14 days. As in the SCCOPE trial, this was associated with a modestly shorter hospitalization (7 versus 9 days, $p=0.027$).

Despite the very modest benefit demonstrated, the latest GOLD guidelines as well as many clinicians recommend the use of systemic steroids during COPD exacerbations. What remains to be determined is the optimal dose and duration of therapy. The SCCOPE trial used the largest dose of steroids to date (125 mg solumedrol q6h for 3 days, followed by a tapering dose of prednisone), while the Davies trial demonstrated a similar reduction in hospitalization using a much smaller dose. Finally, clinicians who decide to prescribe steroids must be mindful that the *long-term* side effects of corticosteroid therapy, particularly with regard to bone mineral density and peripheral muscle function, remain unquantified.

Antibiotics

The use of antibiotics in AECOPD remains controversial. They are more likely to be useful in patients with increasing symptoms and increased volume or purulence of sputum. Many clinicians also include antibiotics in the treatment of COPD exacerbations. The major trial supporting this practice was published by Anthonisen et al. (246). Anthonisen demonstrated that a 10-day course of antibiotics was of benefit in *outpatient* exacerbations characterized by at least two of the following three findings: increased dyspnea, sputum volume and sputum purulence. The actual magnitude of benefit from antibiotics is uncertain because "dangerously ill" patients were excluded. Furthermore, the major outcome of "treatment success" was defined as absence of symptoms by 21 days—hospitalization or death was not specifically examined.

The optimal choice of antibiotics is unknown. Patients treated in the Anthonisen trial were prescribed TMP-SMX, doxycycline, or amoxicillin at the discretion of the treating physician. Since that time, antibiotic resistance patterns have changed, and both second-generation macrolides (azithromycin) and "respiratory" fluroquinolones (levofloxacin, moxifloxacillin, gatifloxacillin) have become available. These agents offer potentially broader antimicrobial coverage (e.g., against *Mycoplasma*), but it should be emphasized that they have *not* been demonstrated to be *superior* to older antibiotics. Thus, treatment of COPD exacerbations with older antibiotics remains reasonable.

IX. Summary

COPD represents a complex group of disorders that show great pathophysiological and clinical diversity. Given this diversity, rigorous assessment of the individual patient's impairment, disability, and handicap is required to optimize management strategies. A comprehensive management plan is needed to achieve maximal therapeutic impact in the symptomatic COPD patients. Education is a pivotal component. Bronchodilator therapy will maximize volume reduction and improve dyspnea and exercise endurance. Agents such as tiotropium and long-acting beta$_2$ agonists, which provide sustained 24-hr bronchodilatation and volume reduction, represent a definite advance in therapy. Short-acting bronchodilators can be added to long-acting agents to enhance symptom control, but dosages must be individualized. The role of inhaled steroids in the management of advanced COPD is not established. Preliminary information suggests that these agents may be beneficial in alleviating dyspnea and in improving health status in COPD, but the results of ongoing trials are awaited to provide a definitive answer.

Supervised exercise training is the next step in the management of COPD patients and has been shown to significantly increase activity levels and to improve dyspnea and the overall health status of patients. To maintain these benefits, careful follow-up and patients' adherence to a home-based training schedule is imperative. For selected individuals, other interventions—such as ambulatory oxygen therapy, anxiolytics or opiates, and lung volume reduction surgery—may be indicated. Prompt detection and aggressive management of exacerbations of COPD are crucial in order to avoid prolonged morbidity, and even mortality.

An individualized, comprehensive approach to management that incorporates combined pharmacological therapies and exercise training can maximize symptom control, exercise capabilities, and health status, even in patients with advanced disease.

References

1. Mannino DM, Brown C, Giovino GA. Obstructive lung disease deaths in the United States from 1979 through 1993. An analysis using multiple-cause mortality data. Am J Respir Crit Care Med 1997; 156:814–818.
2. Thom TJ. International comparisons in COPD mortality. Am Rev Respir Dis 1989; 140:S27–S34.
3. Feinleib M, Rosenberg HM, Collins JG, Delozier JE, Pokras R, Chevarley FM. Trends in COPD morbidity and mortality in the United States. Am Rev Respir Dis 1989; 140:S9–S18.
4. Chen JC, Mannino MD. Worldwide epidemiology of chronic obstructive pulmonary disease. Curr Opin Pulm Med 1999; 5:93–99.
5. Pauwels RA, Buist AS, Calverley PMA, Jenkins CR, Hurd SS. On behalf of the GOLD Scientific Committee. Global strategy for the diagnosis, management and prevention of chronic obstructive pulmonary disease: NHLBI/WHO Global initiative for chronic obstructive lung disease (GOLD) workshop summary. Am J Respir Crit Care Med 2001; 163:1256–1276.
6. O'Donnell DE, Revill S, Webb KA. Dynamic hyperinflation and exercise intolerance in COPD. Am J Respir Crit Care Med 2001; 164:770–777.
7. Pride NB, Macklem PT. Lung mechanics in disease. In: Fishman AP, ed. Handbook of Physiology, Sec 3, Vol III, Part 2: The Respiratory System. Bethesda, MD: American Physiological Society, 1986:659–692.
8. Younes M. Determinants of thoracic excursions during exercise. In: Whipp BJ, Wasserman K, eds. Lung Biology in Health and Disease. Vol 42: Exercise, Pulmonary Physiology and Pathophysiology. New York: Marcel Dekker, 1991:1–65.
9. Stubbing DG, Pengelly LD, Morse JLC, Jones NL. Pulmonary mechanics during exercise in subjects with chronic airflow obstruction. J Appl Physiol 1980; 49:511–515.
10. O'Donnell DE, Lam M, Webb KA. Measurement of symptoms, lung hyperinflation and endurance during exercise in chronic obstructive pulmonary disease. Am J Respir Crit Care Med 1998; 158:1557–1565.
11. Marin JM, Carrizo SJ, Gascon M, Sanchez A, Gallego BA, Celli BR. Inspiratory capacity, dynamic hyperinflation, breathlessness and exercise performance during the 6-minute-walk test in chronic obstructive pulmonary disease. Am J Respir Crit Care Med 2001; 163:1395–1399.
12. O'Donnell DE, Webb KA. Breathlessness in patients with severe chronic airflow limitation: physiologic correlates. Chest 1992; 102:824–831.

13. Sinderby C, Spahija J, Beck J, Kaminski D, Yan S, Comtois N, Sliwinski P. Diaphragm activation during exercise in chronic obstructive pulmonary disease. Am J Respir Crit Care Med 2001; 163:1637–1641.
14. Tantucci C, Duguet A, Similowski T, Zelter M, Derenne JP, Milic-Emili J. Effect of salbutamol on dynamic hyperinflation in chronic obstructive pulmonary disease patients. Eur Respir J 1998; 12:799–804.
15. Eltayara L, Becklake MR, Volta CA, Milic-Emili J. Relationship between chronic dyspnea and expiratory flow limitation in patients with chronic obstructive pulmonary disease. Am J Respir Crit Care Med 1996; 154:1726–1734.
16. Diaz O, Villafranco C, Ghezzo H, Borzone G, Leiva A, Milic-Emili J, Lisboa C. Exercise tolerance in COPD patients with and without tidal expiratory flow limitation at rest. Eur Respir J 2000; 16:269–275.
17. O'Donnell DE, Chau LKL, Bertley JC, Webb KA. Qualitative aspects of exertional breathlessness in chronic airflow limitation: pathophysiologic mechanisms. Am J Respir Crit Care Med 1997; 155:109–115.
18. O'Donnell DE, Webb KA. Exertional breathlessness in patients with chronic airflow limitation: the role of hyperinflation. Am Rev Respir Dis 1993; 148:1351–1357.
19. Meek PM, Schwartzstein RMS, Adams L, Altose MD, Breslin EH, Carrieri-Kohlman V, Gift A, Hanley MV, Harver A, Jones PW, Killian K, Knobel A, Lareau S, Mahler DA, O'Donnell DE, Steele B, Stuhlbarg M, Title M. Dyspnea mechanism, assessment and management: a consensus statement (American Thoracic Society). Am J Respir Crit Care Med 1999; 159:321–340.
20. O'Donnell DE. Exertional breathlessness in chronic respiratory disease. In: Mahler DA, ed. Lung Biology in Health and Disease. Vol III: Dyspnea. New York: Marcel Dekker, 1998:97–147.
21. Killian KJ, Campbell EJM. Dyspnea. In: Roussos C, Macklem PT, eds. Lung Biology in Health and Disease. Vol 29 (Part B): The Thorax. New York: Marcel Dekker, 1985:787–828.
22. Altose M, Cherniack N, Fishman AP. Respiratory sensations and dyspnea: perspectives. J Appl Physiol 1985; 58:1051–1054.
23. Chen Z, Eldridge FL, Wagner PG. Respiratory associated rhythmic firing of midbrain neurones in cats: relation to level of respiratory drive. J Appl Physiol 1991; 437:305–325.
24. Chen Z, Eldridge FL, Wagner PG. Respiratory-associated thalamic activity is related to level of respiratory drive. Respir Physiol 1992; 90:99–113.
25. Davenport PW, Friedman WA, Thompson FJ, Franzen O. Respiratory-related cortical potentials evoked by inspiratory occlusion in humans. J Appl Physiol 1986; 60:1843–1948.
26. Gandevia SC, Macefield G. Projection of low threshold afferents from human intercostal muscles to the cerebral cortex. Respir Physiol 1989; 77:203–214.
27. Homma I, Kanamara A, Sibuya M. Proprioceptive chest wall afferents and the effect on respiratory sensation. In: Von Euler C, Katz-Salamon M, eds. Respiratory Psychophysiology. New York: Stockton Press, 1988:161–166.
28. Banzett RB, Lansing RW, Reid MB, Adams L, Brown R. "Air hunger" arising from increased P_{CO_2} in mechanically ventilated quadriplegics. Respir Physiol 1989; 76:53–68.
29. Altose MD, Syed I, Shoos L. Effects of chest wall vibration on the intensity of dyspnea during constrained breathing. Proc Int Union Physiol Sci 1989; 17:288.

30. Matthews PBC. Where does Sherrington's "muscular sense" originate: muscles, joints, corollary discharge? Annu Rev Neurosci 1982; 5:189–218.
31. Roland PE, Ladegaard-Pederson, HA. A quantitative analysis of sensation of tension and kinaesthesia in man. Evidence for peripherally originating muscular sense and a sense of effort. Brain 1977; 100:671–692.
32. Noble MIM, Eisele JH, Trenchard D, Guz A. Effect of selective peripheral nerve blocks on respiratory sensations. In: Porter R, ed. Breathing: Hering-Breyer Symposium. London: Churchill, 1970:233–246.
33. Zechman FR Jr, Wiley RL. Afferent inputs to breathing: respiratory sensation. In: Fishman AP, ed. Handbook of Physiology. Sec 3, Vol II, Part 2: The Respiratory System. Bethesda MD: American Physiological Society, 1986:449–474.
34. Banzett RB, Dempsey JA, O'Donnell DE, Wamboldt MZ. Symptom perception and respiratory sensation in asthma. Am J Respir Crit Care Med 2000; 162:1178–1182.
35. Kukorelli T, Namenyi J, Adam G. Visceral afferent projection areas in the cortex representation of the carotid sinus receptor area. Acta Physiol Acad Sci 1969; 36:261–263.
36. O'Donnell DE, Sanii R, Younes M. Improvements in exercise endurance in patients with chronic airflow limitation using CPAP. Am Rev Respir Dis 1988; 138:1510–1514.
37. Belman MJ, Botnick WC, Shin JW. Inhaled bronchodilators reduce dynamic hyperinflation during exercise in patients with chronic obstructive pulmonary disease. Am J Respir Crit Care Med 1996; 153:967–975.
38. Chrystyn H, Mulley BA, Peake MD. Dose response relation to oral theophylline in severe chronic obstructive airways disease. Br Med 1988; 297:1506–1510.
39. O'Donnell DE, Lam M, Webb KA. Spirometric correlates of improvement in exercise performance after anticholinergic therapy in COPD. Am J Respir Crit Care Med 1999; 160:542–549.
40. Martinez FJ, Montes de Oca M, Whyte RI, Stetz J, Gay SE, Celli BR. Lung-volume reduction improves dyspnea, dynamic hyperinflation and respiratory muscle function. Am J Respir Crit Care Med 1997; 155:1984–1990.
41. Laghi F, Jurban A, Topeli A, Fahey PH, Garrity F Jr, Archids JM, DePinto DJ, Edwards LC, Tobin MJ. Effect of lung volume reduction surgery on neuromechanical coupling of the diaphgram. Am J Respir Crit Care Med 1998; 157:475–483.
42. O'Donnell DE, Bertley J, Webb KA, Conlan AA. Mechanisms of relief of exertional breathlessness following unilateral bullectomy and lung volume reduction surgery in advanced chronic airflow limitation. Chest 1996; 110:18–27.
43. Petrof BJ, Calderini E, Gottfried SB. Effect of CPAP on respiratory effort and dyspnea during exercise in severe COPD. J Appl Physiol 1990; 69:178–188.
44. Barbara JA, Roca J, Ramirez J, Wagner PD, Usetti P, Rodriquez-Roisin R. Gas exchange during exercise in mild chronic obstructive pulmonary disease. Am Rev Respir Dis 1991; 144:520–525.
45. Dantzker DR, D'Alonzo GE. The effect of exercise on pulmonary gas exchange in patients with severe chronic obstructive pulmonary disease. Am Rev Respir Dis 1986; 134:1135–1139.
46. Dillard TA, Piantadosi S, Rajagopal KR. Prediction of ventilation at maximal exercise in chronic airflow obstruction. Am Rev Respir Dis 1985; 132:230–235.

47. O'Donnell DE, McGuire M, Samis L, Webb KA. Effects of general exercise training on ventilatory and peripheral muscle strength and endurance in chronic airflow limitation. Am J Respir Crit Care Med 1998; 157:1489–1497.

48. Begin P, Grassino A. Inspiratory muscle dysfunction and chronic hypercapnia in chronic obstructive pulmonary disease. Am Rev Respir Dis 1991; 143:905–912.

49. Burrows B, Earle RH. Course and prognosis of chronic obstructive lung disease: a prospective study of 200 patients. N Engl J Med 1969; 280:397–404.

50. O'Donnell DE, D'Arsigny C, Fitzpatrick M, Webb KA. Exercise hypercapnia in advanced chronic obstructive pulmonary disease. Am J Respir Crit Care Med 2002; 166:663–668.

51. O'Donnell DE, McGuire M, Samis L, Webb KA. The impact of exercise reconditioning on breathlessness in severe chronic airflow limitation. Am J Respir Crit Care Med 1995; 152:2005–2013.

52. O'Donnell DE, Bain DJ, Webb KA. Factors contributing to relief of exertional breathlessness during hyperoxia in chronic airflow limitation. Am J Respir Crit Care Med 1997; 155:530–535.

53. Light RW, Muro JR, Sato RI, Stansbury DW, Fischer CE, Brown SE. Effects of oral morphine on breathlessness and exercise tolerance in patients with chronic obstructive pulmonary disease. Am Rev Respir Dis 1989; 139:126–133.

54. Gosker HR, Wouters EF, Van der Vusse GJ, Schols AM. Skeletal muscle dysfunction in chronic obstructive pulmonary disease and chronic heart failure: underlying mechanisms and therapy perspectives. Am J Clin Nutr 2000; 71:1033–1047.

55. Casaburi R. Skeletal muscle dysfunction in chronic obstructive pulmonary disease. Med Sci Sports Exerc 2001; 33(suppl 7):S662–S670.

56. Killian KJ, Leblanc P, Martin DH, Summers E, Jones NL, Campbell EJM. Exercise capacity and ventilatory, circulatory and symptom limitation in patients with chronic airflow limitation. Am Rev Respir Dis 1992; 146:935–940.

57. Bernard S, Leblanc P, Whittom F, Carrier G, Jobin J, Belleau R, Maltais F. Peripheral muscle weakness in patients with chronic obstructive pulmonary disease. Am J Respir Crit Care Med 1998; 158:629–634.

58. Wilson DO, Rogers RM, Wright EC, Anthonisen NR. Body weight in chronic obstructive pulmonary disease: the National Institutes of Health intermittent positive pressure breathing trial. Am Rev Respir Dis 1989; 139:1435–1438.

59. Gosselink R, Trooster T, Decramer M. Peripheral muscle weakness contributes to exercise limitation in COPD. Am J Respir Crit Care Med 1996; 153:976–980.

60. Whittom F, Jobin J, Simard PM, Leblanc P, Simard C, Bernard S, Belleau R, Maltais F. Histochemical and morphological characteristics of the vastus lateralis muscle in patients with chronic obstructive pulmonary disease. Med Sci Sports Exerc 1998; 30:1467–1474.

61. Jakobsson P, Jorfeldt L, Henriksson J. Metabolic enzyme activity in the quadriceps femoris muscle in patients with severe chronic obstructive pulmonary disease. Am J Respir Crit Care Med 1995; 151:374–377.

62. Jobin J, Maltais F, Doyon JF, Leblanc P, Simard PM, Simard AA, Simard C. Chronic obstructive pulmonary disease: capillarity and fiber-type characteristics of skeletal muscle. J Cardiopulm Rehab 1998; 18:432–437.

63. Casaburi R. Deconditioning. In: Fishman AP, ed. Lung Biology in Health and Disease: Pulmonary Rehabilitation. New York: Marcel Dekker, 1996:213–230.

64. Casaburi R. Exercise training in chronic obstructive lung disease. In: Casaburi R, Petty TL. eds. Principles and Practice of Pulmonary Rehabilitation. Philadelphia: Saunders, 1993:204–224.

65. Cooper CB. Determining the role of exercise in patients with chronic obstructive pulmonary disease. Med Sci Sports Exerc 1995; 27:147–157.

66. Casaburi R, Porszasz J, Burns MR, Carithers ER, Chang RS Y, Cooper CB. Physiologic benefits of exercise training in rehabilitation of patients with severe chronic obstructive pulmonary disease. Am J Respir Crit Care Med 1997; 115:1541–1551.

67. Wilson JR, Martin JL, Schwartz D, Ferraro N. Exercise intolerance in patients with chronic heart failure: role of impaired nutritive flow to skeletal muscle. Circulation 1984; 69:1079–1087.

68. Green HR. Myofibrillar composition and mechanical function in mammalian skeletal muscle. In: Shepard RJ, ed. Sports Science Reviews. Champaign, IL: Human Kinetic Publishers, 1992:43–64.

69. Semple PD, Bestall GH, Watson WS, Hume R. Hypothalamic-pituitary dysfunction in respiratory hypoxia. Thorax 1981; 36:605–609.

70. Semple PD, Bestall GH, Watson WS, Hume R. Serum testosterone depression associated with hypoxia in respiratory failure. Clin Sci 1989; 58:105–106.

71. Semple PD, Watson WS, Bestall GH, Bethel MIF, Grant JK, Hume R. Diet, absorption, and hormone studies in relation to body weight in obstructive airways disease. Thorax 1979; 34:783–788.

72. Takabatake N, Nakamura H, Mingmihaba O, Inage M, Inoue S, Kagaya S, Yamaki M, Tomoike H. A novel pathophysiologic phenomenon in cachexic patients with chronic obstructive pulmonary disease. Am J Respir Crit Car Med 2001; 163:1314–1319.

73. Heunks KMA, Vina J, Van Herwaarden CLA, Folgering MTM, Gimeno A, Dekhuizen PNR. Xanthine oxidase is involved in exercise-induced oxidative stress in chronic obstructive pulmonary disease. Am J Physiol 1999; 277:R1697–R1704.

74. Vina J, Severa E, Acensi M, Sastre J, Pallardo JS, Ferrero JS, Garcia-de-la-Asuncion J, Anton V, Marin J. Exercise causes blood glutathione oxidation in chronic obstructive pulmonary disease and prevention by O_2 therapy. J Appl Physiol 1996; 81(5):2198–2202.

75. Fletcher CM. The clinical diagnosis of pulmonary emphysema: an experimental study. Proc Res Soc Med 1952; 45:577–584.

76. Fletcher CM, Elmes PC, Wood CH. The significance of respiratory symptoms and the diagnosis of chronic bronchitis in a working population. Br Med 1959; 1:257–266.

77. Mahler DA, Guyatt GH, James PW. Clinical measurement of dyspnea. In: Mahler DA, ed. Lung Biology in Health and Disease. Vol III: Dyspnea. New York: Marcel Dekker, 1998:149–198.

78. Mahler D, Weinberg D, Wells C, Feinstein A. The measurement of dyspnea: contents, interobserver agreement and physiologic correlates of new new clinical ideas. Chest 1984; 85:751–758.

79. Mahler D, Rosiello R, Harver A, Lentine T, McGovern J, Daubenspeck J. Comparison of clinical dyspnea ratings and physiological measurements of respiratory sensation in obstructive pulmonary disease. Am Rev Respir Dis 1987; 135:1229–1233.

80. Mahler D, Harver A, Rosiello R, Daubenspeck J. Measurement of respiratory sensation in interstitial lung disease. Chest 1989; 96:767–771.
81. Stokes WA. A treatise on the diagnosis and treatment of diseases of the chest. Part 1: Diseases of the Lung and Windpipe. London: The New Sydenham Society 1837:168–169.
82. Stubbing D, Campbell EJM. The physical examination of the chest. Med Clin North Am 1982; 21:2041–2044.
83. O'Donnell DE. Assessment of bronchodilator efficacy in symptomatic COPD: is spirometry useful? Chest 2000; 117:42–47.
84. O'Donnell DE, Forkert L, Webb KA. Evaluation of bronchodilator response in patients with "irreversible" emphysema. Eur Respir J 2001; 18:914–920.
85. Borg GAV. Psychophysical basis of perceived exertion. Med Sci Sports 1982; 14:377–381.
86. Gift AG. Validation of a vertical visual analogue scale as a measure of clinical dyspnea. Rehab Nurs 1989; 14:313–325.
87. Johnson BD, Weisman IM, Zeballos RJ, Beck KC. Emerging concepts in the evaluation of ventilatory limitation during exercise: the exercise tidal flow-volume loop. Chest 1999; 116:488–503.
88. McGavin CR, Artvinli M, et al. Dyspnea, disability, and distance walked: comparison of estimates of exercise performance in respiratory disease. Br Med J 1978; 2:241–243.
89. Singh SJ, Morgan MDL. Development of a shuttle walking test of disability in patients with chronic airways obstruction. Thorax 1992; 47:1019–1024.
90. Frontera WR, Hughes VA, Dallal GE, Evans WJ. Reliability of isokinetic muscle strength testing in 45- to 78-year-old men and women. Arch Phys Med Rehabil 1993; 74:1181–1185.
91. Danneskiold-Samsoe B, Kofod V, Munter J, Grimby G, Schnohr P, Jensen G. Muscle strength and functional capacity in 78–81 year old men and women. Eur J Appl Physiol 1984; 52:310–314.
92. Aniansson A, Grimby G, Rundgren A. Isometric and isokinetic quadriceps muscle strength in 70-year-old men and women. Scand J Rehab Med 1989; 12:161–168.
93. Guyatt GH, Berman LB, Townsend M, Pugsley SO, Chambers LW. A measure of quality of life for clinical trials in chronic lung disease. Thorax 1987; 42:773–778.
94. Jones PW, Quirk JH, Baveystock CM. Littlejohn T. A self-complete measure of health status for chronic airflow limitation. Am Rev Respir Dis 1992; 145:1321–1327.
95. Lareau S, Carriere-Kohlman V, Janson-Bjerklie S, Roos PJ. Development and testing of the Pulmonary Functional Status and Dyspnea Questionnaire (PFSDQ). Heart Lung 1994; 23:242–250.
96. Weaver TE, Narsavage GL. Physiological and psychological variables related to functional status in COPD. Nurs Res 1992; 41:286–291.
97. Guyatt GH, Townsend M, Puglsey SO, Keller JL, Short HD, Taylor DW, Newhouse MT. Bronchodilators in chronic airflow limitation. Effects on airway function, exercise capacity and quality of life. Am Rev Respir Dis 1987; 135:1069–1074.
98. Jones PW, Bosh TK. Quality of life changes in COPD patients treated with salmeterol. Am J Respir Crit Care Med 1997; 155:1283–1289.

99. Mahler DA, Donohue JF, Barber RA, Goldman MD, Gross NJ, Wisniewski ME, Yancey SW, Zakes BA, Rickard KA, Anderson WH. Efficacy of salmeterol in the treatment of COPD. Chest 1999; 115:957–965.

100. Cooper JD, Trulock EP, Triantafillou AN, et al. Bilateral pneumectomy (volume reduction) for chronic obstructive pulmonary disease. J Thorac Cardiovasc Surg 1995; 109:106–119.

101. Tougaard L, Krone T, Sorknaes A, Ellegaard H. Economic benefits of teaching patients with chronic obstructive pulmonary disease about their illness. The PASTMA Group. Lancet 1992; 339:1517–1520.

102. Bourbeau J, Julien M, Rouleau M, Maltais F, Beaupre A, Begin R, Renzi P, Lacasse Y, Belleau R. Impact of an integrated rehabilitative self-management program on health status: A multicentre randomized control trial. Am J Respir Crit Care Med 2000; 163:A56, A254.

103. Ries AL, Kaplan RM, Limberg TM, Prewitt LM. Effects of pulmonary rehabilitation on physiologic and psychosocial outcomes in patients with chronic obstructive pulmonary disease. Ann Intern Med 1995; 122:823–832.

104. Spence DPS, Hay JG, Pearson MG, Calverley PMA. Oxygen desaturation and breathlessness during corridor walking in chronic obstructive lung disease. Effect of oxitropium bromide. Thorax 1993; 48:1145–1150.

105. Hay JG, Stone P, Carter J, Church S, Eyre-brook A, Pearson M, Woodcock A, Calverley P. Bronchodilator reversibility, exercise performance and breathlessness in stable chronic obstructive pulmonary disease. Eur Respir J 1992; 5:659–664.

106. Mahler DA, Mathay RA, Synder PE, Wells CK, Loke J. Sustained release theophylline reduces dyspnea in non-reversible obstructive airways disease. Am Rev Respir Dis 1985; 131:22–25.

107. Papiris S, Galavotti V, Sturani C. Effects of beta agonists on breathlessness and exercise tolerance in patients with chronic obstructive pulmonary disease. Respiration 1986; 49:101–108.

108. Vathenen AS, Britton JR, Ebden P, Cookson JB, Wharrad HJ, Tattersfield AE. High-dose inhaled albuterol in severe chronic airflow limitation. Am Rev Respir Dis 1988; 138:850–855.

109. Gross NJ, Petty TL, Friedman M, Skorodin MS, Silvers GW, Donohue JF. Dose response to ipratropium as a nebulized solution in patients with chronic obstructive pulmonary disease. A three-center study. Am Rev Respir Dis 1989; 139:1188–1191.

110. Easton PA, Jadue C, Dhingra S, Anthonisen NR. A comparison of the bronchodilating effects of a beta-2 adrenergic agent (albuterol) and an anticholinergic agent (ipratropium bromide), given by aerosol alone or in sequence. N Engl J Med 1986; 315:735–739.

111. Higgins BG, Powell RM, Cooper S, Tattersfield AE. Effect of salbutamol and ipratropium bromide on airway calibre and bronchial reactivity in asthma and chronic bronchitis. Eur Respir J 1991; 4:415–420.

112. Jenkins SC, Heaton RW, Fulton TJ, Moxham J. Comparison of domiciliary nebulized salbutamol and salbutamol from a metered-dose inhaler in stable chronic airflow limitation. Chest 1987; 91:804–807.

113. COMBIVENT Inhalation Aerosol Study Group. In chronic obstructive pulmonary disease, a combination of ipratropium and albuterol is more effective than either agent alone. An 85-day multicenter trial. Chest 1994; 105:1411–1419.

114. The COMBIVENT Inhalation Solution Study Group. Routine nebulized ipratropium and albuterol together are better than either alone in COPD. Chest 1997; 112:1514–1521.

115. Gross N, Tashkin D, Miller R, Oren J, Coleman W, Linberg S. Inhalation by nebulization of albuterol-ipratropium combination is superior to either agent alone in the treatment of chronic obstructive pulmonary disease. Dey Combination Solution Study Group. Respiration 1998; 65:354–362.

116. Dahl R, Geefhorst LAPM, Nowak D, Nonikov V, Byrne AM, Thomson M, Till D, Della G. CIOPPA. Inhaled formoterol dry powder versus ipratropium bromide in chronic obstructive pulmonary disease. Am J Resp Crit Care Med 2001; 164:778–784.

117. O'Donnell DE, Webb KA. Mechanisms of improved exercise performance in response to salmeterol therapy in COPD. Am J Respir Crit Care Med 2002; 165:A61.

118. Jones PW, Koch P, Menijoge SS, Witek TJ. The impact of COPD exacerbations on health related quality of life is attenuated by tiotropium. Am J Respir Crit Care Med 2001; 163:A771.

119. Casaburi R, Mahler DA, Jones PW, Wanner A, San Pedro G, ZuWallack RL, et al. A long term evaluation of once daily inhaled tiotropium in COPD. Eur Respir J 2002; 19(2):217–224.

120. Vincken W, Van Noord JA, Greefhoest APM, Bantage T, Kesten S, Korducki L, Cornellisen PJ. Improvement in health status in patients with COPD during 1 year treatment with tiotropium. Eur Respir J 2002; 19(2):209–216.

121. O'Donnell DE, Magnussen H, Aguilaniu B, Gerken F, Hamilton A, Fluge T. Spiriva (Tiotropium) improves exercise tolerance in COPD. Am J Respir Crit Care Med 2002; 165:A98.

122. O'Donnell DE, Magnussen H, Aguilaniu B, Make B, Fluege T, Hamilton A. Spiriva (Tiotropium) reduces exertional dyspnea in COPD. Am J Respir Crit Care Med 2002; 165:B27.

123. Mahler DA, Matthay RA, Snyder PE, Wells CK, Loke J. Sustained-release theophylline reduces dyspnea in nonreversible obstructive airway disease. Am Rev Respir Dis 1985; 131(1):22–25.

124. McKay SE, Howie CA, Thomson AH, Whiting B, Addis GJ. Value of theophylline treatment in patients handicapped by chronic obstructive lung disease. Thorax 1993; 48(3):227–232.

125. ZuWallack R, Mahler D, Riley J. Salmeterol plus theophylline combination therapy in the treatment of COPD. Chest 2001; 119:1661–1670.

126. Van Andel AE, Reisner C, Menjoge SS, Witek TJ. Analysis of inhaled corticosteroid and oral theophylline use among patients with stable COPD from 1987 to 1995. Chest 1999; 340:1941.

127. Confalonieri M, Mainardi E, Della Porta R, Bernorio S, et al. Inhaled cortiosteroids reduce neutrophillic bronchial inflammation in patients with chronic obstructive pulmonary disease. Thorax 1998; 53:583.

128. Culpitt SV, Maziak W, Loukidis S, Nightingale JA, et al. effect of high dose inhaled steroid on cells, cytokines, and proteases in induced sputum in chronic obstructive pulmonary disease. Am J Respir Crit Care Med 1999; 160:1635.

129. Keatings VM, Jatakanon A, Worsdell YM, Barnes PJ. Effects of inhaled and oral glucocorticoids on inflammatory indices in asthma and COPD. Am J Respir Crit Care Med 1997; 155:542.

130. Thompson AB, Mueller MB, Heires AJ, et al. Aerosolized beclomethasone in chronic bronchitis. Am Rev Respir Dis 1992; 146:389.

131. Harding SM, Freedman S. A comparison of oral and inhaled steroids in patients with chronic airways obstruction: features determining response. Thorax 1978; 33:214.

132. Shim CS, Williams MH. Aerosol beclomethasone in patients with steroid responsive chronic obstructive pulmonary disease. Am J Med 1983; 78:655.

133. Toogood JH, Baskerville J, Errington N, et al. Determinants of the response to beclomethasone aerosol at various dosage levels: a multiple regression analysis to identify clinically useful predictors. J Allergy Clin Immunol 1977; 60:367.

134. Paggiaro PL, Dahl R, Bakran I, et al. Multicentre randomized placebo-controlled trial of inhaled fluticasone propionate in patients with chronic obstructive pulmonary disease. Lancet 1998; 351:773.

135. Vestbo J, Sorenson T, Lange P, et al. Long-term effect of inhaled inhaled budesonide in mild and moderate chronic obstructive pulmonary disease; a randomized controlled trial. Lancet 1999; 353:1948.

136. Pauwels RA, Lofdahl C, Laitinen LS, et al. Long-term treatment with inhaled budesonide in persons with mild chronic obstructive pulmonary disease who continue smoking. N Engl J Med 1999; 340:1948.

137. Burge PS, Calverley PMA, Jones PW, et al. Randomized, double blind, placebo controlled study of fluticasone propionate in patients with moderate to severe chronic obstructive pulmonary disease: the ISOLDE trial. Br Med J 2000; 320:1297.

138. Lung Health Study Research Group. Effect of inhaled triamcinolone on the decline in pulmonary function in chronic obstructive pulmonary disease. N Engl J Med 2000; 343:1902.

139. Casaburi R. Exercise training in chronic obstructive lung disease. In: Casaburi R, Petty TL. eds. Principles and Practice of Pulmonary Rehabilitation. Philadelphia: Saunders, 1993:204.

140. Strijbos JW, Sluiter JH, Postma DS, Gimeno F, Koeter GH. Objective and subjective performance indicators in COPD. Eur Respir J 1989; 2:666–669.

141. Reardon J, Awad E, Normandin E, Vale F, Clark B, ZuWallack RL. The effect of comprehensive outpatient pulmonary rehabilitation on dyspnea. Chest 1994; 105:1046–1052.

142. Cockroft AE, Saunders MJ, Berry G. Randomized controlled trial of rehabilitation in chronic respiratory disability. Thorax 1981; 36:200–203.

143. Goldstein RS, Gork EH, Stubbing D, Avendano MA, Guyatt GH. Randomized controlled trials of respiratory rehabilitation. Lancet 1994; 344:1394–1397.

144. Lacasse Y, Wong E, Guyatt GH, King D, Cook DJ, Goldstein RS. Meta-analysis of respiratory rehabilitation in chronic obstructive pulmonary disease. Lancet 1996; 348:1115–1119.

145. Ries AL, Kaplan RM, Limberg TM, Prewitt LM. Effects of pulmonary rehabilitation on physiologic and psychosocial outcomes in patients with chronic obstructive pulmonary disease. Ann Intern Med 1995; 122:823–832.

146. O'Donnell DE, McGuire M, Samis L, Webb KA. Effects of general exercise training on ventilatory and peripheral muscle strength and endurance in chronic airflow limitation. Am J Respir Crit Care Med 1998; 157:1489–1497.

147. Casaburi R, Patessio A, Ioli F, Zanaboni S, Donner CF, Wasserman K. Reduction in exercise lactic acidosis and ventilation as a result of exercise training in obstructive lung disease. Am Rev Respir Dis 1991; 143:9–18.

148. Maltais F, Leblanc P, Simard C, Jobin J, Berube C, Bruneau J, Carrier L, Belleau R. Skeletal muscle adaptation to endurance training in patients with chronic obstructive pulmonary disease. Am J Respir Crit Care Med 1996; 154:442–447.

149. Casaburi R, Porszasz J, Burns MR, Carithers ER, Chang RSY, Cooper CB. Physiologic benefits of exercise training in rehabilitation of patients with severe chronic obstructive pulmonary disease. Am J Respir Crit Care Med 1997; 155:1541–1551.

150. Martinez FJ, Couser JJ, Celli BR. Respiratory response to arm elevation in patients with chronic airflow obstruction. Am Rev Respir Dis 1991; 143:476–480.

151. Martin TW, Zeballos RJ, Weisman IM. Gas exchange during maximal upper extremity exercise. Chest 1991; 99:420–425.

152. Epstein S, Breslin E, Roa J, Celli B. Impact of unsupported arm training and ventilatory muscle training on the metabolic and ventilatory consequences of unsupported arm elevation and exercise in patients with chronic airflow obstruction. Am Rev Respir Dis 1991; 143:A-81.

153. Ries AL, Ellis B, Hawkins RW. Upper extremity exercise training in chronic obstructive pulmonary disease. Chest 1988; 93:688–692.

154. Simpson K, Killian K, McCartney N, Stubbing DG, Jones NL. Randomized controlled trial of weight-lifting exercise in patients with chronic airflow limitation. Thorax 1992; 47:70–75.

155. Faling LJ. Pulmonary rehabilitation—physical modalities. Clin Chest Med 1986; 7:599–618.

156. Tiep BL, Burns M, Kao D, Madison R, Herrera J. Pursed lip breathing training using ear oximetry. Chest 1986; 90:218–221.

157. Sinclair JD. The effect of breathing exercises in pulmonary emphysema. Thorax 1955; 10:246–249.

158. Becklake MR, McGregor M, Goldman HI, Braudo JL. A study of the effects of physiotherapy in chronic hypertrophic emphysema using lung function tests. Dis Chest 1954; 26:180–191.

159. Williams IP, Smith CM, McGavin CR. Diaphragmatic breathing training and walking performance in chronic airways obstruction. Br J Dis Chest 1982; 76:164–166.

160. Gosselink RA, Wagenaar RC, Rijswijk H, Sargeant AJ, Decramer ML. Diaphragmatic breathing reduces efficiency of breathing in patients with chronic obstructive pulmonary disease. Am J Respir Crit Care Med 1995; 151:1136–1142.

161. Rodenstein DO, Stanescu. Absence of nasal airflow during pursed-lip breathing: the soft palate mechanisms. Am Rev Respir Dis 1983; 128:716–718.

162. Thoman R, Stoker G, Ross J. The efficacy of pursed lip breathing in patients with chronic obstructive pulmonary disease. Am Rev Respir Dis 1966; 93:100–106.

163. O'Donnell DE, Sanii R, Anthonisen NR, Younes M. Expiratory resistive loading in patients with severe chronic airflow limitation: an evaluation of ventilatory mechanics and compensatory responses. Am Rev Respir Dis 1987; 136:102–107.

164. Kim J, Larson J, Covey M, Vitalo C, Alex C, Patel M. Inspiratory muscle training in patients with chronic obstructive pulmonary disease. Nurs Res 1993; 42:356–362.

165. Smith L, Cook D, Guyatt G, Madhaven J, Oxman A. Respiratory muscle training in chronic airflow limitation: a meta-analysis. Am Rev Respir Dis 1992; 145:533–529.

166. Belman MJ, Shadmehz R. Targeted resistive ventilatory training in chronic pulmonary disease. J Appl Physiol 1988; 65:2726–2735.

167. Bellemare F, Bigland-Ritchie B. Assessment of human diaphgram strength and activation using phrenic nerve stimulation. Respir Physiol 1984; 58:263–267.

168. Polkey MI, Kyroussis D, Hamnegarad C.-H, Mills GH, Green M, Moxham J. Diaphragm strength in chronic obstructive pulmonary disease. Am J Respir Crit Care Med 1996; 154:1310–1317.

169. Similowsky T, Yan S, Gauthier AP, Macklem PT, Bellemere F. Contractile properties of the human diaphragm during chronic hyperinflation. N Engl J Med 1991; 325:917–923.

170. Harver A, Mahler DA. Targeted inspiratory muscle training improves respiratory muscle function and reduces dyspnea in chronic obstructive pulmonary disease. Ann Intern Med 1989; 111:117–124.

171. Kim J, Larson J, Covey M, Vitalo C, Alex C, Patel M. Inspiratory muscle training in patients with chronic obstructive pulmonary disease. Nurs Res 1993; 42:356–362.

172. Griffiths TL, Burr ML, Campbell IA, et al. Results at one year of outpatient multidisciplinary pulmonary rehabilitation: A randomized controlled trial. Lancet 2000; 335:362–368.

173. Report of the Medical Research Council Working Party. Long term domiciliary oxygen therapy in chronic hypoxic cor pulmonale complicating chronic bronchitis and emphysema. Lancet 1981; 1:681–686.

174. Nocturnal Oxygen Therapy Trial Group. Continuous or nocturnal oxygen therapy in hypoxemic chronic obstructive lung disease: a clinical trial. Ann Intern Med 1980; 93:391–398.

175. Chronos N, Adams L, Guz A. Effect of hyperoxia and hypoxia on exercise-induced breathlessness in normal subjects. Clin Sci 1988; 74:531–537.

176. Lane R, Cockcroft A, Adams L, Guz A. Arterial oxygen saturation and breathlessness in patients with chronic obstructive airways disease. Clin Sci 1987; 72:693–698.

177. O'Donnell DE, Bain DJ, Webb KA. Factors contributing to relief of exertional breathlessness during hyperoxia in chronic airflow limitation. Am J Respir Crit Care Med 1997; 155:530–535.

178. Seinburn CR, Wakefield JM, Jones PW. Relationship between ventilation and breathlessness during exercise in chronic obstructive airways disease is not altered by prevention of hypoxemia. Clin Sci 1984; 67:515–519.

179. Webb KA, D'Arsigny C, O'Donnell DE. Exercise response to added oxygen in patients with COPD and variable gas exchange abnormalities. Am J Respir Crit Care Med 2001; 163:A269.

180. Woodcock AA, Gross ER, Geddes DM. Oxygen relieves breathlessness in "pink puffers." Lancet 1981; 1:907–909.

181. Libby DM, Bisco WA, King TKC. Relief of hypoxia-related bronchoconstriction by breathing 30 percent oxygen. Am Rev Respir Dis 1981; 123:171–175.

182. Bye PTP, Esau SA, Levy RO, Shiner RJ, Macklem PT, Martin JG, Pardy RL. Ventilatory muscle function during exercise in air and oxygen patients with chronic airflow limitation. Am Rev Respir Dis 1985; 132:236–240.

183. Dean NC, Brown JK, Himelman RB, Doherty JJ, Gold WM, Stuhlbarg MS. Oxygen may improve dyspnea and endurance in patients with chronic obstructive pulmonary disease and only mild hypoxemia. Am Rev Respir Dis 1992; 148:941–945.

184. Somfay A, Porszasz J, Lee SM, Casaburi R. Dose-response effect of oxygen on hyperinflation and exercise endurance in nonhypoxaemic COPD patients. Eur Respir J 2001; 18:77–84.

185. Bruera E, de Stoutz N, Velasco-Leiva A, Schoeller T, Hanson J. Effects of oxygen on dyspnoea in hypoxaemic terminal cancer patients. Lancet 1993; 342:13–14.

186. Ventafridda V, Spoldi E, De Conno F. Control of dyspnea in advanced cancer patients (letter). Chest 1990; 98:1544–1545.

187. Light RW, Muro JR, Sato RI, Stansbury DW, Fischer CE, Brown SE. Effects of oral morphine on breathlessness and exercise tolerance in patients with chronic obstructive pulmonary disease. Am Rev Respir Dis 1989; 139:126–133.

188. Santiago TV, Johnson J, Riley DJ, Edelman NH. Effects of morphine on ventilatory response to exercise. J Appl Physiol 1979; 47:112–118.

189. Weil JV, McCullough RE, Kline JS, Sodal IE. Diminished ventilatory response to hypoxia and hypercapnia after morphine in normal man. N Engl J Med 1975; 292:1103–1106.

190. Sackner MA. Effects of hydrocodone bitartrate on breathing pattern of patients with chronic obstructive pulmonary disease and restrictive lung disease. Mt Sinai Med J 1984; 51:222–226.

191. Stark RD, Morton PB, Sharman P, Percival PG, Lewis JA. Effects of codeine on the respiratory responses to exercise in healthy subjects. Br J Clin Pharmacol 1983; 15:355–359.

192. Supinski GS, DiMarco A, Bark H, Chapman K, Clary S, Altose M. Effect of codeine on the sensations elicited by loaded breathing. Am Rev Respir Dis 1990; 141:1516–1521.

193. Young IH, Daviskas E, Keena VA. Effect of low dose nebulised morphine on exercise endurance in patients with chronic lung disease. Thorax 1989; 44:387–390.

194. Woodcock AA, Gross ER, Gellert A, Shah S, Johnson M, Geddes DM. Effects of dihydrocodeine, alcohol, and caffeine on breathlessness and exercise tolerance in patients with chronic obstructive lung disease and normal blood gases. N Engl J Med 1981; 305:1611–1616.

195. Woodcock AA, Johnson MA, Geddes DM. Breathlessness, alcohol and opiates. N Engl J Med 1982; 306:1363–1364.

196. Johnson MA, Woodcock AA. Dihydrocodeine for breathlessness in "pink puffers." Br Med J 1983; 286:675–677.

197. Eisneer N, Luce P, Denman W, West C. Effect of oral diamorphine on dyspnea in chronic obstructive pulmonary disease (COPD). Am Rev Respir Dis 1990; 141:A323.

198. Eisner N, Denman WT, West C, Luce P. Oral diamorphine: Lack of effect on dyspnoea and exercise tolerance in the "pink puffer" syndrome. Eur Respir J 1991; 4:926–931.

199. Stark RD, Gambles SA, Lewis JA. Methods to assess breathlessness in healthy subjects: a critical evaluation and application to analyze the acute effects of diazepam and promethazine on breathlessness induced by exercise or by exposure to raised levels of carbon dioxide. Clin Sci 1981; 61:429–439.

200. Rice KL, Kronenberg RS, Hedemark LL, Niewoehner DE. Effects of chronic administration of codeine and promethazine on breathlessness and exercise tolerance in patients with chronic airflow obstruction. Br J Dis Chest 1987; 81:287–292.
201. Leung R, Hill P, Burdon J. Effect of inhaled morphine on the development of breathlessness during exercise in patients with chronic lung disease. Thorax 1996; 51:596–600.
202. Chau LKL, Webb KA, O'Donnell DE. Relief of exertional breathlessness with nebulized morphine sulfate in patients with chronic lung disease. Am J Respir Crit Care Med 1996; 153:A656.
203. Saunders C, Baines M. Living with Dying: The Management of Terminal Disease, 2nd ed. Oxford, England: Oxford University Press, 1989.
204. Kinzel T. Symptom control in geriatric patients with terminal cancer: Pain, Nausea, and Vomiting. Geriatrics 1988; 43:83–84, 87–89.
205. Storey P. Symptom control in advanced cancer. Semin Oncol 1994; 21:748–753.
206. Roberts DK, Thorne SE, Pearson C. The experience of dyspnea in late-stage cancer. Patients' and nurses' perspectives. Cancer Nurs 1993; 16:310–320.
207. Foley KM. Clinical tolerance to opioids. In: Bassbaun AI, Beeson JM, eds. Towards a New Pharmacotherapy of Pain. Dahlem Konferenzen. Chichester, England: Wiley, 1991:181–204.
208. Mitchell HP, Murphy K, Minty K, Guz A, Patterson SC, Minty PS, Rosser RM. Diazepam in the treatment of dyspnoea in the "pink puffer" syndrome. Q J Med 1980; 49:9–20.
209. Woodcock AA, Gross ER, Geddes DM. Drug treatment of breathlessness: contrasting effects of diazepam and promethazine in pink puffers. Br Med J 1981; 283:343–346.
210. Man GCW, Hsu K, Sproule BJ. Effect of alprazolam on exercise and dyspnea in patients with chronic obstructive pulmonary disease. Chest 1986; 90:832–836.
211. Singh NP, Despars JA, Stansbury DW, Avalos K, Light RW. Effects of buspirone on anxiety levels and exercise tolerance in patients with chronic airflow obstruction and mild anxiety. Chest 1993; 103:800–804.
212. Argyropoulou P, Patakas D, Koukou A, Vasiliadis P, Georgopoulos D. Buspirone effect on breathlessness and exercise performance in patients with chronic obstructive pulmonary disease. Respiration 1993; 60:216–220.
213. FitzGerald MX, Keelan PJ, Cugell DW, Gaensler EA. Long term results of surgery for bullous emphysema. J Thorac Cardiovas Surg 1974; 68:566–587.
214. Pearson MG, Ogilvie C. Surgical treatment of emphysematous bullae—late outcome. Thorax 1983; 38:134–137.
215. Pride NB, Barter CE, Hugh-Jones P. The ventilation of bullae and the effect of their removal on thoracic gas volumes and tests of overall pulmonary function. Am Rev Respir Dis 1973; 107:83–98.
216. Ohta M, Nakahara K, Yasumitsu T, et al. Prediction of post-operative performance status in patients with giant bullae. Chest 1992; 101:668–673.
217. Nissen RA conservative operation of air cysts of the lung. Rocky Mtn Med J 1945; 40:595.
218. O'Donnell DE. Volume reduction surgery in patients with chronic airflow limitation: a physiological rationale. Semin Respir Crit Care Med 1996; 17:509–516.

219. Brantigan OC, Mueller E. Surgical treatment of pulmonary emphysema. Am Surg 1957; 23:789–804.
220. Wakabayashu A. Thorascopic laser penumoplasty in the treatment of diffuse bullous emphysema. Ann Thorac Surg 1995; 60:936–942.
221. Yusen RD, Trulock EP, Lefrak SS, et al. Volume reduction surgery patient selection criteria and clinical profiles. Chest 1995; 108:96S.
222. Orens JB, Krasna MJ, McKay KJ, et al. The physiological changes at rest and during exercise following lung reduction surgery for emphysema. Chest 1995; 108:96S.
223. Sciurba FC, Keenan RJ, Landreneau RJ, et al. Increased elastic recoil: a mechanism of improvement following lung reduction surgery for diffuse emphysema. Am J Respir Crit Care Med 1995; 1551:A12.
224. Pierce JA, Growdon JH. Physical properties of the lungs in giant cyst. N Engl J Med 1962; 267:169–173.
225. Gelb AF, Gold WM, Nadel JA. Mechanisms limiting airflow in bullous lung disease. Am Rev Respir Dis 1973; 107:571–578.
226. Laros CD, Gelissen JH, Bergstein PGM, et al. Bullectomy for giant bullae in emphysema. J Thorac Cardiovas Surg 1986; 91:63–70.
227. O'Donnell DE, Webb KA, Chau L, et al. Mechanisms of relief of exertional breathlessness following unilateral bullectomy and lung volume reduction surgery for emphysema. Chest 1996; 110:18–27.
228. Traveline JM, Paddonizio V, Criner G. Effect of bullectomy on diaphragmatic strength. Am J Respir Crit Care Med 1995; 152:1697–1701.
229. Rodriquez-Roisen R. Towards a consensus definition for COPD exacerbation. Chest 2000; 117:3985–4015.
230. Connors AF Jr, Dawson NV, Thomas C, Harrell FE Jr, Desbiens N, Fulkerson WJ, et al. Outcomes following acute exacerbation of severe chronic obstructive lung disease. The SUPPORT Investigators (Study to Understand Prognoses and Preferences for Outcomes and Risks of Treatments) [published erratum appears in Am J Respir Crit Care Med 1997; 155:386]. Am J Respir Crit Care Med 1996; 154:959–967.
231. Kong GK, Belman MJ, Weingarten S. Reducing length of stay for patients hospitalized with exacerbation of COPD by using a practice guideline. Chest 1997; 111:98–94.
232. Fuso L, Incalzi RA, Pistelli R, Muzzolon R, Valente S, Pagiliari G, et al. Predicting mortality of patients hospitalized for acutely exacerbated chronic obstructive pulmonary disease. Am J Med 1995; 98:272–277.
233. Seneff MG, Wagner DP, Wagner RP, Zimmerman JE, Knaus WA. Hospital and 1-year survival of patients admitted to intensive care units with acute exacerbation of chronic obstructive pulmonary disease. JAMA 1995; 274:1852–1857.
234. Seemungel TA, Donaldson GC, Paul EA, Bertall JC, Jeffries DJ, Wedzicha JA. Effect of exacerbation on quality of life in patients with chronic obstructive pulmonary disease. Am J Respir Crit Care Med 1998; 157:1418–1422.
235. Seemungal TA, Haper-Owens R, Blowmik A, Jeffries DJ, Wedzicha JA. Time course and recovery of exacerbations in patients with chronic obstructive pulmonary disease. Am J Respir Crit Care Med 2000; 161:1608–1613.
236. Friedman M, Serby C, Menoyoge S, Douglas Wilson JD, Hilleman DE, Witek JJ. Pharmaco-economic evaluation of a combination of Ipratropium plus

albuterol compared with Ipratropium alone and albuterol alone in COPD. Chest 1999; 115:635–641.

237. Karpel JP. Bronchodilator responses to anticholinergic and beta-adrenergic agents in acute and stable COPD. Chest 1991; 99:871.

238. Berry RB, Shinto RA, Wong FH, et al. Nebulizer vs spacer for bronchodilator delivery in patients hospitalized for acute exacerbations of COPD. Chest 1989; 96:1241.

239. Hodder RV, Calcutt LE, Leech JA. Metered dose inhaler with spacer is superior to wet nebulization for emergency room treatment of acute, severe asthma. Chest 1988; 94(suppl 1):52S.

240. Salmeron S, Brochard L, Mal H, et al. Nebulized versus intravenous albuterol in hypercapnic acute asthma. A multicenter double-blind randomized study. Am J Respir Crit Care Med 1994; 149:466.

241. Rice KL, Leatherman JW, Duane PG, et al. Aminophylline for acute exacerbations of chronic obstructive pulmonary disease. Ann Intern Med 1987; 107:305.

242. Seidenfield J, Jones W, Moss R, et al. Intravenous aminophylline in the treatment of acute bronchospastic exacerbations of chronic obstructive pulmonary disease. Ann Emerg Med 1984; 13:248.

243. Albert RK, Martin TR, Lewis SW. Controlled clinical trial of methyprednisolone in patients with chronic bronchitis and acute respiratory insufficiency. Ann Intern Med 1980; 92:753.

244. Niewoehner DE, Erbland ML, Deupre RH. Effect of systemic glucocorticoids on exacerbations of chronic obstructive pulmonary disease. N Engl J Med 1999; 340:1941.

245. Davies L, Angus RM, Calverley PMA. Oral corticosteroids in patients admitted to hospital with exacerbations of chronic obstructive pulmonary disease: a prospective randomized controlled trial. Lancet 1999; 354:456.

246. Anthonisen NR, Manfreda J, Warren CPW, et al. Antibiotic therapy in exacerbations of chronic obstructive pulmonary disease. Ann Intern Med 1987; 106:196.

247. O'Donnell DE, D'Arsigny C, Webb KA. Effect of hypoxia on ventilatory limitation during exercise in advanced chronic obstructive pulmonary disease. Am J Respir Crit Care Med 2001; 163:892–898.

248. O'Donnell DE. Dyspnea in advanced chronic obstructive pulmonary disease. J Heart Lung Transplant 1998; 17:544–554.

Table 4 Typical Abnormalities During Exercise in COPD

Significant dyspnea and leg discomfort
Reduced peak $\dot{V}_{O_2}$ and work rate
Low maximal heart rate
Elevated submaximal ventilation
Low peak ventilation
High ratio of ventilation to maximal ventilatory capacity ($\dot{V}_E$/MVC)
Blunted V_T response to exercise, with increased breathing frequency
High deadspace (V_D/V_T)
Variable arterial oxygen desaturation
Pa_{CO_2} usually normal but may increase
Reduced dynamic IC with exercise (i.e., dynamic hyperinflation)
Reduced IRV at low work rates
High V_T/IC ratios at low work rates

information is arguably important in the assessment of mechanisms of exercise intolerance in a given patient. In this regard, exercise flow-volume loops can provide a noninvasive assessment of dynamic mechanics and allow greater refinement in the evaluation of the ventilatory constraints to exercise (6,87) (Fig. 2).

Serial IC measurements can be used to track end-expiratory lung volume (EELV) during exercise (Figs. 2 and 3). This approach is based on the reasonable assumption that TLC does not change appreciably during exercise in COPD and that reductions in dynamic IC must, therefore, reflect increases in EELV or dynamic hyperinflation (DH) (9). However, regardless of any possible changes in TLC with exercise, progressive reduction of an already diminished resting IC means that V_T becomes positioned closer to the actual TLC and the upper alinear extreme of the respiratory system's pressure-volume relationship, where there is increased elastic loading of the respiratory muscles. We have recently shown that IC measurements during constant-load cycle exercise are both highly reproducible and responsive in patients with severe COPD provided that due care is taken in their measurement (10).

Changes in the dynamic volume components during exercise can be measured by a combination of serial IC and tidal volume measurements: end-inspiratory lung volume (EILV) can be calculated by adding EELV to V_T (Fig. 3). The operating lung volumes during exercise dictate the length-tension and the force-velocity characteristics of the ventilatory muscles and influence breathing pattern and the quality and intensity of dyspnea. Moreover, dynamic volume measurements give clear information about the extent of mechanical restriction during exercise in COPD (Figs. 2 and 3). Inspiratory reserve volume (IRV) during exercise, in particular, provides an indication of the existing constraints on V_T expansion. Similarly, the reserves of inspiratory and expiratory flow can be evaluated by measuring the difference between tidal flow rates and those generated at the same volume during maximal maneuver (Fig. 2).

E. Field Tests of Exercise Performance

A number of exercise test protocols are available and include tests of functional disability, such as timed walking distances and combined tests of physiological impairment and disability using incremental or constant-load protocols during cycle ergometry or treadmill testing. These various tests provide different but complementary information for the purpose of clinical assessment; the choice of test depends on the type of clinical information required.

Timed Walking Distances

Timed walking distance tests are the most popular and widely used exercise tests in clinical practice. The 6-min walking distance (6 MWD), in particular, has been shown to be a simple, reproducible test and is an acceptable general measure of functional disability in COPD patients (88). No normative population data are available for 6 MWD, so comparison of exercise performance across individuals is not possible at present. To ensure satisfactory test-retest reproducibility with this field test, care must be taken in the conduct of the test to account for learning effects with repeated testing and the strong influence of patient motivation on test performance. Timed walking distances have the disadvantage that the "work rate" cannot be controlled: work rate may be highly variable between tests, thus confounding comparisons.

Physiological measurements, other than heart rate and arterial oxygen saturation, are difficult to perform during corridor walking and little data are available on the validity of Borg scaling of symptoms and of IC measurements during this 6-min test. The 6 MWD has been repeatedly shown to have satisfactory responsiveness following interventions such as exercise training, volume reduction surgery, and lung transplantation in COPD, but this test may be less sensitive for assessment of bronchodilator therapy or inhaled anti-inflammatory agents. There is currently no consensus as to the quantification or stratification of disability in COPD using the 6 MWD, nor is it clear what improvement in the 6 MWD constitutes a clinically meaningful response to interventions. Six-min treadmill walking, which facilitates concurrent physiological measurement, and the shuttle test (where work rate is better controlled) are currently being tested as alternatives to the traditional 6-min walk test and may prove to be superior (89).

Submaximal Exercise Endurance Testing

Constant-load, submaximal exercise tests—with measurements of dynamic ventilatory mechanics, symptom intensity and endurance time—may have wider application than incremental exercise testing or field walking tests for the purposes of therapeutic evaluation. We have recently shown that constant-load cycle exercise, conducted at approximately 60% of the predetermined maximal work rate, was highly reproducible when measured on four occasions over an 8-week period of clinical stability in 29 patients with advanced COPD (10). Such tests have the potential to provide new insights into the interface between physiological impairment and disability and how both these parameters can be favorably altered by therapeutic interventions.

As already mentioned, quantitative flow-volume-loop analysis during constant-load exercise protocols offers a noninvasive assessment of dynamic ventilatory mechanics. The greater the increase in dynamic IC during exercise following pharmacological or surgical volume reduction, the lesser the inspiratory threshold and elastic load on the inspiratory muscles. Consequently, mechanical restriction and the extent of neuromechanical uncoupling of the respiratory system are improved. It has become clear that even small increases in dynamic IC (on the order of 0.3 to 0.4 L) translate into clinically meaningful improvements in dyspnea and exercise tolerance in severely hyperinflated patients with COPD (6,39).

Exercise endurance time measured during constant-load cycle protocols has been shown to be highly responsive to such interventions as bronchodilators (39), exercise training (47), oxygen therapy (52), volume reduction surgery (42), and noninvasive ventilatory assistance (36), where improvements in the range of 30 to 40% over control have been reported. Preliminary information suggests that acute responses of this magnitude reflect sustained increases of daily activities, but this question requires further study.

F. Peripheral Muscle Strength Testing

In addition to assessment of ventilatory and cardiovascular reserves during CPET, it is also important to assess the status of the peripheral muscles required to perform the task of locomotion. The extent of peripheral muscle weakness has been shown to correlate well with the intensity of perceived exertional leg discomfort (56). As already mentioned, peripheral muscle weakness is not uncommon in advanced COPD and will respond to targeted training of appropriate intensity and duration. There is no consensus as to the most suitable strength test for patients with COPD. We measure isokinetic peak torque (using a Cybex II or LIDO dynamometer). We test the muscles throughout a specified range of motion at a controlled angular velocity of 30, 60 and 90 degrees per second. Similar trials are performed for each muscle group. The highest torque of the trials is recorded for each muscle group at each angular velocity and expressed as a percent of predicted normal (90–92).

G. Measurement of Quality of Life

Comprehensive questionnaires have recently been developed that are designed to evaluate the impact of diseases such as COPD on quality of life (93–96). These health-related quality-of-life instruments permit a rigorous evaluation of the far reaching implications of chronic dyspnea and other respiratory symptoms on mood and psychological well-being, impairment, handicap, disability, and lifestyle restriction in individual patients (93–96). Reliability and validity estimates have been published for a number of health-related quality-of-life questionnaires, and these have been used increasingly in the evaluation of therapeutic interventions such as pulmonary rehabilitation (93–96), volume reduction surgery (100), and short-and long-acting bronchodilators (97–99). Although these questionnaires provide valuable comprehensive clinical information, their administration is time-consuming. They are currently used in the clinical trial setting and not routinely in daily clinical practice. In the future, the development of more simplified, abbreviated quality-of-life questionnaires may prove to have broader clinical utility.

IV. Management

A. Education

Patient education has been recognized by the GOLD Consensus Committee as a pivotal component in the management of COPD (5). Current management paradigms for COPD are physician-centered, "reactive" in nature, and primarily based on pharmacological therapy. For advanced symptomatic COPD, a more comprehensive, "proactive" multidisciplinary approach that addresses the physical, psychological and social underpinnings of this chronic disease state is likely more appropriate. There is now preliminary evidence that structured educational programs increase knowledge about COPD, improve quality of life, and result in a reduction in health service utilization (101,102). In a recent study, Bourbeau et al. (102) show that an educational program delivered by a trained case manager (with close follow-up of patients) can result in significantly reduced hospital emergency visits, unscheduled office visits, and hospitalizations over a 1-year period. However, education alone does not improve exercise tolerance or exertional dyspnea (103) (Fig. 6). To improve dyspnea and exercise performance, supervised educational programs should incorporate individualized exercise training. Future studies are needed to determine the health impact and economic feasibility of supervised, long-term, home-based and community-based exercise programs. Components of an educational program for advanced COPD are provided in Table 5.

B. Bronchodilator Therapy

Until recently, an arbitrary increase in $FEV_{1.0}$ has been used as a primary indicator of bronchodilator efficacy. Currently, new therapeutic agents are more rigorously evaluated in terms of their impact on ventilatory mechanics, disability, and handicap (Fig. 7).

Bronchodilator therapy is the first step in the management of patients with symptomatic COPD. All classes of bronchodilator therapy (i.e., inhaled

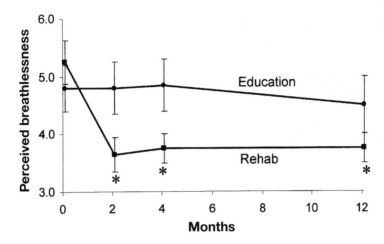

Figure 6 The effects of a pulmonary rehabilitation program versus education only on perceived breathlessness in COPD ($^{*}p < 0.05$). (From Ref. 103.)

beta$_2$ agonists, inhaled anticholinergics, and oral theophyllines) have been shown to improve exertional dyspnea and increase exercise capacity in COPD patients when tested in placebo-controlled studies (36–38,97,104–107). The mechanisms of these beneficial effects are complex and not fully elucidated. From the available literature on the topic, a few generalizations are possible (36–38,97). First, meaningful improvement in symptoms, activity levels, and quality of life occur in the presence of modest or no changes in $FEV_{1.0}$ after bronchodilator therapy. Second, the single laboratory bronchodilator reversibility test is not predictive of symptomatic responses to that agent. Third, different patients respond differently to different classes of bronchodilators or to a single class of bronchodilators over time. Fourth, combination bronchodilator therapy may have synergistic effects on respiratory symptoms in COPD. Fifth, the mode of delivery and doses of bronchodilators must be carefully individualized for maximal benefit.

Our understanding of the mechanisms by which bronchodilators can potentially relieve exertional dyspnea and improve exercise endurance has recently increased. Bronchodilators improve airway function and reduce the resistive and elastic loads on the respiratory muscles. Belman et al. (37), in an elegant mechanical study, showed that relief of dyspnea following albuterol (salbutamol) therapy in advanced COPD correlated well with reduction in operational lung volumes as well as a reduction in inspiratory effort required for a given tidal volume change, the latter being an index of neuromechanical coupling of the respiratory system. In that study, important reductions in lung volume occurred in the presence of only minimal changes in $FEV_{1.0}$. Similarly, Chrystyn et al. (38) showed that improvement in exercise endurance (6 MWD) following incremental oral theophylline therapy was associated in a dose-

Table 5   Components of an Education Program

Smoking cessation
Basic information: pathophysiology
Rationale for medical Rx
Effective inhaler technique
Self-management plan
Coping skills development
Strategies to alleviate dyspnea
Decision making re AECOPD
Advanced directives/end-of-life issues
Identify educational resources

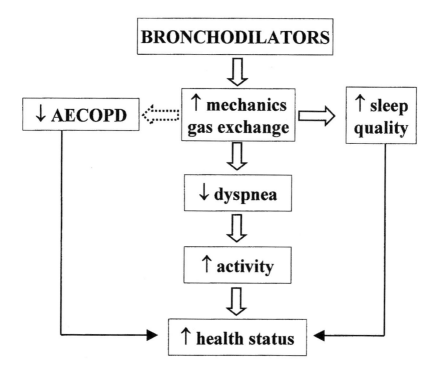

Figure 7   By improving respiratory mechanics and/or gas exchange, bronchodilators may improve dyspnea, activity levels, health status or quality of life, and sleep quality in COPD. Improvements in mechanics and/or gas exchange may also lead to reductions in the frequency and/or severity of acute exacerbations in COPD (AECOPD).

response manner, with the reduction in resting plethysmographic FRC and trapped gas volume (plethysmographic versus helium-derived lung volumes). Again in this study, there was little change in the postbronchodilator $FEV_{1.0}$. We have shown (39), in a placebo-controlled study, that relief of exertional dyspnea and improved exercise endurance following acute anticholinergic therapy [nebulized ipratropium bromide (IB) 500 μg] in advanced COPD correlated well with improvement in dynamic IC measurements, which reflect dynamic changes in dynamic EELV. Changes in IC-derived measures such as EILV, IRV, and the V_T/IC ratio also correlated well with reduced exertional dyspnea measured by the Borg scale. Because of the bronchodilator-induced increase in expiratory flow rates over the tidal volume range, patients could maintain the same or greater ventilation at lower operational lung volumes with a more efficient breathing pattern and lesser degrees of mechanical restriction during exercise (39) (Fig. 8). This translated into reduced dyspnea and a delay in ventilatory limitation, with subsequent improvement in exercise endurance, by an average of 32% over control values (Fig. 8). Increased IC and IRV following ipratropium meant that V_T at end-exercise was positioned on the lower, more linear, portion of the respiratory system's pressure-volume relationship, where there is reduced elastic and inspiratory threshold loading of the inspiratory muscles. Therefore, less pressure is required for a greater tidal volume response after ipratropium compared with placebo.

Short-Acting Bronchodilators—Practical Considerations

Although the guidelines of the American Thoracic Society (ATS) for the management of COPD recommend high dosages of short-acting bronchodilators [e.g., ipratropium bromide (20 μg), four to six puffs at intervals of 4 to 6 hr], dose-response relationships, at least using the $FEV_{1.0}$ as the outcome measure, are relatively flat in COPD (108,109). However, despite the lack of scientific evidence, clinical experience has shown that greater symptom control can be achieved with higher dosages of anticholinergics in selected patients. The nebulized route of delivery has not been shown to be superior to the metered-dose inhaler (MDI) with spacer device in terms of the $FEV_{1.0}$ response in stable COPD patients (112). However, patients with advanced COPD often express a personal preference for the wet nebulizer over the MDI. For patients who have low maximal inspiratory pressures because of hyperinflation and who are unable to hold their breath for the requisite 8 to 10 sec following an MDI inhalation, the nebulized route may be preferable. Decisions about the optimal route of delivery should be made on an individual basis. Combination products (e.g., ipratropium bromide + albuterol) have been shown to have greater effects on the $FEV_{1.0}$ than either agent given alone and are more convenient for the patient (113–115).

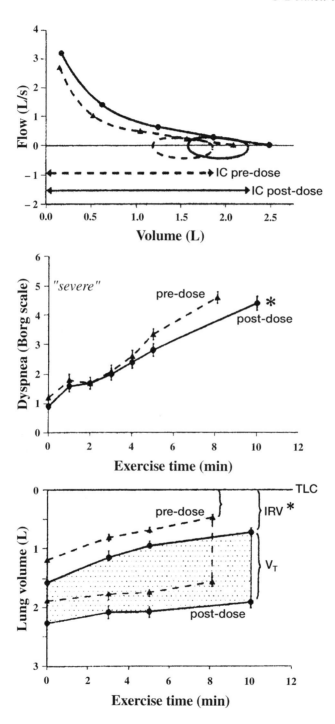

Table 6 Attributes of Bronchodilators in COPD

	Salmeterol	Tiotropium
Improve lung mechanics	✓	✓
Relieve/reduce dyspnea	✓	✓
Improve health status	✓	✓
Reduce frequency and/or severity of exacerbations	✓	✓
Improve exercise tolerance	?	✓
Modify disease progression	✗	✗
Few side effects	✓	✓

Long-Acting Bronchodilators

Long-acting beta$_2$ agonists (LABA), such as salmeterol and formoterol, provide sustained 24-hr bronchodilatation and therefore have a theoretical advantage over multiple short-acting bronchodilator dosing regimes. These agents may also improve sleep quality and relieve troublesome early-morning symptoms. Moreover, the long-term mechanical improvements as a result of sustained volume reduction (to a level that is seen after surgical volume reduction) may improve inspiratory muscle function and exercise capacity to a greater extent than multiple short-acting bronchodilator dosing (116) (Table 6). In a 12-week randomized trial in 780 patients with COPD who received formoterol (12 or 24 µg), placebo, or ipratropium (40 µg four times daily), formoterol (in both dosages) was superior to ipratropium with respect to symptom relief and improved quality of life. In a 12-week study with 411 patients, salmeterol was compared with placebo and ipratropium (99). A significant improvement with salmeterol compared with placebo was seen at four out of six time points, although ipratropium was significantly superior to placebo at all time points (99). Salmeterol has also been shown to improve

Figure 8 Responses to bronchodilator therapy (nebulized ipratropium bromide, 500 µg) are shown. As postdose maximal expiratory flow-volume relationships improve, tidal flow-volume curves at rest can shift to the right—i.e., lung hyperinflation is reduced as reflected by an increased IC (top panel). Exertional dyspnea decreased significantly ($^*p < 0.05$) in response to bronchodilator therapy (middle panel). Operational lung volumes improve in response to bronchodilator therapy—i.e., mechanical constraints on V_T expansion are reduced as IC and IRV are increased significantly ($^*p < 0.05$) (lower panel). (Adapted from Ref. 103.)

quality-of-life measurements as measured by the St. George's Respiratory Questionnaire (SGRQ). In a 16-week placebo-controlled study, 50 and 100 µg of salmeterol given twice daily produced similar improvements in $FEV_{1.0}$. Health status, as measured by the SGRQ total score, however, improved only with the lower dose, possibly because of better tolerability (98). Mean overall changes from baseline in SRGQ scores exceeded the accepted clinically meaningful threshold for the questionnaire (98). Salmeterol has also been shown to favorably affect rates of acute exacerbations in COPD (99). In 20 patients with severe hyperinflated COPD, salmeterol has been shown to acutely improve peak symptom-limited $\dot{V}_{O_2}$ and to relieve exertional dyspnea. These improvements clearly correlated with increased resting and exercise IC (117).

Tiotropium

Tiotropium is a new, once-daily inhaled anticholinergic agent with prolonged M_3-receptor antagonist activity. In a study of over 900 patients, tiotropium (18 µg once daily) significantly improved SGRQ scores compared with baseline and placebo (118). At the end of the year, the differences between tiotropium and placebo (SGRQ impact scores) exceeded the clinically significant threshold of four units ($p < 0.01$). Tiotropium has been compared with placebo and ipratropium in four replicate clinical trials at a dosage of 18 µg daily via Handihaler. Significantly greater improvements of trough $FEV_{1.0}$ and FVC, and morning and evening peak flows were seen with tiotropium with no evidence of tachyphylaxis (119,120). Placebo-controlled and ipratropium-controlled trials have shown that tiotropium treatment resulted in reduced incidence of exacerbations, later onset of first exacerbation, fewer exacerbations per patient per year, delayed onset of first hospitalization due to COPD exacerbations, and fewer hospitalizations per patient per year (119,120).

Transition Dyspnea Index (TDI) focal scores for dyspnea were statistically significantly greater in the tiotropium group compared with the placebo group at all time points (119,120). Similarly, in the ipratropium-controlled studies, mean TDI focal scores were significantly greater in the tiotropium group compared with the ipratropium group at all time points. Between group differences in TDI focal scores in the placebo and ipratropium controlled studies at intervals during the study showed approximately a one-unit difference in the TDI, which is believed to be the minimally clinically significant improvement (119,120). Additional recent studies in 187 patients with COPD have shown significant sustained volume reduction as indicated by a decreased residual volume and improved inspiratory capacity during tiotropium compared with placebo (121,122). These volume improvements correlated with improved exercise endurance and reduced intensity of dyspnea at a standardized work rate. Moreover, exercise endurance, measured by constant-load cycle ergometry, improved progressively over the 42 days of the trial (121,122).

Oral Theophylline

The ATS Guidelines recommend adding sustained-release theophyllines if patients remain breathless despite adequate short-acting inhaled bronchodilators. Oral theophyllines have been shown to reduce breathlessness and improve exercise tolerance in COPD. These improvements appear to be associated with reduction in thoracic gas volumes in a dose-dependent manner (38). A small open-label study in patients with poorly reversible bronchoconstriction found an average increase in the TDI focal score of 2.5 following sustained-release theophylline therapy (123). Improvements of this magnitude are likely to be clinically meaningful. A study by McKay et al. (124) in 15 COPD patients using inhaled beta$_2$ agonists and ipratropium plus placebo, low-dose theophylline (9.1 ± 2.3 mg/L), or high dose theophylline (16.8 ± 4.2 mg/L) for a total of 7 weeks found minor improvements in $FEV_{1.0}$ and FVC but significant improvements in dyspnea ($p > 0.05$) in the higher-dose group. ZuWallack et al. (125) conducted a randomized, double-blind, double-dummy, parallel-group trial in 943 patients with COPD. Patients were randomly assigned to receive salmeterol (42 µg twice daily) alone or in addition to oral theophylline for 12 weeks. Combination treatment with salmeterol plus theophylline provided significantly ($p < 0.05$) greater improvements in pulmonary function and symptoms ($p < 0.05$) and significantly fewer COPD exacerbations ($p < 0.023$). Patients benefited from the combination treatment without a resulting increase in adverse sequelae. These findings collectively justify a trial of added oral theophyllines to achieve serum levels of 10 to 20 µg/mL in symptomatic COPD patients. The potential advantage of theophylline over short-acting beta$_2$ agonists is that it provides 24-hr bronchodilatation and delivery to the peripheral bronchi is assured. However, intolerable side effects often preclude their routine use.

Summary—Bronchodilators

The primary aim of bronchodilator therapy is to improve symptoms and exercise performance. Sustained pharmacological lung volume reduction is one factor that has been linked to improvements in these outcomes (Table 6). In patients with persistent symptoms, who require frequent short-acting bronchodilators, tiotropium or a long-acting beta$_2$ agonist should be prescribed. There are currently insufficient information to recommend combination therapy of tiotropium with LABA or with inhaled corticosteroid-LABA combinations. However, an additive or synergistic benefit is anticipated for these combinations. If tiotropium is selected, then further symptom control can be achieved by adding a short acting beta$_2$ agonist, either in regular dosing or on an as-needed basis. If salmeterol or formoterol is prescribed, then combined ipratropium-albuterol (taken regularly or when required) should maximize symptom control. Oral theophylline remains a third-line agent but can be added to LABA to enhance symptom control in selected patients.

C. Inhaled Steroids

Although neither the GOLD guidelines nor the previous ATS recommendations include inhaled corticosteroids (ICS) as part of *first-line* therapy in COPD, studies have noted that almost 50% of patients with COPD will be prescribed ICS (126). Part of this practice may be due to the failure of clinicians to recognize that the inflammatory processes in COPD and asthma are distinct. While there is clear evidence in asthma that treatment with ICS results in both a reduction in airway inflammation and a clinical improvement, the evidence supporting this practice in COPD has been more modest. Physicians treating patients with COPD must weigh this modest benefit with the cost of potentially lifelong treatment and risk of adverse events, acknowledging that, in patients with extreme functional limitation from severe COPD, even small improvements may be clinically relevant.

Effect of ICS on Markers of Inflammation

If ICS does indeed modify the inflammatory process associated with COPD, then one would logically be able to measure the effect on markers of inflammation. Indeed, several studies have attempted to do so. The major weaknesses of these studies include small patient numbers, variable treatment periods, and heterogeneity in the choice of inflammatory markers. Typically, 20 or fewer COPD patients were assessed for periods between 2 and 8 weeks. A wide variety of inflammatory markers were studied, ranging from number of sputum neutrophils (127) to metalloproteinase levels (128) to interleukin (IL)-8 and tumor necrosis factor (TNF)-alpha levels (129) to a "bronchitis index" [based on bronchoscopy and bronchoalveolar lavage (BAL) results] (139). Not surprisingly, the results of these studies are varied, with some showing a biochemical "benefit" from ICS (127,132) but others not demonstrating any evidence of reduced inflammation. Interpreting the negative results is difficult, as the findings may reflect either a lack of benefit from ICS or inadequacy of the markers employed to measure inflammation. Conversely, one may not be able to extrapolate positive results from laboratory testing to clinical outcomes. At this point, the only clear conclusion from these studies is that they have been unable to definitively demonstrate or exclude a benefit for ICS in COPD.

Effect of ICS on Disease Progression

Most ICS trials include measurement of $FEV_{1.0}$ as a marker of disease progression. Although it could easily be argued that $FEV_{1.0}$ is, at best, a crude predictor of individual functional limitation in COPD, it does correlate with mortality risk and is widely available. Early studies were limited by small patient numbers (133,134), biased patient selection [preselection of patients with steroid-responsive disease (134)], and/or inclusion of asthmatic as well as COPD patients (135). The last 4 years, however, have seen the publication of several large, well-designed randomized placebo-controlled trials examining the effect of ICS on $FEV_{1.0}$.

The first major trial was by the International COPD Study Group (Paggiaro) (136). This trial enrolled 281 patients with a wide range of severity ($FEV_{1.0}$ 35–90%). The treatment arm was given fluticasone 500 μg twice daily. Follow-up was limited to 6 months. At that time, there was a 9.4% (0.15-L) difference in $FEV_{1.0}$ between the two treatment arms.

The Copenhagen City Lung Study was the next major trial (135). In contrast to the Paggiaro study, it enrolled 290 patients with disease of mild to moderate severity (the average postbronchodilator $FEV_{1.0}$ was 86% of predicted). Patients were treated with a total daily dose of 1200 μg budesonide for 6 months followed by 800 μg for 30 months. The average rate of decline in $FEV_{1.0}$ was 41.8 and 45.1 mL/year for the untreated and treated arms, respectively, which was not significantly different. The EUROSCOP trial included much larger numbers ($n = 912$) of current smokers, but included only patients with mild to moderate COPD (mean $FEV_{1.0}$ 77% predicted) (135). Again, no significant difference in $FEV_{1.0}$ was noted after 3 years treatment with 800 μg of budesonide per day.

The ISOLDE study is arguably the most relevant to this chapter, as it included the patients with relatively more severe disease than those in the other trials: the mean $FEV_{1.0}$ in the study population was 50% of predicted (137). However, even this study excluded patients with very severe disease ($FEV_{1.0} < 0.8$ L). This study, as well, failed to demonstrate any significant alteration in the decline of $FEV_{1.0}$ with ICS (fluticasone, 500 μg twice daily).

The most recent ICS trial is the Lung Health Study (138), which enrolled 1116 patients with mainly moderate COPD (mean $FEV_{1.0}$ 64% predicted). Treatment with 1200 μg per day of triamcinolone did not offer any benefit in $FEV_{1.0}$. Thus, the findings of the four largest ICS trials to date suggest that ICS does not have any major impact on $FEV_{1.0}$.

Effect of ICS on COPD Exacerbations

It can be argued that a reduction in frequency of exacerbations is more clinically relevant than small changes in $FEV_{1.0}$. This may be particularly true in patients with severe disease, who are more likely to require medical attention and hospitalization with even small changes in spirometric measurements. Most of the above trials recorded the number of exacerbations as either a primary or secondary endpoint. Unfortunately, the term *exacerbation* was defined principally by the need to seek medical attention without any specific criteria.

The number of COPD exacerbations was the primary endpoint in the International COPD Study Group trial. There was no significant difference between ICS and placebo in total number of exacerbations, although there were less combined "moderate" and "severe" exacerbations (defined as requiring treatment by family physician and hospitalization, respectively).

These results were somewhat contradicted in the Lung Health Study, which showed that ICS reduced ambulatory visits but did not impact on hospitalization. In the Copenhagen study, there was no difference between number of COPD exacerbations in the ICS arm versus placebo. In both cases, the frequency of exacerbation was low (0.36 per patient per year), likely reflecting the mild disease in the study population. Frequency of exacerbations was not measured in the EUROSCOP trial.

The first large study to demonstrate a reduction in total exacerbations was the ISOLDE study, which, as mentioned above, included patients with more severe disease than the other studies. ISOLDE defined an exacerbation as a "worsening of respiratory symptoms that required treatment with oral steroids or antibiotics, or both, as judged by the general practitioner." An important weakness of this study was that 43% of the treatment arm and 53% of the placebo arm withdrew during the trial; the most common reason for withdrawal was "frequent" exacerbations (*frequent* was not defined). Despite this potential bias against ICS, the investigators still noted a statistically significant reduction in the frequency of exacerbations (0.99 versus 1.32 per year). This finding was accompanied by a slowing of the decline in health status (assessed by questionnaire). Although the withdrawal of patients with frequent exacerbations makes generalization of this result difficult, the ISOLDE study raises the possibility that ICS may be beneficial in COPD patients with frequent exacerbations.

Adverse Effects

Given that the potential benefit of ICS (reduction in frequency of exacerbations) is small, the decision to add ICS to therapy must take into consideration the possibility of adverse effects. Because patients with COPD are often prescribed short courses of systemic steroids as well, it is somewhat difficult to assess the frequency of adverse events attributable purely to ICS. Oral candidiasis and hoarseness are probably the most common adverse effects from ICS, each occurring in less than 5% of treated patients over 6 months (134). Despite the relatively low systemic absorption of ICS, there is a potential for systemic side effects. Increased bruising was noted in the ISOLDE study (137). Laboratory evidence of adrenal suppression as also been noted (134), but clinical adrenal crises have not been reported. Of arguably greatest importance is the risk of osteoporosis: the Lung Health Study was the first large ICS trial to demonstrate a significant difference in bone density associated with ICS (138). The clinical relevance of this in terms of fracture risk remains undefined (and probably underestimated), as long-term follow-up of COPD patients on ICS is not available.

ICS—Summary

In summary, for patients with severe COPD, ICS may reduce the frequency of exacerbations. This conclusion is essentially based on the findings of two studies (137,138). There is no evidence that progression of disease, at least measured by $FEV_{1.0}$, is altered by ICS alone, although there may be a slowing of the decline in health status. The evidence demonstrating a synergistic effect with the combination of ICS and LABA is appealing, although the magnitude of benefit remains modest. This benefit must be weighed against a risk of adverse events, particularly of osteoporosis—a risk of unknown magnitude— as well as the cost of lifelong treatment. In patients with severe disease, in whom exacerbations are frequent and potentially associated with hospitaliza- tion and loss of independence, ICS (perhaps with LABA) may be a worthwhile adjunct to multimodality therapy. Several questions regarding ICS and COPD remain. The optimal dose is unknown: 500 µg of flucticasone twice daily was used in the ISOLDE trial, but a smaller dose may offer similar clinical benefit and less systemic absorption. Ideally, one would like to be able to predict which patients potentially stand to benefit from ICS or to clearly assess a clinical response to ICS on an individual basis, but neither is possible for the present.

D. Exercise Training

Patients who, despite optimized combination pharmacotherapy, have persis- tent activity-related dyspnea and exercise curtailment should be encouraged to undergo exercise training. The aim of exercise training is to break the vicious cycle of skeletal muscle deconditioning, progressive dyspnea, and immobility so as to improve symptoms and activity levels and restore patients to the highest level of independent function. All symptomatic patients should be encouraged to engage in regular activity and to avoid the inevitable drift toward an inactive lifestyle. Formal exercise training is generally provided within the context of a comprehensive, multidisciplinary pulmonary rehabilita- tion program that includes education, psychosocial support, occupational therapy, and nutritional advice. It is now well established that the exercise training component of the rehab program is pivotal in explaining the benefits of improved exercise capacity and reduced dyspnea. In this regard, Ries et al. (130) randomized 119 COPD patients to a comprehensive educational program alone or to a pulmonary rehabilitation program that incorporated supervised exercise training. In contrast to the "education group," where minimal improvement occurred, the subgroup randomized to exercise training showed highly significant improvements in exercise endurance, symptom-limited peak $\dot{V}_{O_2}$, and chronic activity-related dyspnea (103) (Fig. 6).

Initial skepticism about the value of exercise training has now yielded to a general acceptance of the beneficial effects of this modality as an effective symptom-relieving strategy in patients with advanced COPD. Certainly there is now abundant evidence for important subjective and objective benefits as a result of exercise training, at least in the short term. Casaburi pooled the results of 37 uncontrolled studies to evaluate the effects of aerobic training on exercise capacity in 933 patients with COPD (average $FEV_{1.0} = 1.1$ L) (139). Despite vast differences in exercise training protocols, patients almost invariably achieved meaningful improvements in exercise performance and activity levels. Several recent controlled trails have provided unequivocal evidence of clinical benefit. Strijbos et al. (140) randomized patients to a 12-week pulmonary rehabilitation program with exercise ($n = 30$) or no treatment ($n = 15$): exertional dyspnea ratings fell significantly in the exercise group and not in control. Reardon et al. (141) similarly showed that patients ($n = 10$) randomized to a 6-week exercise training program significantly improved exertional dyspnea and treadmill exercise duration as well as chronic dyspnea measured by the TDI; whereas no improvements were evident in those randomized to control (delayed treatment). Cockcroft et al. (142) randomized dyspneic patients to a treatment group (i.e., 6 weeks of exercise training) and the usual care group who received no exercise training. After 6 weeks, 2 of 16 control patients and 16 of 18 treated patients improved dyspnea, 12-min walk distance, and peak oxygen uptake. Goldstein et al. (143) showed that patients randomized to an 8-week inpatient intensive multimodality exercise program significantly improved exercise endurance (i.e., 6 MWD), dyspnea, and quality of life, whereas no significant benefits were found in untreated patients. Moreover, the improvement in exercise endurance persisted at least over the 6-month period of observation in the study.

Two recent metanalyses examined the effectiveness of pulmonary rehabilitation, including exercise training, and confirmed the clinical benefits. Lacasse et al. (144) analyzed the results of 14 randomized control trials and found significant improvements in dyspnea, exercise performance (6 MWD increased by an average of 55.7) and health-related quality-of-life indices. Cambach et al. (145) combined the results of 18 acceptable pulmonary rehabilitation studies and reported overall significantly beneficial effects in the 6 MWD and all four categories of the Chronic Respiratory Questionnaire.

Mechanisms of Improved Dyspnea Following Exercise Training

Physiological mechanisms of improved dyspnea and exercise performance are not fully understood. Mechanisms include (1) reduced ventilatory demands secondary to improved aerobic capacity or increased efficiency (146–149), (2) increased inspiratory muscle strength and endurance (146), (3) improved breathing pattern with a greater efficiency of CO_2 elimination (146,149), and (4) habituation to dyspnea or increased tolerance of dyspneogenic sensory perturbations.

Peripheral Muscle Training

Most rehabilitation programs incorporate specific strength training of the peripheral muscles. Exercise training has been shown to improve peripheral muscle function and perceived leg discomfort in both moderate and severe COPD (146–149). Measurable improvements in peripheral muscle function, including strength and endurance, have been consistently reported (147,146). Quadriceps muscle biopsies have confirmed increased aerobic enzyme

5

Role of Physiological Assessment in Advanced Interstitial Lung Disease

IDELLE M. WEISMAN

William Beaumont Army Medical Center
El Paso, and
University of Texas Health
    Science Center at San Antonio
San Antonio, Texas, U.S.A.

**JOSEPH P. LYNCH III and
FERNANDO J. MARTINEZ**

University of Michigan
Ann Arbor, Michigan, U.S.A.

Interstitial lung diseases (ILDs) are a heterogeneous group of disorders with varying histological appearances characterized by a disruption of the pulmonary parenchyma (1). Although the incidence is difficult to estimate with accuracy, Coultas and colleagues completed an epidemiological study in a New Mexico county suggesting an overall incidence of 31.5 per 100,000 in males and 26.1 per 100,000 in females (2). Importantly, pulmonary fibrosis and idiopathic pulmonary fibrosis (IPF) together accounted for 46.2% of all ILDs in males and 44.2% of those in females.

As a consequence of progressive lung destruction and increasing ventilatory, circulatory, and skeletal muscle impairment, structural and functional reserves are reduced and exercise intolerance and exertional dyspnea inexorably proceed becoming more prominent and disabling in patients with advanced interstitial lung disease. Given their important clinical consequences, this chapter reviews resting and exercise physiological assessment in patients with advanced ILD, focusing on current scientific knowledge and technical advances, emerging concepts in exercise limitation, and the clinical implications and potential applications of such assessment in patient management. The role of clinical exercise testing in functional assessment/monitoring in clinical decision analysis is also discussed.

I. Physiological Abnormalities

Physiological assessment, which includes a functional or exercise component, is increasingly utilized in clinical practice in order to optimize patient management and provide answers to questions not available from resting pulmonary function tests. Importantly, resting pulmonary and cardia function testing cannot reliably predict exercise performance and functional capacity ($\dot{V}_{O_2}$ peak) in individual patients with ILD (3–5). Furthermore, in advanced disease, pulmonary function parameters may be remarkably similar among the different disease categories. FVC, FEV_1, and total lung capacity (TLC) have been inconsistent predictors of $\dot{V}_{O_2}$max in patients with ILD. Although patient with abnormally low (<70% predicted) resting carbon monoxide diffusing capacity (DL_{CO}) are likely to experience abnormal exercise gas exchange, DL_{CO} is a poor predictor of gas exchange abnormalities during exercise in patients with ILD (3,4–6) and asbestos exposure (5). Even though exertional dyspnea is a common symptom in patients with ILD, exercise often stops due to leg discomfort, chest pain, or fatigue rather than dyspnea (7–9). Furthermore, exercise limitation in most patients is thought to be multifactorial (10–14). Importantly, resting cardiopulmonary measurements are unable to prioritize/ quantitate exercise-limiting factors important for reducing symptoms, initiating/monitoring therapeutic interventions, and potentially improving quality of life for patients with advanced ILD. Finally, subjective measures of a patient's quality of life reveal a stronger correlation with exercise tolerance than with either spirometry or oxygenation in patients with COPD (15); such information in patients with ILD remains incompletely characterized. Last, maximal exercise testing can be safely performed in the vast majority of patients (12,16,17).

Exercise testing has been felt to be uniquely well suited to the evaluation of patients with interstitial lung disease. Several clinical exercise testing modalities are available for functional assessment and include 6-min walk tests (6MWT), graded exercise testing, and cardiopulmonary exercise testing. The 6MWT is practical, simple to perform, and does not require high-tech equipment or advanced technical training (18–20). It addresses the global and integrated submaximal (and for some possibly even maximal) exercise response, but it is unable to provide specific information on the function of each contributing organ system involved in exercise and of the mechanism of exercise limitation (20). Standard cardiac exercise stress tests primarily endeavor to identify ischemic heart disease and generally cannot define underlying pathophysiology in patients with exercise intolerance of nonischemic origin (21–25). The diagnostic potential of standard exercise testing can be enhanced by the concurrent measurement of respiratory gas exchange.

Cardiopulmonary exercise testing (CPET) involves the measurement of oxygen uptake ($\dot{V}_{O_2}$), carbon dioxide output ($\dot{V}_{C_{O_2}}$), and minute ventilation ($\dot{V}_E$) in addition to monitoring 12-lead electrocardiography (ECG), blood pressure, and pulse oximetry (SpO_2) during a symptom-limited exercise tolerance test.

Measurement of arterial blood gases provides important information on pulmonary gas exchange. CPET is valuable in identifying mechanisms of exercise limitation (i.e., heart, lungs, blood, and/or skeletal muscles) and in detecting early disease. As CPET is reported to be safe in patients with pulmonary hypertension and significant arterial desaturation due to primary pulmonary hypertension, a similar safety profile would be anticipated for patients with advanced ILD (12,16,17,26). Indications for cardiopulmonary exercise testing in patients with ILD appear in Table 1.

For clinical exercise testing purposes, electronically braked cycle ergometry is preferable, although treadmill testing is an acceptable alternative if quantitation of work is not critical. Symptom-limited incremental exercise protocols with increases in work intensity of 5 to 25 W/min are widely used. Ideally, exercise should last 8 to 12 min; however, in advanced disease, it is likely that lesser durations of exercise will be achieved. Recently, constant work protocols (based on peak CPET results) have become popular, especially in assessing therapeutic interventions (7,8,27) and for corroborating pulmonary gas exchange when an arterial catheter is not an option (28). Computerized exercise systems permit an impressive number of variables to be measured during CPET (Table 2).

For patients with ILD, pulmonary gas exchange variables maybe particularly helpful, especially when tests of arterial blood gases are being performed. The reproducibility of CPET measurements in patients with ILD is generally good as assessed by Marciniuk et al., who studied six patients with ILD (three with IPF) during three maximal exercise studies over a 28-day period (29). The coefficient of variation was quite acceptable for maximal $\dot{V}_{O_2}$ (5.3%) and oxygen saturation (2.5%). The reader is referred to other sources for a more thorough evaluation of CPET methodology, equipment, and protocols (12,17,23,24) and the current approach to interpretation of CPET results (12,22).

In general, for patients with early or occult ILD, CPET is efficacious in the early detection of subtle pulmonary gas exchange abnormalities not revealed by routine testing. This is important in establishing a timely diagnosis,

Table 1 Indications for Cardiopulmonary Exercise Testing in ILD

Objective assessment of symptoms
Detection of early (occult) gas exchange abnormalities
Overall assessment/monitoring of pulmonary gas exchange
Determination of magnitude of hypoxemia and for O_2 prescription
Determination of potential exercise limiting factors
Documentation of therapeutic responses
Specific clinical applications
Exercise evaluation and prescription for pulmonary rehabilitation
Evaluation for impairment-disability
Evaluation for lung or heart-lung transplantation

Table 2 Measured and Derived Variables and Indices During Cardiopulmonary Exercise Testing

Variables[a]	Noninvasive	Invasive (ABGs)
Work	Work Rate	
Metabolic	$\dot{V}_{O_2}$, $\dot{V}_{CO_2}$, R, AT (also known as LT)	Lactate
Cardiovascular	HR, ECG, BP, O_2 pulse, $\Delta HR/\Delta \dot{V}_{O_2}$	
Ventilatory	$\dot{V}_E$, V_T, f_b, $\dot{V}_E/MVV$, IC, V_T/IC, EELV, EILV, EILV/TLC	
Pulmonary gas exchange	SpO_2, $\dot{V}_E/\dot{V}_{CO_2}$, $\dot{V}_E/\dot{V}_{O_2}$ $P_{ET}O_2$, $P_{ET}CO_2$	SaO_2, PaO_2, $PAO_2 - PaO_2$, V_D/V_T
Acid base		pH, $PaCO_2$, HCO_3^-
Symptoms	Dyspnea, leg fatigue, chest pain	

[a] Abnormality of a variable does not necessarily define exercise limitation in that category.

Key: ABGs, arterial blood gases; $\dot{V}_{O_2}$, oxygen uptake; $\dot{V}_{CO_2}$, carbon dioxide output; R, respiratory exchange ratio; AT, anaerobic threshold; LT, lactate threshold; hr, heart rate; ECG, electrocardiogram; BP, blood pressure; O_2 pulse, oxygen pulse; $\dot{V}_E$, expired minute ventilation; V_T, tidal volume; f_b, breathing frequency; $\dot{V}_E/MVV$, ventilatory reserve; $P_{ET}O_2$, end-tidal pressure of oxygen; $P_{ET}CO_2$, end-tidal pressure of carbon dioxide; IC, inspiratory capacity; V_T/IC, ratio of tidal volume to inspiratory capacity; EELV, end-expiratory lung volume; EILV, end-inspiratory lung volume; SpO_2, pulse oximetry; $\dot{V}_E/\dot{V}_{CO_2}$, ventilatory equivalent for carbon dioxide; $\dot{V}_E/\dot{V}_{O_2}$, ventilatory equivalent for oxygen; SaO_2, arterial oxygen saturation; PaO_2, arterial oxygen tension; $PAO_2 - PaO_2$, alveolar-arterial oxygen pressure difference; V_D/V_T, ratio of physiological dead space to tidal volume; pH, hydrogen ion concentration; $PaCO_2$, arterial carbon dioxide tension; HCO_3^-, bicarbonate.

Source: Modified from Ref. 11.

accurate physiological severity assessment, as well as permitting the monitoring of therapeutic interventions (3,4,6,30–37). Whether CPET, in particular exercise pulmonary gas exchange, has prognostic value for IPF is controversial and requires additional investigation (38,39).

The role of CPET in evaluating patients with interstitial lung disease for pulmonary rehabilitation and for patient selection/monitoring pre-and post–lung transplantation remains incompletely characterized and underutilized in patients with ILD and requires additional prospective evaluation. Currently, both the 6MWT and CPET are used for functional assessment. A 6MWT is a useful tool in the assessment of when to list patients for transplantation, with 6MWD < 400 m predicting death with a sensitivity of 0.80, specificity of 0.27, positive predictive value of 0.27, and negative predictive value of 0.91 (40). The six minute walk distance and SpO_2 desaturation but not exertional dyspnea correlated with baseline lung function variables using stepwise multiple regression analysis in 40 patients with ILD (41). Recent work in patients with primary pulmonary hypertension has confirmed that reductions in $\dot{V}_{O_2}$ peak reflect reduced cardiac output and functional capacity and that CPET and 6MWT test provide complementary information in the evaluation of these patients (26).

Whether a 6MWT and/or CPET should be used depends on the questions being asked and the available resources; both provide complementary albeit different information (11,12,20). It is likely that 6MWT results will *not* replace CPET in circumstances in which information not available from 6MWT results is necessary for clinical decision making. This includes determination of etiology of exercise limitation, need for an individualized exercise prescription (for pulmonary rehabilitation prior to transplantation), system-based monitoring of therapeutic interventions including effect(s) of pulmonary rehabilitation and transplantation, and gauging capacity for physical work, which are important for disability impairment evaluation. In general, 6MWT results are too imprecise under these circumstances, as recently noted in clinical commentary on 6MWT in cardiac patients (42). Additional prospective evaluation in patients with ILD is required.

A. Pathophysiology

The majority of ILDs share common physiological abnormalities (43) (Table 3).

A restrictive ventilatory defect is typically reflected by a downward and rightward shift of the static expiratory pressure-volume curve. The lung recoil is increased over the range of the inspiratory capacity with a reduction of total lung capacity (TLC) and vital capacity (44–46); the coefficient of retraction (pleural pressure at TLC/lung volume at TLC) is elevated compared to normal subjects (30,44). The mechanisms for these changes in compliance are multifactorial and include loss of lung volume (46–49), reduced alveolar distensibility (47,50–54), reduced alveolar size (50,55), and increased surface tension due to abnormalities of surfactant (56,57).

Table 3 Patterns of Physiological Abnormalities in Selected Interstitial Lung Diseases

Disease	FVC	FEV$_1$/FVC	DL$_{CO}$	TLC	Exercise P(A−a)$_{O_2}$
Idiopathic pulmonary fibrosis	↓ ↔	↑ ↔	↓	↓ ↔	↑ ↑
Connective tissue disease	↓ ↑ ↔	↑ ↔ ↓	↓	↓ ↔	↑ ↔
Sarcoidosis	↓ ↔	↑ ↔ ↓	↓ ↔	↓ ↔	↑ ↔
Langerhans cell histiocytosis	↓ ↔	↑ ↔ ↓	↓	↔ ↑	↑

Key: FVC = forced vital capacity; FEV$_1$, forced expiratory volume in 1 sec; DL$_{CO}$ diffusing capacity; TLC, total lung capacity; P(A−a)$_{O_2}$, alveolar–arterial oxygen tension gradient. ↑, increase; ↓, decrease; ↔, remain the same.
Source: Ref. 401.

B. Flows and Lung Volumes

Typically static lung volumes are reduced in ILDs. The vital capacity (VC) is reduced to a greater extent than the functional residual capacity (FRC) (43). In compiling data from several reported series, Gottlieb and Snider reported a mean reduction in FRC to 79% predicted compared with a reduction in VC to 63% and TLC to 72% predicted (58). Both the tidal volume and inspiratory capacity are reduced, with the ratio of V_T to IC (V_T/IC) increased compared to normal subjects (8) (Fig. 1). The TLC, determined by the balance between lung and chest wall recoil and inspiratory muscle strength, is usually less severely affected due to the normal or near normal chest wall recoil and the preserved inspiratory muscle function in most patients (51,58,59). The residual volume (RV) is well preserved in most cases and the RV/TLC ratio is frequently increased (58,60–65). Airway function, defined by spirometric measurements, is usually well preserved in ILD, although airflow obstruction may be frequent in sarcoidosis (66–79) and rheumatoid arthritis (80–82). Conflicting reports using more sophisticated testing have been published regarding small airway

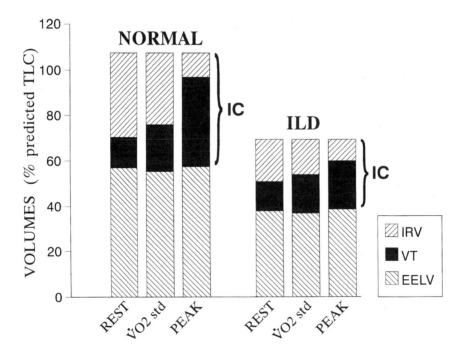

Figure 1 Operational lung volumes at rest at a standardized $\dot{V}_{O_2}$ of 50% predicted maximum ($\dot{V}_{O_2}$max), and at peak exercise in normal subjects and in patients with ILD. Values are mean ± SE. TLC, total lung capacity; IRV, inspiratory reserve volume; EELV, end-expiratory lung volume. Inspiratory capacity (IC) is significantly reduced in patients with ILD ($p < 0.01$). (From Ref. 8.)

function (65,83,84). Unfortunately, the abnormalities are not specific and the magnitude of the changes varies widely from patient to patient.

Two groups have described atypical physiological presentations in patients with IPF with preserved lung volumes (85,86). Cherniack and colleagues confirmed a higher FVC and TLC in smokers than never smokers (85). Similarly, Doherty et al. examined a group of 48 patients with cryptogenic fibrosing alveolitis, of which 21 demonstrated a normal VC ($>80\%$ predicted)(86). Those with preserved VC were more likely to be male (76 versus 48%) current smokers (57 versus 22%) and to have a heavier lifetime history of cigarette smoking (38 versus 25 pack-years). The TLC was also significantly higher in the group with preserved VC (90.1 versus 64.7% predicted). Importantly, there was no difference in prognosis or treatment between the two groups; high-resolution computed tomography (HRCT) confirmed a similar degree of pulmonary fibrosis in the two groups, although concomitant emphysema was much more likely in the group with a preserved VC (86 versus 19%). It is evident that superimposed smoking can alter the typical physiological presentation of IPF.

C. Gas Exchange

Diffusing capacity (DL_{CO}) is typically reduced in ILD to a greater extent than the lung volume at which it is measured (65). In addition, the diffusing capacity appears to be decreased to a greater extent with IPF than for other ILDs (4,87). For example, Dunn et al. noted a DL_{CO} of 45% predicted in 21 patients with IPF compared with 79% predicted in 20 patients with sarcoidosis, despite similar lung volumes (87). A similar difference was noted in DL_{CO}/alveolar volume (VA) (54 versus 97% predicted).

D. Exercise Capacity

Exercise Limitation

Many factors contribute to exercise limitation in patients with advanced ILD (Table 4). Current scientific knowledge appreciates that exercise limitation or low $\dot{V}_{O_2}$max achieved in patients with advanced respiratory illness is complex, usually multifactorial, and as such not limited by any single component of the O_2 transport/utilization process but rather by their collective quantitative interaction (12). Although several factors may be involved, one factor often predominates, possibly because of its multisystem impact (i.e., hypoxemia) with variable contributions to exercise intolerance from the other factors. Presently, the magnitude of each factor's relative contribution to exercise intolerance in patients with advanced ILD remains incompletely characterized.

Multiple factors contribute to the increased ventilatory requirement during exercise in patients with advanced ILD (Table 5). Importantly, whereas ventilatory constraint(s) (limitation) have traditionally been thought to be primarily exercise-limiting in patients with ILD, recent work has suggested that

Table 4   Mechanisms of Exercise Limitation in Advanced ILD

Respiratory
   Pulmonary gas exchange impairment
   Arterial hypoxemia
   Inefficient ventilation
   Increased dead-space ventilation
   Ventilatory mechanical dysfunction
   Respiratory muscle dysfunction
Circulatory
   Reduced stroke volume
   Abnormal heart rate response
   Abnormal pulmonary (pulmonary hypertension) and systemic circulation
   Hemodynamic consequences of increased intrapleural pressures
   Abnormal blood (anemia, carboxyhemglobin)
Peripheral factors
   Skeletal muscle dysfunction
   Neuromuscular dysfunction
   Peripheral circulatory abnormalities
Malnutrition, medication effects
Deconditioning
Perceptual symptoms
   Dyspnea, leg fatigue, generalized fatigue
Environmental
Motivation, psychosocial effects

Exercise limitation is multifactorial

Source: Adapted from Ref. 22.

Table 5   Factors Contributing to Increased Ventilatory Requirements During Exercise in Patients with Advanced ILD

Increased dead-space ventilation (V_D/V_T)
Inefficient ventilation
Hypoxemia
Early-onset metabolic acidosis
Pulmonary hypertension
Nonchemical stimuli (lung receptors)
Increased central drive

---

hypoxemia, not respiratory mechanics, appears to be the predominant factor contributing to exercise limitation during incremental exercise (27,88). In the first of two noteworthy studies, supplemental O_2 (60%) was administered to 7 patients with ILD and impaired room air exercise performance manifested by ↓ $\dot{V}_{O_2}$ peak, ↓ peak work rate, and SaO_2 ↓ 11%. Supplemental O_2 sufficient to prevent arterial desaturation resulted in significant improvement in exercise performance ($\uparrow \dot{V}_{O_2}$ peak, $\uparrow$ peak work, $\uparrow$ anaerobic threshold), which the authors suggested, most likely resulted from increasing O_2 delivery to exercising muscles. Also, despite improvement of mean $\dot{V}_{O_2}$ peak by about 20% with supplemental O_2, $\dot{V}_{O_2}$ peak was still only 67% of predicted, suggesting that other factors were involved and presumably that exercise limitation was multifactorial.

A subsequent study that evaluated the impact of supplemental O_2 (60%) and added dead space in 7 patients with ILD corroborated that hypoxemia and not mechanics limits exercise in ILD (88). Additionally, exercise tidal flow-volume loop analysis of 7 patients with ILD has also suggested that respiratory mechanics were not the cause of exercise limitation (7) (see "Exercise Ventilatory Mechanics," below). However, a cautionary note is offered. From a clinical perspective, some patients with ILD, perhaps early in their disease or with different subtypes, appear predominantly ventilatory-limited (12)(see case #4 of Ref. 12). Whether these patients will develop circulatory limitation as hypoxemia continues due to progressive parenchymal and vascular destruction remains unknown. Current knowledge would suggest that despite the excessive respiratory muscle function burden associated with advanced ILD, respiratory muscle fatigue, if present, is apparently not an important factor in exercise limitation (27,88–90).

A recent provocative retrospective analysis of 42 patients with ILD suggested that exercise limitation is primarily due to pulmonary circulatory pathophysiology rather than ventilatory mechanics. (91). Reduced peak $\dot{V}_{O_2}$ values were more often due to pulmonary vascular disease than impaired ventilatory mechanics, as measured during incremental exercise. The degree of circulatory dysfunction was proportional to the severity of underlying lung disease. Although based on suboptimal data analysis, the pathophysiological discussion highlighting the importance of impaired O_2 transport in exercise limitation in patients with ILD is attractive (91), especially when coupled with the data from the hypoxemia/supplemental O_2 studies cited previously (27,88). It is possible that the improvement in peak $\dot{V}_{O_2}$ with supplemental O_2 is partly due to improvement in pulmonary hemodynamics or cardiovascular function, as evidenced by the improvement in peak $\dot{V}_{O_2}$ being strongly correlated with resting DL_{CO} (27). Prospective studies designed to answer questions of circulatory dysfunction as the predominant exercise-limiting factor in ILD are required. These studies should include analysis of ILD subtypes, including the impact of disease severity and progression. (Can patients present as ventilatory-or combined ventilatory/circulatory-limited and progress to circulatory-limited, or do patients usually remain circulatory-limited? Are outcomes different for those who are circulatory-limited versus ventilatory limited?)

Abnormal symptom perception (especially breathlessness, leg/general fatigue, etc.) is an important stated cause of exercise cessation in patients with advanced ILD (see "Dyspnea," below). This may be associated with apparent nonphysiological limitation to exercise ($\dot{V}_E/MMV < 85\%$, peak heart rate $< 85\%$ or 15 beats). Evaluating submaximal trending of exercise responses, especially heart rate responses (see "Cardiovascular Abnormalities," below), in this challenging scenario can be helpful. Deconditioning, peripheral muscle dysfunction, and nutritional status (12,92–94) are increasingly recognized to be important cocontributors to exercise limitation in patients with chronic lung disease, including patients with advanced ILD. A vicious cycle of (progressive) symptoms, especially dyspnea and fatigue, leads to a reduction in physical activity and increasing deconditioning. This is compounded by episodes of decompensation often requiring steroids, weight loss, malnutrition, loss of muscle mass, and consequent skeletal muscle dysfunction and mental depression. Although an extensive and expanding database on theses topics are available for patients with chronic heart failure and chronic obstructive pulmonary disease (COPD), because of similarities due to chronic respiratory illness, application to patients with advanced ILD may also be possible. Additional work is required.

Typical Exercise Responses in Patients with Advanced ILD

Although underlying etiology may vary, functional physiological assessment in patients with advanced ILD reveals common pathophysiological character-istics usually associated with severe often end-stage lung disease and its adverse multisystem impact. This is in contrast to functional ILD assessment performed at an earlier stage, in which a spectrum of respiratory (restrictive mechanical and pulmonary gas exchange) and cardiovascular abnormalities may be observed; whether the predominance of any particular pattern reflects differences in disease severity and/or ILD subtypes (see below) is unknown. Typical CPET responses in patients with advanced ILD appear in Table 6. An illustrative case study including tabular and graphic data appear in Table 7 and Figure 2, respectively.

Patients with advanced ILD exhibit reduced maximal or peak aerobic capacity ($\dot{V}_{O_2}$ peak), maximal work rate (WR_{peak}), and submaximal exercise endurance compared to age-and sex-matched normal subjects (3,29,32,95–97). The reduction in aerobic capacity ($\dot{V}_{O_2}$ max) is related to resting pulmonary function, including FEV_1 (% predicted), total lung capacity (% predicted), and DL_{CO} (% predicted) and can be useful for disability (functional capacity to perform physical work) assessment in patients with advanced ILD (32,98). Resting DL_{CO} may be the best correlate of $\dot{V}_{O_2}$ max in patients with ILD ($r = 0.76$, $p < 0.001$) (91). However, despite significant correlation between these resting indices and $\dot{V}_{O_2}$ max, results of routine pulmonary function testing alone may not be sufficiently reliable in predicting or quantitating exercise responses, exercise limitation, or disability in the individual patient, as noted previously (3,99–103). This may be particularly important in patients with nonventilatory reasons for stopping exercise (104).

Table 6 Typical CPET Responses in Advanced ILD[a]

Symptoms: dyspnea, leg discomfort, generalized fatigue
↓ Aerobic capacity ($\dot{V}_{O_2}$) peak, ↓ work
↓ Anaerobic threshold (AT)
Abnormal pulmonary gas exchange
    ↑ $\dot{V}_E/\dot{V}_{CO_2}$ and ↑ $\dot{V}_E/\dot{V}_{O_2}$ responses
    ↓ Pa_{O_2}, ↑ P_AO_2–PaO_2, ↓ Sa_{O_2}
    ↑/↔ V_D/V_T responses
    ↔ $PaCO_2$ and ↔ $P_{ET}CO_2$
Abnormal cardiovascular responses
    ↓ Peak heart rate, ↑ HR at submaximal $\dot{V}_{O_2}$ (abnormal HR-$\dot{V}_{O_2}$) relationship,
    $\Delta HR/\Delta \dot{V}_{O_2} > 50$
    ↓ O_2 pulse
    ECG abnormalities: RVH, RAE, RAD, RBBB
Abnormal ventilatory responses
    ↓ $\dot{V}_E$ peak, ↑ submaximal $\dot{V}_E$ (abnormal $\dot{V}_E$ versus $\dot{V}_{O_2}$ and $\dot{V}_E$ versus $\dot{V}_{CO_2}$
    relationships)
    Normal or ↑ $\dot{V}_E$/MVV (no ventilatory reserve)
    ↓ V_T, ↑ f_b, (or blunted V_T response)
    ↓ IC, ↑ V_T/IC, ↔ EELV, ↑ EILV/TLC

Key: CPET, cardiopulmonary exercise testing; ILD, interstitial lung diseases; ↑, increase; ↓, decrease; ↔, remain the same; RVH, right ventricular hypertrophy; RAE, right atrial enlargement; RAD, right axis deviation; RBBB, right bundle branch block.
[a] See text for discussion.

Table 7 Maximal Cardiopulmonary Incremental Exercise Test in a Patient with Biopsy-Proven Interstital Pulmonary Fibrosis

JH, 56-year-old Caucasian Male. Height, 175 cm; Weight, 83 kg; Diagnosis: biopsy proven IPF. FVC, L 3.02 (66%) FEV1, L 2.59 (40%); DLCO, mL/min/mmHg, 15.48 (53%); TLC, L 4.53 (67%); MVV calc, L/min 141 (40x FEV$_1$). Reason for testing: Evaluation for exercise intolerance, progressive exertional dyspnea, and desaturation. Protocol: 20 w/min incremental cycle ergometry to volitional exhaustion.

Variable	Peak	% Predicted	Variable	Rest	Peak
Work rate (W)	140	68%	SaO_2, %	94%	85%
$\dot{V}_{O_2}$, L/min	1.34	55%	SpO_2, %	96%	86%
AT, L/min	0.94	(38%)[a]>0.97	PaO_2, mmHg	84	56
$\Delta \dot{V}_{O_2}/\Delta WR$ L/min/w	6.8	N (>8.29)	$PaCO_2$, mmHg	40	38
HR, bpm	145	83%	pH	7.40	7.34
$\Delta HR/\Delta \dot{V}_{O_2}$ bpm/L/min	72	<50	$P_AO_2 - P_aO_2$, mmHg	5	55
O_2 pulse, mL/beat	9.2	66%	V_D/V_T	0.51	0.53
$\dot{V}_E$, L/min	83	59%[b]			
f_b, br/min	47	<60	**Stop:** fatigue 10/10 (BORG		
$\dot{V}_E/\dot{V}_{CO_2}$, at AT	45	<34	Scale)		
RER	1.10				

[a] AT as percent of $\dot{V}_{O_2}$ peak predicted.
[b] $\dot{V}_E$ peak/MVV (%).

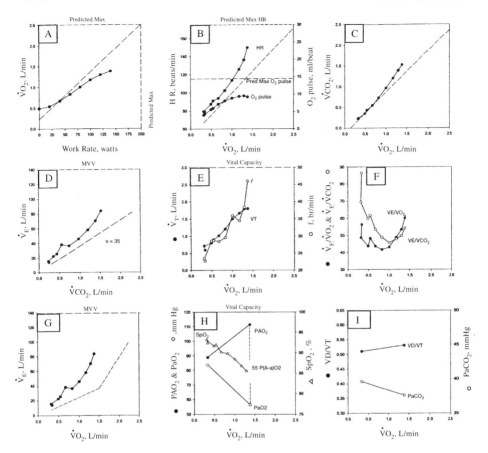

Figure 2 J.H.—Graphic representation of a maximal, incremental cardiopulmonary exercise test in a subject with biopsy-proven interstitial pulmonary fibrosis. These graphic data are 1-minute interval averaged. The results are compared with calculated reference values obtained from several sources (dashed lines). (A) Plot oxygen uptake ($\dot{V}_{O_2}$) versus work rate reveals a reduced aerobic capacity ($\dot{V}_{O_2}$ peak), work rate (W), and markedly abnormal $\dot{V}_{O_2}$-WR relationship: (B) Plot of heart rate (HR) versus $\dot{V}_{O_2}$ reveals a hypercirculatory pattern ($\uparrow\Delta HR/\Delta\dot{V}_{O_2}=72$, normal <50), evidenced by elevated HR responses at submaximal levels of $\dot{V}_{O_2}$. The control population for this ILD cohort group achieved a maximal HR = 82% predicted. This patient achieved HR = 83% predicted, suggesting apparent physiological (circulatory) limitation. The O_2 pulse was reduced. (C) Plot of $\dot{V}_{CO_2}$ (carbon dioxide production) versus $\dot{V}_{O_2}$ (modified V-slope) reveals a low anaerobic threshold; (D) Plot of minute ventilation ($\dot{V}_E$) versus carbon dioxide output ($\dot{V}_{CO_2}$) demonstrates an abnormal slope (lower 95% CI < 34) with significant ventilatory reserve at peak exercise. (E) A blunted tidal volume (V_T) increase and increased respiratory frequency (f) versus $\dot{V}_{O_2}$ reveals a rapid shallow breathing pattern, (F) Ventilatory equivalents for O_2 ($\dot{V}_E/\dot{V}_{O_2}$) and CO_2 ($\dot{V}_E/\dot{V}_{CO_2}$) versus $\dot{V}_{O_2}$ are abnormally high throughout exercise, reflecting inefficient ventilation due mostly to increased dead-space ventilation. (G) Minute ventilation ($\dot{V}_E$) versus $\dot{V}_{O_2}$ demonstrates a hyperventilatory response and significant ventilatory reserve at peak exercise. (H)

Exercise Ventilatory Mechanics

The impaired resting ventilatory mechanics (reduced operational lung volumes/ capacities, increased elastic recoil at FRC, and reduced compliance—all reflections of abnormal pressure-volume relationships) exacerbate respiratory demand–capacity relationships during exercise (24,105,106).

Demand Versus Capacity

Factors contributing to the increased ventilatory demand during exercise in patients with advanced ILD include increased ventilatory requirements (Table 5) associated with the increased metabolic demand as well as body weight, mode of testing, etc. (107). These factors are responsible for the marked increase in submaximal minute ventilation (abnormal $\dot{V}_E$–$\dot{V}_{O_2}$ relationship), but with reduced maximal minute ventilation (Figs. 2 and 3b). Ventilatory capacity estimated from direct measurement of the MVV or calculated (FEV$_1$ 40) is reduced mostly due to abnormal ventilatory mechanics but may also be affected by ventilatory muscle function, genetics, aging, and the multisystem impact of chronic disease (94,107,108). Mechanical ventilatory limitation ($\dot{V}_{Emax}$ approaching or exceeding ventilatory capacity) may or may not occur, with the latter more likely in patients with advanced ILD, especially IPF (7,27,88,109). Consequently, the ventilatory reserve, an index of ventilatory demand ($\dot{V}_{Emax}$) to ventilatory capacity (MVV), may be reduced (high V_E/ MVV) or normal. Interestingly, in patients with sarcoidosis, the ventilatory reserve is often reduced, especially in patients with higher radiographic stages of disease (110), in those with symptoms (111), and in those with poorer pulmonary function (112).

Exercise Tidal Flow–Volume Loop Analysis, Negative Expiratory Technique

Alternatively, exercise tidal flow–volume loop analysis provides a visual index of ventilatory constraint by aligning (for comparison) flow-volume loops obtained during exercise with maximal resting flow–volume loops (extFVL/ MFVL) (107,113). The volume and flow-rate differences between the exercise tidal flow – volume loop and MFVL curve maybe useful for determining

---

Arterial O_2 tension (PaO_2), alveolar–arterial O_2 gradient difference PA_{O_2}–Pa_{O_2}, SpO_2, and SaO_2 versus $\dot{V}_{O_2}$ demonstrates no hypoxemia, normal PA_{O_2}–Pa_{O_2}, SpO_2, and SaO_2 at rest with hypoxemia ($\Delta PaO_2 = \downarrow 28$ mmHg), an abnormally widened PA_{O_2}–Pa_{O_2} ($\uparrow$ to 55 mmHg, normal <35 mmHg) and significant desaturation ($SpO_2 \downarrow \Delta 10$ mmHg decreasing throughout exercise) and at peak exercise. (I) Physiological dead space to tidal volume ratio (V_D/V_T) and arterial C_{O_2} tension ($PaCO_2$) versus $\dot{V}_{O_2}$ reveals an abnormal increase in V_D/V_T from rest to exercise and a Pa_{CO_2} response that is only slightly changed. Consequently, the acid-base status at peak exercise reveals a metabolic acidosis without the appropriate respiratory compensation. Exercise stopped due to fatigue 10/10 (Borg scale).

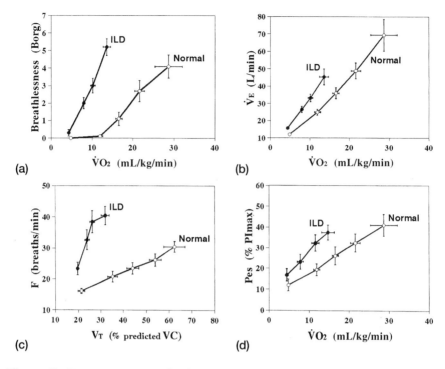

Figure 3 Responses to exercise in normal subjects and patients with ILD. (a) Dyspnea. (b) Minute ventilation ($\dot{V}_E$). (c) Breathing pattern [breathing frequency (f)]. (d) Esophageal pressure (Pes). Values are means $\pm$SE. Borg, Borg scale; $\dot{V}_{O_2}$, O_2 uptake; V_T, tidal volume; PI_{max}, maximal inspiratory pressure. Pes measurements were obtained in only 8 of 12 patients with ILD. All slopes are significantly greater (p, 0.05) in patients with ILD than in normal subjects. (From Ref. 8.)

ventilatory limitation (constraint). A recent study of seven patients with ILD using exercise tidal flow–volume loop analysis revealed that patients were not breathing near their maximal ventilatory capacity and that respiratory mechanics were not exercise-limiting (7). Interestingly, patients who stop exercise due to dyspnea ($n = 4$) experience significant expiratory flow limitation, increased EELV (see below), abnormal inspiratory flow loops, and less arterial desaturation compared to those who stop due to leg fatigue ($n = 3$) (Fig. 4) (7). This implies that expiratory flow limitation in some ILD patients contributes to the dyspnea of exercise, although additional studies would be necessary to corroborate these findings (7). However, using the negative expiratory pressure (NEP) technique, in which a negative pressure (5–10 cm) at the mouth is applied during expiration and then determining whether ventilation increases, failed to show evidence of obstruction when applied in patients with ILD (114).

Because of lung volume constraints on V_T expansion, patients with advanced ILD exhibit a rapid shallow breathing pattern during exercise, with

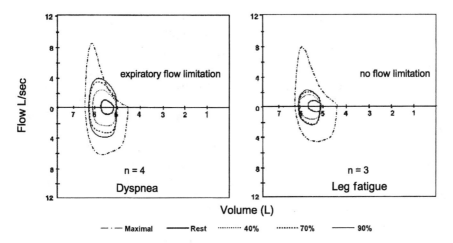

Figure 4 Maximal and exercise tidal flow-volume loops in patients with ILD. Left: Patients who stopped secondary to dyspnea. Right: Patients who stopped due to leg fatigue. Minimal change was observed in EELV in both groups, with the group complaining of dyspnea demonstrating significant expiratory flow limitation. (From Ref. 7.)

increases in minute ventilation achieved mostly by increases in respiratory frequency, with low V_T and minimal changes in end-expiratory lung volume (EELV) (TLC-IC = EELV) compared to normal subjects (7,8,95,116) (Figs. 1, and 3c). Usually, V_T increases during exercise by encroaching upon IRV and ERV, resulting in increases in end-inspiratory lung volume (EILV) and decreases in EELV, respectively (7,8,117) (Fig. 1). As a result of increased elastic recoil at FRC, ERV is reduced and the blunted V_T increase occurs through encroachment on IRV. Consequently, V_T represents a greater percentage of a blunted IC increase (V_T/IC) from rest and compared to normal subjects (7,8) (Fig. 1). The IC as an index of operational lung volumes during exercise can be measured utilizing either spirometry or exercise tidal flow volume loop–maximal flow-volume loop analysis (7,107,117). Peak V_T/VC is usually although not invariably normal (118,119). Abnormal lung mechanics and the increased elastic load associated with lung fibrosis (120) as well as increased afferent reflexes originating from the lung and/or chest wall have been suggested as the reasons for increased respiratory drive and consequent increased ventilatory requirements seen in these patients (121) (Table 5).

The rapid shallow breathing strategy during exercise correlates with disease severity (120,122) and may contribute to the impressive exertional dyspnea that patients with ILD experience by breathing at a higher lung volume (↑ EILV/TLC), thereby increasing the elastic work of the respiratory muscles (7,8); it may minimize the work of breathing by possibly enabling the respiratory muscles to maintain force development without (diaphragmatic) fatigue (95), and does not appear to be significantly affected by morphine administration (123) or by supplemental O_2 administration (27,88).

Finally, it is well appreciated that at rest, patients with ILD adapt a rapid shallow breathing pattern, as normal subjects do not. This is thought to be due to the combined influences of altered mechanical constraints and increased central output from the respiratory controller for CO_2, thereby avoiding hypercapnia and excessive dead space ventilation; thus it minimizes respiratory effort and reduces dyspnea. The impact of departing from this pattern and whether patients with restrictive lung disease can do it volitionally—and, furthermore, what the effects on dyspnea would be—was addressed in a recent well-designed study (124). In that study, breathing pattern was nonobstructively monitored over 1 hr in 10 patients with restrictive lung disease and 7 controls and then, on a separate day, dyspnea was monitored (Borg scale) while all subjects copied different tidal volumes and respiratory frequencies. Small variations from average resting tidal volume caused marked increases in dyspnea in patients, and the relationship was parabolic ($r^2 = 0.97$; $p < 0.001$), demonstrating that patients with restrictive lung disease adopt a rather monotonous (tightly constrained) breathing pattern, probably as a deliberate strategy to avoid dyspnea (124). This is consistent with what is observed during exercise.

Pulmonary Gas Exchange

Patients with advanced ILD will usually have resting hypoxemia and a widened P_AO_2–PaO_2, which is exacerbated during exercise, with consequent impressive arterial desaturation, reduced Pa_{O_2}, and abnormal increases in P_AO_2–PaO_2 observed (3,4,6,32,125,126). Multiple mechanisms—including ventilation perfusion ($\dot{V}/\dot{Q}$) mismatching, O_2 diffusion limitation, and low mixed venous PO_2—have been shown to contribute to the abnormally increased (P_AO_2–PaO_2) (125,127,128). Whereas earlier explanation emphasized diffusion limitation for the "alveolar-capillary block syndrome" (129), current understanding based on the multiple inert gas exchange technique emphasizes the importance of $\dot{V}/\dot{Q}$ mismatching and quantifies the contribution of limited O_2 diffusion to (P_AO_2–PaO_2) at rest at 19%, increasing to only 40% with exercise (125). Earlier work had reported 30% with exercise (127).

$\dot{V}/\dot{Q}$ mismatching results from pulmonary vascular involvement and is clinically manifest by two patterns: high $\dot{V}/\dot{Q}$ mismatch, associated with capillary destruction and consequent increased V_D/V_T, and inefficient ventilation ($\dot{V}_E/\dot{V}_{CO_2}$) or low $\dot{V}/\dot{Q}$ mismatch, resulting from rapid transit times through unaffected areas ("shunt-like effects"), with reduced PaO_2 and widened (P_AO_2–PaO_2). Although high $\dot{V}/\dot{Q}$ abnormalities occur more commonly and correlate better with $\dot{V}_{O_2}$max, most patients with ILD (65%) possess both high and low $\dot{V}/\dot{Q}$ abnormalities (91). Hypoxemia in patients with ILD may also be a consequence of right-to-left intracardiac shunting through a patent foramen ovale resulting from increased right-sided heart pressures (23).

Exercise P_AO_2–PaO_2 has been reported to best correlate with histological index in patients with pneumoconiosis and or interstitial pneumonia (130) and to correlate strongly with cellularity and fibrosis in patients with IPF when resting and peak exercise Pa_{O_2} did not (30). The increase in (P_AO_2–PaO_2) with exercise in IPF has also been shown to correlate with DL_{CO} and $DL/\dot{V}A$ (% predicted) (38). In another study of 15 patients with IPF, $DL/\dot{V}A$ (% predicted) correlated with extent of $\dot{V}/\dot{Q}$ mismatching, extent of O_2 diffusion limitation, and exercise P_AO_2–PaO_2 (125). Interestingly, in that study, patients with higher vascular tone (as determined by supplemental O_2 breathing release from hypoxic vasoconstriction) demonstrated better overall $\dot{V}/\dot{Q}$ matching, as has previously been reported in patients with primary pulmonary hypertension (131). The clinical implications, as speculated by the authors, were that patients with early IPF and less anatomic derangement of the pulmonary vasculature would be more capable of adjusting $\dot{V}/\dot{Q}$ matching to maintain normal or near normal Pa_{O_2}, whereas in more advanced disease (greater fibrosis), the pulmonary circulation progressively loses this ability as pulmonary hypertension develops, with consequent marked worsening of pulmonary gas exchange; furthermore, the impact of a worsening $\dot{V}/\dot{Q}$ during exercise would be amplified because of the greater fall in mixed venous Pa_{O_2}, shorter transit times, and shorter residence time for O_2 equilibrium (125).

Exercise arterial desaturation has been shown to correlate with resting DL_{CO} measurements in patients with ILD (132). Although the prediction of exercise desaturation from resting DL_{CO} measurements in patients with ILD may not be consistently reliable (6,133,134), patients with DL_{CO} below 70% are more likely to desaturate (6). When DL_{CO} is less than 50% predicted, patients are more likely to develop pulmonary hypertension and an abnormally widened P_AO_2–PaO_2 during exercise (64). Cor pulmonale usually occurs with $DL_{CO} < 30\%$. The exercise impairment reported in patients with Langerhans cell granulomatosis is purportedly due to pulmonary vascular dysfunction and is reflected in resting DL_{CO} correlating with $\dot{V}_{O_2}max$, W_{max}, P_AO_2–PaO_2 and V_D/V_T exercise responses (135).

Exercise-induced hypoxemia may impair performance not only by increasing ventilatory requirements with consequent abnormal ventilatory and dyspnea responses (see "Dyspnea," below) but perhaps also by adversely impacting myocardial and circulatory function during exercise. Several mechanisms have been proposed (see "Cardiovascular Abnormalities" and "Exercise Limitation," below). These include the following:

1. Reduction of O_2 transport via hypoxic vasoconstriction (and the attendant increase in right ventricular afterload), resulting in a reduction in right ventricular ejection fraction) (136). Consequently, right ventricular end-diastolic volume increases and the interventricular septum abnormally shifts leftward—impacting left ventricular compliance, diastolic filling, myocardial contractility, left ventricular stroke volume and thereby reducing cardiac output.

This phenomenon is thought due to ventricular interdependence and has been reported in patients with right ventricular pressure and volume overload (137).

2. Hypoxemia during exercise significantly correlates with pulmonary hypertension (138,139) and purportedly exacerbates resting pulmonary hypertension, thus increasing morbidity in patients with ILD (139–141).
3. Exercise-induced hypoxemia lowers the O_2 content of blood, thereby reducing oxygen pulse and $\dot{V}_{O_2}$max.
4. Patients with exercise-induced hypoxemia may experience an additional cardiac stress as hypoxia increases heart rate, supposedly through the stimulation of circulating catecholamines (142), thereby increasing the possibility of myocardial ischemia.

Supplemental O_2 breathing has been suggested for relieving myocardial ischemia and improving exercise performance in patients with exercise-induced hypoxemia (143). The major functional consequence of arterial hypoxemia during exercise in patients with advanced ILD is that it may result in reduced O_2 transport to exercising muscles (32,140,144,145) and to the heart (143). The impressive improvement in exercise performance with supplemental O_2 breathing suggests that arterial hypoxemia and, in turn, reduced O_2 transport to exercising muscles are major contributing factors to exercise limitation in patients with ILD (see "Exercise Limitation," above (27)).

Inefficient Ventilation

The ventilatory equivalent for $\dot{V}_{CO_2}$ ($\dot{V}_E/\dot{V}_{CO_2}$) is a good noninvasive estimator of efficiency of ventilation. Inefficient ventilation manifested by increased $\dot{V}_E/\dot{V}_{CO_2}$ responses due primarily to increased V_D/V_T and excessive ventilation due to hypoxemia and mechanoreceptor stimulation are usually observed throughout exercise and contribute to the increased ventilatory requirement associated with advanced ILD (Table 5). Failure of V_D/V_T responses to decrease normally with exercise is anticipated; usually, V_D/V_T either remains the same or increases as a reflection of severe $\dot{V}/\dot{Q}$ mismatching (21,23,24,32,38,125). V_D/V_T determined noninvasively using $P_{ET}CO_2$ yields unreliable results (146). The $PaCO_2$ usually remains unchanged from rest but may increase or decrease (32). Consequently, the acid-base status at peak exercise often reveals a mixed disturbance: metabolic acidosis without the appropriate respiratory compensation or metabolic acidosis and metabolic alkalosis (see illustrative case study, Table 7, Fig. 2).

Cardiovascular Abnormalities

Cardiovascular abnormalities during exercise are common and reflect predominantly pulmonary vascular and right ventricular dysfunction, but they may also include left ventricular dysfunction. The development of pathological circulatory limitation may depend on several factors, including specific ILD entity, severity of underlying pulmonary parenchymal and pulmonary vascular involvement, the time course of disease progression—including pulmonary hypertension—and ultimately the heart's inability to maintain adequate cardiac output in the face of increased pulmonary hypertension, progressive hypoxemia, and worsening mechanical derangement. Pulmonary hypertension is common in advanced ILD, present both at rest and during exercise and reflecting usually severe disease. Consequently, the elevation of pulmonary artery pressures with exercise can be impressive despite the administration of supplemental O_2 (142,147). Because of ventricular interdependence, patients with severe pulmonary disease and pulmonary hypertension manifest reduced right ventricular ejection fraction and abnormal leftward bowing of the interventricular septum, resulting in reduced left ventri cular ejection fraction, which may improve with transplantation (137,148).

The $HR-\dot{V}_{O_2}$ relationship reveals higher HR values at rest and at submaximal levels of $\dot{V}_{O_2}$ in patients versus normal subjects (95). Alternatively, this relationship can be expressed as the heart rate response ($\Delta HR/\Delta\dot{V}_{O_2}$ between maximal and baseline values, normal < 50) (149). In patients with advanced ILD, a hypercirculatory heart rate response pattern ($\Delta HR/\Delta\dot{V}_{O_2} > 50$) is often revealed (Fig. 2). Low peak HR responses are usually observed, especially in more severe disease, as exercise terminates early. Because of symptom limitation, physiological limitation may not be achieved. Abnormal heart rate responses are often accompanied by a reduced stroke volume (122,140,150), electrocardiographic abnormalities (151), and evidence of biventricular dysfunction (136,150). Cardiovascular dysfunction may result from both hypoxemia (as noted previously) and the increased intrapleural pressures that are often seen in patients with deranged respiratory mechanics associated with ILD (105,106). Both preload (reduced left ventricular filling) and increased left ventricular afterload effects may result (152,153). The O_2 pulse is reduced, which may reflect several factors, including reduced stroke volume, hypoxemia, and deconditioning. Early-onset metabolic acidosis with a low anaerobic threshold (AT) commonly occurs and most probably reflects pulmonary vascular circulatory dysfunction (O_2 transport) (91) as well as contributions from skeletal muscle dysfunction and deconditioning (O_2 utilization) (12). Interestingly, one group has recently confirmed that impaired exercise performance in patients with scleroderma was related to the presence of pulmonary hypertension (154).

Dyspnea

As with other chronic cardiorespiratory disorders, dyspnea is a prominent symptom contributing to premature exercise termination in many patients with ILD, with leg fatigue and generalized fatigue reported in others (10,155). Ratings of exertional dyspnea using three different measurement tools have been validated for use in patients with ILD during exercise and have been shown to significantly correlate with resting DL_{CO} (8) and impaired exercise pulmonary gas exchange (156). More recent work reported by O'Donnell et al. (JAP) using the Borg scale (157) has expanded our understanding of the relationship between exertional dyspnea, mechanical derangements, and reduced exercise capacity by referencing dyspnea ratings to physiological variables during incremental and constant work exercise in 12 patients with ILD and 12 age-matched normal subjects (8). The Borg oxygen uptake ($\dot{V}_{O_2}$) slope was used as an index of exertional dyspnea and revealed significant differences between groups, with earlier onset and greater exertional dyspnea noted at submaximal values of $\dot{V}_{O_2}$ in patients with ILD (Fig. 3a); a more rapid shallow breathing pattern (Fig. 3c) was also observed, as was greater inspiratory effort during exercise in patients with ILD than in normal subjects. This was evidenced by the elevated slope of the relationship between esophageal pressure/maximal inspiratory pressure [(Pes)/ PI_{max}] and $\dot{V}_{O_2}$ (percent predicted) (Fig. 3d). Previous work had also reported that exertional dyspnea was significantly related to increased ventilatory effort and increased muscle work in patients with ILD (7,155).

In this noteworthy study by O'Donnell et al., both qualitative and quantitative differences in exertional dyspnea between groups were observed (8). Although both groups describe increased "work and/or effort" and "heaviness of breathing," only patients with ILD (as opposed to normal subjects) used the following descriptors at the end of exercise: "unsatisfied inspiratory effort," "increased inspiratory difficulty," and "rapid breathing." At symptom-limited peak exercise, when dyspnea intensity and inspiratory effort (esophageal pressure to maximal inspiratory pressure ratio or Pes/PI_{max}, percent predicted) were similar, the distinct qualitative differences between groups were attributed to the differences in ventilatory demand and ventilatory mechanics—i.e., reduced inspiratory capacity, heightened awareness of mechanical constraint on tidal volume expansion ($\uparrow Pes/V_T$), and tachypnea (see "Ventilatory Mechanics," above) in patients with ILD. Importantly, different physiological factors appeared to contribute to the intensity of exertional dyspnea in each group. The best correlate of the Borg-$\dot{V}_{O_2}$ slope was the resting V_T/IC in patients with ILD ($r = 0.58$, $p < 0.05$), while in normal subjects it was the slope of Pes/PI_{max}-$\dot{V}_{O_2}$ ($r = 0.60$, $p < 0.05$), suggesting that in patients with ILD, exertional dyspnea is more likely related to mechanical constraints on volume expansion than to indices of inspiratory effort. Additional work in this area is required.

II. Clinical Applications

Pulmonary function testing is often used and recommended in the management of patients with ILD (158,159). Potential clinical applications include (1) aiding in diagnosis, (2) establishing disease severity, (3) defining prognosis, and (4) monitoring response to therapy and disease progression. Given the enormous number of ILDs (>150) (160,161), a review of all ILDs is beyond the scope of this text. In this review, we discuss in detail salient physiological features of several of the most common interstitial lung diseases presenting in advanced stages, including idiopathic pulmonary fibrosis, pulmonary fibrosis complicating connective tissue disorders, sarcoidosis, and eosinophilic granuloma.

A. Pulmonary Function Testing and Differential Diagnosis in ILDs

Physiological presentation of ILDs are not specific, particularly in patients with advanced disease. PFT data should be used in conjunction with clinical, radiographic, and histological information. In patients with appropriate symptoms, PFTs can serve as early diagnostic tools. In a report of 44 dyspneic patients with normal chest radiographs and biopsy-proven ILD, decreases in DL_{CO} were observed in 73%, while reductions in VC or TLC were noted in 57 and 16% of patients, respectively (162). Interestingly, pulmonary function tests may be abnormal even in patients with a normal HRCT. One group noted abnormal PFTs (FVC mean 72% and $DL_{CO}/\dot{V}A$ mean 72% predicted) in three patients with normal HRCT scans and open lung biopsies demonstrating ILD (163). Resting PFTs may be normal in the early phases of IPF (62,164). Risk and colleagues identified two patients with biopsy-proven IPF who had normal pulmonary mechanics and a $DL_{CO} > 70\%$ predicted; however, $P(A-a)_{O_2}$ at rest and exercise was abnormal (6).

Several groups have tried to differentiate ILDs based upon patterns of physiological aberrations (65). Residual volume is often elevated in asbestosis (165), silicosis (166) and hypersensitivity pneumonia (167) but is normal or reduced in IPF/UIP (65). Gas exchange (as assessed by DL_{CO}) is disproportionately reduced in IPF/UIP compared to sarcoidosis or asbestosis, even at comparable lung volumes (87,168). Unfortunately, there is considerable overlap in these findings, which limits the practical clinical value of these differences.

Several groups have highlighted the importance of histological classification of pulmonary fibrosis, with a survival advantage reported for nonspecific interstitial pneumonia (NSIP), desquamative interstitial pneumonia (DIP), and respiratory bronchiolitis interstitial lung disease (RBILD) compared to UIP (169–174). It appears that the physiological patterns are similar between UIP and NSIP (Table 8). In both UIP and NSIP, decreased lung volumes and DL_{CO} are noted (170–174). One group reported no difference between these two entities in spirometry or DL_{CO}, but the TLC was lower in UIP (170); the latter finding has been confirmed by others (175). Others found slightly greater impairment in DL_{CO} in UIP compared to NSIP (171,174,176). In contrast, some investigators have reported no significant differences in TLC or DL_{CO} between NSIP and UIP (173,174).

Differences in CPET response(s) may be noted between different specific ILD types (4,122). Patients with interstitial pulmonary fibrosis (IPF) experience a greater degree of arterial desaturation and abnormal pulmonary

Table 8 Physiological Patterns of Usual Interstitial Pneumonitis and Nonspecific Interstitial Pneumonia

Study		Number of patients	FVC (% pred)	TLC (% pred)	DL_{CO} (% pred)	PaO_2
Nagai et al. (171)	NSIP	31	74	—	56	70
	UIP	64	70	—	44	76
Daniil et al. (173)	NSIP	15	73	72	44	74
	UIP	15	74	66	44	69
Bjoraker at al. (170)	NSIP	14	80	76	50	—
	UIP	63	79	68	48	—
Nicholson et al. (174)	NSIP	28	71	—	39	10.6 KPA
	UIP	37	72	—	44	10.8 KPA
Flaherty et al. (175)	Fibrotic NSIP	28	73	78	51	—
	Cellular NSIP	5	72	78	69	—
	UIP	106	67	73	51	—

Key: NSIP, Non-specific interstitial pneumonia; UIP, usual interstitial pneumonia.
Source: Modified from Ref. 401.

gas exchange during exercise than do patients with sarcoidosis (87) and those with cryptogenic fibrosing alveolitis, scleroderma type (139,177). A similar degree of desaturation from rest to exercise in patients with UIP (92% rest versus 85% exercise) and NSIP (93 versus 83%) has been reported (170,174). Although patients with ILD have traditionally been thought to be ventilatory-limited, a recent retrospective analysis has suggested that circulatory factors may be primarily exercise-limiting (91). It would appear that patients with IPF (141,178) may be more likely circulatory-limited, as are those with scleroderma (179) and patients with cryptogenic fibrosing alveolitis, scleroderma type (139,177). However, this provocative concept requires additional work for IPF and for other ILD entities. Some investigators have suggested that patients with sarcoidosis may have disproportionate cardiovascular abnormalities due to associated left-and right-sided myocardial involvement (136,150,180). Additional investigation is necessary. The coexistence of a high $\dot{V}_E/MVV$ (no Ventilatory reserve [VR]) and cardiovascular abnormalities and limitations may signal the presence of combined exercise limitation.

III. Idiopathic Pulmonary Fibrosis

Idiopathic pulmonary fibrosis (IPF) is the prototype of ILDs manifesting themselves with restrictive physiology and impaired gas exchange (160,181): it is associated with the histopathological pattern of usual interstitial pneumonia (UIP) (160,169,181). Recent reviews emphasize that other idiopathic interstitial pneumonias (IIPs) share clinical and physiological features that mimic UIP but have a better prognosis and are far more responsive to therapy (160,169). Current recommendations from international consensus statements restrict the term *IPF* to patients with idiopathic UIP (160,161). In the following discussion, we use the term *UIP* when patients in published series were specifically classified as UIP (not simply IPF or CFA). For general discussion, we use the term *IPF/UIP* to emphasize the fact that the *clinical entity* IPF should be restricted to patients with the *histopathological pattern* of UIP.

A. Pulmonary Function Testing and Diagnosing IPF/UIP

IPF/UIP patients characteristically exhibit reduced lung volumes, normal or increased expiratory flow rates, increased FEV_1/FVC ratio, and reduced DL_{CO}(160,182,183). Hypoxemia or a widened $P(A-a)_{O_2}$, accentuated by exercise, is a cardinal feature of IPF (160,182,183). Impairments in gas exchange (DL_{CO}) and oxygenation may be evident early in the course of the disease, even when spirometry and lung volumes are normal (87). The reduced DL_{CO} reflects loss of pulmonary capillary volume ventilation as well as perfusion abnormalities (160). A restrictive defect is characteristic of IPF/UIP, but lung volumes may be normal if emphysema coexists (86,182,184). In this context, DL_{CO} and oxygenation are disproportionately reduced (86,182,184). Cardiopulmonary exercise testing (CPET) demonstrates hypoxemia; widened $A-aO_2$ gradient; reduced oxygen consumption ($\dot{V}_{O_2}$); increased dead space (V_D/V_T); increased minute ventilation for the level of oxygen consumption; high-frequency, low-tidal-volume breathing pattern; and a low O_2 pulse (8,27,183).

B. Pulmonary Function Testing and Disease Severity

IPF is a heterogeneous disorder with varying degrees of inflammation and fibrosis (63,185). Several investigators have examined the potential for physiological measurements to differentiate between fibrosis and inflammation (31,85,186–188). Gaensler et al. noted a "fair correlation" between histological severity of IPF on open-lung biopsies and physiological indices (130). Crystal and colleagues noted a "good" correlation between fibrosis and the coefficient of retraction and the change in exercise PaO_2 and $P(A-a)O_2$ but a "poor" correlation with spirometry, lung volumes, DL_{CO}, or resting gas exchange in 18 patients with IPF (164). In a more detailed analysis, Fulmer and colleagues described a semiquantitative histological analysis of open lung biopsies in 23 patients with IPF (30). Physiological studies performed included spirometry, lung volumes, DL_{CO}, static volume–pressure relationships, and steady-state exercise gas exchange. Most parameters of lung distensibility correlated with the extent of fibrosis but *not* with cellularity. Spirometry, lung volumes and DL_{CO} correlated poorly with histological abnormality, but exercise gas exchange [PaO_2 and $P(A-a)O_2$], corrected for achieved $\dot{V}_{O_2}$, correlated best with histological fibrosis and, to a lesser extent, cellularity (30). In another study of 14 untreated patients with IPF and 7 with pneumoconioses, gas transfer and lung volumes correlated with the extent of fibrosis and cellular infiltration; however, physiological parameters could not discriminate alveolitis from fibrosis (189). Cherniack et al. used a complex semiquantitative histological scoring system in 96 patients with IPF (85). No significant correlations were noted between histological fibrosis and any physiological parameter. However, the DL_{CO} correlated with "desquamation" of cells within the alveolar space. Significant differences were noted between morphological-physiological correlations in never smokers and ever smokers. Exercise gas exchange correlated with histological fibrosis only in never smokers.

Watters et al. developed a composite score incorporating clinical (dyspnea), radiographic (chest radiograph), and physiological parameters—i.e., the CRP score (31). The physiological component of the CRP included spirometric measures, lung volume (thoracic gas volume), DL_{CO} corrected for alveolar volume, and resting and exercise PaO_2 corrected for achieved $\dot{V}_{O_2}$. The CRP score correlated better with a semiquantitative histological total pathology score. A more recent study from the same institution suggests that a modified CRP scoring system incorporating additional clinical features and radiological findings provided improved correlations with histopathological abnormality (190).

Among pulmonary functional parameters, DL_{CO} correlates better with extent of disease on HRCT scans than lung volumes or spirometry (39,177). British investigators analyzed HRCT scans in 68 patients with CFA; 14 had concomitant emphysema (177). Extent of fibrosing alveolitis and emphysema on CT were independent determinants of functional impairment. Among the 14 patients with emphysema, lung volumes (FVC and TLC) were preserved and DL_{CO} and PaO_2 were reduced. In patients without emphysema on CT, the extent of disease on CT correlated with percent predicted DL_{CO} ($r = -0.68$), oxygenation desaturation with exercise ($r = 0.64$), and the physiological component of the CRP score ($r = -0.62$); spirometry or lung volumes were less helpful (177). Another study of 39 patients with IPF observed moderate correlations between global extent of lung involvement on HRCT, with DL_{CO} ($r = -0.40$, $p = 0.03$) and FVC ($r = -0.46$, $p = 0.003$) (39). In addition, the extent of ground-glass opacities (GGO) correlated with FVC ($r = -0.58$, $p = 0.0001$) (39). Both the extent of GGO and overall global extent of disease on CT correlated with PaO_2 at peak exercise. Another study of 38 patients with pulmonary fibrosis associated with Hermansky-Pudlak syndrome observed similar correlations between the extent of disease on HRCT and FVC ($r = -0.66$) and DL_{CO} ($r = -0.66$) (191). Unfortunately, such global physiological correlations are of doubtful clinical value in individual patients.

C. Pulmonary Function Testing and Prognosis in Idiopathic Pulmonary Fibrosis

The value of physiological studies in predicting prognosis or responsiveness to therapy is limited (65). Physiological parameters provide only a rough estimate of severity of disease but cannot accurately discriminate inflammation from fibrosis (85,87,189). Severe derangements in physiological tests (e.g., PFTs, gas exchange, oxygenation) predict a worse prognosis and lower survival rates (39,185,192–197). Numerous studies cited higher mortality rates when FVC or DL_{CO} were severely impaired. However, the thresholds for predicting higher mortality vary. For FVC, values associated with higher mortality included $< 67\%$ predicted (192) $< 60\%$ predicted (62) $> 10\%$ decrease in VC in 1 year (195). Others studies cited worse survival when DL_{CO} was severely impaired, but the cutoff points for DL_{CO} included $<30\%$ predicted (198), $< 45\%$ predicted (62,64), $< 39\%$ predicted (199), and $>20\%$ decrease in 1 year (195). It is of interest that one group reported reductions in $DL_{CO} < 45\%$ predicted to be associated with an increased incidence of pulmonary hypertension (200). Changes in TLC are less predictive of prognosis or survival, but some studies cited higher mortality rates when TLC was $< 78\%$ predicted (184) or $< 80\%$ predicted (201). In a study of 56 patients with IPF, parameters associated with worse survival included (1) an initial FVC $< 60\%$ predicted, (2) $DL_{CO} < 40\%$ predicted, (3) mean pulmonary artery pressure $> 30\,mmHg$, or (4) age over 40 years at first symptoms (62). A retrospective study of 244 patients with CFA noted that decreased FVC was an independent predictor of increased mortality (202). Another retrospective study of 99 patients with IPF treated with corticosteroids ($+/-$azathioprine), suggested that survival was worse in patients with a pretherapy TLC $< 78\%$ predicted or VC $< 83\%$ predicted (184). Interestingly, DL_{CO}, PaO_2 at rest, $P(A-a)O_2$ and PaO_2 with exercise did not predict survival in that series (184). Increased FEV_1/FVC ratio has also been associated with diminished survival (203). Some investigators have suggested that changes in oxygen saturation with exercise correlated with subsequent disease progression in IPF (38,182). Most recently, one group identified patients with IPF/UIP referred for lung transplantation ($n = 115$) and examined baseline clinical, physiological, and radiological features that predicted 2-year survival (199). A $DL_{CO} < 39\%$ predicted and increased fibrotic abnormality on HRCT of the chest were the best predictors of survival (199). The presence of greater lung stiffness appears to provide additional predictive value (204).

In summary, prognosis appears poorer in patients with severe decreases in FVC, TLC, DL_{CO} or oxygenation but the correlations are inexact. Recent studies suggest that HRCT may be superior to physiological parameters in ascertaining prognosis or responsiveness to therapy (194,205). A predominant ground-glass pattern on HRCT scan predicts a high rate of responsiveness to corticosteroid therapy, whereas "reticular" or "honeycomb" patterns predict a low rate of responsiveness to therapy (39,177,194,206). Gay et al. prospectively examined 38 patients with biopsy-proven IPF (194). Using receiver operating characteristic curve analysis, only semiquantitative estimates of HRCT and histological fibrosis predicted survival. Importantly, no physiological parameter was predictive, nor did there parameters enhance the ability of HRCT to predict prognosis. A recent study has confirmed the predictive value of semiquantitative HRCT estimates of fibrotic abnormality but noted that the DL_{CO} % predicted added predictive value to the HRCT findings (199).

D. Pulmonary Function Testing and Monitoring Response to Therapy and Disease Progression

PFTs are frequently used in clinical practice to determine disease progression and response to therapy. Given the limited morphological-physiological correlations described earlier and the need for simple, patient-friendly diagnostic studies, most clinicians rely on spirometry, lung volumes, DL_{CO}, and measurement of arterial oxygenation. To understand the threshold of change in these parameters, which may be clinically significant, one needs first to appreciate the variability of these physiological indices.

The American Thoracic Society has provided detailed guidelines standardizing spirometric measurement (207). The variability in FVC is well defined among normal subjects and patients with pulmonary disease (207). In addition, recent guidelines provide standardization for DL_{CO} (208). Despite these standards, significant variability remains. Kangalee and Abboud reported inter- and intralaboratory variability in testing of a single, normal subject during a 13-year period (209). The coefficient of variation was lowest for spirometry and for intralaboratory testing. Variability was significant greater for TLC and DL_{CO}, particularly in the interlaboratory measurement of DL_{CO}. Care must be taken in interpreting serial physiological studies, particularly the DL_{CO} (210). As such, most investigators define clinically significant changes in spirometry for patients with IPF as a change in FVC > 10 to 15% (185,192,195,198,201,211–213) and 20% for DL_{CO} (65,195,198,211,212). Data on the reproducibility of exercise testing in IPF patients are sparse.

Pulmonary function tests are valuable in the serial evaluation of patients with IPF/UIP. Stack et al. noted an improved survival in IPF patients demonstrating an early rise in FVC > 10% with corticosteroid therapy (213). Augusti and colleagues performed serial PFTs in 19 patients with IPF (214); a decrease in FVC, TLC, or DL_{CO} by 1.5 years was noted in patients who continued to progress during the 3 years of follow-up. Van Oortegem et al. retrospectively reviewed 25 patients with IPF; improvement in FVC or DL_{CO} after 3 months of therapy predicted stability or improvement during long-term follow-up (215). Hanson et al. described 58 IPF patients who survived at least 1 year from the initiation of therapy and had serial spirometry (195). Survival was better in patients with an improved or unchanged FVC at 1 year compared to patients exhibiting a 10% reduction in FVC. Similarly, survival was worse among patients experiencing 20% decline in DL_{CO} after 1 year of therapy. The concordance between both of these studies was good; no patient with improved

FVC had a fall DL_{CO}. Interestingly, measurement of resting or exercise oxygenation provided no incremental value. Xaubet et al. followed 23 patients with IPF for a mean of 7.5 months after initial assessment (39). The overall extent of abnormality in HRCT correlated with changes in DL_{CO} ($r = -0.57$) and FVC ($r = -0.51$).

The clinical, radiological, physiological (CRP) score represents a potentially more accurate method for assessing response to therapy in IPF. Response is defined as 10-point drop in CRP; stability, < 10-point change; nonresponse (NR), 10-point rise in CRP (31). One group has recently identified that responders or stable patients (based on CRP score) after 3 months of corticosteroid therapy had an improved long-term survival compared to NR (216). Unfortunately, the CRP is cumbersome and has not been validated. Direct comparisons between CRP scoring and simpler pulmonary function testing are required.

IV. Collagen Vascular Diseases

Pulmonary complications of collagen vascular diseases (CVDs) are protean and are important causes of morbidity and mortality (161,217). The spectrum of histopathological disorders includes UIP, NSIP, cellular or follicular bronchiolitis, bronchiolitis obliterans (with or without organizing pneumonia), alveolar hemorrhage, and pulmonary vasculitis (161,217–219). Pulmonary fibrosis—indistinguishable clinically, physiologically, and radiographically from IPF/UIP—can complicate each of the CVDs (220). Although the course of pulmonary fibrosis complicating CVD (CVD-FA) is more indolent than that of IPF (220), severe and even fatal respiratory failure can result. Optimal therapy of CVD-FA remains controversial, but corticosteroids and immuno-suppressive or cytotoxic agents have been used with success (221,222).

A. Progressive Systemic Sclerosis (Scleroderma)

Scleroderma [or progressive systemic sclerosis (PSSc)] is a systemic disease that causes fibrosis (sclerosis) and vasculopathy of skin, kidney, gastrointestinal tract (particularly esophagus), muscle, heart, and lung (223). Although the disease usually progresses indolently over years, it can rarely exhibit a more fulminant course. Chronic interstitial lung disease and pulmonary hypertension are common features, occurring in more than three-quarters of patients with PSSc (217,224). Less common pulmonary manifestations include recurrent aspiration pneumonia (among patients with severe esophageal dysmotility), bronchiolitis obliterans, pulmonary hemorrhage, and bronchioloalveolar cell carcinoma (217,224). Fibrosing alveolitis is a common cause of death due to PSSc (217,225,226), with postmortem studies documenting pulmonary fibrosis in 74 to 100% of patients with PSSc (227,228). Given this high frequency of lung involvement, pulmonary function has been studied by many investigators over the past several decades.

B. Pulmonary Function Testing and Diagnosis

Published data evaluating PFTs in patients with scleroderma are extensive (61,229–246). Interstitial lung disease (fibrosing alveolitis) is more common in patients with diffuse PSSc compared than in those with the more limited CREST (calcinosis, Raynaud's phenomenon, esophageal dysfunction, sclerodactyly, and telangiectasia) variant. Skin involvement in CREST is limited to the distal extremities; severe visceral involvement is mild or absent (247). The most characteristic features of FA in PSSc include reductions in DL_{CO} and lung volumes. Decreases in TLC were noted in 32 to 67% of patients with PSSc; decreases in FVC in 11 to 77% of patients (223). In one report of 101 patients with PSSc (17 localized, 84 systemic), PFTs were normal in 54%; mild, moderate, and severe restrictive defects were observed in 26, 10 and 10% respectively (229). In general, increasing severity of PSSc is associated with worse lung function. Owens et al. contrasted PFTs in 88 patients with CREST variant with tests obtained from 77 patients with diffuse PSSc (236). Mean FVC was lower in patients with diffuse PSSC (87% predicted) compared to patients with CREST (94% predicted); the DL_{CO} was lower in patients with CREST, which likely reflects pulmonary hypertension—more common in patients with the CREST variant (223). Similarly, pulmonary dysfunction is worse in patients with PSSc compared to patients with systemic lupus erythematosus or rheumatoid arthritis (239). Reduced muscle strength has been suggested as a cause of pulmonary dysfunction in PSSc (248,249). In PSSc patients with a history of smoking, a depressed DL_{CO} but preserved TLC were noted (177).

Isolated decrease in DL_{CO} is common (177,237,238,245,246,250,251) and is the most sensitive of the static PFT parameters in detecting lung involvement in scleroderma (233,252,253). Some investigators have suggested that a decreased DL_{CO} is more likely in smokers (254). In a review of 815 patients with scleroderma seen at the University of Pittsburgh between January 1972 and December 1987, a total of 339 (42.6%) had a restrictive defect; 152 (19%) had an *isolated* reduction in DL_{CO} (<80% predicted) (237). Among the patients with only a decrement in DL_{CO}, 11% developed pulmonary hypertension (which was ultimately fatal in all patients). Pulmonary hypertension is more frequent in patients with $DL_{CO} < 55\%$ predicted or FVC (% predicted)/ DL_{CO} (% predicted) ratio >1.4. Previous reports (238) suggested that DL_{CO} is a sensitive marker of pulmonary vascular involvement (177,255). However, decreases in DL_{CO} can also reflect parenchymal involvement (256). Interestingly, DL_{CO} may vary with changes in ambient temperature (257). This may be caused by reduced perfusion following cold exposure (i.e., an intrapulmonary correlate to Raynaud's phenomenon) (258). Some investigators have cited a high frequency of airway disease in patients with PSSc (242,244,245), but this may reflect a concomitant history of cigarette smoking (61,243).

Routine PFTs may miss PSSc patients with mild parenchymal lung disease. In a prospective study of 34 patients with PSS, chest radiographs were abnormal in 29% of patients with normal PFTs (234). More sophisticated physiological measurements are more sensitive in identifying parenchymal lung disease. Pistelli et al. reported abnormal lung compliance in 17 of 18 patients with PSS, including three with normal DL_{CO}; 10 patients had reduced lung volumes (241). Others have reported that static lung compliance may be a more sensitive marker for defining decreased lung function in PSS (244,259,260). Static lung compliance is higher in smokers with PSSc (254). Exercise impairment is common in scleroderma patients; this is often associated with elevated ventilatory response(177,232,261–263). CPETs are often normal, even in patients with normal pulmonary mechanics. In one study, 78 patients were evaluated. CPET was performed in 12 patients with PSS with normal DL_{CO}; exercise V_D/V_T was abnormal in 12; in 9 patients, widened $P(A - a)_{O_2}$ was noted during exercise (263) (Fig. 5). When parenchymal or pulmonary vascular disease is suspected but routine PFTs are normal, CPET may be useful.

C. Pulmonary Function Testing and Disease Severity

Numerous investigators examined correlations between measures of disease severity and physiological testing. In 34 PSSc patients who had open-lung biopsies, inverse correlations were found between DL_{CO} and the degree of interstitial fibrosis ($r = -0.46$) and loss of lung architecture ($r = -0.40$) on open lung biopsy (77). British investigators evaluated the pattern and extent of HRCT abnormalities in 59 patients with PSSc without overt pulmonary hypertension to determine correlations with spirometry, lung volumes, DL_{CO}, exercise gas exchange, and CRP scores (177). DL_{CO} correlated better with HRCT than spirometry, lung volumes, or exercise values. In a separate study, correlations between FVC and DL_{CO} and HRCT were found in patients with

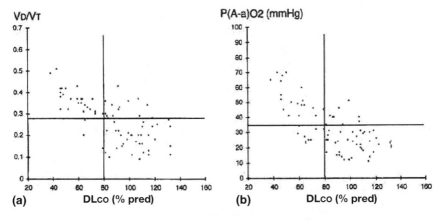

Figure 5 (a) Correlation between resting, baseline DL_{CO} (% predicted), and V_D/V_T in 78 patients with systemic sclerosis. (b) Correlation between resting, baseline DL_{CO} (% predicted) and $p(P_A–PaO_2)$ in 78 patients with systemic sclerosis. (From Ref. 263.)

IPF or PSSc (177). HRCT correlated with exercise gas exchange in patients with IPF but not PSSc; greater impairments in gas exchange during exercise were noted in patients with IPF. A similar finding, albeit with lower correlation coefficients (DL_{CO} versus HRCT, $r = -0.50$ and TLC versus HRCT, $r = -0.39$), was documented by another group (264). Others confirmed good correlations between DL_{CO} and HRCT ($r = 0.70$) and a better correlation between VC and HRCT ($r = 0.83$) (265). Abnormal cell profiles on bronchoalveolar lavage (BAL) increase as the DL_{CO} decreases (266). Lower DL_{CO} and FVC correlate with worsening radiographic and histopathological derangements. DL_{CO} and FVC appear to be the optimal physiological parameters to gauge disease severity in PSSc patients, although HRCT may better serve this role.

D. Pulmonary Function Testing and Prognosis in PSS

The prognosis of scleroderma is closely tied to the development of visceral disease, including renal, cardiac, and pulmonary involvement (223,225,267–269). Five-year survival ranges from 17 to 45% in PSSc patients with pulmonary involvement (220,240,270–273). Several groups have examined the ability of PFTs to predict long-term survival. Peters-Golden et al. identified the DL_{CO} as most predictive of survival in 71 patients followed for a mean of 5 years (240). Five-year survival was only 9% among patients with a $DL_{CO} < 40\%$ predicted compared to 75% survival when the DL_{CO} exceeded 40% of predicted values (Fig. 6). An obstructive ventilatory pattern was also associated with a lesser 5-year survival (240). A separate group has recently validated that a $DL_{CO} < 40\%$ predicted adversely impacts survival (274). Similar results in a larger cohort of patients with PSSc has also been reported (275). Another study cited 5-year survival in PSSc patients with fibrosing alveolitis (FA) of 17% (220). Survival in PSSc-FA is better than patients with IPF with comparable degrees of pulmonary dysfunction, even when matched for extent and pattern of disease on HRCT (220). In a multivariable analysis, a threshold of $> 50\%$ predicted for DL_{CO} was an independent predictor of survival. Similarly, a recent multivariable model identified the presence of proteinuria, an elevated sedimentation rate and a $DL_{CO} < 70\%$ predicted as most predictive of survival in 280 patients with scleroderma (276). The importance of a $DL_{CO} < 70\%$ predicted has been confirmed by a large Canadian study (267).

The pathophysiological basis for the influence of DL_{CO} on survival may reflect its correlation with pulmonary vascular involvement (237). Severe reductions in FVC is associated with worse survival. In one retrospective study of 890 patients with PSSc, 10-year survival was worse in patients with $FVC < 50\%$ predicted compared to patients than moderate (FVC 50–75% predicted) or mild restriction ($FVC > 75\%$ predicted) (235). In this series of patients, 116 (14%) had severe disease; 40% of deaths were directly attributed to restrictive lung disease and in 27% lung involvement was a major contributing factor. These data were incorporated in a disease severity scale for PSSc (277). In this project, an international study group developed an

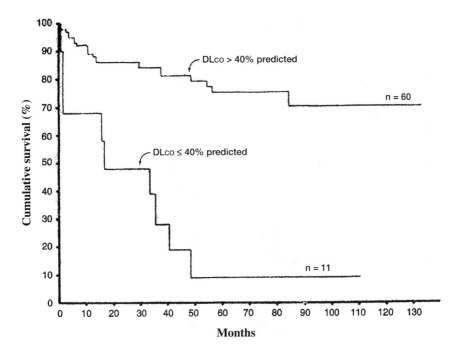

Figure 6 Cumulative survival function in patients with systemic sclerosis who had a DL_{CO} above and below 40% predicted. A significantly lower survival is noted in patients with $DL_{CO} < 40\%$ predicted ($p < 0.01$). (From Ref. 240.)

organ-specific disease severity scale. For lung involvement, the FVC, DL_{CO}, radiographic and clinical data were incorporated into a multivariable model, as illustrated in Table 9. In both cohorts (1980–1987 and 1988–1993) mortality increased as the severity of lung disease worsened. A modification of this system has recently been validated (273).

E. Pulmonary Function Tests and Monitoring Response to Therapy and Disease Progression

Several groups have examined serial PFTs in patients with PSSc. The conclusions have varied, in part depending on the nature of the study (retrospective versus prospective), the type of patient studied (limited versus diffuse scleroderma), the severity of pulmonary disease at baseline, and differences in clinical parameters (disease duration, treatment, demographic variables) (222,235,237,245,246,252–254,278–280). There is substantial heterogeneity in serial changes during follow-up. In an early study, Colp et al. followed 16 patients with PSSc for a mean of 4.6 years; lung volumes or DL_{CO} fell in only three patients (279). Others noted similar findings (246). In contrast, Bagg and Hughes noted gradual progression of restrictive abnormality (253). A

Table 9 Lung Severity Scale and Cumulative Survival Rates for Severity Grades 0–4 for 1980–1987 and 1988–1993 Cohorts of the University of Pittsburgh Databank Patients

Severity grade	Variable	Cumulative survival to death [a]	
		At 5 years 1980–1987 ($n = 579$)	At 5 years 1988–1993 ($n = 680$)
0 (none)	DL_{CO} 80% +, or FVC 80% +, or fibrosis (radiographic) absent, or PHT absent, or bibasilar rales absent	$n = 206$, 86%	$n = 256$, 86%
		} $p < 0.0001$	} $p = 0.12$
1 (mild)	DL_{CO} 70–80%, or FVC 70–80%, or bibasilar rales present, or fibrosis present, PHT mild	$n = 189$, 70%	$n = 147$, 81%
		} $p = 0.008$	} $p = 0.61$
2 (moderate)	DL_{CO} 50–69%, or FVC 50–69%	$n = 51$, 90%	$n = 126$, 84%
		} $p = 0.48$	} $p < 0.0001$
3 (severe)	$DL_{CO} < 50\%$, or FVC < 50%, or PHT moderate or severe	$n = 40$, 85%	$n = 92$, 61%
		} $p < 0.0001$	} $p = 0.017$
4 (end-stage)	O_2 required	$n = 93$, 43%	$n = 59$, 36%
Trend for all 5 survival curves		$p < 0.0001$	$p < 0.0001$

[a] Each p value represents the difference between the two survival curves overall rather than only at 5 years. DL_{CO}, diffusing capacity of carbon monoxide, % predicted; PHT, pulmonary (arterial) hypertension; FVC, forced vital capacity, % predicted.
Source: Ref. 277.

similar gradual progression was reported by Schneider et al., who performed serial PFTs in 38 patients followed over a mean of 63 months (278). The overall trend was of a slowly progressive restrictive defect; the mean rate of loss in FVC was more than three times the normal rate of FVC loss. Interestingly, the drop in DL_{CO} was similar to the expected normal loss. In the 27 patients who had serial measurements of both FVC and DL_{CO}, these parameters were normal or improved in only 3 patients. The same group performed serial PFTs in 24 patients followed for approximately 5 years (245). The mean rate of change for pulmonary function was not different than normal; substantial variability was noted with changes in DL_{CO}, lung volumes, and spirometry occurring independent of each other (245). Interestingly, in the study of Steen et al., DL_{CO} rose by > 20% in approximately half of 73 patients followed for a mean of 5.4 years after initial evaluation; DL_{CO} normalized in 27% during the follow-up period.

Two recent prospective studies examined serial change in pulmonary function. In one study of 61 patients, annual rates of change in PFTs included FVC (-51 mL/year); TLC (-66 mL/year); DL_{CO} (-1.29 mL/min/mmHg per year) (254). During the 3.1 years of follow-up, few patients changed from initially normal to abnormal results and the average symptoms did not appear to progress. The initial lung function had no significant influence on the subsequent rate of change. In a larger group of 176 patients, most of whom had limited disease (71%), DL_{CO} normalized in 16%; 44% of patients with an initially normal PFTs developed an isolated reduction in DL_{CO} (280). Few patients with an initially isolated reduction in DL_{CO} (the most frequent initial physiological pattern) progressed to restrictive pulmonary disease.

Although the course of FA complicating PSSc is usually indolent, some patients exhibit a more rapid course. Factors associated with a deteriorating course and increased risk of pulmonary hypertension include peripheral vascular involvement, digital pitting or ulcerations, severe Raynaud's phenomenon, and a history of smoking (245,281). The presence of increased neutrophils on BAL (a surrogate marker of alveolitis) has been associated with an accelerated loss of lung function (252,282) and more extensive fibrosis on HRCT (220). While controlled randomized therapeutic trials have not been done, favorable responses have been noted with corticosteroids or immuno-suppressive agents (220,235,283). One retrospective study cited greater improvement in vital capacity in PSSc patients treated with cyclophosphamide (CP) compared to D-penicillamine, corticosteroids, no therapy, or immuno-suppressive agents other than CP (235). In a prospective open trial, PFTs improved in 14 of 18 patients treated with oral CP (2–2.5 mg/kg/day) plus prednisone (283). Therapy may improve pulmonary function in a subset of PSSc patients with alveolitis. In a recent study, serial changes in pulmonary function and survival were assessed in 103 scleroderma patients who had BAL or lung biopsy (222). Cyclophosphamide was administered to 39 patients with initial "alveolitis" (by BAL or lung biopsies); 30 with alveolitis did not receive cytotoxic therapy; 34 patients had no evidence of alveolar inflammation at initial visit (222). Change in DL_{CO}, FVC, and survival were worse in untreated patients with alveolitis. While randomized controlled trials are essential to determine optimal therapy, these data support a trial of cytotoxic or immunosuppressive therapy for a subset of patients with a deteriorating course or surrogate markers of alveolitis (e.g., by HRCT or BAL). Since the natural history of FA in PSSc is highly variable, longitudinal measurements of PFTs are essential to monitor the course. Since spirometric and gas exchange variables may change independently of each other, it is wise to monitor both spirometry and DL_{CO} serially.

V. Rheumatoid Arthritis

Pleuropulmonary complications of rheumatoid arthritis (RA) are protean and include fibrosing alveolitis (FA) (also termed rheumatoid lung disease), obliterative bronchiolitis, lymphocytic infiltration of small airways, pleural effusions, rheumatoid nodules, pulmonary vasculitis, pulmonary hypertension, bronchiectasis, and infectious or toxic complications of cytotoxic drug therapy (217,284–286). The presence of FA in RA varies widely (3–41%) among published studies, which reflects heterogeneous patient populations and different methods to detect disease (217). Aberrations in HRCT scans have been cited in 19 to 52% of patients with RA, even in the absence of pulmonary symptoms (287–290). The presence of extent of FA does not correlate with the extent, duration, or activity of the articular or systemic components (217). The course of FA complicating RA (i.e., rheumatoid lung disease) is usually indolent, but 1 to 4% of patients developed severe, disabling FA (217). Treatment of rheumatoid lung disease is similar to FA complicating other collagen vascular diseases (CVDs).

A. Pulmonary Function Testing and Diagnosis

Pulmonary function tests reveal restrictive defects or reduced DL_{CO} in 10 to 40% of patients with RA, even in the absence of specific symptoms (286,288,291,292). This is particularly true in advanced disease. Abnormalities in milder disease have been identified by numerous groups. Banks et al. contrasted 342 patients with RA from a university hospital rheumatology clinic with 265 controls from other outpatient clinics (291). A mild restrictive defect was noted in the RA cohort, particularly among nonsmokers; the DL_{CO} was decreased in 27% of RA patients. Seven patients had clearly defined interstitial disease. Similarly, in a prospective study of 155 RA patients and 55 control subjects, a restrictive component and low DL_{CO} were more common among patients with RA (293). Several investigators noted reductions in DL_{CO} (up to 40% of patients in some series) (294–296), but the confounding effect of cigarette smoking could not be excluded in many patients (297–299). Gabbay et al. examined 36 adults with newly diagnosed RA (joint symptom duration < 2 years) from hospital or community practices (288). Chest radiographs, HRCT, PFTs, HRCT, BAL, and ^{99m}Tc-DTPA nuclear scanning were prospectively assessed. Abnormalities consistent with ILD were noted in 58% of patients; PFTs were consistent with ILD in 22%; BAL and HRCT were abnormal in 52 and 33% of patients, respectively. Cervantes-Perez et al. prospectively examined 140 patients with RA, 25 of whom had open-lung biopsies (300). Twelve patients had normal lung function (DL_{CO} not measured) despite an abnormal lung biopsy in eight. Bronchoscopic and radiographic techniques appear to be more sensitive in identifying ILD in RA patients. In an effort to predict ILD in RA (defined as abnormal BAL findings), 58 nonsmoking patients were studied by Popp et al. (301). Abnormalities on BAL cell profiles were detected in 42 patients (73%) (i.e., >15% lymphocytes, >3% neutrophils, or >250,000 cells per milliliter); by logistic regression analysis, male gender, a lower FVC and changes in several laboratory parameters were associated with an increased likelihood of ILD. Both FVC and DL_{CO} are useful in detecting ILD in RA patients, but smoking history may be a confounding factor. Respiratory muscle abnormality has also been identified in patients with RA (302,303). Most recently, a prospective study of 150 patients with RA underwent HRCT and PFT (290). A total of 28 patients (19%) exhibited HRCT features of FA; 7 demonstrated an FVC < 80% predicted and 23 a $DL_{CO} < 75\%$ predicted. Interestingly, 52% of patients without FA demonstrated a reduced DL_{CO}. As such, the sensitivity and specificity of pulmonary function tests in RA remains unclear. HRCT may be more more sensitive in identifying ILD in this patient population.

Although controversial, airway disease has been the most frequent physiological aberration in some studies of RA. Bronchiolar abnormalities are well described in these patients (304). In a prospective study of female never smokers with RA, airflow obstruction was documented by spirometry in 50% (81). In a prospective case-control study comparing 100 RA patients and 88 control subjects, airflow obstruction was noted in 16% of nonsmoking RA patients compared with none of the controls (82). In contrast, Sassoon and colleagues suggested that airway dysfunction in RA likely reflected factors other than the RA (84). Two groups examined airway function physiologically and radiographically. Cortet et al. studied 64 patients with spirometry, DL_{CO}, and HRCT (83). Small airway dysfunction was present in 13% of patients; the most frequent radiographic correlates were bronchiectasis (30%), pulmonary nodules (28%), and air trapping (25%). In a similar study, abnormalities of HRCT were noted in 35 of 50 patients (70%) (80). Airflow obstruction was noted in 9 (18%), as defined by a reduced FEV_1/FVC and small airway disease in an additional 5 patients by more sensitive tests. The prevalence of airway hyperreactivity was higher in RA patients (55%) compared to controls (16%) in one study (305). Radiological confirmation of bronchiectasis was noted in 12 of 150 patients prospectively studied using HRCT (290).

B. Pulmonary Function Testing and Disease Severity

The heterogeneity limits the ability to establish clear cut conclusions regarding disease severity (223). In an unselected cohort of patients with RA and known lung disease ($n = 336$), multivariable analysis was utilized to identify abnormality in pulmonary function tests (FVC $< 80\%$, $n = 42$ or $DL_{CO} < 80\%$ predicted, $n = 64$) (306). Age, male gender, smoking history, and measures of RA activity were related to abnormal pulmonary function testing. The association between increased RA joint disease and greater decrease in FVC and TLC was also noted by Hyland and colleagues (293). In contrast, others found no correlation with decrease in DL_{CO} and multiple clinical indices (298) or with the presence of small airways disease (84).

C. Pulmonary Function Testing and Prognosis

The significant clinical heterogeneity impairs the ability to define clear prognostic factors in rheumatoid lung disease (223). In two studies, the survival of patients with rheumatoid arthritis and ILD was decreased by 3.5 to 4.9 years (296,307). Hakala examined all RA patients hospitalized between 1978 and 1982 in Finland (296). Among 57 patients hospitalized with ILD, 8 had probable drug-induced disease and 49 had pulmonary fibrosis attributed to RA. Five-year survival in the latter group was only 39%; progressive pulmonary fibrosis was the cause of death in 80% of these patients. Patients who died had a lower FVC at the time of admission (62% predicted) compared to survivors (78% predicted); DL_{CO} was similar in both groups (51 versus 53% predicted). It is evident that a rough correlation exists between low FVC and increased mortality. One group has recently suggested that $DL_{CO} < 54\%$ predicted at presentation is 80% sensitive and 93% specific in defining progressive RA-associated FA (308).

D. Pulmonary Function Testing and Monitoring Response
to Therapy and Disease Progression in RA

Longitudinal changes in PFTs were reported by Linstow et al. (309). This group examined 63 RA patients with an initial normal FVC (102% predicted) but a mildly decreased DL_{CO} (70% predicted) over 8 years of follow-up. Interestingly, FVC decreased slightly (to 95 % predicted) whereas DL_{CO} rose (to 85% predicted). No correlation was noted between changes in pulmonary function and drug therapy. Similarly, others noted little effect of methotrexate therapy on pulmonary function (spirometry, lung volumes, and DL_{CO}) over a mean treatment period of several years (310,311). In contrast, Dayton et al. noted a mild increase in RV during an average period of 4.4 years of low-dose methotrexate therapy (312). Little change was noted in other lung volumes, spirometry, or DL_{CO}. In contrast, others noted mild decrements in FVC (2.2%) and DL_{CO}/VA (4.8%) during methotrexate therapy; these changes did not predict the development of methotrexate pneumonitis (incidence of 3.2%)

(313). In contrast, a clinically significant decrement in DL_{CO} (11%) was noted in 42 RA patients treated with varying treatment regimens; the 28 patients treated with D-penicillamine experienced a less severe decrement in DL_{CO} (7%) (314). We believe spirometry and DL_{CO} are the most useful parameters to assess and follow the course of ILD in RA patients (223).

VI. Polymyositis and Dermatomyositis

Pleuropulmonary complications of polymyositis (PM) or dermatomyosisis (DM) are protean and include fibrosing alveolitis (FA), respiratory failure secondary to neuromuscular weakness, aspiration pneumonia due to weakness of the pharyngeal musculature, diaphragmatic paresis or dysfunction, obliterative bronchiolitis, and opportunistic infections (217,219). Fibrosing alveolitis complicates PM or DM in 3 to 10% of patients (217). Interestingly, the histopathological picture of nonspecific interstitial pneumonia is much more frequent in this disease, likely accounting for the improved survival noted with interstitial disease complicating this disorder (315). The severity of FA does not correlate with the course of the muscle disease or systemic features (217,316). Serological markers identify patients at greatest risk for FA. Circulating antibodies to the enzyme histidyl-tRNA-synthetase (anti-Jo1, anti-PL7, and anti-PL-12) or KJ are present in a majority of patients with PM or DM *with* FA but in < 20% of patients with PM or DM *without* FA (217,316). The presence of Jo-1–positive antibodies does not appear to impact survival in patients with associated ILD (315). Clinical features and management of FA complicating DM or PM are similar to those of other CVDs (217).

VII. Overlap Syndrome and Mixed Connective Tissue Disease

Overlap syndrome is characterized by clinical manifestations overlapping with two or more of the five major CVDs [e.g., PSSc, RA, PM, DM, or systemic lupus evy them atosus (SLE)] (217). Mixed connective tissue disease (MCTD) displays overlapping features of CVDs, high-titer circulating antibodies (anti-RNP) to a ribonuclease-sensitive extractable nuclear antigen (ENA), and a speckled antinuclear antibody (ANA) (217,317). Pulmonary complications occur in up to 85% of patients with MCTD. Of these, FA and pulmonary hypertension are the most common and important (217,318). Fibrosing alveolitis develops in 25 to 85% of patients with MCTD during the course of the disease (217,317). The clinical expression of FA complicating MCTD is variable. Treatment is similar to FA complicating other CVDs.

VIII. Sjögren's Syndrome

Sjögren's syndrome (SS) is characterized by lymphocytic infiltration and destruction of exocrine glands and symptoms of xerostomia and/or xeropthalmia (sicca syndrome). SS may occur as a primary syndrome (pSS) or as a secondary syndrome (sSS) in the context of a specific autoimmune disorder (e.g., RA, SLE, PM, DM, or PSS_C) (217). Pulmonary manifestations of primary and secondary SS include FA, lymphoid interstitial pneumonia (LIP), lymphoproliferative disorders (pseudolymphoma or lymphoma), xerotrachea, pleural effusions, and bronchiolitis obliterans with organizing pneumonia (BOOP) (217). The reported incidence of FA complicating SS ranges from 9 to 55%, reflecting variations in the diagnostic testing and populations studied (217,319–322). PFTs are abnormal in 25 to 44% of patients with SS (217,319–322). In one recent study of 37 consecutive patients with primary Sjögren's syndrome and normal chest radiographs, abnormal HRCT images were noted in 24 (65%) (323). Interestingly, HRCT was normal in four patients with abnormal pulmonary function, while pulmonary function was normal in seven patients with abnormal HRCT. As such, PFT and HRCT are likely complementary in the identification of pulmonary disease complicating Sjögren's syndrome. The course of FA complicating SS is variable, and treatment is not well defined.

IX. Sarcoidosis

Sarcoidosis, a multisystemic granulomatous disease of uncertain etiology, involves the lung or intrathoracic lymph nodes in more than 90% of patients (324–327). The clinical spectrum of sarcoidosis is protean, but pulmonary manifestations predominate (324,328). Extrapulmonary involvement is common and may be the presenting or dominant feature (328,329). The histological hallmark of sarcoidosis is non necrotizing (noncaseating) granulomata, characterized by multinucleated giant cells, epithelioid cells, mononuclear phagocytes, and lymphocytes (325). Chest radiographs are abnormal in more than 90% of patients with sarcoidosis (324,325). The most characteristic feature is bilateral hilar lymphadenopathy (BHL) with or without concomitant right paratracheal lymph node enlargement (324,325). Parenchymal infiltrates are present in 25 to 50% of patients (324,325). The clinical course is variable. Spontaneous remissions occur in nearly two-thirds of patients, but the course is chronic in 10 to 30% (328). Chronic sarcoidosis involving lungs or extrapulmonary organs can be debilitating; fatalities occur in 1 to 4% of patients (324,325). Treatment of sarcoidosis is controversial (327). Corticosteroids are the mainstay of therapy for patients with symptomatic or progressive disease. Short-term responses are often dramatic, but relapses are common with cessation or taper of the drug. Immunosuppressive or cytotoxic drugs have been used in patients refractory to or intolerant of corticosteroids

(327). Long-term efficacy of any form of therapy has not been proven. Lung transplantation is an option for patients with end-stage sarcoidosis (330).

X. Pulmonary Function Tests in Sarcoidosis

A. Pulmonary Function Testing and Diagnosis in Sarcoidosis

PFTs in sarcoidosis typically reveal a restrictive pattern with a reduction in the DL_{CO} (87,324), although one study suggested that airflow limitation may be the most common abnormality in newly diagnosed patients (77). Lung function is often normal in patients with lower radiographic stages of disease (324,331). Abnormality in PFTs are detected in approximately 20% of patients with radiographic stage I sarcoidosis but are present in 40 to > 70% of patients with interstitial infiltrates (stage II, III, or IV)(74,324,332–337). In the setting of a negative chest radiograph (stage 0), several groups noted decreased in FVC in 15 to 25% of patients and in DL_{CO} in 25 to 50% (67,74,77). Interestingly, in 4 patients with a normal CT scan, 3 had abnormal spirometry and reduced DL_{CO} (338). Reductions in DL_{CO} is most sensitive of the easily available diagnostic studies (339,340).

Measurement of lung compliance has been performed in research settings (70,75,341–344) and may be a sensitive measure of parenchymal involvement (345). Only 4 of 18 patients with stage I radiographic disease had a normal VC, DL_{CO} and lung compliance in one early study (346). Similarly, in one series, 20% of patients with reduced compliance had normal VC and TLC (345). However, measurement of compliance has no clinical value in individual patients. Aberrations in CPET have been cited in up to 47% of patients with sarcoidosis (principally ventilatory limitation or increased V_D/V_T with exercise (112,180). In one study 4 of 14 patients with stage 0 or I sarcoidosis displayed ventilatory limitation during exercise (110). In a separate study, 4 of 14 *asymptomatic* subjects exhibited ventilatory limitation (111). In a study of 23 patients with mild pulmonary sarcoidosis (6 had normal VC and DL_{CO}), CPETs were abnormal in 9 of 20 (45%) evaluable patients, including 2 patients with normal PFTs (180). Miller and colleagues performed CPET in 30 sarcoidosis patients with normal spirometry; DL_{CO} was normal in 21 and 13 had normal chest radiographs (112). Ventilatory abnormalities during maximal exercise testing were detected in 14 patients (47%) (112). CPET abnormalities (e.g., excessive ventilation to oxygen consumption and abnormal V_D/V_T), were noted in 8 of 9 patients with a low DL_{CO} compared to 11 of 21 with a normal DL_{CO}. A widened $P(A - a)_{O_2}$ gradient was seen predominantly in patients with reduced DL_{CO} (112). Similarly, in a series of 32 patients, exercise-induced desaturation correlated with resting DL_{CO}; patients with a baseline $DL_{CO} < 55\%$ predicted had a greater fall in Pa_{O_2} during exercise (347). Most recently, Medinger et al. examined, retrospectively, PFT and CPET results in 48 patients with biopsy-proven sarcoidosis (348). Interestingly, for patients with the least radiographic disease, the physiological measures most significantly associated with radiographic stage were $\Delta P(A-a)O_2$ and $\Delta P(A-a)O_2/\Delta \dot{V}O_2$. CPET is more sensitive that static PFTs in assessing work capacity (344), but its practical value is limited.

Airway involvement in sarcoidosis was first recognized in 1941, when Benedict reported an asthma-like picture in a young patient with sarcoidosis who had bronchoscopic evidence of mucosal infiltration with epithelioid granulomas (349). Subsequent studies noted airway obstruction in one-third or more of patients with pulmonary parenchymal involvement (69,77,350,351). Airway obstruction in sarcoidosis may be attributed to various mechanisms, including narrowing of the bronchial wall due to either granulomatous lesion or fibrotic scarring (69,350,352,353), compression by enlarged lymph nodes, airway distortion due to pulmonary fibrosis (76,353), small airway disease, or bronchial hyperreactivity (66,68,71–73,77). Small airways disease is common in sarcoidosis. In one study of 18 patients with restrictive lung disease and parenchymal infiltrates on chest radiographs, all 18 displayed abnormal airway function by at least one test (73). One study of 107 patients with newly diagnosed sarcoidosis noted that airflow limitation, characterized by decreased FEV_1/FVC ratio, was the most common physiological abnormality, present in 61 patients (57%) (77). Reductions in DL_{CO} were noted in 29 (27%); only 7 (6%) had a restrictive defect (77).

Importantly, in patients with greater degrees of fibrotic parenchymal distortion, more severe abnormalities in large airway obstruction may be present (74,79,354). In the study of Sharma et al., severe decrements in FEV_1/FVC were seen in patients with stage II/III (15%) or stage IV disease (33%)(74). Corticosteroids may be efficacious in patients with endobronchial sarcoidosis and airflow obstruction (78). However, progressive airflow obstruction may occur. Coates and Neville retrospectively analyzed 32 patients with intrathoracic sarcoidosis (16 smokers); airflow obstruction (defined as $FEV_1/FVC < 0.70$) was noted in 1 of 6 nonsmokers and 6 and 16 smokers at presentation (355). After a mean of 4 years of follow-up (range 1–21 years), 10 of 16 smokers and 5 of 16 nonsmokers had persistent airflow obstruction by spirometry.

Increased airway hyperactivity in response to methacholine challenge has been documented in sarcoid patients (356–358). Bechtel et al. reported exaggerated bronchial hyperreactivity to methacholine in 50% of patients with stage I and stage II sarcoidosis (357). Clinically this may result in chronic hacking cough. The exact mechanism of this bronchial hyperreactivity is not clear, but it may reflect granulomatous inflammation involving the bronchial mucosa. Fridman et al. demonstrated granulomata in bronchial mucosal biopsies in 63% of patients with sarcoidosis (359). Similarly Shorr et al. noted that all sarcoid patients with airway hyperreactivity demonstrated abnormal endobronchial findings compared to similar bronchoscopic findings in only 45.5 % of sarcoid patients without airway hyperreactivity (360). The relationship of this airway hyperreactivity and subsequent abnormalities in airway function remains undefined.

B. Pulmonary Function Testing and Disease Severity in Sarcoidosis

Several studies have examined correlation between PFTs and various pathological, chest radiographic, CT, and BAL parameters. Correlations between physiological and pathological abnormalities are imprecise (331). In one early study, granuloma density correlated with tidal volume, minute ventilation, and increased anatomic dead space (343). A subsequent study demonstrated a weak but significant correlation between reduction in DL_{CO} and the degree of parenchymal lung change (as assessed by percutaneous needle biopsies) (361). In a complex study that assessed approximately 80 histological features from open-lung biopsy specimens, the "mean interstitial cell index" correlated with FVC ($r = -0.37$) and DL_{CO} ($r = -0.38$)(362). Huang et al. evaluated pathological-physiological correlations in 81 sarcoidosis patients who had open-lung biopsies (363). DL_{CO} correlated with the presence of granulomata, interstitial pneumonitis, and overall lung pathology. Reductions in FVC correlated only with the overall lung pathology. Despite some rough correlations, these diverse studies affirm that physiological parameters are unable to predict the histological severity of disease (340,343,361–363).

Numerous authors correlated pulmonary function in sarcoidosis with semiquantitative chest radiography. Using a modification of the International Labor Organization (ILO) classification scheme in 211 patients with sarcoidosis, McLoud et al. found that radiographic severity correlated best with FVC ($r = -0.49$) and DL_{CO} ($r = -0.32$) (340). Others found similar modest correlations (364,365). A review of conventional CTs performed in 27 sarcoid patients noted that nodular opacities correlated with less severe dyspnea and larger lung volumes than predominantly irregular opacities ($p < 0.05$) (365). CT provided superior pictorial display than chest radiographs but was no better than chest radiography in estimating functional or clinical impairment (365). Brauner et al. found moderate to poor correlations between either HRCT or chest radiography and pulmonary function (366). Other investigators corroborated that the extent of disease on CT correlated poorly with functional impairment (367). Radiographic-physiological correlations are improved when HRCT using semiquantitative scoring systems are applied (365,368). Semiquantitative scores from CT demonstrated inverse correlations with FVC ($r = -0.81$) and, to a lesser extent, with DL_{CO}($r = -0.49$) (338). More recently, Hansell et al. confirmed inverse correlations between the FVC, FEV_1, FEV_1/FVC and DL_{CO} and reticular pattern on HRCT (369). Few other radiographic features correlated with physiological parameters. Another study found that reticular and fibrotic abnormalities on HRCT correlated modestly with physiological aberrations, but mass opacities or confluence did not (370). More recently, Abehsera et al. have confirmed that TLC, VC, and DL_{CO} were significantly lower in sarcoid patients with honeycomb pattern on HRCT, while the FEV_1 was lower in patients with bronchial distortion (371). These various studies suggest that the extent and pattern of HRCT correlate roughly with physiological parameters. However, direct measurement of physiological parameters is required to extent the degree of pulmonary functional impairment.

C. Pulmonary Function Testing and Prognosis in Sarcoidosis

The natural history of sarcoidosis is heterogeneous. Most patients stabilize or improve over time, but 10 to 30% develop progressive pulmonary dysfunction (324). Most well-defined adverse prognostic factors are clinical in nature (328). Numerous authors have examined the role of baseline physiological measurements to predict long-term outcome. Maña et al. examined multiple parameters collected at baseline and their correlation with persistent disease activity over follow-up (372). Using Cox proportional-hazard modeling, variables that independently influenced the persistence of activity over time included age >40 years [relative risk (RR) of 1.67], Angiotensin converting enzyme (ACE) level (RR 1.45), male sex (RR 1.8), and FVC $<80\%$ predicted (RR 2.17). Some studies have suggested improved response to corticosteroids among patients with low DL_{CO} (341), but most studies found that pulmonary functional parameters cannot predict long-term outcome (373–376). In a separate study, reduced DL_{CO} discriminated between patients who worsened compared to those who remained stable or improved (377). Not surprisingly, mortality due to sarcoidosis is higher among patients displaying more severe physiological impairment (378).

D. Pulmonary Function Testing and Monitoring Response to Therapy and Disease Progression in Sarcoidosis

Although the predictive value of baseline PFTs is limited, sequential studies are important to follow the course of the disease. PFTs provide quantifiable, objective measures of the evolution of disease (and assess response to therapy). Numerous studies have shown that the vital capacity improves more frequently than the DL_{CO} (379–381), TLC (344), or arterial oxygenation (331). Importantly, the VC and DL_{CO} share a common direction of change in over two-thirds of patients; discordant changes occur in fewer than 5% of patients (331,382). Given the variability of DL_{CO} and the expense of full lung volumes (by helium dilution or body plethysmographic techniques), spirometry and flow-volume loops are the most useful and cost-effective parameters to use in following the course of the disease. Additional studies—such as DL_{CO}, TLC, or gas exchange—have a role in selected patients. Criteria for assessing "response" or improvement have not been validated. However, most investigators define a change in FCV >10 to 15% or $DL_{CO} >20\%$ as significant (65,331,383–385). Responses to therapy are often evident within 6 to 12 weeks of initiation of therapy. In some patients, improvement in FVC may be seen within 3 weeks of therapy (Fig. 7) (386).

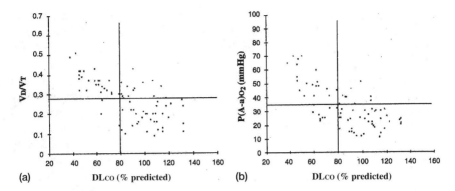

Figure 7 Rate of improvement in vital capacity in 11 patients related to the duration of steroid treatment. (From Ref. 386.)

XI. Langerhans Cell Histiocytosis (Pulmonary Eosinophilic Granuloma)

Langerhans cell histiocytosis (LCH) (also termed Langerhans cell granulomatosis or pulmonary eosinophilic granuloma) is a rare disease of unknown etiology occurring almost exclusively in cigarette smokers (136,387–393). Predominant symptoms include cough, dyspnea, and pneumothorax (135,387,390–393). HRCT scans in LCH are distinctive, and reveal numerous thin-walled cysts, preferentially involving the upper and middle lung zones (136,366,392,393).

A. Pulmonary Function Testing and Diagnosis in Langerhans Cell Histiocytosis

Aberrations in PFTs are noted in > 80% of patients with LCH, Typical features include reductions in DL_{CO} (70–80%) and lung volumes (50–70%), normal or increased FEV_1/FVC ratio, increased RV, and impaired gas exchange (135,388,390–393). PFTs are normal in 15 to 20% of patients (389,390–393). Reductions in DL_{CO} are most frequent and may reflect involvement or destruction of lung parenchyma or pulmonary capillaries (135). Pure restrictive or mixed obstructive-restrictive patterns may be observed (135,388,390,391). A pure obstructive defect with reduced FEV_1/FVC ratio is uncommon (135). Obstruction defects may reflect cigarette smoking, concomitant emphysema, or bronchiolar obstruction that results from the peribronchiolar distribution of the inflammatory and fibrotic lesions (388). As the disease progresses, cysts and bullous disease may develop, resulting in air trapping or airflow obstruction (389,391). Air trapping (increased RV) is noted in nearly 50% of patients with pulmonary LCH but hyperinflation (TLC > 110%) is uncommon (135,394). Cardiopulmonary exercise tests in LCH demonstrate reductions in exercise tolerance, maximal workload, oxygen consumption, and anaerobic threshold; worsening gas exchange, and increased ratio of dead space to tidal volume (V_D/V_T) with exercise (135,393). Crausman et al. performed CPET in 23 patients with LCH (135). Two subsets were identified on the basis of elastic recoil. The coefficient of elastic recoil was increased in 12; restriction was present in 11 of these 12. In contrast, 10 had normal elastic recoil and relatively preserved lung function. However, exercise capacity was limited in both groups (workload $53\% +/- 3\%$). The baseline V_D/V_T ratio or its response to exercise was abnormal in 16 of 23 patients, suggesting pulmonary vascular disease. Strong correlations were found between overall exercise performance (% predicted V_{O_2} max) and indices of vascular involvement: i.e., DL_{CO} ($r = 0.68$, $p = 0.0004$), baseline V_D/V_T (-0.65; $p0.001$); exercise V_D/V_T ($r = -0.67$, $p = 0.0004$). Similar correlations were noted when exercise performance was measured by maximal workload achieved. Vascular dysfunction likely plays the major role in limiting exercise capacity, but impaired pulmonary mechanics, airflow obstruction, or hypoxemia may contribute. A recent study of 21 patients with advanced pulmonary LCH referred for lung transplantation confirmed the importance of pulmonary vascular lesions in this disease (394). Among 21 patients in whom PFTs were performed, the dominant aberration was a reduced DL_{CO} (mean 27% of predicted); other salient features included reduced FEV_1 (mean 46% predicted); reduced PaO_2 (mean 53 mmHg), increased RV (mean 166% predicted), and normal TLC (mean 95% predicted). Pulmonary hypertension was present in all patients (mean PA pressure was 59 mmHg), and was *independent* of other pulmonary functional parameters. Histopathology of lung in 12 patients revealed a proliferative vasculopathy involving muscular arteries and veins. The degree of pulmonary hypertension was greater in LCH compared to patients with chronic obstructive pulmonary disease (COPD) or idiopathic pulmonary fibrosis (IPF) with more severe parenchymal destruction (394). In patients with LCH, no correlations were found between FEV_1, FEV_1/FVC, DL_{CO}, PaO_2, $PaCO_2$, and mean pulmonary artery pressure (Ppa), cardiac index (CI), or total pulmonary vascular resistance (TPVRi) (all $p > 0.1$). Conversely, in patients with COPD Ppa correlated with FEV_1/FVC ($r = 0.38$, $p = 0.03$) and there was a trend for TPVRi to correlate with Pa_{O_2} ($r = -0.035$, $p = 0.06$). In patients with IPF, TPVRi correlated with TLC ($r = 0.67$, $p = 0.01$). These data suggest that pulmonary hypertension in LCH reflects a primary vasculopathy and is independent of small airways and lung parenchymal injury.

B. Pulmonary Function Testing and Prognosis in Langerhans Cell Histiocytosis

Although data are limited, severe impairment in DL_{CO} or VC has been associated with a worse prognosis (389,395,396). In one retrospective study of 45 patients with pulmonary LCH, factors associated with diminished survival by univariate analysis included older age at diagnosis, lower FEV_1/FVC ratio, high RV/TLC (>0.33), and use of corticosteroids (395). By multivariate analysis, only older age and lower FEV_1/FVC ratio were associated with diminished survival. A recent large, retrospective study identified multiple features influencing survival in univariate analysis (397). These features included a lower FEV_1, a higher RV, a lower FEV_1/FVC ratio, and a reduced DL_{CO}. After adjusting for expected survival at 10 years based on life expectancy in the general population, a lower DL_{CO}, lower FEV_1, and higher RV maintained predictive ability. As such, physiological studies can be used to establish prognosis in eosinophilic granuloma.

C. Pulmonary Function Testing and Monitoring Response to Therapy and Disease Progression

Serial PFTs are advised to monitor the course of the disease. Due to its rarity and variable natural history, optimal therapy for pulmonary LCH is controversial. Given the central role of cigarette smoking in its pathogenesis (390,398,399), the disease stabilizes or improves in more than two-thirds of patients following cessation of smoking (135,389–393). In 15 to 31% of patients, the disease progresses, with worsening lung function (135,389–393). Fatality rates range from 6 to 27% (135,389–393). The impact of treatment is unknown (389–391,395). Lung transplantation is an option for patients with end-stage pulmonary LCH (393,400).

XII. Summary

Physiological assessment, which includes resting pulmonary function testing, is valuable in the optimal management of patients with ILD and advanced ILD. Although it has been suggested that HRCT is superior to physiological parameters in defining prognosis or responsiveness to therapy for patients with IPF (194,199), DL_{CO} % predicted appears to have added predictive value to the HRCT findings (199). Furthermore, this is consistent with other studies, which have demonstrated that FVC and DL_{CO} are the physiological parameters that best reflect global extent of disease in IPF using HRCT as a gold standard. Resting pulmonary function testing is likewise of considerable relevance in the clinical decision-making process of other ILD subtypes, possibly reflecting that in advanced stages, a remarkable similarity in pulmonary function parameters occurs. Therefore serial pulmonary function testing is advised to monitor therapy and disease progression in IPF and other ILD subtypes. Prognostic capabilities notwithstanding, resting physiological and radiological modalities, however, maybe inadequate in providing answers to clinically relevant questions in the individual patient.

It is reasonable, therefore, that functional physiological assessment may then be appropriate in the management of patients with advanced ILD. This may be especially germane for the determination of exercise limitation, which is multifactorial (10–14) in patients with chronic respiratory illness and reflects multisystem problems. Importantly, resting cardiopulmonary measurements are unable to prioritize/quantitate exercise-limiting factors important for reducing symptoms, initiating/monitoring therapeutic interventions, and potentially improving quality of life for patients with advanced ILD. Additionally, since health status assessment (HRQOL) reveals a stronger correlation with exercise tolerance than with either spirometry or oxygenation in patients with other chronic cardiorespiratory disorders, a *functional* assessment maybe useful in more optimally managing patients with advanced ILD. Additional studies in patients with ILD and advanced ILD are necessary, including which functional modality—i.e., 6-min walk test or CPET—may be most helpful. The clinical questions being asked and the available resources will likely be key. Constant work-cycle ergometry has been shown to be significantly more sensitive than 6-min walk tests in evaluating therapeutic interventions.

Appreciating that 1) pulmonary gas exchange abnormalities during exercise have been a good maker of morphologic severity in patients with IPF (30) and 2) DL_{CO} and $\Delta PAO_2 - PaO_2$ maybe useful prognostic indicators of SaO_2 over time in IPF (38), and 3) furthermore, that $\downarrow PaO_2$ during exercise showed a significant association with the extent of ground-glass appearance on HRCT and overall lung involvement (39), the importance of *routinely* measuring exercise pulmonary gas exchange in patients with ILD remains uncertain, especially as it relates to cost and technical requirements. In general, functional evaluation has been underutilized in patients with ILD and advanced ILD, especially in the areas of pulmonary rehabilitation, transplantation, and health status evaluation. Further studies will be necessary to establish the role of physiological functional assessment and its potential for enhanced patient management and improved quality of life in individual patients with advanced ILD.

References

1. Schwarz MI. Approach to the understanding, diagnosis, and management of interstitial lung disease. In: Schwarz M, King T Jr, eds. Interstitial Lung Disease. Hamilton, Ontario, Canada: Decker, 1998:3–30.
2. Coultas DB, Zumwalt RE, Black WC, Sobonya RE. The epidemiology of interstitial lung diseases. Am J Respir Crit Care Med 1994; 150:967–972.
3. Bye PT, Anderson SD, Woolcock AJ, Young IH, Alison JA. Bicycle endurance performance of patients with interstitial lung disease breathing air and oxygen. Am Rev Respir Dis 1982; 126:1005–1012.
4. Keogh BA, Lakatos E, Price D, Crystal RG. Importance of the lower respiratory tract in oxygen transfer. Exercise testing in patients with interstitial and destructive lung disease. Am Rev Respir Dis 1984; 129:S76–S80.
5. Sue DY, Oren A, Hansen JE, Wasserman K. Diffusing capacity for carbon monoxide as a predictor of gas exchange during exercise. N Engl J Med 1987; 316:1301–1306.

6. Risk C, Epler GR, Gaensler EA. Exercise alveolar-arterial oxygen pressure difference in interstitial lung disease. Chest 1984; 85:69–74.

7. Marciniuk DD, Sridhar G, Clemens RE, Zintel TA, Gallagher CG. Lung volumes and expiratory flow limitation during exercise in interstitial lung disease. J Appl Physiol 1994; 77:963–973.

8. O'Donnell DE, Laurence KL Chau TP, Webb KA. Qualitative aspects of exertional dyspnea in patients with interstitial lung disease. J Appl Physiol 1998; 84:2000–2009.

9. Hamilton AL, Killian KJ, Summers E, Jones NL. Muscle strength, symptom intensity, and exercise capacity in patients with cardiorespiratory disorders. Am J Respir Crit Care Med 1995; 152:2021–2031.

10. Jones NL, Killian KJ. Exercise limitation in health and disease. N Engl J Med 2000; 343:632–641.

11. Weisman IM, Zeballos RJ. Clinical exercise testing. Clin Chest Med 2001; 22:679–701.

12. American Thoracic Society, American College of Chest Physicians. Statement on cardiopulmonary exercise testing. Am J Respir Crit Care Med 2003; 167:211–277.

13. Wagner PD. Determinants of maximal oxygen transport and utilization. Annu Rev Physiol 1996; 58:21–50.

14. Dempsey JA, Babcock MA. An integrative view of limitations to muscular performance. Adv Exp Med Biol 1995; 384:393–399.

15. Curtis JR, Deyo RA, Hudson LD. Pulmonary rehabilitation in chronic respiratory insufficiency. 7. Health-related quality of life among patients with chronic obstructive pulmonary disease. Thorax 1994; 49:162–170.

16. Sun XG, Hansen JR, Oudiz RJ, Wasserman K. Exercise pathophysiology in patients with primary pulmonary typertension. Circulation 2001; 104:429–435.

17. Beck KC, Weisman IM. Methods for cardiopulmonary exercise testing. In: Weisman IM, Zeballos RJ, eds. Clinical Exercise Testing, Progress in Respiratory Research, Vol. 32. Basel: Karger, 2002:43–59.

18. Guyatt GH, Thompson PJ, Berman LB, Sullivan MJ, Townsend M, Jones NL, Pugsley SO. How should we measure function in patients with chronic heart and lung disease? J Chronic Dis 1985; 38:517–524.

19. Guyatt GH, Townsend M, Keller J, Singer J, Nogradi S. Measuring functional status in chronic lung disease: conclusions from a randomized control trial. Respir Med 1991; 85 (Suppl B):17–21; discussion 33–37.

20. American Thoracic Society. ATS Statement: guidelines for the six-minute walk test. Am J Respir Crit Care Med 2002; 166:111–117.

21. Weisman IM, Zeballos RJ. An integrated approach to the interpretation of cardiopulmonary exercise testing. Clin Chest Med 1994; 15:421–445.

22. Weisman IM, Zeballos RJ. An integrative approach to the interpretation of cardiopulmonary exercise testing. In: Weisman IM, Zeballos RJ, eds. Clinical Exercise Testing, Progress in Respiratory Research, Vol. 32. Basel: Karger, 2002; 300–322.

23. Wasserman, K, Hansen JE, SUE, DY, Whipp BJ, Cusaburi, Principles of exercise testing and interpretation 3rd ed. Philadelphia: Lippincott Williams & Wilkins, 1999.

24. Jones NL. Clinical Exercise Testing, 4th ed. Philadelphia: Saunders, 1997.

25. ACC/AHA. Guidelines for Exercise Testing: a report of the American College of Cardiology/American Heart Association Task Force on Practice Guidelines (Committee on Exercise Testing). J Am Coll Cardiol 1997; 30:260–311.

26. Miyamoto S, Nagaya N, Satoh T, Kyotani S, Sakamaki F, Fujita M, Nakanishi N, Miyatake K. Clinical correlates and prognostic significance of six-minute walk test in patients with primary pulmonary hypertension. Comparison with cardiopulmonary exercise testing. Am J Respir Crit Care Med 2000; 161:487–492.

27. Harris-Eze AO, Sridhar G, Clemens RE, Gallagher CG, Marciniuk DD. Oxygen improves maximal exercise performance in interstitial lung disease. Am J Respir Crit Care Med 1994; 150:1616–1622.

28. Zeballos RJ, Weisman IM, Connery SM. Comparison of pulmonary gas exchange measurements between incremental and constant work exercise above the anaerobic threshold. Chest 1998; 113:602–611.

29. Marciniuk DD, Watts RE, Gallagher CG. Reproducibility of incremental maximal cycle ergometer testing in patients with restrictive lung disease. Thorax 1993; 48:894–898.

30. Fulmer JD, Roberts WC, von Gal ER, Crystal RG. Morphologic-physiologic correlates of the severity of fibrosis and degree of cellularity in idiopathic pulmonary fibrosis. J Clin Invest 1979; 63:665–676.

31. Watters LC, King TE, Schwarz MI, Waldron JA, Stanford RE, Cherniack RM. A clinical, radiographic, and physiologic scoring system for the longitudinal assessment of patients with idiopathic pulmonary fibrosis. Am Rev Respir Dis 1986; 133:97–103.

32. Marciniuk DD, Gallagher CG. Clinical exercise testing in interstitial lung disease. Clin Chest Med 1994; 15:287–303.

33. Martinez FJ, Stanopoulos I, Acero R, Becker FS, Pickering R, Beamis JF. Graded comprehensive cardiopulmonary exercise testing in the evaluation of dyspnea unexplained by routine evaluation. Chest 1994; 105:168–174.

34. Orens JB, Becker FS, Lynch JP III, Christensen PJ, Deeb GM, Martinez FJ. Cardiopulmonary exercise testing following allogeneic lung transplantation for different underlying disease states. Chest 1995; 107:144–149.

35. Weisman IM, Zeballos RJ. Clinical evaluation of unexplained dyspnea. Cardiologia 1996; 41:621–634.

36. Medinger AE, Khouri S, Rohatgi PK. Sarcoidosis: the value of exercise testing. Chest 2001; 120:93–101.

37. King TE Jr, Tooze JA, Schwarz MI, Brown KR, Cherniack RM. Predicting survival in idiopathic pulmonary fibrosis: scoring system and survival model. Am J Respir Crit Care Med 2001; 164:1171–1181.

38. Agusti C, Xaubet A, Agusti AG, Roca J, Ramirez J, Rodriguez-Roisin R. Clinical and functional assessment of patients with idiopathic pulmonary fibrosis: results of a 3 year follow-up. Eur Respir J 1994; 7:643–650.

39. Xaubet A, Agusti C, Luburich P, Roca J, Monton C, Ayuso MC, Barbera JA, Rodriguez-Roisin R. Pulmonary function tests and CT scan in the management of idiopathic pulmonary fibrosis. Am J Respir Crit Care Med 1998; 158:431–436.

40. Kadikar A, Maurer J, Kesten S. The six-minute walk test: a guide to assessment for lung transplantation. J Heart Lung Transplant 1997; 16:313–319.

41. Chetta A, Aiello M, Foresi A, Marangio E, D'Ippolito R, Castagnaro A, Olivieri D. Relationship between outcome measures of six-minute walk test and baseline

lung function in patients with interstitial lung disease. Sarcoidosis Vasc Diffuse Lung Dis 2001; 18:170–175.

42. Nohria A, Eldrin L, Warner Stevenson L. Medical management of advanced heart failure. JAMA 2002; 287:628–639.

43. O'Donnell DE. Physiology of interstitial lung disease. In: Schwarz M, King T Jr, eds. Interstitial Lung Disease. Hamilton, Ontario, Canada: Decker, 1998:51–70.

44. Schlueter DP, Fink JN, Sosman AJ. Pulmonary function in pigeon breeders' disease: a hypersensitivity pneumonitis. Ann Intern Med 1969; 70:457–470.

45. Glaister DH, Schroter RC, Sudlow MF, Milic-Emili J. Bulk elastic properties of excised lungs and the effect of a transpulmonary pressure gradient. Respir Physiol 1973; 17:347–364.

46. Gibson CJ, Edmonds JP, Hughes GR. Diaphragm function and lung involvement in systemic lupus erythematosus. Am J Med 1977; 63:926–932.

47. Finucane KE. Lung volumes and distensibility. Aust N Z J Med 1984; 14:790–793.

48. de Troyer A, Yernault JC. Inspiratory muscle force in normal subjects and patients with interstitial lung disease. Thorax 1980; 35:92–100.

49. West J, Alexander J. Studies on respiratory mechanics and the work of breathing in pulmonary fibrosis. Am J Med 1959; 27:529–544.

50. Thompson PW, James IT, Wheatcroft S, Pownall R, Barnes CG. Circadian rhythm of serum cytidine deaminase in patients with rheumatoid arthritis during rest and exercise. Ann Rheum Dis 1989; 48:502–504.

51. Gibson GJ, Pride NB, Davis JN, Loh LC. Pulmonary mechanics in patients with respiratory muscle weakness. Am Rev Respir Dis 1977; 115:389–395.

52. Colebatch HJ, Ng CK, Nikov N. Use of an exponential function for elastic recoil. J Appl Physiol 1979; 46:387–393.

53. Knudson RJ, Kaltenborn WT. Evaluation of lung elastic recoil by exponential curve analysis. Respir Physiol 1981; 46:29–42.

54. Mead J. Mechanical properties of the lung. Physiol Rev 1961; 41:281–330.

55. Haber PS, Colebatch HJ, Ng CK, Greaves IA. Alveolar size as a determinant of pulmonary distensibility in mammalian lungs. J Appl Physiol 1983; 54:837–845.

56. McCormack FX, King TE Jr, Voelker DR, Robinson PC, Mason RJ. Idiopathic pulmonary fibrosis. Abnormalities in the bronchoalveolar lavage content of surfactant protein A. Am Rev Respir Dis 1991; 144:160–166.

57. Robinson PC, Watters LC, King TE, Mason RJ. Idiopathic pulmonary fibrosis. Abnormalities in bronchoalveolar lavage fluid phospholipids. Am Rev Respir Dis 1988; 137:585–591.

58. Gottlieb D, Snider G, Phan S, et al. Lung Function in Pulmonary Fibrosis. New York: Marcel Dekker, 1995.

59. Nava S, Rubini F. Lung and chest wall mechanics in ventilated patients with end stage idiopathic pulmonary fibrosis. Thorax 1999; 54:390–395.

60. Yernault JC, de Jonghe M, de Coster A, Englert M. Pulmonary mechanics in diffuse fibrosing alveolitis. Bull Physiopathol Respir (Nancy) 1975; 11:231–244.

61. Bjerke RD, Tashkin DP, Clements PJ, Chopra SK, Gong Jr H, Bein M. Small airways in progressive systemic sclerosis (PSS). Am J Med 1979; 66:201–209.

62. Jezek V, Fucik J, Michaljanic A, Jeskova L. The prognostic significance of functional tests in kryptogenic fibrosing alveolitis. Bull Eur Physiolpathol Respir 1980; 16:711–720.

63. Carrington CB, Gaensler EA, Coutu RE, FitzGerald MX, Gupta RG. Natural history and treated course of usual and desquamative interstitial pneumonia. N Engl J Med 1978; 298:801–809.

64. Tukiainen P, Taskinen E, Holsti P, Korhola O, Valle M. Prognosis of cryptogenic fibrosing alveolitis. Thorax 1983; 38:349–355.

65. O'Donnell DE, Lam M, Webb KA. Measurement of symptoms, lung hyperinflation, and endurance during exercise in chronic obstructive pulmonary disease. Am J Respir Crit Care Med 1998; 158:1557–1565.

66. Scano G, Monechi GC, Stendardi L, LoConte C, Van Meerhaeghe A, Sergysels R. Functional evaluation in Stage I pulmonary sarcoidosis. Respiration 1986; 49:195–203.

67. Renzi G, Dutton RE. Pulmonary function in diffuse sarcoidosis. Respiration 1974; 31:124–136.

68. Dutton RE, Renzi PM, Lopez-Majano V, Renzi GD. Airway function in sarcoidosis: Smokers vs nonsmokers. Respiration 1982; 43:164–173.

69. Stjernberg N, Thunell M. Pulmonary function in patients with endobronchial sarcoidosis. Acta Med Scand 1984; 215:121–126.

70. Bradvik I, Wollmer P, Simonsson B, Albrechtsson U, Lyttkens K, Jonson B. Lung mechanics and their relationship to lung volumes in pulmonary sarcoidosis. Eur Respir J 1989; 2:643–651.

71. Radwan L, Grebska E, Koziorowski A. Small airways function in pulmonary sarcoidosis. Scand J Respir Dis 1978; 59:37–43.

72. Argyropoulou PK, Patakas DA, Louridas GE. Airway function in stage I and stage II pulmonary sarcoidosis. Respiration 1984; 46:17–25.

73. Levinson RS, Metzger LF, Stanley NN, Kelsen SG, Altose MD, Cherniack NS, Brody JS. Airway function in sarcoidosis. Am J Med 1977; 62:51–59.

74. Sharma OP, Johnson R. Airway obstruction in sarcoidosis. A study of 123 nonsmoking black American patients with sarcoidosis. Chest 1988; 94:343–346.

75. McCarthy DS, Sigurdson M. Lung function in pulmonary sarcoidosis. Ir J Med Sci 1978; 147:413–419.

76. Miller A, Teirstein AS, Jackler I, Chuang M, Siltzbach LE. Airway function in chronic pulmonary sarcoidosis with fibrosis. Am Rev Respir Dis 1974; 109:179–189.

77. Harrison BD, Shaylor JM, Stokes TC, Wilkes AR. Airflow limitation in sarcoidosis—a study of pulmonary function in 107 patients with newly diagnosed disease. Respir Med 1991; 85:59–64.

78. Lavergne F, Clericki C, Sadoun D, Brauner MW, Battesti JP, Valeyre D. Airway obstruction in bronchial sarcoidosis. Outcome with treatment. Chest 1999; 116:1194–1199.

79. Cieslicki J, Zych D, Zielinski J. Airways obstruction in patients with sarcoidosis. Sarcoidosis 1991; 8:42–44.

80. Perez T, Remy-Jardin M, Cortet B. Airways involvement in rheumatoid arthritis. Clinical, functional, and HRCT findings. Am J Respir Crit Care Med 1998; 157:1658–1665.

81. Radoux V, Menard HA, Begin R, Decary F, Koopman WJ. Airways disease in rheumatoid arthritis patients. One element of a general exocrine dysfunction. Arthritis Rheum 1987; 30:249–256.

82. Vergnenegre A, Pugnere N, Antonini MT, Arnaud M, Melloni B, Treves R, Bonnaud F. Airway obstruction and rheumatoid arthritis. Eur Respir J 1997; 10:1072–1078.

83. Cortet B, Perez T, Roux N, Flipo RM, Duuesnoy B, Delcambre B, Remy-Jardin M. Pulmonary function tests and high resolution computed tomography of the lungs in patients with rheumatoid arthritis. Ann Rheum Dis 1997; 56:596–600.

84. Sassoon CSH, McAlpine SW, Tashkin DP, Baydur A, Quismoro FP, Mongan ES. Small airways function in nonsmokers with rheumatoid arthritis. Arthritis Rheum 1984; 27:1218–1226.

85. Cherniack RM, Colby TV, Flint A, Thurlbeck WM, Waldron JA, Ackerson L, Schwarz MI, King TE. Correlation of structure and function in idiopathic pulmonary fibrosis. Am J Respir Crit Care Med 1995; 151:1180–1188.

86. Doherty MJ, Pearson MG, O'Grady EA, Pellegrini V, Calverley PMA. Cryptogenic fibrosing alveolitis with preserved lung volumes. Thorax 1997; 52:998–1002.

87. Dunn TL, Watters LC, Hendrix C, Cherniack RM, Schwarz MI, King TE Jr. Gas exchange at a given degree of volume restriction is different in sarcoidosis and idiopathic pulmonary fibrosis. Am J Med 1988; 85:221–224.

88. Harris-Eze AO, Sridhar G, Clemens RE, Zintel TA, Gallagher CG, Marciniuk DD. Role of hypoxemia and pulmonary mechanics in exercise limitation in interstitial lung disease. Am J Respir Crit Care Med 1996; 154:994–1001.

89. Gallagher CG, Hof VI, Younes M. Effect of inspiratory muscle fatigue on breathing pattern. J Appl Physiol 1985; 59:1152–1158.

90. Gallagher CG, Younes M. Breathing pattern during and after maximal exercise in patients with chronic obstructive lung disease, interstitial lung disease, and cardiac disease, and in normal subjects. Am Rev Respir Dis 1986; 133:581–586.

91. Hansen JE, Wasserman K. Pathophysiology of activity limitation in patients with interstitial lung disease. Chest 1996; 109:1566–1576.

92. Mancini DM, Walter G, Reichek N, Lenkinski R, McCully KK, Mullen JL, Wilson JR. Contribution of skeletal muscle atrophy to exercise intolerance and altered muscle metabolism in heart failure. Circulation 1992; 85:1364–1373.

93. Troosters T, Gosselink R, Decramer M. Deconditioning and principles of training. In: Weisman IM, Zeballos RJ, eds. Clinical Exercise Testing, Progress in Respiratory Research. Basel: Karger, 2002; 60–71.

94. Gosker HR, Uszko-Lencer NHMK, Wouters EF, van der Vusse GJ, Schols AM. Muscular alterations in chronic obstructive pulmonary disease and chronic heart failure at rest and during exercise. In: Weisman IM, Zeballos RJ, eds. Clinical Exercise Testing, Progress in Respiratory Research. Basel: Karger, 2002:18–29.

95. Burdon JG, Killian KJ, Jones NL. Pattern of breathing during exercise in patients with interstitial lung disease. Thorax 1983; 38:778–784.

96. Marciniuk DD, Watts RE, Gallagher CG. Dead space loading and exercise limitation in patients with interstitial lung disease. Chest 1994; 105:183–189.

97. Anderson SD, Bye PT. Exercise testing in the evaluation of diffuse interstitial lung disease. Aust N Z J Med 1984; 14:762–768.

98. Markovitz GH, Cooper CB. Exercise and interstitial lung disease. Curr Opin Pulm Med 1998; 4:272–280.

99. Cotes JE. Lung Function: Assessment and Application in Medicine, 5th ed. Oxford, UK: Blackwell Scientific Publications, 1993.

100. Cotes JE, Zejda J, King B. Lung function impairment as a guide to exercise limitation in work-related lung disorders. Am Rev Respir Dis 1988; 137:1089–1093.

101. Smith DD. Pulmonary impairment/disability evaluation: controversies and criticisms. Clin Pulm Med 1995; 2:334–343.

102. Sue DY. Exercise testing in the evaluation of impairment and disability. Clin Chest Med 1994; 15:369–387.

103. Epler GR, Saber FA, Gaensler EA. Determination of severe impairment (disability) in interstitial lung disease. Am Rev Respir Dis 1980; 121:647–659.

104. Sue DY. Evaluation of impairment and disability: the role of cardiopulmonary exercise testing. In: Weisman IM, Zeballos RJ, eds. Clinical Exercise Testing, Progress in Respiratory Research. Basel: Karger, 2002:217–230.

105. Pride N, Macklem PT. Lung Mechanics in Disease. In: Fishman AP, Macklem PT, Mead J, eds. Handbook of Physiology: The Respiratory System, Mechanics of Breathing. Baltimore: Williams & Wilkins, 1986:659–692.

106. Warren CP, Tse KS, Cherniack RM. Mechanical properties of the lung in extrinsic allergic alveolitis. Thorax 1978; 33:315–321.

107. Johnson BD, Weisman IM, Zeballos RJ, Beck KC. Emerging concepts in the evaluation of ventilatory limitation during exercise: the exercise tidal flow-volume loop. Chest 1999; 116:488–503.

108. Johnson BD. Respiratory system responses to exercise in aging. In: Weisman IM, Zeballos RJ, eds. Clinical Exercise Testing, Progress in Respiratory Research. Basel: Karger, 2002:89–98.

109. Gallagher CG. Exercise limitation and clinical exercise testing in chronic obstructive pulmonary disease. Clin Chest Med 1994; 15:305–336.

110. Athos L, Mohler JG, Sharma OP. Exercise testing in the physiologic assessment of sarcoidosis. Ann N Y Acad Sci 1986; 465:491–501.

111. Matthews JI, Hooper RG. Exercise testing in pulmonary sarcoidosis. Chest 1983; 83:75–81.

112. Miller A, Brown LK, Sloane MF, Bhuptani A, Teirstein AS. Cardiorespiratory responses to incremental exercise in sarcoidosis patients with normal spirometry. Chest 1995; 107:323–329.

113. Babb TG. Mechanical ventilatory constraints in aging, lung disease, and obesity: perspectives and brief review. Med Sci Sports Exerc 1999; 31:S12–S22.

114. Baydur A, Milic-Emili J. Expiratory flow limitation during spontaneous breathing: comparison of patients with restrictive and obstructive respiratory disorders. Chest 1997; 112:1017–1023.

115. Jones N. Determinants of breathing pattern in exercise. In: Wasserman K, Whipp BJ, eds. Exercise. Pulmonary Physiology and Pathophysiology. New York: Marcel Dekker, 1991:99–119.

116. Johnson BD, Beck KC, Zeballos RJ, Weisman IM. Advances in pulmonary laboratory testing. Chest 1999; 116:1377–1387.

117. Yan S, Kaminski D, Sliwinski P. Reliability of inspiratory capacity for estimating end-expiratory lung volume changes during exercise in patients with chronic obstructive pulmonary disease. Am J Respir Crit Care Med 1997; 156:55–59.

118. Jones NL, Rebuck AS. Tidal volume during exercise in patients with diffuse fibrosing alveolitis. Bull Eur Physiopathol Respir 1979; 15:321–328.

119. Gowda K, Zintel T, McParland C, Orchard R, Gallagher CG. Diagnostic value of maximal exercise tidal volume. Chest 1990; 98:1351–1354.

120. Renzi G, Milic-Emili J, Grassino AE. The pattern of breathing in diffuse lung fibrosis. Bull Eur Physiopathol Respir 1982; 18:461–472.
121. Van Meerhaeghe A, Scano G, Sergysels R, Bran M, De Coster A. Respiratory drive and ventilatory pattern during exercise in interstitial lung disease. Bull Physiopathol Respir (Nancy) 1981; 17:15–26.
122. Spiro SG, Dowdeswell IR, Clark TJ. An analysis of submaximal exercise responses in patients with sarcoidosis and fibrosing alveolitis. Br J Dis Chest 1981; 75:169–180.
123. Harris-Eze AO, Sridhar G, Clemens RE, Zintel TA, Gallagher CG, Marciniuk DD. Low-dose nebulized morphine does not improve exercise in interstitial lung disease. Am J Respir Crit Care Med 1995; 152:1940–1945.
124. Brack T, Jubran A, Tobin MJ. Dyspnea and decreased variability of breathing in patients with restrictive lung disease. Am J Respir Crit Care Med 2002; 165:1260–1264.
125. Agusti AG, Roca J, Gea J, Wagner PD, Xaubet A, Rodriguez-Roisin R. Mechanisms of gas-exchange impairment in idiopathic pulmonary fibrosis. Am Rev Respir Dis 1991; 143:219–225.
126. Denison D, Al-Hillawi H, Turton C. Lung function in interstitial lung disease. Semin Respir Med 1984; 6:40–54.
127. Jernudd-Wilhelmsson Y, Hornblad Y, Hedenstierna G. Ventilation-perfusion relationships in interstitial lung disease. Eur J Respir Dis 1986; 68:39–49.
128. Wagner PD. Ventilation-perfusion matching during exercise. Chest 1992; 101:192S–198S.
129. Austrian R, McClement JH, Renzetti AD, Donald AW, Riley RL, Cournand A. Clinical and physiologic features of some types of pulmonary diseases with impairment of alveolar-capillary diffusion: the syndrome of "alveolar-capillary block." Am J Med 1951; 11:667–685.
130. Gaensler EA, Carrington CB, Coutu RE, Fitzgerald MX. Radiographic-physiologic-pathologic correlations in interstitial pneumonias. Prog Respir Res 1975; 8:223–241.
131. Dantzker DR, Bower JS. Pulmonary vascular tone improves $\dot{V}_A/\dot{Q}$ matching in obliterative pulmonary hypertension. J Appl Physiol 1981; 51:607–613.
132. Nordenfelt I, Svensson G. The transfer factor (diffusing capacity) as a predictor of hypoxaemia during exercise in restrictive and chronic obstructive pulmonary disease. Clin Physiol 1987; 7:423–430.
133. Bradvik I, Wollmer P, Blom-Bulow B, Albrechtsson U, Jonson B. Lung mechanics and gas exchange during exercise in pulmonary sarcoidosis. Chest 1991; 99:572–578.
134. Kelley MA, Panettieri RA Jr, Krupinski AV. Resting single-breath diffusing capacity as a screening test for exercise-induced hypoxemia. Am J Med 1986; 80:807–812.
135. Crausman RS, Jennings CA, Tuder RM, Ackerson LM, Irvin CG, King TE Jr. Pulmonary histiocytosis X: pulmonary function and exercise pathophysiology. Am J Respir Crit Care Med 1996; 153:426–435.
136. Baughman RP, Gerson M, Bosken CH. Right and left ventricular function at rest and with exercise in patients with sarcoidosis. Chest 1984; 85:301–306.
137. Alpert JS. Effect of right ventricular dysfunction on left ventricular function. Adv Cardiol 1986; 34:25–34.

138. Hawrylkiewicz I, Izdebska-Makosa Z, Grebska E, Zielinski J. Pulmonary haemodynamics at rest and on exercise in patients with idiopathic pulmonary fibrosis. Bull Eur Physiopathol Respir 1982; 18:403–410.

139. Weitzenblum E, Ehrhart M, Rasaholinjanahary J, Hirth C. Pulmonary hemodynamics in idiopathic pulmonary fibrosis and other interstitial pulmonary diseases. Respiration 1983; 44:118–127.

140. Bush A, Busst CM. Cardiovascular function at rest and on exercise in patients with cryptogenic fibrosing alveolitis. Thorax 1988; 43:276–283.

141. Enson Y, Thomas HM III, Bosken CH, Wood JA, Leroy EC, Blanc WA, Wigger HJ, Harvey RM, Cournand A. Pulmonary hypertension in interstitial lung disease: relation of vascular resistance to abnormal lung structure. Trans Assoc Am Physicians 1975; 88:248–255.

142. Davidson D, Stalcup SA, Mellins RB. Systemic hemodynamics affecting cardiac output during hypocapnic and hypercapnic hypoxia. J Appl Physiol 1986; 60:1230–1236.

143. Morrison DA, Stovall JR. Increased exercise capacity in hypoxemic patients after long-term oxygen therapy. Chest 1992; 102:542–550.

144. Agusti AG, Roca J, Rodriguez-Roisin R, Xaubet A, Agusti-Vidal A. Different patterns of gas exchange response to exercise in asbestosis and idiopathic pulmonary fibrosis. Eur Respir J 1988; 1:510–516.

145. Krishnan BS, Marciniuk DD. Cardiorespiratory responses during exercise in interstitial lung disease. In: Weisman IM, Zeballos RJ, eds. Clinical Exercise Testing, Progress in Respiratory Research, Vol. 32. Basel: Karger, 2002:186–199.

146. Lewis DA, Sietsema KE, Casaburi R, Sue DY. Inaccuracy of noninvasive estimates of V_D/V_T in clinical exercise testing. Chest 1994; 106:1476–1478.

147. Widimsky J, Riedel M, Stanek V. Central haemodynamics during exercise in patients with restrictive pulmonary disease. Bull Eur Physiopathol Respir 1977; 13:369–379.

148. Vizza CD, Lynch JP, Ochoa LL, Richardson G, Trulock EP. Right and left ventricular dysfunction in patients with severe pulmonary disease. Chest 1998; 113:576–583.

149. Eschenbacher WL, Mannina A. An algorithm for the interpretation of cardiopulmonary exercise tests. Chest 1990; 97:263–267.

150. Gibbons WJ, Levy RD, Nava S, Malcolm I, Marin JM, Tardif C, Magder S, Lisbona R, Cosio MG. Subclinical cardiac dysfunction in sarcoidosis. Chest 1991; 100:44–50.

151. Shah NS, Velury S, Mascarenhas D, Spodick DH. Electrocardiographic features of restrictive pulmonary disease, and comparison with those of obstructive pulmonary disease. Am J Cardiol 1992; 70:394–395.

152. Pinsky MR. Effects of changing intrathoracic pressure on the normal and failing heart. In: Lenfant C, Scharf SM, Cassidy SS, eds. Lung Biology in Health and Disease, Heart-Lung Interactions in Health and Disease. New York: Marcel Dekker, 1989:839–878.

153. Rodarte JR, Rehder K. Dynamics of respiration. In: Fishman AP, Macklem PT, Mead J, eds. *Handbook of Physiology: The Respiratory System, Mechanics of Breathing.* Baltimore: Williams & Wilkins, 1986:131–144.

154. Morelli S, Ferrante L, Sgreccia A, Eleuteri ML, Perrone C, De Marzio P, Balsano F. Pulmonary hypertension is associated with impaired exercise peformance in patients with systemic sclerosis. Scand J Rheumatol 2000; 29:236–242.

155. Leblanc P, Bowie D, Summers E, Jones N, Killian K. Breathlessness and exercise in patients with cardiorespiratory disease. Am Rev Respir Dis 1986; 133:21–25.

156. Mahler D, Harver A, Rosielly R, Daubenspeck J. Measurement of respiratory sensation in interstitial lung disease. Evaluation of clinical dyspnea ratings and magnitude scaling. Chest 1989; 96:767–771.

157. Borg GA. Psychophysical bases of perceived exertion. Med Sci Sports Exerc 1982; 14:377–381.

158. Reynolds HY. Diagnostic and management strategies for diffuse interstitial lung disease. Chest 1998; 113:192–202.

159. Johnston IDA, Prescott BJ, Chalmers JC, Rudd RM. British Thoracic Society study of cryptogenic fibrosing alveolitis: current presentation and initial management. Thorax 1997; 52:38–44.

160. King TE Jr. Approach to the patient with interstitial lung disease. In: Rose B, ed. Up To Date. Wellesley, MA: American Thoracic Society; 2000.

161. British Thoracic Society. The diagnosis, assessment, and treatment of diffuse parenchymal lung disease in adults: British thoracic society recommendations. Thorax 1999; 54:S1–S30.

162. Epler GR, McLoud TC, Gaensler EA, Mikus JP, Carrington CB. Normal chest roentgenograms in chronic diffuse infiltrative lung disease. N Engl J Med 1978; 298:934–939.

163. Orens JB, Kazerooni EA, Martinez FJ, Curtis JL, Gross BH, Flint A, Lynch JP III. The sensitivity of high-resolution CT in detecting idiopathic pulmonary fibrosis proved by open lung biopsy. A prospective study. Chest 1995; 108:109–115.

164. Crystal RG, Fulmer JD, Roberts WC, Moss ML, Line BR, Reynolds HY. Idiopathic pulmonary fibrosis. Clinical, histologic, radiographic, physiologic, scintigraphic, cytologic, and biochemical aspects. Ann Intern Med 1976; 85:769–788.

165. Williams R, Hugh-Jones P. The significance of lung function changes in asbestosis. Thorax 1960; 15:109–119.

166. Bohadana AB, Peslin R, Poncelet B, Hannhart B. Lung mechanical properties in silicosis and silicoanthracosis. Bull Eur Physiopathol Respir 1980; 16:521–532.

167. William JV. Pulmonary function in patients with farmer's lung. Thorax 1963; 18:255–263.

168. Augusti AGN, Roca J, Rodriguez-Roisin R, Xaubet A, Agusti-Vidal A. Different patterns of gas exchange response to exercise in asbestosis and idiopathic pulmonary fibrosis. Eur Respir J 1988; 1:510–516.

169. Katzenstein ALA, Myers JL. Idiopathic pulmonary fibrosis. Clinical relevance of pathologic classification. Am J Respir Crit Care Med 1998; 157:1301–1315.

170. Bjoraker JA, Ryu JH, Edwin MK, Myers JL, Tazelaar HD, Schroeder DR, Offord KP. Prognostic significance of histopathologic subsets in idiopathic pulmonary fibrosis. Am J Respir Crit Care Med 1998; 157:199–203.

171. Nagai S, Kitaichi M, Itoh H, Nishimura K, Colby TV. Idiopathic nonspecific interstitial pneumonia/fibrosis: comparison with idiopathic pulmonary fibrosis and BOOP. Eur Respir J 1998; 12:1010–1019.

172. Cottin V, Donsbeck AV, Revel D, Loire R, Cordier JF. Nonspecific interstitial pneumonia. Individualization of a clinicopathologic entity in a series of 12 patients. Am J Respir Crit Care Med 1998; 158:1286–1293.

173. Daniil ZD, Gilchrist FC, Nicholson AG, Hansell DM, Harris J, Colby TV, duBois RM. A histologic pattern of nonspecific interstitial pneumonia is associated with a better prognosis than usual interstitial pneumonia in patients with cryptogenic fibrosing alveolitis. Am J Respir Crit Care Med 1999; 160:899–905.

174. Nicholson AG, Colby TV, du Bois RM, Hansell DM, Wells AU. The prognostic significance of the histologic pattern of interstitial pneumonia in patients presenting with the clinical entity of cryptogenic fibrosing alveolitis. Am J Respir Crit Care Med 2000; 162:2213–2217.

175. Flaherty KR, Toews GB, Travis WD, Colby TV, Kazerooni EA, Gross BH, Jain A, Strawderman RL III, Paine R, Flint A, Lynch JP III, Martinez FJ. Clinical significance of histological classification of idiopathic interstitial pneumonia. Eur Respir J 2002; 19:275–283.

176. Park JS, Lee KS, Kim JS, Park CS, Suh YL, Choi DL, Kim KJ. Nonspecific interstitial pneumonia with fibrosis: Radiographic and CT findings in seven patients. Radiology 1995; 195:645–648.

177. Wells AU, Hansell DM, Rubens MB, Cailes JB, Black CM, du Bois RM. Functional impairment in lone cryptogenic fibrosing alveolitis and fibrosing alveolitis associated with systemic sclerosis: a comparison. Am J Respir Crit Care Med 1997; 155:1657–1664.

178. Sturani C, Papiris S, Galavotti V, Gunella G. Pulmonary vascular responsiveness at rest and during exercise in idiopathic pulmonary fibrosis: effects of oxygen and nifedipine. Respiration 1986; 50:117–129.

179. Sudduth CD, Strange C, Cook WR, Miller KS, Baumann M, Collop NA, Silver RM. Failure of the circulatory system limits exercise performance in patients with systemic sclerosis. Am J Med 1993; 95:413–418.

180. Sietsema KE, Kraft M, Ginzton L, Sharma OP. Abnormal oxygen uptake responses to exercise in patients with mild pulmonary sarcoidosis. Chest 1992; 102:838–845.

181. Rhew DC, Riedinger MS, Sandhu M, Bowers C, Greengold N, Weingarten SR. A prospective, multicenter study of a pneumonia practice guideline. Chest 1998; 114:115–119.

182. Wells AU, King AD, Rubens MB, Cramer D, du Bois RM, Hansell DM. Lone cryptogenic fibrosing alveolitis: a functional-morphologic correlation based on extent of disease on thin-section computed tomography. Am J Respir Crit Care Med 1997; 155:1367–1375.

183. Flaherty KR, Martinez FJ. The role of pulmonary function testing in pulmonary fibrosis. Curr Opin Pulm Med 2000; 6:404–410.

184. Erbes R, Schaberg T, Loddenkemper R. Lung function tests in patients with idiopathic pulmonary fibrosis. Are they helpful for predicting outcome? Chest 1997; 111:51–57.

185. Turner-Warwick M, Burrows B, Johnson A. Cryptogenic fibrosing alveolitis: clinical features and their influence on survival. Thorax 1980; 35:171–180.

186. Fulmer JD, Roberts WD, Crystal RG. Diffuse fibrotic lung disease: a correlative study. Chest 1976; 69(suppl):263–265.

187. Keogh BA, Crystal RG. Pulmonary function testing in interstitial pulmonary disease. What does it tell us? Chest 1980; 78:856–865.

188. Kanengiser LC, Rapoport DM, Epstein H, Goldring RM. Volume adjustment of mechanics and diffusion in interstitial lung disease. Lack of clinical significance. Chest 1989; 96:1036–1042.

189. Chinet T, Jaubert F, Dusser D, Danel C, Chretien J, Huchon GJ. Effects of inflammation and fibrosis on pulmonary function in diffuse lung fibrosis. Thorax 1990; 45:675–678.

190. King Jr TE, Tooze JA, Schwarz MI, Brown K, Cherniack RM. Predicting survival in idiopathic pulmonary fibrosis: scoring system and survival model. Am J Respir Crit Care Med 2001; 164:1181–2001.

191. Brantly M, Avila NA, Shotelersuk V, Lucero C, Huizing M, Gahl WA. Pulmonary function and high-resolution CT findings in patients with an inherited form of pulmonary fibrosis, Hermansky-Pudlak syndrome, due to mutations in HPS-1. Chest 2000; 117:129–136.

192. Rudd RM, Haslam PL, Turner-Warwick M. Cryptogenic fibrosing alveolitis: relationships of pulmonary physiology and bronchoalveolar lavage to response to treatement and prognosis. Am Rev Respir Dis 1981; 124:1–8.

193. Wells A. Clinical usefulness of high resolution computed tomography in cryptogenic fibrosing alveolitis. Thorax 1998; 53:1080–1087.

194. Gay SE, Kazerooni EA, Toews GB, Lynch JP III, Gross BH, Cascade PN, Spizarny DL, Flint A, Schork MA, Whyte RI, Popovich J, Hyzy R, Martinez FJ. Idiopathic pulmonary fibrosis. Predicting response to therapy and survival. Am J Respir Crit Care Med 1998; 157:1063–1072.

195. Hanson D, Winterbauer RH, Kirtland SH, Wu R. Changes in pulmonary function test results after 1 year of therapy as predictors of survival in patients with idiopathic pulmonary fibrosis. Chest 1995; 108:305–310.

196. Hubbard R, Johnston I, Britton J. Survival in patients with cryptogenic fibrosing alveolitis. A population-based cohort study. Chest 1998; 113:396–400.

197. Douglas WW, Ryu JH, Schroeder DR. Idiopathic pulmonary fibrosis. Impact of oxygen and colchicine, prednisone, or no therapy on survival. Am J Respir Crit Care Med 2000; 161:1172–1178.

198. Raghu G, Mageto YN, Lockhart D, Schmidt RA, Wood DE, Godwin JD. The accuracy of the clinical diagnosis of new-onset idiopathic pulmonary fibrosis and other interstitial lung disease: a prospective study. Chest 1999; 116:1168–1174.

199. Mogulkoc N, Brutsche MH, Bishop PW, Greaves SM, Horrocks AW, Egan JJ. Pulmonary function in idiopathic pulmonary fibrosis and referral for lung transplantation. Am J Respir Crit Care Med 2001; 164:103–108.

200. Panos RJ, Mortenson RL, Niccoli SA, King TE. Clinical deterioration in patients with idiopathic pulmonary fibrosis: causes and assessment. Am J Med 1990; 88:396–404.

201. Johnson MA, Kwan S, Snell NJC, Nunn AJ, Darbyshire JH, Turner-Warwick M. Randomized controlled trial comparing prednisolone alone with cyclophosphamide and low dose prednisolone in combination in cryptogenic fibrosing alveolitis. Thorax 1989; 44:280–288.

202. Hubbard R, Venn A, Smith C, Cooper M, Johnston I, Britton J. Exposure to commonly prescribed drugs and the etiology of cryptogenic fibrosing alveolitis: a case-control study. Am J Respir Crit Care Med 1998; 157:743–747.

203. Schwartz DA, vanFossen DS, Davis CS, Helmers RA, Dayton CS, Burmeister LF, Hunninghake GW. Determinants of progression in idiopathic pulmonary fibrosis. Am J Respir Crit Care Med 1994; 149:444–449.

204. King TE Jr, Schwarz MI, Brown K, Tooze JA, Colby TV, Waldron JA Jr, Flint A, Thurlbec W, Cherniack RM. Idiopathic pulmonary fibrosis: relationship between histopathologic features and mortality. Am J Resp Crit Care Med 2001; 164:1025–1032.

205. Wells AU, Hansell DM, Rubens MB, Cullinan P, Black CM, du Bois RM. The predictive value of appearances on thin-section computed tomography in fibrosing alveolitis. Am Rev Respir Dis 1993; 148:1076–1082.

206. Wells AU, Rubens MB, DuBois RM, Hansell DM. Serial CT in fibrosing alveolitis: prognostic significance of the initial pattern. AJR 1993; 161:1159–1165.

207. American Thoracic Society. Lung function testing: selection of reference values and interpretative strategies. Am Rev Respir Dis 1991; 144:1202–1218.

208. American Thoracic Society. Single-breath carbon monoxide diffusing capacity (transfer factor)—recommendations for a standard technique. 1995 Update. Am Rev Respir Crit Care Med 1993; 152:2185–2198.

209. Kangalee KM, Abboud RT. Interlaboratory and intralaboratory variability in pulmonary function testing. A 13-year study using a normal biologic control. Chest 1992; 101:88–92.

210. Crapo RO. Carbon monoxide diffusing capacity (transfer factor). Semin Respir Crit Care Med 1998; 19:335–347.

211. Douglas WW, Ryu JH, Swensen SJ, Offord KP, Shroeder DR, Caron GM, DeRemee RA. Colchicine versus prednisone in the treatment of idiopathic pulmonary fibrosis. A randomized prospective study. Am J Respir Crit Care Med 1998; 158:220–225.

212. Raghu G, DePaso WJ, Cain K, Hammar SP, Wetzel CE, Dreis DF, Hutchinson J, Pardee NE, Winterbauer RH. Azathioprine combined with prednisone in the treatement of idiopathic pulmonary fibrosis: A prospective double-blind, randomized, placebo-controlled clinical trial. Am Rev Respir Dis 1991; 144:291–296.

213. Stack BHR, Choo-Kang YFJ, Heard BE. The prognosis of cryptogenic fibrosing alvcolitis. Thorax 1972; 27:535–542.

214. Augusti C, Xaubet A, Agusti AGN, Roca J, Ramirez J, Rodriguez-Roisin R. Clinical and functional assessment of patients with idiopathic pulmonary fibrosis: results of a 3-year follow-up. Eur Respir J 1994; 7:643–650.

215. van Oortegem K, Wallaert B, Marquette CH, Ramon P, Perez T, Lafitte JJ, Tonnel AB. Determinants of response to immunosuppressive therapy in idiopathic pulmonary fibrosis. Eur Resir J 1994; 7:1950–1957.

216. Flaherty KE, Wald J, Blavais M, Weisman IM, Zeballos RJ, Zisman D, Rubenfire M, Martinez FJ. Unexplained exertional limitation: Characterization in a large cohort discovered to have mitchondrial myopathy. Am J Respir Crit Care Med 2001; 164:425–432.

217. Lynch JP, Orens JB, Kazerooni EA. Collagen vascular disease. In: Sperber M, ed. Diffuse Lung Disease: A Comprehensive Clinical-Radiological Overview. London: Springer-Verlag, 1999; 325–355.

218. Lynch JP, Flint A, Belperio J. et al. Bronchiolar complication of connective tissue disorder. Semin Respir Crit Care Med 1999; 20:149–168.

219. Tazelaar HD, Viggiano RW, Pickersgill J, Colby TV. Interstitial lung disease in polymyositis and dermatomyositis. Clinical features and prognosis as correlated with histologic findings. Am Rev Respir Dis 1990; 141:727–733.

220. Wells AU, Cullinan P, Hansell DM, Rubens MB, Black CM, Newman-Taylor AJ, Du Bois RM. Fibrosing alveolitis associated with systemic sclerosis has a better prognosis than lone cryptogenic fibrosing alveolitis. Am J Respir Crit Care Med 1994; 149:1583–1590.

221. Davas EM, Peppas C, Maragou M, Alvanou E, Hondros D, Dantis PC. Intravenous cyclophosphamide pulse therapy for the treatment of lung disease associated with scleroderma. Clin Rheumatol 1999; 18:455–461.

222. White W, Moore W, Wigley FM, Xiao HQ, Wise RA. Cyclophosphamide is associated with pulmonary function and survival benefit in patients with scleroderma and alveolitis. Ann Intern Med 2000; 132:947–954.

223. King TE. Connective tissue disease. In: Schwarz MI, King TE, eds. Interstitial Lung Disease. Hamilton, Ontario, Canada: Decker, 1998:451–505.

224. Cheema GS, Quismorio FP Jr. Interstitial lung disease in systemic sclerosis. Curr Opin Pulm Med 2001; 7:283–290.

225. Steen VD, Medsger TA Jr. Severe organ involvement in systemic sclerosis with diffuse scleroderma. Arthritis Rheum 2000; 43:2437–2444.

226. Hesselstrand R, Scheja A, Akesson A. Mortality and causes of death in a Swedish series of systemic sclerosis patients. Ann Rheum Dis 1998; 57:682–686.

227. D'Angelo WA, Fries FJ, Masi AT, Shulman LE. Pathologic observations in systemic sclerosis (scleroderma): a study of fifty-eight autopsy cases and fifty-eight matched controls. Am J Med 1969; 46:428–440.

228. Weaver AL, Divertie MB, Titus JL. Pulmonary scleroderma. Dis Chest 1968; 54:490–498.

229. Konig G, Luderschmidt C, Hammer C, Adelmann-Grill B, Braun-Falco O, Fruhmann G. Lung involvement in scleroderma. Chest 1984; 85:318–324.

230. Adhikari PK, Bianchi FA, Boushy SF, et al. Pulmonary function in scleroderma. Am Rev Respir Dis 1962; 86:546–550.

231. Hughes DTD, Lee FI. Lung function in patients with systemic slerosis. Thorax 1963; 18:16–20.

232. Ritchie B. Pulmonary function in scleroderma. Thorax 1964; 19:28–36.

233. Wilson RJ, Rodnan GP, Robin ED. An early pulmonary physiologic abnormality in progressive systemic sclerosis (diffuse scleroderma). Am J Med 1964; 36:361–369.

234. Spagnolatti L, Zoia MC, Volpini E, Convertino G, Fulgoni P, Corsico A, Vitulo P, Cerveri I. Pulmonary function in patients with systemic sclerosis. Monaldi Arch Chest 1997; 52:4–8.

235. Steen VD, Conte C, Owens GR, Medsger TA. Severe restrictive lung disease in systemic sclerosis. Arthritis Rheum 1994; 37:1283–1289.

236. Owens GR, Fino GJ, Herbert DL, Steen VD, Medsger TA, Pennock BE, Cottrell JJ, Rodnan GP, Rogers RM. Pulmonary function in progressive systemic sclerosis. Comparison of CREST syndrome variant with diffuse scleroderma. Chest 1983; 84:546–550.

237. Steen VD, Graham G, Conte C, Owens GR, Medsger TA Jr. Isolated diffusing capacity reduction in systemic sclerosis. Arthritis Rheum 1992; 35:765–770.

238. Stupi AM, Steen VD, Owens GR, Barnes EL, Rodnan GP, Medsger TA. Pulmonary hypertension in the CREST syndrome variant of systemic sclerosis. Arthritis Rheum 1986; 29:515–524.

239. Laitinen O, Salorinne Y, Poppius H. Respiratory function in systemic lupus erythematosus, scleroderma, and rheumatoid arthritis. Ann Rheum Dis 1973; 32:531–535.

240. Peters-Golden M, Wise RA, Hochberg MC, Stevens MB, Wigley FM. Carbon monoxide diffusing capacity as predictor of outcome in systemic sclerosis. Am J Med 1984; 77:1027–1034.

241. Pistelli R, Maini CL, Fuso L, Muzzolon R, Bonetti MG, Incalzi RA, Giordano A, Paoletti S. Pulmonary involvement in progressive systemic sclerosis: A multidisciplinary approach. Respiration 1987; 51:296–306.

242. Guttadauria M, Ellman H, Emmanuel G, Kaplan D, Diamond H. Pulmonary function in scleroderma. Arthritis Rheum 1977; 20:1071–1079.

243. Kostopoulos C, Rassidakis A, Sfikakis PP, Anotiades L, Mavrikakis M. Small airways dysfunction in systemic sclerosis. A controlled study. Chest 1992; 102:875–881.

244. Blom-Bulow B, Jonson B, Brauer K. Lung function in progressive systemic sclerosis is dominated by poorly compliant lungs and stiff airways. Eur J Respir Dis 1985; 66:1–8.

245. Peters-Golden M, Wise RA, Schneider PD, Hochberg MC, Stevens MB, Wigley FM. Clinical and demographic predictors of loss of pulmonary function in systemic sclerosis. Medicine (Baltimore) 1984; 63:221–231.

246. Abramson MJ, Barnett AJ, Littlejohn GO, Smith MM, Hall S. Lung function abnormalities and decline in spirometry in scleroderma: an overrated danger? Postgrad Med J 1991; 67:632–637.

247. Yousem SA. The pulmonary pathologic manifestations of the CREST syndrome. Hum Pathol 1990; 21:467–474.

248. Sackner MA, Akgun N, Kimbel P, Lewis DH. The pathophysiology of scleroderma involving the heart and respiratory system. Ann Intern Med 1964; 60:611–630.

249. Medsger TAJ, Rodnan GP, Moossy J, Vester JW. Skeletal muscle involvement in progressive sytemic sclerosis (scleroderma). Arthritis Rheum 1968; 11:554–568.

250. Edelson JD, Hyland RH, Ramsden M, Chamberlain D, Kortan P, Meindok HO, Klein MH, Braude AC, Lee P, Rebuck AS. Lung inflammation in scleroderma: Clinical, radiographic, physiologic and cytopathological features. J Rheumatol 1985; 12:957–963.

251. Arroliga AC, Podell DN, Matthay RA. Pulmonary manifestations of slceroderma. J Thorac Imaging 1992; 7:30–45.

252. Witt C, Borges AC, John M, Fietze I, Baumann G, Krause A. Pulmonary involvement in diffuse cutaneous systemic sclerosis: bronchoalveolar fluid granulocytosis predicts progression of fibrosing alveolitis. Ann Rheum Dis 1999; 58:635–640.

253. Bagg LR, Hughes DT. Serial pulmonary function tests in progressive systemic sclerosis. Thorax 1979; 34:224–228.

254. Greenwald GI, Tashkin DP, Gong H, Simmons M, Duann S, Furst DE, Clements P. Longitudinal changes in lung function and respiratory symptoms in progressive systemic sclerosis. Prospective study. Am J Med 1987; 83:83–92.

255. Ungerer RG, Tashkin DP, Furst D, Clements PJ, Gong H, Bein M, Smith JW, Roberts N, Cabeen W. Prevalence and clinical correlates of pulmonary arterial hypertension in progressive systemic sclerosis. Am J Med 1983; 75:65–74.

256. Diot E, Giraudeau B, Maillot F, Diot P. Decrease in DL_{CO} in systemic sclerosis correlates with acceleration of DTPA clearance. Eur Respir J 1999; 14:728.
257. Emmanuel G, Saroja D, Gopinathan K, et al. Environmental factors and the diffusing capacity of the lung in progressive systemic sclerosis. Chest 1976; 69:304–306.
258. Furst DE, Davis JA, Clements PJ, et al. Abnormalities of pulmonary vascular dynamics and inflammation in early progressive systemic sclerosis. Arthritis Rheum 1981; 24:1403–1408.
259. Gupta D, Aggarwal AN, Sud A, Jindal SK. Static lung mechanics in patients of progressive systemic sclerosis without obvious pulmonary involvement. Indian J Chest Dis Allied Sci 2001; 2:97–101.
260. Sud A, Gupta D, Wanchu A, Jindal SK, Bambery P. Static lung compliance as an index of early pulmonary disease in systemic sclerosis. Clin Rheum 2001; 20:177–180.
261. Godfey S, Bluestone R, Higgs BE. Lung function and the response to exercise in systemic sclerosis. Thorax 1969; 24:427–434.
262. Blom-Bulow B, Jonson B, Bauer K. Factors limiting exercise performance in progressive systemic sclerosis. Semin Arthritis Rheum 1983; 13:174–181.
263. Schwaiblmair M, Behr J, Fruhmann G. Cardiorespiratory responses to incremental exercise in patients with systemic sclerosis. Chest 1996; 110:1520–1525.
264. Diot E, Boissinot E, Asquier E, Guilmot JL, Lemarie E, Valat C, Diot P. Relationship between abnormalities on high-resolution CT and pulmonary function in systemic sclerosis. Chest 1998; 114:1623–1629.
265. Pignone A, Matucci-Cerinic M, Lombardi A, Fedi R, Fargnoli R, De Dominicis R, Cagnoni M. High resolution computed tomography in systemic sclerosis. Real diagnostic utilities in the assessment of pulmonary involvement and comparison with other modalities of lung investigation. Clin Rheum 1992; 11:465–472.
266. Domagala-Kulawik J, Hoser G, Doboszynska A, Kawiak J, Droszcz W. Interstitial lung disease in systemic sclerosis: comparison of BALF lymphocyte phenotype and DLCO impairment. Respir Med 1998; 92:1295–1301.
267. Scussel-Lonzetti L, Joyal F, Raynaud JP, Roussin A, Rich E, Goulet JR, Raymond Y, Senecal JL. Predicting mortality in systemic sclerosis. Analysis of a cohort of 309 French Canadian patients with emphasis on features at diagnosis as predictive factors for survival. Medicine (Baltimore) 2002; 81:154–167.
268. Ferri C, Valentini G, Cozzi F, Sebastiani M, Michelassi C, La Montagna G, Bullo A, Cazzato M, Tirri E, Storino F, Giuggioli D, Cuomo G, Rosada M, Bombardieri S, Todesco S, Tirri G, (SIR-GSSSc). The Systemic Sclerosis Study Group of the Italian Society of Rheumatology. Systemic sclerosis. Demographic, clinical and serologic features and survival in 1,012 Italian patients. Medicine (Baltimore) 2002; 81:139–153.
269. MacGregor AJ, Canavan R, Knight C, Denton CP, Davar J, Coghlan J, Black CM. Pulmonary hypertension in systemic sclerosis: risk factors for progression and consequences for survival. Rheumatology 2001; 40:453–459.
270. Medsger TAJ, Masai AT, Rodnan GP, et al. Survival with systemic sclerosis (scleroderma). Ann Intern Med 1971; 75:369–376.
271. Bennett R, Bluestone R, Holt PJL, Bywaters EGL. Survival in scleroderma. Ann Rheum Dis 1971; 30:581–588.

272. Eason RJ, Tan PL, Gow PJ. Progressive systemic sclerosis in Auckland: a ten year review with emphasis on prognostic features. Aust N Z J Med 1981; 11:657–662.

273. Giersson AJ, Wollheim FA, Akesson A. Disease severity of 100 patients with systemic sclerosis over a period of 14 years: using a modified Medsger scale. Ann Rheum Dis 2001; 60:1117–1122.

274. Jacobsen S, Ullman S, Shen GQ, Wiik A, Halberg P. Influence of clinical features, serum antinuclear antibodies, and lung function on survival of patients with systemic sclerosis. J Rheumatol 2001; 28:2454–2459.

275. Altman RD, Medsger Jr TA, Bloch DA, Michel BA. Predictors of survival in systemic sclerosis (scleroderma). Arthritis Rheum 1991; 23:403–413.

276. Bryan C, Knight C, Black CM, Silman AJ. Prediction of five-year survival following presentation with scleroderma. Development of a simple model using three disease factors at first visit. Arthritis Rheum 1999; 42:2660–2665.

277. Medsger Jr TA, Silman AJ, Steen VD, Black CM, Akesson A, Bacon PA, Harris CA, Jablonska S, Jayson MIV, Jimenez SA, Krieg T, Leroy EC, Maddison PJ, Russell ML, Schachter RK, Wollheim FA, Zacharaie H. A disease severity scale for systemic sclerosis: development and testing. J Rheumatol 1999; 26:2159–2167.

278. Schneider PD, Wise RA, Hochberg MC, Wigley FM. Serial pulmonary function in systemic sclerosis. Am J Med 1982; 73:385–394.

279. Colp CR, Riker J, Williams MH Jr. Serial changes in scleroderma and idiopathic interstitial lung disease. Arch Intern Med 1973; 132:506–515.

280. Jacobsen S, Halberg P, Ullman S, Hoier-Madsen M, Petersen J, Mortensen J, Wiik A. A longitudinal study of pulmonary function in Danish patients with systemic sclerosis. Clin Rheum 1997; 16:384–390.

281. Groen H, Wichers G, ter Borg EJ, van der Mark TW, Wouda AA, Kallenberg CG. Pulmonary diffusing capacity disturbances are related to nailfold capillary changes in patients with Raynaud's phenomenon with and without an underlying connective tissue disease. Am J Med 1990; 89:34–41.

282. Silver RM, Miller KS, Kinsella MB, Smith EA, Schabel SI. Evaluation and management of scleroderma lung disease using bronchoalveolar lavage. Am J Med 1990; 88:470–476.

283. Akesson A, Scheja A, Lundin A, Wollheim FA. Improved pulmonary function in systemic sclerosis after treatment with cyclophosphamide. Arthritis Rheum 1994; 37:729–735.

284. Toews GB, Lynch JP III. Methotrexate in sarcoidosis. Am J Med Sci 1990; 300:33–36.

285. Helmers R, Galvin J, Hunninghake GW. Pulmonary manifestations associated with rheumatoid arthritis. Chest 1991; 100:235–238.

286. Roschmann RA, Rothenberg RJ. Pulmonary fibrosis in rheumatoid arthritis: a review of clinical features and therapy. Semin Arthritis Rheum 1987; 16:174–185.

287. Fujii M, Adachi S, Shimizu T, Hirota S, Sako M, Kono M. Interstitial lung disease in rheumatoid arthritis: assessment with high-resolution computed tomography. J Thorac Imaging 1993; 8:54–62.

288. Gabbay E, Tarala R, Will R, Carroll G, Adler B, Cameron D, Lake FR. Interstitial lung disease in recent onset rheumatoid arthritis. Am J Respir Crit Care Med 1997; 156:528–535.

289. McDonagh J, Greaves M, Wright AR, Heycock C, Owen JP, Kelly C. High resolution computed tomography of the lungs in patients with rheumatoid arthritis and interstitial lung disease. Br J Rheumatol 1994; 33:118–122.

290. Dawson JK, Fewins HE, Desmond J, Lynch MP, Graham DR. Fibrosing alveolitis in patients with rheumatoid arthritis as assessed by high resolution computed tomography, chest radiography, and pulmonary function tests. Thorax 2001; 56:622–627.

291. Banks J, Banks C, Cheong B, Umachandran V, Smith AP, Jessop JD, Pritchard MH. An epidemiological and clinical investigation of pulmonary function and respiratory symptoms in patients with rheumatoid arthritis. Q J Med 1992; 85:307–308.

292. Anaya JM, Diethelm L, Ortiz LA, Gutierrez M, Citera G, Welsh RA, Espinoza LR. Pulmonary involvement in rheumatoid arthritis. Semin Arthritis Rheum 1995; 24:242–254.

293. Hyland RH, Gordon DA, Broder I, Davies GM, Russell ML, Hutcheon MA, Reid GD, Cox DW, Corey PN, Mintz S. A systematic controlled study of pulmonary abnormalities in rheumatoid arthritis. J Rheumatol 1983; 10.

294. Frank ST, Weg JG, Harkleroad LE, Fitch RF. Pulmonary dysfunction in rheumatoid disease. Chest 1973; 63:27–34.

295. Popper MS, Bogdonoff ML, Hughes RL. Interstitial rheumatoid lung disease. Chest 1972; 62:243–249.

296. Hakala M. Poor prognosis in patients with rheumatoid arthritis hospitalized for interstitial lung fibrosis. Chest 1988; 93:114–118.

297. Westedt ML, Hazes JMW, Breedveld FC, Sterk PJ, Dijkman JH. Cigarette smoking and pulmonary diffusion defects in rheumatoid arthritis. Rheumatol Int 1998; 18:1–4.

298. Davidson C, Brooks AGF, Bacon PA. Lung function in rheumatoid arthritis. A clinic survey. Ann Rheum Dis 1974; 33:293–297.

299. Oxholm P, Bundgaard A, Birk Madsen E, Manthorpe R, Vejlo Rasmussen F. Pulmonary function in patients with primary Sjogren's syndrome. Rheumatol Int 1982; 2:179–181.

300. Cervantes-Perez P, Toro-Perez AH, Rodriguez-Jurado P. Pulmonary involvement in rheumatoid arthritis. JAMA 1980; 243:1715–1719.

301. Popp W, Rauscher H, Ritschka L, Braun O, Scherak O, Kolarz G, Zwick H. Prediction of interstitial lung involvement in rheumatoid arthritis. The value of clinical data, chest roentgenogram, lung function, and serologic parameters. Chest 1992; 102:391–394.

302. Gorini M, Ginanni R, Spinelli A, Duranti R, Andreotti L, Scano G. Inspiratory muscle strength and respiratory drive in patients with rheumatoid arthritis. Am Rev Respir Dis 1990; 142:289–294.

303. Cimen OB, Deviren SD, Yorgancioglu ZR. Pulmonary function tests, aerobic capacity, respiratory muscle strength and endurance of patients with rheumatoid arthritis. Clin Rheum 2001; 20:168–173.

304. Hayakawa H, Sato A, Imokawa S, Toyoshima M, Chida K, Iwata M. Bronchiolar disease in rheumatoid arthritis. Am J Respir Crit Care Med 1996; 154:1531–1536.

305. Hassan WU, Keaney NP, Holland CD, Kelly CA. Bronchial reactivity and airflow obstruction in rheumatoid arthritis. Ann Rheum Dis 1994; 53:511–514.

306. Saag KG, Kolluri S, Koehnke RD, Georgou TA, Rachow JW, Hunninghake GW, Schwartz DA. Rheumatoid arthritis lung disease. Determinants of radiographic and physiologic abnormalities. Arthritis Rheum 1996; 39:1711–1719.

307. Turner-Warwick M, Evans RC. Pulmonary manifestations of rheumatoid disease. Clin Rheum Dis 1977; 3:549–564.

308. Dawson JK, Fewins HE, Desmond J, Lynch MP, Graham DR. Predictors of progression of HRCT diagnosed fibrosing alveolitis in patients with rheumatoid arthritis. Ann Rheum Dis 2002; 61:517–521.

309. Linstow M, Ulrik CS, Kriegbaum NJ, Backer V, Oxholm P. An 8-year follow-up study of pulmonary functon in patients with rheumatoid arthritis. Rheumatol Int 1994; 14:115–118.

310. Beyeler C, Jordi B, Gerber NJ, Hof VI. Pulmonary function in rheumatoid arthritis treated with low-dose methotrexate: a longitudinal study. Br J Rheumatol 1996; 35:446–452.

311. Dawson JK, Graham DR, Desmond J, Fewins HE, Lynch MP. Investigation of the chronic pulmonary effects of low-dose oral methotrexate in patients with rheumatoid arthritis: a prospective study incorporating HRCT scanning and pulmonary function tests. Rheumatology 2002; 41:262–267.

312. Dayton CS, Schwartz DA, Sprince NL, Yagla SJ, Davis CS, Koehnke RK, Furst DE, Hunninghake GW. Low-dose methotrexate may cause air trapping in patients with rheumatoid arthritis. Am J Respir Crit Care Med 1995; 151:1189–1193.

313. Cottin V, Tebib J, Massonnet B, Souquet PJ, Bernard JP. Pulmonary function in patients receiving long-term low-dose methotrexate. Chest 1996; 109:933–938.

314. Haerden J, Coolen L, Dequeker J. The effect of D-penicillamine on lung function parameters (diffusing capacity) in rheumatoid arthritis. Clin Exp Rheumatol 1993; 11:509–513.

315. Douglas WW, Tazelaar HD, Hartman TE, Decker PA, Schroeder DR, Ryu JH. Polymyositis-dermatomyositis–associated interstitial lung disease. Am J Resp Crit Care Med 2001; 164:1182–1185.

316. Marguerie C, Bunn CC, Beynon HL, Bernstein RM, Hughes JM, So AK, Walport MJ. Polymyositis, pulmonary fibrosis and autoantibodies to aminoacyl-tRNA synthetase enzymes. Q J Med 1990; 77:1019–1038.

317. Sullivan M, Genter F, Savvides M, Roberts M, Myers J, Froelicher V. The reproducibility of hemodynamic, electrocardiographic, and gas exchange data during treadmill exercise in patients with stable angina pectoris. Chest 1984; 86:375–382.

318. Jolliet P, Thorens JB, Chevrolet JC. Pulmonary vascular reactivity in severe pulmonary hypertension associated with mixed connective tissue disease. Thorax 1995; 50:96–97.

319. Papathanasiou MP, Constantopoulos SH, Tsampoulas C, Drosos AA, Moutso-poulos HM. Reappraisal of respiratory abnormalities in primary and secondary Sjögren's syndrome. A controlled study. Chest 1986; 90:370–374.

320. Dalavanga YA, Constantopoulos SH, Galanopoulou V, Zerva L, Moutsopoulos HM. Alveolitis correlates with clinical pulmonary involvement in primary Sjögren's syndrome. Chest 1991; 99:1394–1397.

321. Kelly C, Gardiner P, Pal B, Griffiths I. Lung function in primary Sjögren's syndrome: a cross sectional and longitudinal study. Thorax 1991; 46:180–183.

322. Deheinzelin D, Capelozzi VL, Kairalla RA, Barbas Filho JV, Saldiva PH, de Carvalho CR. Interstitial lung disease in primary Sjögren's syndrome. Clinical-pathological evaluation and response to treatment. Am J Respir Crit Care Med 1996; 154:794–799.

323. Uffman M, Kiener HP, Bankier AA, Baldt MM, Zontsich T, Herold CJ. Lung manifestation in asymptomatic patients with primary Sjögren syndrome: assessment with high resolution CT and pulmonary function tests. J Thorac Imaging 2001; 16:282–289.

324. Lynch JP, Kazerooni EA, Gay SE. Pulmonary sarcoidosis. Clin Chest Med 1997; 18:755–785.

325. American Thoracic Society. Statement on sarcoidosis. Am J Respir Crit Care Med 1999; 160:736–755.

326. Newman LS, Rose CS, Maier LA. Sarcoidosis. N Engl J Med 1997; 336:1224–1234.

327. Baughman RP, Sharma OP, Lynch JP III. Sarcoidosis: is therapy effective? Semin Respir Infect 1998; 13:255–273.

328. Costabel U. Sarcoidosis: clinical update. Eur Respir J 2001; 18(suppl 32):56S–68S.

329. Lynch JP III, Sharma OP, Baughman RP. Extrapulmonary sarcoidosis. Semin Respir Infect 1998; 13:229–254.

330. Nunley DR, Hattler B, Keenan RJ, Iacono AT, Yousem S, Ohori NP, Dauber JH. Lung transplantation for end-stage pulmonary sarcoidosis. Sarcoidosis Vasc Diffuse Lung Dis 1999; 16:93–100.

331. Winterbauer RH, Hutchinson JF. Use of pulmonary function tests in the management of sarcoidosis. Chest 1980; 78:640–647.

332. Bistrong HW, Tenney RD, Sheffer AL. Asymptomatic cavitary sarcoidosis. JAMA 1970; 213:1030–1032.

333. Neville E, Walker AN, James DG. Prognostic factors predicting the outcome of sarcoidosis: an analysis of 818 patients. Q J Med 1983; 52:525–533.

334. Romer FK. Presentation of sarcoidosis and outcome of pulmonary changes. Dan Med Bull 1982; 29:27–32.

335. Sharma OP. Pulmonary sarcoidosis and corticosteroids. Am Rev Respir Dis 1993; 147:1598–1600.

336. Winterbauer RH, Belic N, Moores KD. Clinical interpretation of bilateral hilar adenopathy. Ann Intern Med 1973; 78:65–71.

337. Miller A, Chuang M, Teirstein AS, Siltzbach LE. Pulmonary function in stage I and II pulmonary sarcoidosis. Ann N Y Acad Sci 1976; 278:292–300.

338. Bergin CJ, Bell DY, Coblentz CL, Chiles C, Gamsu G, MacIntyre NR, Coleman RE, Putman CE. Sarcoidosis: correlation of pulmonary parenchymal pattern at CT with results of pulmonary function tests. Radiology 1989; 171:619–624.

339. Saumon G, Georges R, Loiseau A, Turiaf J. Membrane diffusing capacity and pulmonary capillary blood volume in pulmonary sarcoidosis. Ann N Y Acad Sci 1976; 278:284–291.

340. McLoud TC, Epler GR, Gaensler EA, Burke GW, Carrington CB. A radiographic classification of sarcoidosis. Physiologic correlation. Invest Radiol 1982; 17:129–138.

341. Sharma OP, Colp C, Williams MH Jr. Course of pulmonary sarcoidosis with and without corticosteroid therapy as determined by pulmonary function studies. Am J Med 1966; 41:541.

342. Holmgren A, Svanborg N. Studies on the cardiopulmonary function in sarcoidosis: I. Cases with bilateral lymph node enlargement and radiographically normal lungs. Acta Med Scand 1961; 170 (suppl 366):5–38.

343. Young RC, Carr C, Shelton TG, Mann M, Ferrin A, Laurey JR, Harden KA. Sarcoidosis: relationship between changes in lung structure and function. Am Rev Respir Dis 1967; 95:224–238.

344. Bradvick I, Wollmer P, Blom-Bulow B, Albrechtsson U, Johnson B. Lung mechanics and gas exchange in steroid treated pulmonary sarcoidosis. A seven year follow-up. Sarcoidosis 1991; 8:105–114.

345. Bradvick I. Use of lung function tests in sarcoidosis. Sarcoidosis Vasc Diffuse Lung Dis 1996; 13:59–62.

346. Sharma OP, Colp C, Williams MH. Pulmonary function studies in patients with bilateral sarcoidosis of hilar lymph nodes. Arch Intern Med 1966; 117:436–439.

347. Karetzky M, McDonough M. Exercise and resting pulmonary function in sarcoidosis. Sarcoidosis Vasc Diffuse Lung Dis 1996; 13:43–49.

348. Medinger AE, Khouri S, Rohatgi PK. Sarcoidosis. The value of exercise testing. Chest 2001; 120:93–101.

349. Benedict EH, Castelman B. Sarcoidosis with bronchial involvement: report of case with bronchoscopic and pathological observations. N Engl J Med 1941; 224:186–189.

350. McCann BG, Harrison BD. Bronchiolar narrowing and occlusion in sarcoidosis correlation of pathology with physiology. Respir Med 1991; 85:282–292.

351. Sharma OP, Badr A. Sarcoidosis: diagnosis, staging, and newer diagnostic modalities. Clin Pulm Med 1994; 1:18–26.

352. Udwadia ZF, Pilling JR, Jenkins PF, Harrison BD. Bronchoscopic and bronchographic findings in 12 patients with sarcoidosis and severe or progressive airways obstruction. Thorax 1990; 45:272–275.

353. Benatar SR, Clark TJ. Pulmonary function in a case of endobronchial sarcoidosis. Am Rev Respir Dis 1974; 110:490–496.

354. Miller A, Teirstein AS, Chuang MT. The sequence of physiologic changes in pulmonary sarcoidosis: Correlation with radiographic stages and response to therapy. Mt Sinai J Med 1977; 44:852–865.

355. Coates R, Neville E. The development of airways obstruction in sarcoidosis among smokers and non-smokers. Sarcoidosis 1993; 10:115–117.

356. Manresa Presas F, Romero Colomer P, Rodriguez Sanchon B. Bronchial hyperreactivity in fresh stage I sarcoidosis. Ann N Y Acad Sci 1986; 465:523–529.

357. Bechtel JJ, Starr T, Dantzker DR, Bower JS. Airway hyperreactivity in patients with sarcoidosis. Am Rev Respir Dis 1981; 124:759–761.

358. Ohrn MB, Skold CM, van Hage-Hamsten M, Sigurdardottir O, Zetterstrom O, Eklund A. Sarcoidosis patients have bronchial hyperreactivity and signs of mast cell activation in their bronchoalveolar lavage. Respiration 1995; 62:136–142.

359. Fridman OH, Blaugrund SM, Siltzbach LE. Biopsy of the bronchial wall as an aid in diagnosis of sarcoidosis. JAMA 1963; 183:646–650.

360. Schorr AF, Torrington KG, Hnatiuk OW. Endobronchial involvement and airway hyperreactivity in patients with sarcoidosis. Chest 2001; 120:881–886.

361. Young RL, Loudon RE, Krumholz RA, Harkleroad LE, Branam GE, Weg JG. Pulmonary sarcoidosis: I. Pathologic considerations. Am Rev Respir Dis 1968; 97:997–1008.

362. Carrington CB, Gaensler EA, Mikus JP, Schachter WA, Burke GW, Goff AM. Structure and function in sarcoidosis. Ann N Y Acad Sci 1976; 278:265–283.
363. Huang CT, Heurich AE, Rosen Y, Moon S, Lyons HA. Pulmonary sarcoidosis: roentgenographic, functional, and pathologic correlations. Respiration 1979; 37:337–345.
364. Lin YH, Haslam PL, Turner-Warwick M. Chronic pulmonary sarcoidosis: relationship between lung lavage cell counts, chest radiograph, and results of standard lung function tests. Thorax 1985; 40:501–507.
365. Muller NL, Mawson JB, Mathieson JR, Abboud R, Ostrow D, Champion P. Sarcoidosis: correlation of extent of disease at CT with clinical, functional, and radiographic findings. Radiology 1989; 171:613–618.
366. Brauner MW, Grenier P, Mouelhi MM, Mompoint D, Lenoir S. Pulmonary histiocytosis X: evaluation with high-resolution CT. Radiology 1989; 172:255–258.
367. Remy-Jardin M, Remy J, Deffontaines C, Duhamel A. Assessment of diffuse infiltrative lung disease: comparison of conventional CT and high-resolution CT. Radiology 1991; 181:157–162.
368. Remy-Jardin M, Giraud F, Remy J, Wattinne L, Wallaert B, Duhamel A. Pulmonary sarcoidosis: role of CT in the evaluation of disease activity and functional impairment and in prognosis assessment. Radiology 1994; 191:675–680.
369. Hansell DM, Milne DG, Wilsher ML, Wells AU. Pulmonary sarcoidosis: morphologic associations of airflow obstruction at thin-section CT. Radiology 1998; 209:697–704.
370. Muers MF, Middleton WG, Gibson GJ, Prescott RJ, Mitchell DN, Connolly CK, Harrison BDW. A simple radiographic scoring method for monitoring pulmonary sarcoidosis: relations between radiographic scores, dyspnoea grade and respirsatory function in the British Thoracic Society Study of Long-Term Corticosteroid Treatment. Sarcoidosis Vasc Diffuse Lung Dis 1997; 14:46–56.
371. Abehsera M, Valeyre D, Grenier P, Jaillet H, Battesti JP, Brauner MW. Sarcoidosis with pulmonary fibrosis: CT patterns and correlation with pulmonary function. AJR Am J Roentgenol 2000; 174:1751–1757.
372. Maña J, Salazar A, Pujol R, Manresa F. Are the pulmonary function tests and the markers of activity helpful to establish the prognosis of sarcoidosis? Respiration 1996; 63:298–303.
373. Lieberman J, Schleissner LA, Nosal A, Sastre A, Mishkin FS. Clinical correlations of serum angiotensin-converting enzyme (ACE) in sarcoidosis. A longitudinal study of serum ACE, 67-gallium scans, chest roentenograms, and pulmonary function. Chest 1983; 84:522–528.
374. Finkel R, Teirstein AS, Levine R, Brown LK, Miller A. Pulmonary function tests, serum angiotensin-converting enzyme levels, and clinical findings as prognostic indicators in sarcoidosis. Ann N Y Acad Sci 1986; 465:665–671.
375. Keogh BA, Hunninghake GW, Line BR, Crystal RG. The alveolitis of pulmonary sarcoidosis. Evaluation of natural history and alveolitis-dependent changes in lung function. Am Rev Respir Dis 1983; 128:256–265.
376. Colp C. Sarcoidosis: course and treatment. Med Clin North Am 1977; 61:1267–1278.

377. Drent M, Jacobs JA, De Vries J, Lamers RJS, Liern IH, Wouters EFM. Does the cellular bronchoalveolar lavage fluid profile reflect the severity of sarcoidosis? Eur Respir J 1999; 13:1338–1344.

378. Baughman RP, Winget DP, Bowen EH, Lower EE. Predicting respiratory failure in sarcoidosis patients. Sarcoidosis Vasc Diffuse Lung Dis 1997; 14:154–158.

379. Johns CJ, MacGregor MI, Zachary JB, Ball WC. Extended experience in the long-term corticosteroid treatment of pulmonary sarcoidosis. Ann N Y Acad Sci 1976; 278:722.

380. Emirgil C, Sobol BJ, Williams MH Jr. Long-term study of pulmonary sarcoidosis: the effect of steroid therapy as evaluated by pulmonary function studies. J Chronic Dis 1969; 22:69.

381. Odlum CM, FitzGerald MX. Evidence that steroids alter the natural history of previously untreated progressive pulmonary sarcoidosis. Sarcoidosis 1986; 3:40–46.

382. Pietinalho A, Tukiainen P, Haahtela T, Persson T, Selroos O. Early treatment of stage II sarcoidosis improves 5-year pulmonary function. Chest 2002; 121:24–31.

383. Lawrence EC, Teague RB, Gottlieb MS, Jhingran SG, Lieberman J. Serial changes in markers of disease activity with corticosteroid treatment in sarcoidosis. Am J Med 1983; 74:747–756.

384. Colp C, Park SS, Williams Jr. MH. Pulmonary function follow-up to 120 patients with sarcoidosis. Ann N Y Acad Sci 1976; 278:301–307.

385. Zaki MH, Lyons HA, Leilop L, Huang CT. Corticosteroid therapy in sarcoidosis. A five-year, controlled follow-up study. N Y State J Med 1987; 87:496–499.

386. Goldstein DS, Williams MH. Rate of improvement of pulmonary function in sarcoidosis during treatment with corticosteroids. Thorax 1986; 41:473–474.

387. Tazi A, Montcelly L, Bergeron A, Valeyre D, Battesti JP, Hance AJ. Relapsing nodular lesions in the course of adult pulmonary Langerhans cell histiocytosis. Am J Respir Crit Care Med 1998; 157:2007–2010.

388. Vassallo R, Ryu JH, Colby TV, Hartman T, Limper AH. Pulmonary Langerhans cell histiocytosis. N Engl J Med 2000; 342:1969–1978.

389. Basset F, Corrin B, Spencer H, Lacronique J, Roth C, Soler P, Battesti JP, Georges R, Chretien J. Pulmonary histiocytosis X. Am Rev Respir Dis 1978; 118:811–820.

390. Travis WD, Borok Z, Roum JH, Zhang J, Feuerstein I, Ferrans VJ, Crystal RG. Pulmonary Langerhans cell granulomatosis (histiocytosis X). A clinicopathologic study of 48 cases. Am J Surg Pathol 1993; 17:971–986.

391. Friedman PJ, Liebow AA, Sokoloff J. Eosinophilic granuloma of lung. Clinical aspects of primary histiocytosis in the adult. Medicine (Baltimore) 1981; 60:385–396.

392. Soler P, Bergeron A, Kambouchner M, Groussard O, Brauner M, Grenier P, Crestani B, Mal H, Tazi A, Battesti JP, Loiseau P, Valeyre D. Is high-resolution computed tomography a reliable tool to predict the histopathological activity of pulmonary Langerhans cell histiocytosis? Am J Respir Crit Care Med 2000; 162:264–270.

393. Brown RE. Pulmonary Langerhans'-cell histiocytosis. N Engl J Med 2000; 343:1654–1655; discussion 1656.

394. Fartoukh M, Humbert M, Capron F, Maitre S, Parent F, Le Gall C, Sitbon O, Herve P, Duroux P, Simonneau G. Severe pulmonary hypertension in histiocytosis X. Am J Respir Crit Care Med 2000; 161:216–223.

395. Delobbe A, Durieu J, Duhamel A, Wallaert B. Determinants of survival in pulmonary Langerhans cell granulomatosis (histiocytosis X). Groupe d'Etude en Pathologie Interstitielle de la Societe de Pathologie Thoracique du Nord. Eur Respir J 1996; 9:2002–2006.

396. Schonfeld N, Frank W, Wenig S, Uhrmeister P, Allica E, Preussler H, Grassot A, Loddenkemper R. Clinical and radiologic features, lung function and therapeutic results in pulmonary histiocytosis X. Respiration 1993; 60:38–44.

397. Vassallo R, Ryu JH, Schroeder DR, Decker PA, Limper AH. Clinical outcomes of pulmonary Langerhans'-cell histiocytosis in adults. N Engl J Med 2002; 346:484–490.

398. Aguayo SM. Determinants of susceptibility to cigarette smoke. Potential roles for neuroendocrine cells and neuropeptides in airway inflammation, airway wall remodeling, and chronic airflow obstruction. Am J Respir Crit Care Med 1994; 149:1692–1698.

399. Mogulkoc N, Veral A, Bishop PW, Bayindir U, Pickering CA, Egan JJ. Pulmonary Langerhans cell histiocytosis: radiologic resolution following smoking cessation. Chest 1999; 115:1452–1455.

400. Etienne B, Bertocchi M, Gamondes JP, Thevenet F, Boudard C, Wiesendanger T, Loire R, Brune J, Mornex JF. Relapsing pulmonary Langerhans cell histiocytosis after lung transplantation. Am J Respir Crit Care Med 1998; 157:288–291.

401. Alhamad EH, Lynch JP III, Martinez FJ. Pulmonary function tests in interstitial lung disease: what role do they have? Clin Chest Med 2001; 22:715–750, ix.

6

Pulmonary Vascular Disease

SEAN P. GAINE

University College Dublin
and Mater Misericordiae Hospital
Dublin, Ireland

I. Introduction

The pulmonary vascular bed provides for the movement of venous blood from the right to the left heart through a low-resistance conduit with a large surface area for intimate contact between blood and alveolar gas. In the normal pulmonary vascular bed, resistance is modulated both by passive factors, such as lung volume, and active factors, such as alveolar oxygen concentration. Disorders of the pulmonary circulation are manifest by an increase in pulmonary vascular resistance, pulmonary hypertension, and the subsequent development of right heart failure. This chapter explores the unique physiology of the pulmonary vascular bed and discusses the effect of pulmonary vascular disease upon rest and exercise physiology.

II. Physiology of the Normal Pulmonary Vascular Bed

A. Pulmonary Vascular Resistance

The equation governing the resistance to blood flow through the pulmonary vascular bed is derived from Ohm's law, which states that the electrical resistance through a circuit is related to the driving force, or voltage, and the electrical current. Similarly, vascular resistance is related to the pressure gradient for flow across the pulmonary vascular bed and the blood flow through the circuit. Since flow is similar in the pulmonary and systemic circulation while the pressure gradient for flow through the systemic circulation is ~ 90 mmHg (upstream minus downstream pressure) and the gradient for the normal pulmonary circulation is only ~ 10 mmHg, it can be seen that the pulmonary vascular resistance is approximately 10% that of the systemic circulation.

However, use of Ohm's law assumes that the relationship of pressure to flow in the pulmonary vascular bed is linear, which would be the case if the circuit were a rigid tube. In a rigid tube with an outflow pressure of zero, the resistance $(\Delta P/\Delta \dot{Q})$ is constant and equal to the slope of a straight line through the origin. However, because pulmonary vessels are distensible, the normal pulmonary vascular bed does not behave like a rigid tube and resistance is not constant over the physiological range of pressure and flow. The diameter and resistance of pulmonary vessels vary with pressure, resulting in a curvilinear relationship between pressure and flow (1). Therefore, the pressure-flow curve is concave to the flow axis with *resistance* defined as the instantaneous slope of this relation. By contrast, true *pulmonary vascular resistance* (PVR) is the slope of a line drawn from any particular point on the pressure flow relation to the origin, or $Ppa - Pla/\dot{Q}T$, where $Ppa = $ pulmonary arterial pressure, $Pla = $ left atrial pressure, and $\dot{Q}T = $ cardiac output [Eq (1)].

$$PVR = \frac{Ppa - Pla}{\dot{Q}t} \qquad\qquad (1)$$

Changes in vascular tone will result in shifts of the pressure-flow relation. However, changes in pulmonary vascular resistance can result from changes in tone or from movement along a nonlinear portion of the pressure flow relation (Fig. 1).

This characteristic of the pulmonary circulation is important to understand when measuring the response of the pulmonary vascular bed to a pharmacological intervention, as is done with a vasodilator trial. Were cardiac output (flow) to increase following administration of a vasoactive drug, such as epoprostenol (due to systemic vasodilation without an effect on the pulmonary vasculature), then the calculated *resistance* could decrease without a shift in the pressure-flow relation. This decrease in *calculated resistance* could be misinterpreted as pulmonary vasodilation, when it was due to the distensibility of the pulmonary circulation. On the other hand, if a pharmacological intervention such as acute administration of adenosine did cause pulmonary vasodilation and also an increase in cardiac output, the pressure-flow could shift such that there was *no change* in the calculated resistance (2,3). However, by taking a number of measurements and plotting the pulmonary vascular pressure-flow relation, the true PVR can be determined.

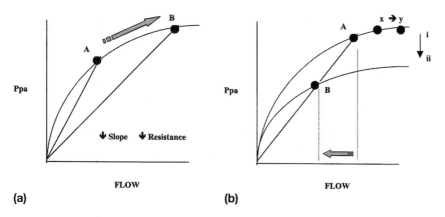

Figure 1 The pressure-flow curve. (a) *Resistance* is defined as the instantaneous slope of this curve. Were cardiac output (flow) to increase following administration of a vasoactive drug (A → B), then the calculated resistance (slope) could decrease without a shift in the pressure-flow relation. This decrease in calculated resistance can be misinterpreted as pulmonary vasodilatation. (b) Pulmonary vascular resistance (PVR). Changes in vascular tone will result in shifts of the pressure flow relation (i → ii). However, changes in pulmonary vascular resistance can result from changes in tone (i → ii) or from movement along a nonlinear portion of the pressure flow relation (x → y). A pharmacological intervention caused a reduction in vascular tone (i → ii) and also a decrease in cardiac output (A → B). While there is *no change* in the calculated resistance (slope), the true pulmonary vascular resistance (PVR) has decreased.

B. Passive Regulation of Pulmonary Vascular Resistance

Recruitment and Distensibility in the Pulmonary Vascular Bed

The pulmonary vascular bed has considerable reserve. While it is a low-pressure, high-flow system at rest, it can, during exercise, accommodate increases in cardiac output of up to four times resting values, with only a small rise in the inflow pressure. This phenomenon occurs by the process of both recruitment and distention. When pulmonary artery pressure is low, many of the pulmonary capillaries are collapsed without flow; however, as pressure and flow increase, capillaries that were previously closed begin to open (recruitment), and vessels that were open widen in diameter (distention). This decrease in pulmonary vascular resistance as pressure increases, through recruitment and distention, contributes to the curvilinear shape of the pressure-flow relation (4).

Effect of Lung Volume on Resistance

Because the pulmonary blood vessels have a relatively small amount of vascular smooth muscle, a low intravascular pressure, and high distensibility, passive factors such as lung volume and respiration have a considerable effect on pulmonary vascular resistance. During respiration, changes in lung inflation affect the diameter of extra-alveolar vessels and of alveolar vessels differently, resulting in a variation in resistance with changes in lung volume. During lung inflation, the extra-alveolar compartment—comprising the arteries, arterioles, veins, and venules—is pulled open by traction of the surrounding elastic lung parenchyma; during lung deflation, these vessels narrow (5,6). By contrast, alveolar vessels are exposed to alveolar pressure and the diameter of these vessels varies indirectly with transpulmonary pressure (alveolar pressure – pleural pressure) and with lung volume. Factors that increase lung volume, such as positive end-expiratory pressure (PEEP), compress alveolar vessels and increase vascular resistance (7).

Effect of Vessel Position on Blood Flow

A four-zone model of pulmonary perfusion has been described, where the relationship between pulmonary arterial pressure (Ppa), pulmonary venous pressure (Ppv), and alveolar pressure (Palv) governs the regional distribution of blood flow in the lungs (8,9). Zone I conditions result in increased alveolar dead space (VD) at the lung apex where blood flow is impeded because Palv exceeds both Ppa and Ppv. In zone II Ppa is greater than both Palv and Ppv, thereby permitting blood flow. However, because Palv remains higher than Ppv in zone II, changes in Ppv do not have an effect on flow or on upstream pressures, thereby producing the characteristics of the so-called waterfall effect or Starling resistor (10,11). Because left atrial pressure is normally well above alveolar pressure, Zone II is limited to the upper third of the lung. In zone III, any influence of Palv is removed, as the pulmonary veins are now below the right atrium and therefore Ppv is greater than Palv. In zone III changes in Ppv will affect flow and have an effect on upstream pressures. During exercise as pulmonary blood flow increases, inflow (Ppa) and outflow (Ppv) pressures increase, thus converting all regions to zone III (12). Finally, zone IV conditions are described at the lung base where is postulated that the observed decrease in blood flow results from increased interstitial pressure (13).

C. Active Regulation of Pulmonary Vascular Resistance

Pulmonary vascular resistance is also regulated by numerous active mechanisms, including alveolar oxygen tension, autonomic innervation, circulating vasoactive mediators, and local endothelial–smooth muscle interaction. In the normal pulmonary vascular bed, acute reduction in *alveolar oxygen tension* (PA_{O_2}) causes pulmonary vasoconstriction of the precapillary arteries, diverting blood to better-ventilated regions and thereby reducing shunt and maintaining efficient ventilation/perfusion ($\dot{V}/\dot{Q}$) matching. Increased [H^+] also causes pulmonary vasoconstriction and can further augment hypoxic vasoconstriction (14). The mechanism of hypoxic pulmonary vasoconstriction remains unknown (15).

While the pulmonary circulation is heavily innervated by the *autonomic nervous system*—which includes adrenergic, cholinergic and nonadrenergic noncholinergic (NANC) systems—the role it plays in regulating the pulmonary circulation appears relatively minor (16,17). Furthermore, the innervation is greatest in the proximal elastic arteries and decreases toward the periphery, suggesting that these nerves modulate pulmonary vascular compliance rather than resistance (16). The indirect effects of the autonomic nervous system on cardiac output or venous return are perhaps more significant in the normal pulmonary circulation.

Pulmonary vascular tone is also influenced by a number of *circulating factors* (18). Direct effect of catecholamines on smooth muscle alpha$_1$ and alpha$_2$ receptors results in vasoconstriction, while vasodilation is mediated by smooth muscle and endothelial beta$_1$ receptors and endothelial alpha$_2$ receptors. Furthermore, both histamine, stored in basophils or lung mast cells, and, serotonin (5-HT), produced locally by circulating platelets, mediate vasoconstriction in the pulmonary circulation.

Complex *local endothelial—smooth muscle interaction* is involved in maintaining low pulmonary vascular tone. Under normal physiological conditions, endothelial cells release predominately relaxing or vasodilator mediators; however, under certain physiological and pathophysiological conditions, the balance may shift towards release of constricting mediators (19,20). The primary endothelium-derived relaxing factors (EDRFs) released by the pulmonary endothelium are nitric oxide (NO) and prostacyclin (PGI$_2$) (21). There does not seem to be much tonic release of NO or PGI$_2$ from the pulmonary endothelium during normal conditions, since inhibition of NO synthase (NOS) or cyclo-oxygenase does not cause an increase in vascular resistance. However, during conditions of high tone, such as during hypoxia, inhibition of NOS or cyclooxygenase potentiates vasoconstrcition, suggesting that PGI$_2$ modulates these responses. The endothelium produces constricting factors (EDCFs), which include endothelin, superoxide anion, and the cyclo-oxygenase–dependent mediators thromboxane and prostaglandin H$_2$. (22). The recent demonstration of a beneficial effect of endothelin antagonist in pulmonary arterial hypertension (PAH) supports a role for excessive local endothelin production in severe PAH (23–25).

III. Pathophysiology of the Pulmonary Vascular Bed

A. Pulmonary Hypertension
Disorders of the Respiratory System and Hypoxemia

Because of the capacity of the pulmonary vasculature to recruit and distend, it takes destruction of more than half of the normal vascular bed to result in an increase PVR. Thus, resection of one normal lung should not increase resistance. Parenchymal lung diseases such as idiopathic pulmonary fibrosis (IPF) or emphysema cause destruction, distortion or compression and loss of blood vessels and result in pulmonary hypertension (26–28). Because of the limited distensibility and recruitabiltiy of blood vessels in these interstitial and airway diseases, pulmonary hypertension may be present only when cardiac output is elevated, as during exercise.

Causes of global hypoxia, which may also cause pulmonary hypertension, include exposure to high altitude, central hypoventilation, and obesity hypoventilation syndrome (29,30). People living at altitudes greater than approximately 10,000 ft (about where alveolar oxygen tension falls below 60–70 mmHg) may have pulmonary hypertension that is mild at rest but can become pronounced with exercise (31). Long-term exposure to altitude causes pulmonary vascular remodeling, which increases resistance, although certain populations have adapted to altitude in a way that protects the pulmonary vasculature from remodeling (32).

Disorders Affecting the Pulmonary Blood Vessels

Disorders that primarily affect the pulmonary arteries and arterioles may cause pulmonary hypertension or elevated PVR by causing obliteration or occlusion of vascular channels. Patients with these disorders often come to medical attention after the pulmonary hypertension becomes severe, with signs of right heart failure. They usually complain of dyspnea on exertion and have little evidence of parenchymal lung disease by radiograph (33).

While the vast majority of patients with pulmonary thromboembolism will not develop pulmonary hypertension, some patients with recurrent thromboemboli that do not resolve adequately may develop pulmonary hypertension due to progressive occlusion of the vasculature. Moser and colleagues have described a syndrome of pulmonary hypertension due to chronic thrombotic occlusion of proximal pulmonary arteries. These patients have symptoms and signs of pulmonary hypertension, including dyspnea on exertion and peripheral edema. Diagnostic evaluation reveals abnormal perfusion scans and angiographically demonstrated thrombi in the main and lobar pulmonary arteries. It is important to diagnose this syndrome, because surgical thrombendarerectomy may be curative (34,35).

Primary pulmonary hypertension (PPH) is a syndrome characterized by a pulmonary arterial vasculopathy in the absence of underlying pulmonary parenchymal or cardiac disease. Patients with this disorder are usually women in their twenties to forties who present to a physician with dyspnea on exertion and fatigue. Typically, at diagnosis symptoms have been present for 1 to 2 years and pulmonary artery pressures are elevated substantially at the time of diagnosis. A familial form of PPH has been described, with autosomal dominant inheritance (36–40). The pathophysiology of primary pulmonary hypertension may relate to dysfunctional endothelium. Endothelium has the capacity produce vasodilator/antithrombotic mediators and vasoconstricting/prothrombotic mediators. In PPH, it is speculated that a dysfunctional endothelium creates an initially reversible increase in vasomotor tone, which chronically will evolve into an irreversible state of elevated resistance due to vascular remodeling (41,42). In addition to chronic vasoconstriction, the increased presence of prothrombotic mediators or decreased presence of antithrombotic mediators will promote platelet aggregation and release of platelet-derived vasoactive mediators (e.g., serotonin), both of which may increase vascular resistance (43,44). Patients with PPH have elevated breakdown products of the potent vasoconstrictors thromboxane and prostaglandin F_{2a} relative to normal subjects and to patients with secondary pulmonary hypertension (45).

IV. Physiology of Exercise in Pulmonary Vascular Disease

The clinical diagnosis of pulmonary hypertension requires a resting mean pulmonary artery pressure of greater than 25 mmHg or a mean pulmonary artery pressure with exercise of greater than 30 mmHg (46). The existence of rest and exercise criteria for the diagnosis of pulmonary hypertension is in keeping with the observation that there is considerable reserve in the pulmonary vascular bed. As a result of this reserve, significant vascular disease may be present before there is sufficient loss of the pulmonary vascular bed to cause resting pulmonary hypertension. Exercise testing may uncover early pulmonary vascular disease by demonstrating the loss of the normal pulmonary vasodilator response to exercise and the inability of the right ventricle to adequately increase pulmonary blood flow for the exercise-related increased O_2 demand. The increased right ventricular work eventually causes pulmonary hypertension to become manifest at rest, at which time cardiac catheterization and/or echocardiography are used to establish the diagnosis. In clinical practice, exercise testing has been used to noninvasively grade functional capacity in patients with PPH; performance on exercise tests has prognostic significance and may be used to evaluate treatment efficacy (47–50).

A. Response to Exercise in Pulmonary Vascular Disease

During cardiopulmonary exercise testing (CPET), work rate is increased incrementally to a symptom-limited maximum while the cardiovascular and respiratory responses to the stress of the increased oxygen requirements ($\dot{V}_{O_2}$) and carbon dioxide output ($\dot{V}_{CO_2}$) are measured. The direct relationship between the $\dot{V}_{O_2}$ and the cardiac output ($\dot{Q}$) is described by the Fick equation [Eq. (2)].

$$\dot{V}_{O_2} = \dot{Q}(CaO_2 - C\dot{V}_{O_2}) \tag{2}$$

Similarly, the ventilatory response ($\dot{V}_E$) to exercise is tightly related to CO_2 output ($\dot{V}_{CO_2}$) (51–53).

In one of the earliest studies of exercise in pulmonary arterial hypertension, symptom-limited exercise was used to compare a control group of normal volunteers with a group of nine patients with PPH (47). The patients with PPH had decreased exercise capacity and a decrease in maximal $\dot{V}_{O_2}$.

Patients in the PPH group with the highest PVR had the greatest compromise and were unable to increase their stroke volume in response to exercise. Subsequently, rest and exercise data were obtained from 11 patients with PPH studied with progressive, upright cycle ergometry and compared with data obtained from 11 matched, sedentary control subjects (49). D'Alonzo and coworkers demonstrated a severe exertional limitation due to cardiovascular factors in individuals with PPH and an inability to maintain appropriate oxygen delivery to the body during exercise. They demonstrated a decrease in peak exercise oxygen consumption and an increase in the regression slope, relating minute ventilation to carbon dioxide output in patients with PPH (49). Mean maximal $\dot{V}_{O_2}$ was significantly lower in the PPH group than in controls. At maximal $\dot{V}_{O_2}$, the minute ventilation ($\dot{V}_E$) was similar; however, while no respiratory impairment was recognized, an exaggerated ventilatory response to exercise at any level of $\dot{V}_{CO_2}$ was found. Furthermore, maximal heart rate and oxygen pulse ($\dot{V}_{O_2}$/heart rate) was significantly higher in the control group. Finally, anaerobic threshold occurred earlier during incremental exercise in the PPH group and correlated with the maximal oxygen pulse achieved in patients with PPH (49).

In a group of 16 patients with PPH, ages ranging from 6 to 35, Rhodes and colleagues demonstrated that exercise capacity was reduced below that predicted for age, height, and gender and was inversely correlated with right atrial pressure, pulmonary artery pressure, and PVR obtained at cardiac catheterization. Mean right atrial pressure correlated best with exercise capacity, while poor exercise capacity identified those PPH patients at high risk for a poor outcome from cardiac catheterization. Furthermore, the investigators demonstrated that performance on exercise testing could predict the response to acute vasodilator drug testing insofar as exercise capacity greater than 75% of the predicted value identified the two patients who had a positive response to acute testing (50).

More recently, 53 patients with PPH were evaluated with right heart catheterization and cycle ergometer CPET studies. Reductions in maximal $\dot{V}_{O_2}$, anaerobic threshold, peak O_2 pulse, rate of increase in $\dot{V}_{O_2}$, and ventilatory efficiency were described. Furthermore, New York Heart Association (NYHA) functional class correlated well with parameters of aerobic function and ventilatory efficiency but less so with resting pulmonary hemodynamics (Figs. 2 and 3) (54).

These studies of exercise in pulmonary vascular disease consistently describe the inability to adequately increase blood flow during exercise, resulting in a reduced maximal $\dot{V}_{O_2}$ and the failure to meet the exercise O_2 requirement. The ventilation of underperfused alveoli results in an increase in dead-space ventilation, manifest by an increase in $\dot{V}_E$ relative to the $\dot{V}_{CO_2}$ during exercise. Furthermore, lactic acidosis occurring relatively early during exercise, along with hypoxemia, acts as additional stimuli to breathing and further contributes to the sensation of dyspnea, even though peak $\dot{V}_E$ is well below the maximal voluntary ventilation (Fig. 4) (55).

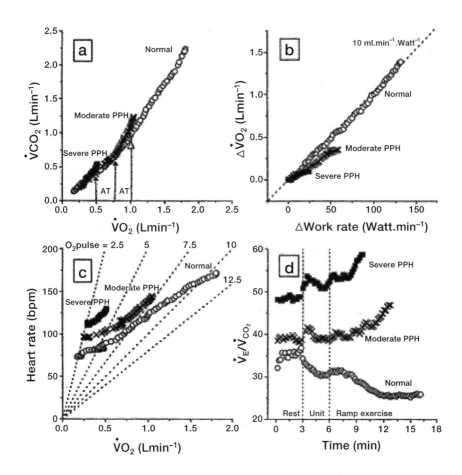

Figure 2 Cardiopulmonary exercise test measurements of two patients with moderate and severe PPH and a normal control subject with similar predicted values. Protocol consisted of 3 min of rest, 3 min of unloaded cycling at 60 rpm (Unl.), and ramp WR of 15, 10, and $5 \, W \cdot min^{-1}$, respectively, to maximal tolerance. (a) CO_2 versus $\dot{V}_{O_2}$ with arrows at the respective AT of each subject. (b) Change in $\dot{V}_{O_2}$ versus change in WR, with dotted line indicating normal slope of $10 \, mL \cdot min^{-1} \cdot W^{-1}$. (c) HR versus $\dot{V}_{O_2}$, with diagonal dotted lines indicating O_2 pulse in $mL \cdot beat^{-1}$. (d) Ventilatory equivalent for CO_2 ($\dot{V}_E/\dot{V}_{CO_2}$) versus time, with vertical dashed lines separating rest, unloaded, and ramp exercise. Characteristic abnormalities of PPH patients depicted are low values for peak $\dot{V}_{O_2}$, AT, peak WR, $\Delta\dot{V}_{O_2}/\Delta WR$, peak HR, and peak O_2 pulse. With PPH, resting $\dot{V}_E/\dot{V}_{CO_2}$ values are elevated and tend to remain relatively constant or increase during exercise, contrasting with lower resting and decreasing $\dot{V}_E/\dot{V}_{CO_2}$ during exercise in normal control subject. Abbreviations: WR; work rate, AT; anaerobic threshold; HR, heart rate. (From Ref. 54.)

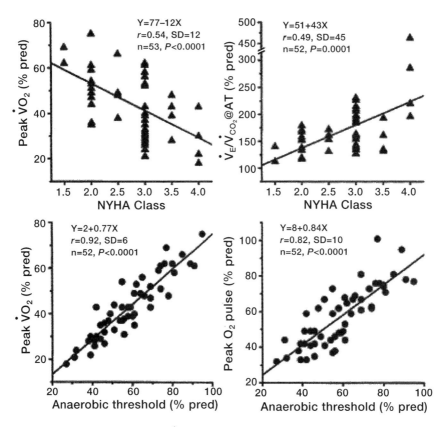

Figure 3 Correlations of peak $\dot{V}_{O_2}$ (percent predicted) and ventilatory equivalent for CO_2 at AT ($\dot{V}_E/\dot{V}_{CO_2}$ at AT) versus NYHA symptom class (top panels) and peak $\dot{V}_{O_2}$ and peak O_2 pulse versus AT (bottom panels) in PPH patients during CPET. All correlations are highly significant. (From Ref. 54.)

The 6-Min Walk Test in Pulmonary Vascular Disease

While cardiopulmonary exercise testing (CPET) with gas exchange can be used to noninvasively measure functional capacity, it can be cumbersome and time-consuming for routine use. On the other hand the 6-min walk test is very simple and reproducible, requiring no expensive equipment; it has been used to assess changes in functional capacity during vasodilator therapy in patients with pulmonary vascular disease (56,57). The 6-min walk test is considered safe because it is a submaximal test and patients are self-limited during exercise (58). The distance walked in 6 min has been shown to correlate closely with peak $\dot{V}_{O_2}$ and $\dot{V}_E-\dot{V}_{CO_2}$ slope in patients with advanced heart failure; it thereby serves as a useful prognostic indicator (Fig. 5) (59,60). In a study of 34 patients with PPH, a distance of less than 300 m was shown to increase mortality risk by 2.4 (61).

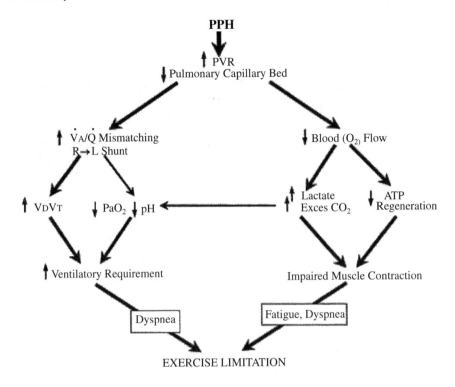

Figure 4 Pathophysiology of exercise limitation in patients with primary pulmonary hypertension (PPH). Arrows show pathways leading to dyspnea, fatigue, and exercise limitation. Abbreviations: PVR, pulmonary vascular resistance; $\dot{V}A/\dot{Q}$, alveolar ventilation/perfusion ratio; V_D/V_T, dead space volume/tidal volume ratio; and Pa_{O_2}, arterial oxygen pressure. (From Ref. 54.)

In one study, the 6-min walk test was performed in 43 patients with PPH, together with cardiopulmonary exercise testing, echocardiography, and right heart catheterization (62). The distance walked significantly decreased in direct proportion to the severity of NYHA functional class. Furthermore, the distance walked correlated with hemodynamic parameters including baseline cardiac output, total pulmonary resistance, and mean right atrial pressure but not with mean pulmonary arterial pressure. The distance walked also correlated strongly with peak $\dot{V}_{O_2}$, oxygen pulse and $\dot{V}_E$–$\dot{V}_{CO_2}$ slope determined by cardiopulmonary exercise testing. Among all the noninvasive parameters measured—including clinical, echocardiographic, and neuro-humoral—only the distance walked in 6 min was independently related to mortality in PPH during a mean follow-up period of 21 ± 16 months (62).

The Effect of Right-to-Left Shunt on the Response to Exercise

A patent foramen ovale (PFO) was demonstrated in 27.3% of 965 autopsy specimens of human hearts from subjects who were evenly distributed by sex

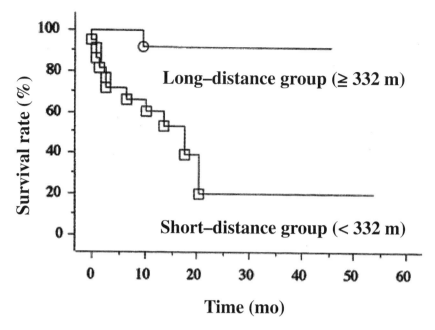

Figure 5 Kaplan-Meier survival curves according to median value of distance walked during the 6-min walk test in patients with primary pulmonary hypertension. Patients walking < 332 m had a significantly lower survival rate than those walking farther (log-rank test, $p < 0.001$). (From Ref. 62.)

and age, with the foramen size increasing with advancing age (63). In normal persons, right-to-left shunting via a patent foramen ovale (PFO) rarely occurs, as left atrial pressure exceeds the right atrial pressure (64). Moreover, because a PFO may be so small or the pressure differences across the septum so minor, shunt blood flow may not be visible by echocardiography, even during a Valsalva maneuver (55).

However, in the setting of abnormally high pulmonary artery pressure and right heart dysfunction, right atrial pressure can exceed left atrial pressure, especially during exercise, and force venous blood through a PFO for a right-to-left shunt. This shunted venous blood not only has a low P_{O_2} but also a high P_{CO_2} and hydrogen ion concentration $[H^+]$, which stimulate systemic arterial chemoreceptors and cause hyperventilation. This compensatory hyperventilation increases CO_2 unloading, thereby maintaining homeostasis of arterial P_{CO_2} and $[H^+]$, despite the exercise-induced right-to-left shunt (65). Consequently, CO_2 unloading from the unshunted pulmonary blood flow increases as alveolar P_{CO_2} falls, but O_2 loading increases less because pulmonary capillary P_{O_2} reaches the flat part of the oxyhemoglobin dissociation curve. Thus, ventilation increases more steeply relative to $\dot{V}_{O_2}$ than $\dot{V}_{CO_2}$, resulting in a greater increase in $\dot{V}_E/\dot{V}_{O_2}$ than $\dot{V}_E/\dot{V}_{CO_2}$. Even at rest, there are distinctly more gas exchange abnormalities (higher $\dot{V}_E/\dot{V}_{O_2}$, $\dot{V}_E/\dot{V}_{CO_2}$, and PET_{O_2} and lower PET_{CO_2} and

Sp_{O_2}) in the shunt than no-shunt groups (Fig. 6). These pre-exercise abnormalities can be attributed to hypoperfusion of well-ventilated lung and probable chronic hyperventilation (54,55).

Effect of Treatment on the Response to Exercise in Pulmonary Hypertension

The treatment of pulmonary vascular disease has advanced over the past decade. In one of the earliest studies describing the effect of treatment on exercise capacity in patients with pulmonary arterial hypertension, D'Alonzo compared hemodynamics obtained at cardiac catheterization with exercise performance in 10 patients with pulmonary hypertension. After 8 weeks of therapy with oral calcium channel blockade, exercise capacity was improved in the patients who had improved hemodynamics (48). However, because only a minority of patients are candidates for long-term calcium channel blocker therapy, epoprostenol, has emerged as the treatment of choice for individuals with advanced pulmonary arterial hypertension (57). In order to determine the efficacy of epoprostenol in a dose that can be administered with minimal side effects, the efficacy of therapy is evaluated by echocardiography (56,66) and/or right-sided heart catheterization (33). However, because of the potential morbidity and cost associated with right-heart catheterization, it has been proposed that exercise testing be used to measure response to therapy (67). A long-term (19.5 $\pm$ 7.5 months) follow-up study of 16 patients with PPH treated with continuous intravenous epoprostenol demonstrated a significant increase in peak $\dot{V}_{O_2}$ and peak O_2 pulse and a trend toward improvement in peak work (Fig. 7) (68). More recently the endothelin antagonist bosentan has emerged as an effective therapy for pulmonary arterial hypertension, with improved hemodynamics and exercise capacity as measured by the 6-min walk test (69).

However, the mechanisms by which continuous intravenous epoprostenol therapy improves exercise tolerance in patients with pulmonary arterial hypertension are unclear. It has been suggested that the decrease in PVR observed following long-term epoprostenol therapy may explain the improved exercise tolerance (70). However, the improvement in exercise tolerance begins within the first few weeks after epoprostenol initiation, antedating changes in resting pulmonary hemodynamics (71). In a study of seven patients with PPH treated with continuous intravenous epoprostenol, hemodynamic variables were unchanged after 6 weeks of therapy. However, by contrast, the 6-min walking distance improved in all patients. Changes in the pressure-flow relationship were also reported. The slope of the mean pulmonary artery pressure versus cardiac index plot (Ppa/CI plot), which is taken as the incremental PVR upstream from the site of the closing pressure, significantly decreased with epoprostenol therapy, suggesting that the improvement in exercise tolerance seen after 6 weeks of epoprostenol therapy may be due to a decrease in incremental pulmonary vascular resistance during exercise (72). Because epoprostenol affected only the slope of the pressure-flow plot without

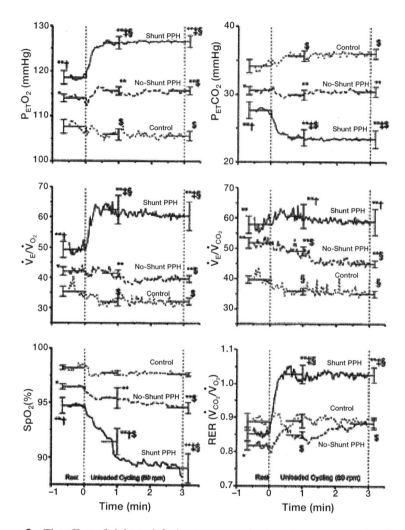

Figure 6 The effect of right-to-left shunts on exercise in pulmonary vascular disease. Average cardiopulmonary exercise test (CPET) responses in the control ($n = 20$), no-shunt-PPH ($n = 39$), and shunt-PPH ($n = 18$) groups during rest and unloaded cycling. Changes in mean PET_{O_2}, PET_{CO_2}, $\dot{V}_E/\dot{V}_{O_2}$, $\dot{V}_E/\dot{V}_{CO_2}$, Sp_{O_2}, and RER are plotted second by second from rest to the end of unloaded exercise. SEE values for the last minute of rest and the periods from 0.5 to 1 min and 2.5 to 3 min of unloaded cycling are also shown. At rest, the $\dot{V}_E/\dot{V}_{CO_2}$ for the PPH groups differ strikingly from the values in the control group; at the end of unloaded cycling, the PET_{O_2}, PET_{CO_2}, $\dot{V}_E/\dot{V}_{O_2}$, Sp_{O_2}, and RER of the shunt and no-shunt groups differ strikingly from each other. Abbreviations: PET_{O_2}, end-tidal O_2; PET_{CO_2}, end-tidal CO_2; RER, carbon dioxide elimination/oxygen consumption ($\dot{V}_{CO_2}/\dot{V}_{O_2}$). $^*p < 0.05$ and $^{**}p < 0.001$ for differences from control group; $\dagger p < 0.05$ and $\ddagger p < 0.001$ for differences between shunt and no-shunt groups for each time period using a two-tailed repeated ANOVA; $\$p < 0.05$ and $\$\$p < 0.001$ for differences from each group's resting values using a paired t-test. (From Ref. 65.)

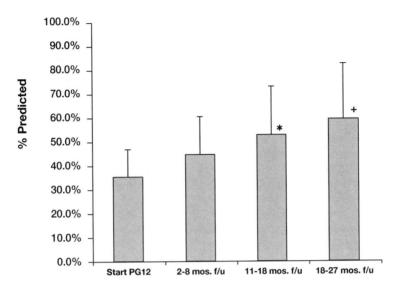

Figure 7 Peak work as percent predicted (mean ± SD) just before starting PGI$_2$ and at three follow-up intervals. *$p < 0.05$; +$p = 0.001$ versus baseline. (From Ref. 68.)

changing resting pressures and flows, the extrapolated pressure intercept, which is commonly taken as the mean, closing pressure increased slightly (Fig. 8) (72). Therefore the slope of multipoint Ppa versus CI curves (true PVR) probably better describes the functional state of the pulmonary vasculature in patients with PPH than a single resistance determination at rest (73–75).

Alternatively, it has been proposed that since decreased perfusion of the ventilated lung—i.e, increased physiological dead space ventilation (V_D/V_T)—results in inefficiency of ventilation, improved perfusion to the ventilated lung resulting from medical therapy might be a useful measure of treatment efficacy. Thus, the $\dot{V}_E/\dot{V}_{CO_2}$ ratio may be useful in measuring the severity of decreased perfusion to the ventilated lung, and the change in $\dot{V}_E/\dot{V}_{CO_2}$ ratio might be useful to evaluate the effectiveness of a drug for treating patients with PPH (67).

B. Exercise-Induced Pulmonary Hypertension

The diagnosis of pulmonary hypertension requires demonstration of an elevated mean pulmonary artery pressure at rest or during exercise (76). Unfortunately, the symptoms of early pulmonary hypertension are nonspecific, resulting in a mean delay in diagnosis of PPH of up to 2 years from symptom onset: as a result, the vast majority of patients have advanced disease unresponsive to conventional oral vasodilators at the time of diagnosis (46,77). Moreover, a significant degree of pulmonary vascular disease can be present before pulmonary hypertension and overt right ventricular dysfunction are evident at rest on echocardiography or catheterization. Therefore conditions of

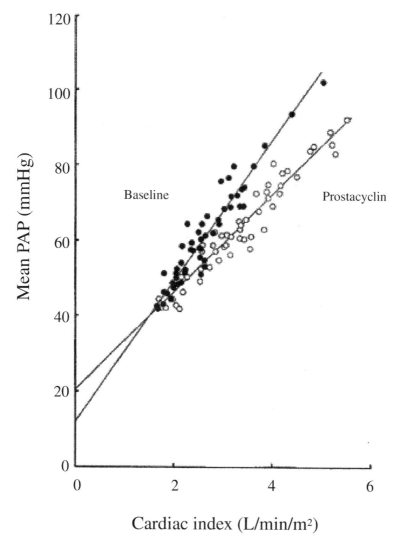

Figure 8 Relation between mean pulmonary artery pressure and cardiac index before (closed circles) and after (open circles) prostacyclin therapy. (From Ref. 72.)

increased pulmonary blood flow, as during exercise, allow for the uncovering of early pulmonary vascular disease (68,78).

Asymptomatic members of two families with familial PPH were studied to determine whether they had an abnormal pulmonary artery systolic pressure (PASP) response on Doppler echocardiography to supine bicycle exercise and to determine whether exercise response might uncover those with the familial PPH mutation and therefore potentially early preclinical disease. Of the 52 family members studied with normal PASP at rest, 14 revealed an abnormal

PASP response to exercise. All 14 of those with this abnormal exercise response, but only 2 of 27 of the remainder with a normal exercise response shared the risk haplotype linked to chromosome 2q31–32 (79). Similarly, there are individuals in whom resting hemodynamics are normal but who develop marked elevations in pulmonary pressure with exercise (80,81). Some of these individuals will undoubtedly have early PPH; however, the natural history of exercise-induced PPH is unknown at present (80). It is conceivable that these patients represent a variant of PPH with a relatively benign natural history. Alternatively, this phenomenon may represent reduced pulmonary vascular compliance of an otherwise normal pulmonary circulation.

Preclinical pulmonary vascular disease may also be exposed by exposure to high altitude. High-altitude pulmonary edema (HAPE) has been described at lower altitudes in individuals with pre-existing conditions affecting the pulmonary circulation. For example, HAPE has been described in patients with an absent right pulmonary artery who had normal pulmonary artery pressures at rest but an abnormal, exaggerated response to exercise (82,83). A recent case report described a patient who had been exposed to anorexigens and who had normal pulmonary artery pressures but developed high altitude pulmonary edema (HAPE) at lower altitude. Supine leg exercise produced a mean pulmonary pressure of 33 mmHg, resulting in the diagnosis of PPH based on exercise catheterization data (31).

The hemodynamic response to exercise may vary with the type of work performed and the muscle groups involved. Arm exercises result in greater increases in heart rate, ventilation, and lactate formation than leg exercises at a comparable degree of oxygen uptake (84,85). The higher ventilatory response to arm exercises does not correlate with the degree of anaerobic work or the concentration of lactate in the arterial blood (86). The systemic vascular resistance remains higher with arm exercises, probably because the inactive large blood vessels of the lower limb muscle fail to dilate. Furthermore, higher sympathetic tone is observed during arm versus leg exercises. Patients with pulmonary vascular disease may complain of dyspnea with upper arm exercises, as in showering or combing hair, sooner than of significant impairment in ambulation. Upper arm exercises in the supine position are an excellent method of determining the response to exercise in individuals during catheterization (86).

The evolution of pulmonary hemodynamics in stable, mild to moderate hypoxemic chronic obstructive lung disease has also been explored. Two right-heart catheterizations were performed at a mean time interval of 6.8 ± 2.9 years in 131 patients. At the time of enrollment, no patient had pulmonary hypertension. However, 76 patients had exercise-induced pulmonary hypertension. Resting and exercising pulmonary artery pressures were independent predictors at the initial catheterization for the subsequent development of pulmonary hypertension. The progression, however, was rather slow, with the average change for the group as a whole being of $+0.4 \, \text{mmHg/year}$ (87).

V. Conclusion

The pulmonary circulation provides a low-resistance conduit with a large surface area for the movement of venous blood from the right to the left heart. Disorders of the pulmonary vascular bed are manifest by an increase in pulmonary vascular resistance and pulmonary hypertension, with the subsequent development of right heart dysfunction and failure. This increase in pulmonary vascular resistance results in the inability to adequately increase blood flow during exercise and results in a reduced maximal $\dot{V}_{O_2}$ and the failure to meet the exercise O_2 requirement. Ventilation during exercise of under-perfused alveoli results in an increase in dead-space ventilation, manifest by an increase in $\dot{V}_E$ relative to the $\dot{V}_{CO_2}$. Furthermore, lactic acidosis occurring relatively early during exercise, along with hypoxemia, acts as additional stimuli to breathing and further contributes to the sensation of dyspnea in pulmonary vascular disease. Measurement of exercise capacity, either with formal CPET or the 6-min walk test, correlates closely with the severity of pulmonary vascular disease and prognosis.

References

1. Roos A, et al. Pulmonary vascular resistance as determined by lung inflation and vascular pressures. J Appl Physiol 1961; 16:77–84.
2. Mitzner W, Huang I. Interpretation of pressure flow curve in the pulmonary vascular bed. In Will J, ed. The Pulmonary Circulation in Health and Disease. Orlando, FL: Academic Press, 1987:215–230.
3. Mitzner W, Wagner E. Pulmonary and bronchial vascular resistance. In: Scharff S, Cassidy S, eds. Heart Lung Interactions in Health and Disease. New York: Marcel Dekker, 1989:45–73.
4. Glazier J, Hughes J, Maloney J. Measurements of capillary dimensions and blood volume in rapidly frozen lungs. J Appl Physiol 1969; 26:65–76.
5. Gil J. Organization of microcirculation of the lung. Annu Rev Physiol 1980; 42:177–186.
6. Lai-Fook S. Perivascular interstitial fluid pressure measured by micropipettes in isolated dog lung. J Appl Physiol 1982; 52:9–15.
7. Howell, J et al. Effect of inflation of the lung different parts of the pulmonary vascular bed. J Appl Physiol 1961; 16:71–76.
8. Dock W. Apical localization of phthsis. Its significance in treatment by prolonged rest in bed. Am Rev Tuberc 1946; 53:297–305.
9. West J, Dollery C, Naimark A. Distribution of blood flow in isolated lung: relation to vascular and alveolar pressures. J Appl Physiol 1964; 19:713–724.
10. Permutt S, Bromberger-Barnea B, Bane H. Alveolar pressure, pulmonary venous pressure, and the vascular waterfall. Med Thorac 1962; 19:239–260.
11. Permutt S, Riley R. Hemodynamics of collapsible vessels with tone. J Appl Physiol 1963; 18:924–932.
12. Levett J, Replogle R. Thermodilution cardiac output: a critical analysis and review of the literature. J Surg Res 1979; 27:392–404.

13. Hughes J, Glazier JB, Maloney JE, West JB. Effect of lung volume on the distribution of pulmonary blood flow in man. Respir Physiol 1968; 4:58–72.
14. Bergofsky E, Lehr D, Fishman A. The effect of changes in hydrogen ion concentration on the pulmonary circulation. J Clin Invest 1962; 41:1492.
15. Ward J, Aaronson P. Mechanisms of hypoxic pulmonary vasoconstriction: can anyone be right? Respir Physiol 1999; 115(3):261–271.
16. Downing S, Lee J. Nervous control of the pulmonary circulation. Annu Rev Physiol 1980; 42:199–210.
17. Widdicombe J, Sterling G. The autonomic nervous system and breathing. Arch Intern Med 1970; 126:311–329.
18. Bergofsky E. Humoral control of the pulmonary circulation. Annu Rev Physiol 1980; 42:221–223.
19. Furchgott RF, Zawadzki JV. The obligatory role of endothelial cells in the relaxation of arterial smooth muscle by acetylcholine. Nature 1980; 288:373–376.
20. Furchgott R, Vanhoutte P. Endothelium-derived relaxing and contracting factors. FASEB J 1989; 3:2007–2018.
21. Vanhoutte P. Other endothelium-derived vasoactive factors. Circulation 1993; 87:v9–v17.
22. Flavahan NA, Vanhoutte PM. Endothelial cell signaling and endothelial dysfunction. Am J Hypertens 1995; 8:28S–41S.
23. Channick R et al. Effects of the dual endothelin receptor antagonist bosentan in patients with pulmonary hypertension: a placebo-controlled study. J Heart Lung Transplant 2001; 20(2):262–263.
24. Giaid A et al. Expression of endothelin-1 in the lungs of patients with pulmonary hypertension. N Engl J Med 1993; 328:1732–1739.
25. Stewart D et al. Increased plasma endothelin-1 in pulmonary hypertension: marker or mediator of disease? Ann Intern Med 1991; 114:464–469.
26. Heath D et al. Pulmonary vascular disease in honeycomb lung. J Pathol Bacteriol 1968; 95:423–430.
27. Timms R, Khaja F, Williams G. Hemodynamic response to oxygen therapy in chronic obstructive pulmonary disease. Ann Intern Med 1985; 102:29–36.
28. Fujii T et al. Role of pulmonary vascular disorder in determining exercise capacity in patients with severe chronic obstructive pulmonary disease. Clin Physiol 1996; 16(5):521–533.
29. Weitzenblum E et al. Daytime pulmonary hypertension in patients with obstructive sleep apnea syndrome. Am Rev Respir Dis 1988; 138:345–349.
30. Kessler R et al. Pulmonary hypertension in the obstructive sleep apnea syndrome: prevalence, causes and therapeutic consequences. Eur Respir J 1996; 9(4):787–794.
31. Naeije R et al. High-altitude pulmonary edema with primary pulmonary hypertension. Chest 1996; 110:286–289.
32. Sharma S. Clinical, biochemical electrocardiographic and noninvasive hemodynamic assessment of cardiovascular status in natives at high to extreme altitudes (3000 m–5000 m) of the Himalaya region. Indian Heart J 1990; 42:375–379.
33. Gaine S. Pulmonary hypertension. JAMA, 2000; 284:3160–3168.
34. Moser KM et al. Thromboendarterectomy for chronic, major vessel thromboembolic pulmonary hypertension: immediate and long term results in 42 patients. Ann Intern Med 1987; 107:560–565.
35. D'Alonzo G, Bower J, Dantzker, DR. Differentiation of patients with primary and thromboembolic pulmonary hypertension. Chest 1984; 85:457–461.

36. Deng Z et al. Familial primary pulmonary hypertension (gene PPH1) is caused by mutations in the bone morphogenetic protein receptor II. Am J Hum Genet 2000; 67(3):737–744.

37. Loyd JE, Newman J. Familial primary pulmonary hypertension: clinical patterns. Am Rev Respir Dis 1984; 129:194–197.

38. Loyd JE et al., Genetic anticipation and abnormal gender ratio at birth in familial primary pulmonary hypertension. Am J Respir Crit Care Med 1995; 152(1):93–97.

39. The International PPH Consortium et al. Heterozygous germline mutations in BMPR-II are the cause of familial primary pulmonary hypertension. Nat Genet 2000; 26(1):81–84.

40. Nichols W et al. Localization of the gene for familial primary pulmonary hypertension to chromosome 2q31–32. Nat Genet 1997; 15(3):277–280.

41. Loscalzo J. Endothelial dysfunction in pulmonary hypertension. N Engl J Med 1992; 327:117–119.

42. Fishman AP. A century of primary pulmonary hypertension. In: Rubin L, Rich S, eds. Primary Pulmonary Hypertension. New York: Marcel Dekker, 1997:1–18.

43. Herve P, et al. Increased plasma serotonin in primary pulmonary hypertension. Am J Med 1995; 99(3):249–254.

44. Nakonechnicov S et al. Platelet aggregation in patients with primary pulmonary hypertension. Blood Coagul Fibrinolysis 1996; 7(2):225–227.

45. Christman B et al. An imbalance between the excretion of thromboxane and prostacyclin metabolites in pulmonary hypertension. N Engl J Med 1992; 327:70–75.

46. Rich S et al. Primary pulmonary hypertension. A national prospective study. Ann Intern Med 1987; 107(2):216–223.

47. Janicki J, Weber KT, Likoff MJ, et al. Exercise testing to evaluate patients with pulmonary vascular disease. Am Rev Respir Dis 1984; 129:93–95.

48. D'Alonzo G, Gianotti L, Dantzker D. Noninvasive assessment of hemodynamic improvement during chronic vasodilator therapy in obliterative pulmonary hypertension. Am Rev Respir Dis 1986, 133:380–384.

49. D'Alonzo G, Gianotti LA, Pohil RL, et al. Comparison of progressive exercise performance of normal subjects and patients with primary pulmonary hypertension. Chest 1987; 92:57–62.

50. Rhodes J et al. Hemodynamic correlates of exercise function in patients with primary pulmonary hypertension. J Am Coll Cardiol 1991; 18:1738–1744.

51. Metra, M, Dei Cas L, Panina G, et al. Exercise hyperventilation in chronic congestive heart failure, and its relation to functional capacity and hemodynamics. Am J Cardiol 1992; 70:622–628.

52. Kleber F, Vietzke G, Wernecke KD, et al. Impairment of ventilatory efficiency in heart failure: prognostic impact. Circulation 2000; 101:2803–2809.

53. Wasserman K, Van Kessel A, Burton GB. Interaction of physiological mechanisms during exercise. J Appl Physiol 1967; 22:71–85.

54. Sun X-G et al. Exercise Pathophysiology in Patients With Primary Pulmonary Hypertension. Circulation 2001; 104(4):429–435.

55. Wasserman K, Hansen JE, Sue DY, et al. Principles of the exercise testing and interpretation, 3rd ed. Baltimore: Lippincott Williams & Wilkins, 1999.

56. Hinderliter AL et al. Effects of long-term infusion of prostacyclin (epoprostenol) on echocardiographic measures of right ventricular structure and function in

primary pulmonary hypertension. Primary Pulmonary Hypertension Study Group. Circulation 1997; 95(6):1479–1486.

57. Barst RJ et al. A comparison of continuous intravenous epoprostenol (prostacyclin) with conventional therapy for primary pulmonary hypertension. The Primary Pulmonary Hypertension Study Group. N Engl J Med, 1996; 334(5):296–302.

58. Woo MA, Moser DK, Stevenson LW, Stevenson WG. Six-minute walk test and heart rate variability: lack of association in advanced stages of heart failure. Am J Respir Crit Care Med 1997; 6:348–354.

59. Cahalin LP, Mathier MA, Semigran MJ, Dec GW, DiSalvo TG. The six-minute walk test predicts peak oxygen uptake and survival in patients with advanced heart failure. Chest 1996; 110:325–332.

60. Roul G, Germain P, Bareiss P. Does the 6-minute walk test predict the prognosis in patients with NYHA class II or III chronic heart failure? Am Heart J 1998; 136:449–457.

61. Paciocco G, Martinez F, Bossone E. Oxygen desaturation on the six-minute walk test an mortality in untreated primary pulmonary hypertension. Eur Respir J 2001; 17:647–652.

62. Miyamoto S et al. Clinical correlates and prognostic significance of six-minute walk test in patients with primary pulmonary hypertension comparison with cardiopulmonary exercise testing. Am J Respir Crit Care Med 2000; 161(2):487–492.

63. Hagen P, Scholz DG, Edwards WD. Incidence and size of patent foramen ovale during the first 10 decades of life: an autopsy study of 965 normal hearts. Mayo Clin Proc 1984; 59:17–20.

64. Lynch J, Schuchard GH, Gross CM, et al. Prevalence of right-to-left atrial shunting in a healthy population: detection by Valsalva maneuver contrast echocardiography. Am J Cardiol 1984; 53:1478–1480.

65. Sun X et al. Gas exchange detection of exercise-induced right-to-left shunt in patients with primary pulmonary hypertension. Circulation 2002; 105:54–60.

66. Shapiro SM et al. Primary pulmonary hypertension: improved long-term effects and survival with continuous intravenous epoerostenol infusion. J Am Coll Cardiol 1997; 30(2):343–349.

67. Ting H, Sun XG, Chuang ML, Lewis DA, Hansen JE. A noninvasive assessment of pulmonary perfusion abnormality in patients with primary pulmonary hypertension. Chest 2001; 119:824–832.

68. Wax D, Garofano R, Barst R. Effects of long-term infusion of prostacyclin on exercise performance in patients with primary pulmonary hypertension. Chest 1999; 116:914–920.

69. Channick R et al. Effects of the dual endothelin receptor antagonist bosentan in patients with pulmonary hypertension: a placebo-controlled study. J Heart Lung Transplant 2001; 20(2):262–263.

70. McLaughlin V et al. Compassionate use of continuous prostacyclin in the management of secondary pulmonary hypertension: a case series. Ann Intern Med 1999; 4:740–743.

71. Rubin LJ et al. Treatment of primary pulmonary hypertension with continuous intravenous prostacyclin (epoprostenol). Results of a randomized trial. Ann Intern Med 1990; 112:485–491.

72. Castelain V et al. Pulmonary artery pressure-flow relations after prostacyclin in primary pulmonary hypertension. Am J Respir Crit Care Med 2002; 165(3):338–340.

73. McGregor M, Sniderman A. On pulmonary vascular resistance: the need for more precise definition. Am J Cardiol 1985; 55:217–221.

74. Fishman A. The respiratory system: circulation and nonrespiratory functions. in Handbook of Physiology. Bethesda, MD: American Physiology Society. 1985:93–166.

75. Kafi S, Melot C, Vachiery JL, Brimioulle S, Naeije R. Partitioning of pulmonary vascular resistance in primary pulmonary hypertension. J Am Coll Cardiol 1998; 31:1372–1376.

76. Rubin L. ACCP consensus statement: primary pulmonary hypertension. Chest, 1987; 104:236–250.

77. Rich S, Kaufmann E, Levy PS. The effect of high doses of calcium-channel blockers on survival in primary pulmonary hypertension. N Engl J Med 1992; 327(2):76–81.

78. Wensel R et al. Effects of hoprost inhalation on exercise capacity and ventilatory efficiency in patients with primary pulmonary hypertension. Circulation 2000; 101:2388.

79. Grünig EBJ, Mereles D, Barth U, Borst MM, Vogt IR, Fischer C, Olschewski H, Kuecherer HF, Kübler W. Abnormal pulmonary artery pressure response in asymptomatic carriers of primary pulmonary hypertension gene. Circulation 2000; 102:1145.

80. Gaine S et al. Unmasking of anorexigen-induced primary pulmonary hypertension by exercise. Am J Respir Crit Care Med 1999; 159:A166.

81. James K et al. Exercise hemodynamic findings in patients with exertional dyspnea. Tex Heart Inst J 2000; 27(2):100–105.

82. Hackett P et al. High-altitude pulmonary edema in persons without the right pulmonary artery. N Engl J Med 1980; 302:1070–1073.

83. Rios B, Driscoll D, McNamara D. High-altitude pulmonary edema with absent right pulmonary artery. Pediatrics 1985; 75:314–317.

84. Asmussen E, Hemmingsen I. Determination of maximum working capacity at different ages in work with the legs or with the arms. Scand J Clin Lab Invest 1958; 10:67–71.

85. Collett M, Liljestrand G. The minute volume of the heart in man during some different types of exercise. Scand Arch Physiol 1924; 45:29–42.

86. Bevegard S, Freyschuss U, Strandell T. Circulatory adaptation to arm and leg exercise in supine and sitting position. J Appl Physiol 1966; 21(1):37–46.

87. Kessler R et al. "Natural history" of pulmonary hypertension in a series of 131 patients with chronic obstructive lung disease. Am J Respir Crit Care Med 2001; 164(2):219–224.

7

Management of Nonbronchiectatic Chronic Obstructive Pulmonary Disease

FERNANDO J. MARTINEZ, STEVEN E. GAY, and KEVIN R. FLAHERTY

University of Michigan
Ann Arbor, Michigan, U.S.A.

Chronic obstructive pulmonary disease (COPD) is defined as a progressive respiratory disease characterized by airflow limitation that is not fully reversible (1,2). This definition includes several distinct pathophysiological conditions, including chronic bronchitis and emphysema. Chronic bronchitis is defined clinically by the presence of a daily, productive cough for more than 3 months with a duration of more than 2 successive years; emphysema is pathologically defined by an enlargement of airspaces (3,4); abnormalities of small airways are frequently seen (5). Importantly, most patients have features of all three of these pathological conditions (4).

The incidence, morbidity, and mortality of COPD continue to rise throughout the world (6). In the United States, COPD affects more than 16 million individuals and is the fourth leading cause of death (6,7). More importantly, of the four most common causes of death in the United States, COPD is the only one that continues to rise in prevalence. Recent estimates suggest that the economic impact of COPD is >$15.5 billion, with the majority ($6.1 billion) spent on hospitalizations. An additional $4.4 billion was estimated to have been spent on physician or other professional fees, $2.5 billion for drug therapy, $1.5 billion for nursing home care, and an additional $1.0 billion for home care services (8).

Table 1 Physiological Approach to Staging Disease Severity in COPD Patients

	Guideline		
Severity of obstruction	British Thoracic Society (14)	American Thoracic Society (1)	Global Initiative for Chronic Obstructive Lung Disease (2)
Mild (I)	60–79% predicted	50–65% predicted	>80% predicted and $FEV_1/FVC < 70\%$
Moderate (II)	40–59% predicted	35–49% predicted	30–80% predicted
Severe (III)	<40% predicted	<35% predicted	<30% predicted

Recently, one group examined these expenditures in a cohort of patients ($n = 413$) with COPD of varying severity followed for a maximum of 60 months (mean 47 ± 10 months) at a university medical center in the United States (8). COPD severity was staged using criteria recently defined by the American Thoracic Society (Table 1) (1). Patients with the most severe COPD (stage III) experienced the highest yearly cost of therapy ($10,812) compared with those with moderate COPD (stage II, $5037) and mild COPD (stage I, $1681). In addition, a separate analysis of a Medicare database from 1992 found per capita expenditures for a Medicare beneficiary with COPD to be 2.4 times that of all beneficiaries (9). The most expensive 10% accounted for almost 50% of all expenditures; higher comorbidity was associated with increased expenditures. The majority of the costs have been attributed to long-term oxygen therapy and hospitalizations (10). Importantly, the indirect costs of COPD in the United States are also staggering, with recent estimates suggesting that increasing severity of COPD is associated with work losses (11).

Data regarding prevalence, morbidity, and economic burden in other parts of the world are more difficult to identify. The Global Burden of Disease Study estimated a worldwide prevalence of COPD in 1990 of 9.34 per 1000 men and 7.33 per 1000 women and estimated that COPD would become the fifth leading cause of disability-adjusted life years lost in 2020, trailing only ischemic heart disease, unipolar major depression, road traffic accidents, and cerebrovascular disease (12,13). The Global Initiative for Chronic Obstructive Lung Disease (GOLD) workshop has presented data on three European countries demonstrating a similar disease burden, ranging from per capita dollar expenditures of $60 to $65 compared with $87 in the United States (2). Clearly COPD represents a major health care problem.

I. Goals of Therapy

COPD is generally a progressive disease, with increasing severity resulting in increasing symptoms, greater impairment in health-related quality of life

(HRQol), more frequent exacerbations, and greater health care costs (8). As such, management should be comprehensive in nature. The GOLD workshop (2) recently recommended an excellent management plan consisting of

Assessing and monitoring disease
Reducing risk factors
Managing stable disease
Managing exacerbations

Furthermore, effective management was stated to include

Preventing disease progression
Alleviating symptoms
Improving exercise tolerance
Improving health status
Preventing and treating complications
Preventing and treating exacerbations
Reducing mortality

The various therapeutic options for the treatment of COPD are discussed in the context of these recommendations.

II. Assessing and Monitoring Disease

A. Diagnosis

The diagnosis of COPD remains a clinical art, particularly as early diagnosis and appropriate staging are important. The broad definition, as suggested by international guidelines, includes a disease of airflow obstruction that is not fully reversible, an appropriate risk factor, and chronic symptoms (cough, sputum production, dyspnea, chest tightness) (1,2,14). Cough is generally one of the first symptoms identified in COPD (15,16), and recent data have suggested that excess sputum production is associated with an excess rate of FEV_1 decline, an increased rate of subsequent hospitalization (17), and a greater impairment in quality of life (18). As such, patients with cough are appropriate candidates for early diagnostic testing to ensure an early diagnosis (19). Similarly, dyspnea is a frequent symptom that tends to be progressive and is important in the genesis of the progressive decline in HRQol (18,20,21). In fact, some investigators have confirmed that quantification of dyspnea adds valuable independent information in stratifying disease severity (20,21).

The physical examination can suggest the presence of wheezing and airflow obstruction but is a crude and insensitive means of detecting more severe disease (3,22,23). In a recent review of 44 studies examining the value of clinical examination in diagnosing airflow obstruction, Holleman and Simel identified no single item or combination of items that ruled out airflow obstruction; objective wheezing, barrel-chest deformity, rhonchi, hyperresonance, subxyphoid apical impulse, and objective measurement of prolonged expiration were the most useful signs in suggesting the presence of airflow obstruction (24). Although forced expiratory time can be helpful in suggesting the presence of disease, judging severity of disease by physical examination is notoriously difficult (3). For example, during an exacerbation in 90 patients with known COPD, only 38% of the physician's estimates of disease severity were accurate; 48% of estimates were high and 14% were low (25).

Given the limitations of the clinical examination, it is evident that confirmation of airflow obstruction is required to assure an accurate diagnosis. Fortunately, this is easily done with spirometry, a widely available, standardized, and relatively inexpensive diagnostic study (19,26). A detailed discussion of the physiological evaluation of patients with suspected airflow obstruction is presented elsewhere in this volume. The presence and extent of bronchoreversibility and its diagnostic value in COPD remains a controversial topic (3). In fact, some degree of bronchoreversibility is often seen in patients meeting diagnostic criteria for COPD (27). Interestingly, some have suggested that bronchoreversibility in the setting of COPD is associated with increased sputum eosinophilia, a picture more typical of asthma (28). Spirometric data are also used to stratify the severity of airflow obstruction. In this way the FEV_1 as a percent of predicted has been utilized to define severe, moderate, and mild disease, as enumerated in Table 1 (1,2,14). These criteria, although arbitrary in nature, identify patient groups with increasing health care costs (8) and progressively worsening HRQol (29).

The role of additional diagnostic testing to identify features of asthma, emphysema, chronic bronchitis, or chronic bronchiolitis in individual patients remains controversial (3). Although asthma is not considered in the diagnosis of COPD, in clinical practice these diseases are not discrete entities and demonstrate significant overlap (5). In fact, Figure 1 illustrates this mix of structural and inflammatory overlap. Interestingly, as noted elsewhere in this volume, increasing attention is being devoted by numerous investigative groups to defining the predominant inflammatory processes involved in the pathogenesis of COPD (5,30–33). Furthermore, these biological differences likely influence the time course of disease. In a sentinel study, one group identified an improved survival and lower rate of decline in FEV_1 over 10 years of follow-up in patients with a clinical diagnosis of asthma compared to those with nonatopic, smoking-related obstructive disease (34). These data suggest that defining subsets of patients with COPD may have prognostic and potential therapeutic value. The optimal approach to the differential diagnosis of patients with COPD remains unclear, although it likely includes the use of advanced radiological techniques, including high-resolution computed tomography (3).

Radiological studies have assumed an increasing role in the evaluation of patients with COPD, particularly computed tomography (CT) (35,36). CT provides excellent visual anatomical detail for detecting, characterizing, and quantitatively determining the severity of emphysema. CT demonstrates

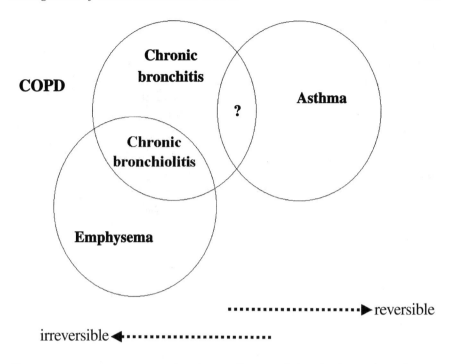

Figure 1 A typical nonproportional Venn diagram of chronic obstructive pulmonary disease (COPD). There is overlap among the most common subsets of COPD, including the extent of bronchoreversibility. (From Ref. 5.)

greater accuracy than chest radiography, while high-resolution CT (HRCT) is more accurate than conventional CT (37,38). Furthermore, emphysema severity on CT correlates well with the pathological severity of emphysema, using either visual scoring systems or quantitative analysis based on Hounsfield unit (HU) threshold measurements (38–42). Similarly, quantitative analysis of emphysema correlates with decreasing diffusing capacity of the lung (DL_{CO}) (43) and is useful in identifying emphysema, usually mild, in patients with an isolated decrement in DL_{CO} (44). Recently, O'Brien et al. identified 110 patients (mean age 66.5 years) who presented to their general practitioner with an episode of acute exacerbation of COPD (45). When patients recovered 2 months later, detailed physiological testing and HRCT were performed. An abnormal spirometry was noted in 88% of the patients; a decreased FEV_1 was confirmed in 70%. Emphysema was present in 51% of the patients, while bronchiectasis was noted in 29%. The influence of such additional diagnostic testing on subsequent medical therapy in individual patients requires further investigation.

B. Monitoring

As COPD is generally a progressive disorder, close serial monitoring is important in optimizing therapeutic interventions (46). Symptomatic monitoring includes quantifying the severity and frequency of cough. In addition, worsening dyspnea strongly influences HRQol in these patients (20,21,29). Similarly, identifying and treating exacerbations of disease are important interventions, as these acute deteriorations in clinical status have a significant effect on pulmonary function, which can take several weeks to recover (47). Furthermore, exacerbations have a significant impact on impaired HRQol in these patients (48,49). The role of serial physiological monitoring remains poorly defined, although serial spirometric monitoring may provide a diagnostic advantage over a single test (19,50). Furthermore, it is important to keep in mind that patients with COPD are at risk of developing other smoking-related illnesses, such as bronchogenic carcinoma and coronary artery disease.

C. Reducing Risk Factors

Cigarette smoking remains the most common risk factor for the development of COPD. As such, smoking cessation is a vital component in a comprehensive approach to the COPD patient. A detailed description is beyond the scope of this work, but comprehensive reviews of the topic have recently been presented (51–53). The Public Health Service Report recommends a five-step program for intervention in smokers (Table 2) (52).

A comprehensive approach to smoking cessation intervention is ideal and should include counseling. Three types have been shown to be effective: practical counseling, social support as part of treatment, and social support arranged outside of treatment (2). Pharmacotherapy has advanced significantly over the past decade. As nicotine is the primary agent leading to addiction (54), an aggressive approach to therapeutic nicotine replacement has proven effective, with many forms available (52,53,55,56). Recent data have suggested that the antidepressants buproprion and nortriptyline increase long-term quit rates (52,53,57).

The importance of smoking cessation has recently been confirmed by the Lung Health Study, a randomized trial of current smokers with borderline to moderate impairment of pulmonary function (58). Approximately 6000 subjects were recruited and followed up to 5 years; half were randomized to an aggressive smoking cessation program plus anticholinergic therapy and the other to usual therapy plus anticholinergic therapy. At least 35% of the subjects were able to quit smoking for extended periods of time, while 22% were able to quit and sustain cessation for 5 years (compared to 6% in the usual-care group). As Figure 2 illustrates, those participants who were able to discontinue smoking and remained sustained quitters exhibited a small increase (of 57 mL) in lung function over the first year, compared to a fall (of 38 mL) in those who continued to smoke. In addition, the sustained quitters had reduced rates of

Table 2 Five-Step Program for Intervention in Smokers

Component	Description of component
ASK	*Systematically identify all tobacco users at every visit.*
	Implement an officewide system ensuring that, for every patient at every clinic visit, tobacco-use status is queried and documented.
ADVISE	*Strongly urge all tobacco users to quit.*
	In a clear, strong, and personalized manner, urge every tobacco user to quit.
ASSESS	*Determine willingness to make a quit attempt.*
	Ask every tobacco user if he or she is willing to make a quit attempt at this time.
ASSIST	*Aid the patient in quitting.*
	Help the patient with a quit plan; provide practical couseling; provide intratreatment social support; help the patient obtain extratreatment social support; recommend use of approved pharmacotherapy except in special circumstances; provide supplementary materials.
ARRANGE	*Schedule follow-up contact.*
	Schedule follow-up contact, either directly or via telephone.

Source: Ref. 52.

FEV_1 decline over the following 4 years (34 mL/year) compared to those who continued to smoke (decline of 63 mL/year).

Although data are more limited, in certain environmental settings exposure to occupational gases or particles as well as indoor and outdoor pollution may be instrumental in the development of COPD (2). Therefore avoidance of these exposures may prove an important intervention to decreasing disease development or progression.

III. Medical Management of the Stable Patient with COPD

Given the global impact of disease in COPD patients, its management must be multifactorial. Early therapeutic interventions were aimed at improving physiological derangement. Therefore many investigators attempted to address treatment response in terms of improvement in airflow limitation, the hallmark of COPD diagnosis (46). Unfortunately, by definition COPD patients do not experience complete reversibility after the administration of bronchodilators. Furthermore, relief of symptoms correlates only weakly with changes in spirometric indices (54). As discussed elsewhere in this volume, recent data have confirmed the importance of lung hyperinflation, particularly with exercise, in the genesis of exertional limitation in patients with COPD (59–63). Therefore alternative physiological techniques are now employed in assessing

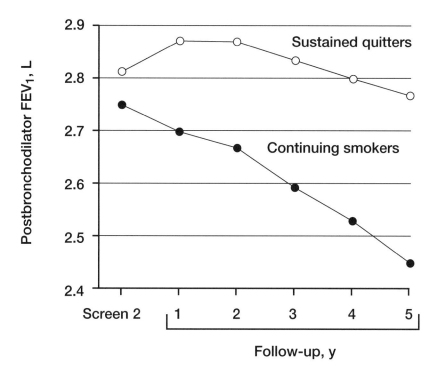

Figure 2 Mean postbronchodilator FEV_1 for participants in the smoking intervention and placebo group who were sustained quitters (open circles) and continuous smokers (closed circles). (From Ref. 58.)

the benefits of specific therapeutic interventions (59). In addition, the GOLD participants, in acknowledging the limitations of relying in single physiological outcomes, have appropriately recommended a more comprehensive approach to the treatment of patients with COPD. Thus therapeutic goals include preventing disease progression, alleviating symptoms, improving exercise tolerance, improving health status, preventing and treating complications, preventing and treating exacerbations, and reducing mortality (2). In discussing available therapeutic alternatives, we attempt, whenever possible in the following discussion, to present a comprehensive assessment of treatment outcomes.

Numerous therapeutic alternatives have been studied and used clinically in COPD patients. These have included medical therapies such as bronchodilators, corticosteroids, and mucolytics. Similarly, nonpharmacologic therapies have included oxygen therapy and pulmonary rehabilitation. Given the improvements in disease staging of COPD patients (1,2,14,46), a stepwise approach has been advocated by many international groups. Figure 3 illustrates the "COPD escalator," showing in the form of a graph a stepwise approach to therapy in COPD. A similar, tabular representation is presented in Table 3, adapted from the GOLD guidelines (2).

A. Bronchodilator Therapy

Bronchodilators have constituted the mainstay of therapy in COPD for many years and remain cornerstones of treatment in all published recommendations. They are used to improve pulmonary function and exercise capacity, relieve symptoms, decrease frequency and severity of exacerbations, improve quality of life, and, ideally, decrease disease progression and mortality. Numerous classes of bronchodilators are currently available for clinical use including anticholinergics, beta agonists, and methylthanxines.

Anticholinergics

The anticholinergic agents are derived from belladonna and other alkaloid plants, which have been used in the treatment of pulmonary disorders for centuries. Over the past several decades, increased knowledge has been accumulated that better defines the cholinergic pathways in the lung. Furthermore, increased selectivity in antimuscarinic agents has created a class of agents with an excellent therapeutic profile (54,64). There are multiple muscarinic receptors in the lung, including periganglionic excitatory (M_1) and smooth muscle (M_3) receptors that stimulate smooth muscle contraction and secretion of mucus (54,65). In contrast, inhibitory postganglionic muscarinic receptors (M_2) can downregulate acetylcholine release and thereby limit the magnitude of vagally mediated bronchoconstriction (54); these M_2 receptors have recently been shown to be functional in patients with stable COPD (66).

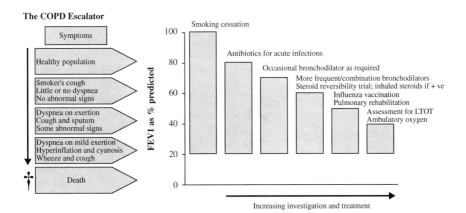

Figure 3 COPD escalator. Summary of the principal components of a management plan for COPD. Note that as disease severity increases, symptoms and signs become more obvious, while the number of treatments used rises. (From Ref. 14.)

Table 3 Therapy at Each Stage of COPD as Adapted from the GOLD Guidelines

Stage	Characteristics	Recommended therapy
All		Avoidance of risk factors Influenza vaccination
0: At risk	Chronic symptoms (cough, sputum) Exposure to risk factors	
I: Mild COPD	$FEV_1/FVC < 70\%$ $FEV_1 \geq 80\%$ predicted	Short-acting bronchodilator as needed
II: Moderate COPD	IIA $FEV_1/FVC < 70\%$ predicted $50\% \leq FEV_1 < 80\%$ predicted With or without symptoms	Regular treatment with one or more bronchodilators Pulmonary rehabilitation Inhaled corticosteroids if significant symptoms and lung function response is evident
	IIB $FEV_1/FVC < 70\%$ $30\% \leq FEV_1 < 50\%$ predicted With or without symptoms	Regular treatment with one or more bronchodilators Pulmonary rehabilitation Inhaled corticosteroids if significant symptoms and lung function response is evident or if repeated exacerbations are present
III: Severe COPD	$FEV_1/FVC < 70\%$ $FEV_1 < 30\%$ predicted or Presence of respiratory failure or right heart failure	Regular treatment with one or more bronchodilators Pulmonary rehabilitation Inhaled corticosteroids if significant symptoms and lung function response is evident or if repeated exacerbations are present Treatment of complications Long-term oxygen therapy if respiratory failure evident Consider surgical therapies

Source: Ref. 2.

Until recently, available anticholinergic agents have been quarternary derivatives of anticholinergic compounds. These compounds do not cross biological barriers easily but, unfortunately, block all muscarinic receptors (54). The new generation of anticholinergic compounds, including tiotropium, exhibit the unique pharmacological property of binding to all muscarinic receptors with varying duration of binding. As such, the slow dissociation from M_3 receptors ($t_{1/2}$ of 35 hr compared to 16 min for ipratropium) and a faster dissociation from M_2 receptors ($t_{1/2}$ of 3.6 hr) creates a functional receptor subtype selectivity of M_3 and M_1 over M_2 receptors (65). These properties and accumulating clinical data (discussed subsequently) have generated increased enthusiasm over their use in COPD patients.

Use of anticholinergics in COPD patients has been demonstrated to yield measurable improvement in airflow, which is at least equal and in many settings better than can be achieved with beta agonists (54,67). Of 38 published studies comparing anticholinergic agents and short-acting beta agonists reviewed by Chapman et al., all but 2 found the anticholinergic agents to be equal and generally superior to short acting beta agonists (68). In addition, several studies have confirmed the ability of anticholinergic drugs to induce bronchodilation even when beta agonists have failed to improve airflow (69,70). Potential reasons for these differences include the predominant effect of anticholinergic agents on central airways versus the more peripheral effect of beta agonists and a decrease in mucus production with anticholinergic therapy (67).

Unfortunately, few studies have administered equivalent doses of anticholinergic agents and beta agonists, making a clear interpretation difficult (67). For example, in stable COPD, two puffs of an anticholinergic drug produce greater bronchodilation than two puffs of a beta agonist, likely representing a dose effect (67).

An additional beneficial effect of anticholinergic therapy includes a longer duration of action in comparison to short-acting beta agonists, as demonstrated by numerous investigators. Braun et al. compared the spirometric effect of ipratropium (two puffs), albuterol (two puffs) and placebo in a group of 25 patients with severe, baseline airflow obstruction (FEV_1 34% predicted) (71). Interestingly, 15 patients did not demonstrate a 15% improvement in FEV_1 after the administration of metaproterenol but experienced improvement after the administration of ipratropium. The long-term effect of anticholinergic therapy has been studied in a systematic review of pooled data from seven randomized controlled trials comparing ipratropium bromide and beta agonists (72). After 3 months of therapy, mean improvement in FEV_1 was significantly higher in the ipratropium arm of the studies (mean 28-mL increase) than the beta agonist studies (mean 1-mL decrease, $p < 0.05$). All seven trials demonstrated a decline in the acute effect of beta agonist treatment with prolonged treatment; five of seven studies demonstrated improvement in the acute effect of ipratropium.

Unfortunately, long-term therapy with ipratropium does not influence progression of COPD (58). Recent studies have defined the role of tiatropium

Table 4 Recent Studies of Tiotropium in COPD Patients

| | | | | Baseline FEV$_1$ (% predicted) | Treatment outcomes | | |
| | | | | | FEV$_1$ | HRQol[a, b] | Exacerbations (% experiencing) |
Study	Agents	Study duration	N				
Casaburi et al. (269)	Tiotropium 18μg qd	92 days	279	39	+0.20 L	NA	16%
	Placebo		191	38	−0.02 L		21.5%
Van Noord et al. (270)	Tiotropium 18μg qd	92 days	191	42	+0.26 L	NA	NA
	Ipratropium 40 μg qid		97	40	+0.18 L		
Casaburi et al. (82)	Tiotropium 18μg qd	1 year	550	39.1	+0.13 L	49%	36%
	Placebo		371	38.1	−0.02 L	30%	42%[c]
Vincken et al. (83)	Tiotropium 18 μg qd	1 year	356	41.9	+0.14 L	52%	35%
	Ipratropium 40 μg qid		179	39.4	−0.03 L	35%	46%[c]

[a] Health-related quality of life.
[b] Percent experiencing a four-unit improvement in St. George's Respiratory Questionnaire.
[c] $p < 0.05$.

in patients with COPD; four comparative studies are presented in Table 4. Dose-ranging studies have suggested a dose of 18 μg/day as optimal from efficacy and safety analyses (73); this dosage resulted in significant short- and long-term bronchodilation (see Table 4). In addition, recent long-term studies have suggested better preservation of bronchodilation with tiotropium compared to ipratropium (Fig. 4).

The response to exercise after anticholinergic therapy has recently been reviewed in a systematic analysis (74). Seventeen studies were described in detail; the majority of studies examining steady-state exercise confirmed a response (three of four single-dose studies and all of three maintenance-dose studies). Of 12 studies, 9 confirmed an effect on maximal exercise capacity. Two published studies have suggested an increasing effect of higher doses on exercise tolerance (75,76). A recent study compared the effect of oxitropium bromide (400 μg) versus placebo in 38 patients with severe COPD (FEV_1 40.8% predicted) (77). Endurance testing proved the most sensitive in detecting the effects of the inhaled anticholinergic agent. The mechanism underlying the benefit in maximal exercise tolerance after inhalation of ipratropium has been defined in a study of 500 μg of nebulized ipratropium versus placebo (78). Although no difference was noted in spirometry, exercise endurance, or exercise dyspnea after placebo administration, improvements were noted after ipratropium. In addition, the change in exercise endurance time and exercise dyspnea correlated best with the change in inspiratory capacity, a measure of dynamic hyperinflation.

In addition to improving pulmonary function and exercise capacity, inhaled anticholinergic agents have been demonstrated to improve symptoms. In the pooled studies described by Rennard et al., significant improvements were noted in dyspnea after ipratropium inhalation in patients who were ex-smokers (72). Similar improvements have been noted in several large studies of ipratropium and long acting beta agonists. In patients with severe COPD (FEV_1 37% predicted) patients treated with either ipratropium or salmeterol experienced similar improvements in transitional dyspnea index (TDI) scores at weeks 2, 4, 6, 8, 10, and 12 (79). In a study with similar methodology, the improvements in dyspnea with ipratropium administration were more modest, only achieving statistical significance from placebo in the first 6 weeks of a 12-week study (80). In contrast, other investigators have not identified a difference in total symptom scores between inhaled ipratropium and placebo (81), potentially reflecting a difference in methodology. Tiotropium has resulted in greater statistical and clinically significant improvements in TDI compared to placebo in a 1-year study (82). Interestingly, tiotropium demonstrated a greater improvement in TDI compared with ipratropium during 1 year of therapy (83).

Improvement in HRQol has been recently described. Mahler et al. noted an improvement in the chronic respiratory disease questionnaire (CRDQ) with ipratropium administration for 12 weeks compared with placebo (79). Interestingly, a similar study did not confirm these findings (80), nor did a recent study utilizing the St. George's respiratory questionnaire (81). Two

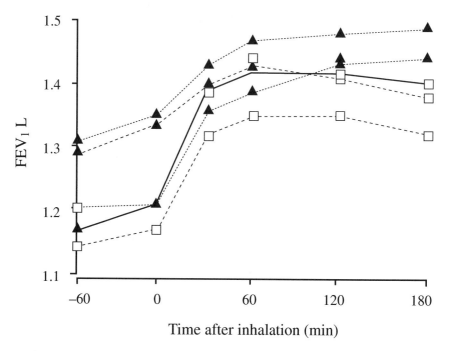

Figure 4 Mean forced expiratory volume in 1 sec (FEV_1) before and during the 3 hr following inhalation of tiotropium (▲) or ipratropium (□) at baseline or day 1 (—) and after 8 days (-----) and 364 days (---). (From Ref. 83.)

studies (Table 4) have confirmed that a greater proportion of patients using tiotropium experiencing clinically significant improvements in HRQol using the St. George's respiratory questionnaire than those using placebo (82) or ipratropium (Fig. 5) (83). Given the important effect of exacerbations on HRQol, the impact of anticholinergic therapy on this outcome has recently been reported. Three groups failed to identify a beneficial effect of ipratropium use, although the definitions of exacerbations varied (79–81). Two long-term studies have confirmed a lower frequency of exacerbation with tiotropium compared to placebo (82) or ipratropium (83) (Table 4). Interestingly, a recent pharmacoeconomic analysis of two placebo-controlled, 3-month-long, randomized studies of ipratropium versus ipratropium plus albuterol or albuterol alone has been published (84). These investigators confirmed a significant decrease in exacerbation frequency in the ipratropium arms that translated into a marked decrease in total treatment costs compared to albuterol alone (Fig. 6). Interestingly, the same group has reported that the use of ipratropium alone or in combination with a beta agonist resulted in a lower total cost of care for patients with stages I to III COPD (8). On the basis of these data, these investigators have suggested a pharmacological algorithm to therapy in COPD patients emphasizing the early use of an anticholinergic agent. Given the further advantages noted with tiotropium, it is expected that a similar if not greater pharmacoeconomic advantage will be seen with this anticholinergic agent.

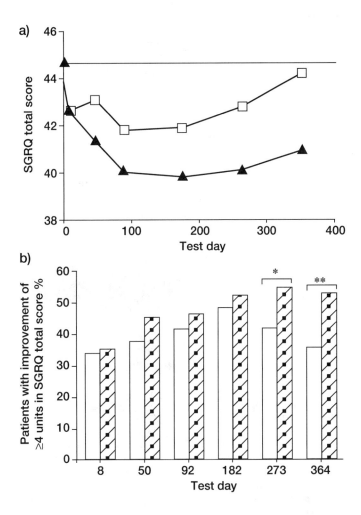

Figure 5 (a) Mean St. George's Respiratory Questionnaire (SGRQ) total score over 1 year for the tiotropium (▲) and ipratropium (□) groups (——— baseline). (b) Proportion of patients with an improvement in SGRQ total score of ≥ four units for the tiotropium (✐) and ipratropium (□) groups during the 1-year study. $^*p < 0.05$; $^{**}p < 0.001$. (From Ref. 83.)

Beta Adrenergic Agonists

Although there is little sympathetic innervation of airway smooth muscle, sympathomimetics have been documented to be efficacious and, until recently, have been the mainstay of COPD management (54). Detailed discussions of the effects of short- and long-acting beta agonists have recently been published (67,74,85–87). In addition, alternative mechanisms for these long-acting agents have recently been detailed (88).

B. Short-Acting Beta Agonists

Short-acting beta agonists have been evaluated in numerous studies and have been shown to cause bronchodilation, although the magnitude of this effect has been highly variable (67). A recent review of the effects of bronchodilators on exercise capacity described the results reported in 14 such studies demonstrating a change in FEV_1 ranging from 93 to 240 mL (74). Some of this variability is inherent to individual patient variability. One large study demonstrated that more than two-thirds of COPD patients who had a $\leq 10\%$ increase in FEV_1 after an inhaled bronchodilator at baseline demonstrated an increase $\geq 15\%$ at some time during the 3-year trial (89). An additional source of variability lies in the dose of beta agonist administered; higher doses may result in further increases in FEV_1 (67), although this may be seen in only a minority of patients (90). Unfortunately, higher dosing may be associated with tremor, tachycardia, and tachyphylaxis (54). The available beta agonists differ in the time of onset,

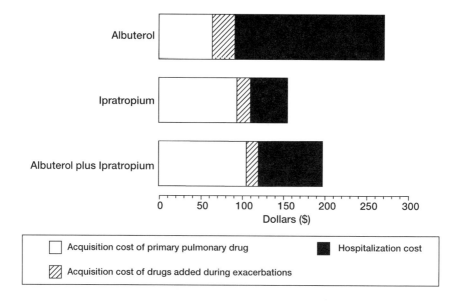

Figure 6 Total treatment costs over the 85-day follow-up period for the three treatment groups. (From Ref. 84.)

degree of beta$_2$-receptor selectivity, and the duration of onset, as outlined in Table 5. A recent prospective study has confirmed the value of short-acting beta agonists as "as needed" medications, in contrast to regular use (91). In a randomized, double-blind, placebo-controlled crossover trial in 53 COPD patients, Cook et al. randomized patients (mean FEV$_1$ 33.6% predicted) in a crossover fashion to inhaled albuterol (200 µg four times per day) versus placebo; all patients received regular ipratropium bromide, beclomethasone, and open-label inhaled albuterol as needed. The patients in the regular-use arm used twice as much albuterol as those in the "as needed" arm. Despite this greater use of short-acting beta agonist, there were no differences in spirometry, quality of life, symptoms, or 6-min walk distance. These data are important, as regular use of short-acting beta agonists has been associated with tachyphylaxis of spirometric improvement (72). Whether "as needed" use negates this phenomenon is not clear. These data support the role of short-acting beta agonists as rescue therapy, as outlined in the recent GOLD guidelines (2).

A recent systematic review of 14 studies described the effects of short-acting beta agonists on exercise capacity (74). Steady-state exercise improved in approximately half of the studies, although lesser improvements were noted in maximal exercise tests. Furthermore, recent studies have confirmed that improvements noted in exercise capacity after beta agonist inhalation relate to improved dynamic hyperinflation (92) or improved right-heart function (93). Similarly, contradictory data have been published regarding changes in HRQol. Guyatt et al. reported that inhaled salbutamol improved HRQol, as measured by the chronic respiratory questionnaire (CRQ), in 19 COPD patients (94). In contrast, quality-of-life scores were not improved in 207 COPD patients (mean FEV$_1$ 34.1% predicted) treated with nebulized albuterol (95). Additional data are required to reconcile these differences.

C. Long-Acting Beta Agonists

Recently, beta agonists with a prolonged duration of action have become clinically available (see Table 5). The effects noted with these agents has been the source of recent, detailed reviews (67,85–87). These agents have been documented to result in significant bronchodilation in COPD patients (85). Although the onset of action of salmeterol appears to be somewhat shorter than with other inhaled beta agonists or inhaled anticholinergic agents, its duration of action has been longer than the comparators with the exception of inhaled formoterol and oral bambuterol, which are similar (86). These data must be interpreted with caution, as significant interpatient variability has been reported. For example, in a single-blind crossover study of salbutamol (200 µg), salmeterol (50 µg), formoterol (24 µg), and placebo in 16 COPD patients (mean FEV$_1$ 39.3% predicted), a similar time of onset to improvement of FEV$_1$ by 15% was noted among the beta agonists (96). Interestingly, the onset of action was more rapid with inhaled formoterol in 9 patients, while it was more rapid

Table 5 Properties of Inhaled Beta Agonists

Agent	Dose per puff (mg)	Beta receptor selectivity		Time to onset (min)	Time to peak effect (min)	Duration of action (hr)
		Beta$_1$	Beta$_2$			
Short-acting agents						
Albuterol	90	+	++++	5–15	30–90	4–6
Metaproterenol	650	+	+++	5–15	10–60	1–3
Pirbuterol	200	+	+++	5–10	30–60	3–5
Terbutaline	200	+	++++	5–30	60–120	3–6
Long-acting agents						
Formoterol	12	+	++++	36–60	60–120	10–14
Salmeterol	21	+	++++	30–60	60–180	10–14

in 5 patients after inhaled salmeterol. Recently, formoterol and salbutamal have been shown to result in a similar onset of bronchodilation (97,98). The potency of salmeterol and formoterol seem to be similar (85). One recent study has suggested that salmeterol has greater potency than formoterol in patients with severe COPD (mean FEV_1 21.5% predicted) (99), while another suggested similar results in a less severely ill population (mean FEV_1 35.4% predicted) (100). Therefore some have suggested that formoterol is more active in mild to moderate COPD while salmeterol is more active in patients with severe disease (85). Interestingly, treatment with salmeterol does not preclude a further bronchodilator response to salbutamol (101,102).

Several large studies have examined the role of long-acting beta agonists during long-term therapy in COPD patients. Some of these studies are enumerated in Table 6. The studies of Mahler et al. (79) and Rennard et al. (80) used a similar format in comparing salmeterol with ipratropium bromide. In both studies the majority of patients experienced acute bronchoreversibility to albuterol challenge. The peak improvement in FEV_1 was similar between both bronchodilators, although the duration of effect was longer with salmeterol (Fig. 7). In both studies, although the peak effect was less in patients without bronchoreversibility to albuterol, significant bronchodilation was noted with both ipratropium and salmeterol in contrast to placebo. These data support the data of others, confirming that the absence of acute bronchoreversibility to short-acting beta agonists does not preclude physiological improvement with long-acting beta agonists (103). Similar findings were noted by Dahl and colleagues, who compared two doses of formoterol with ipratropium and placebo (81). Both doses of formoterol exhibited a greater area under the curve for FEV_1 response than placebo and ipratropium; ipratropium demonstrated a statistically significant bronchodilation compared with placebo.

An improvement in symptoms is a consistent finding in these studies of long acting beta agonists. Both Mahler et al. (79) and Rennard et al. (80) confirmed an improvement in dyspnea with both salmeterol and ipratropium. These data expand earlier data confirming a reduction in dyspnea with resistive breathing after the administration of salmeterol (104). Similarly, Dahl and colleagues noted an improvement in global symptom scores with both formoterol doses compared to placebo; a significant improvement for the dose of 14 µg bid compared to ipratropium ($p = 0.009$) was noted, while the improvement with the dose of 24 µg bid approached significance ($p = 0.06$). Despite improvement in symptoms, neither Mahler et al. or Rennard et al. were able to demonstrate an improvement in 6-min walk distance. These findings are consistent with the findings of other studies (105,106). As reviewed by Liesker et al., minor changes have been noted in studies of maximal exercise testing (74). One group has suggested an improved distance walked with salmeterol and ipratropium compared to placebo, while the time to recovery of Sa_{O_2} after exercise was improved with both bronchodilators (107). A separate group has noted a greater inspiratory capacity during submaximal exercise with salmeterol versus ipratropium 6 hr after dosing, although the IC was

Table 6 Blinded, Controlled Studies of Long-Acting Beta Agonist Therapy > 12 Weeks in Duration in COPD Patients

Study	Agent	N	Study duration	Baseline FEV$_1$	FEV$_1$	Results			
						Beta agonist (puffs per day)	Total HRQol score	Patients with clinically significant Δ	Percent with exacerbation
Boyd et al. (106)	SM 50 µg bid	229	16 weeks	1.31 L		NR	NR	NR	21%
	SM 100 µg bid	218		1.23 L					25%
	Pl	227		1.31 L					26%
Mahler et al. (79)	SM 42 µg bid	135	12 weeks	42.1% pred	SM > IP > Pl	2.0	7.1[a]	46%[a]	20.7%
	IP 36 µg qid	133		37.0% pred		2.4	6.8[a]	39%[a]	30.8%
	Pl	143		40.8% pred		NR	2.1	27%	32.9%
Rennard et al. (80)	SM 42 µg bid	132	12 weeks	1.22 L	SM = IP > Pl	1.8[a]	10.3	465	28.8
	IP 36 µg qid	138		1.28 L		2.1[a]	9.2	41%	26.8
	Pl	135		1.30 L		2.6	6.8	38%	30.4
Dahl et al. (81)	FM 12 mg bid	194	12 weeks	1.33 L (46 %pred)	FM 12 = FM 24	1.2[a]	41.7[a]	NR	NR
	FM 24 mg bid	192		1.31 L (45 %pred)	FM 12/FM 24 > Pl	1.7[a]	43.5[a]	NR	NR
	IP 40 mg qid	194		1.29 L (45 %pred)	FM 12/FM 24 > IP	2.0[b]	47.2[c]	NR	NR
	Pl	200		1.29 L (44 %pred)	IP > Pl	2.5	46.8	NR	NR

Study	Treatment	n	Duration	FEV1	Comparison				
Zuwallack et al. (153)	SM 42 μg bid	310	12 weeks	40.1% pred	SM + Theo > SM >	1.8	+ 7.6	45%	18.1%
	SM + Theo	313		40.8% pred	Theo	1.5	+ 12.7	54%	12.8%[d]
	Theo	315		40.7% pred		2.0	+ 8.6	42%	19.7%
Cazzola et al. (102)	SM + FP	20	12 weeks	~ 1.15 L	SM = SM + FP 250, SM + FP 500,	NR	NR	NR	NR
	250 mg bid	20		~ 1.14 L					
	SM + FP				SM + Theo				
	500 mg bid								
	SM + Theo	20		~ 1.17 L					
		20		~ 1.22 L					

[a] $p < 0.05$ compared to placebo.

[b] $p < 0.05$ compared to FM12 and FM24.
[c] $p < 0.05$ compared to FM 12.
[d] $p < 0.05$ SM + Theo versus Theo.

Key: NR, not reported; HRQol, health-related quality of life; FM, formoterol; BAL, bronchoalveolar lavage; TRI; triamcinolone; SM, salmeterol; IP, ipratropium; Pl, placebo; L, liter; Theo, theophylline; FP, fluticasone propionate.

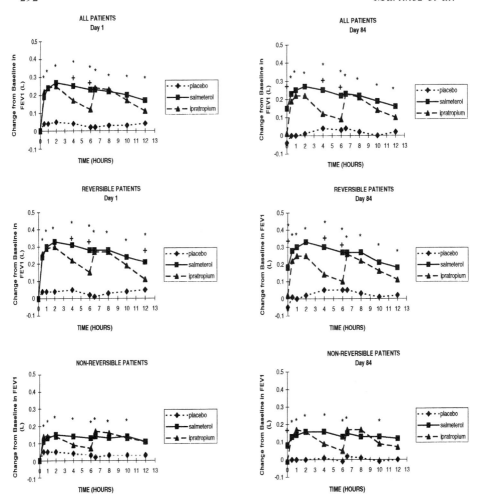

Figure 7 Change from baseline was analyzed within each group and by responsivity strata over a 12-hr period of serial pulmonary function testing at day 1 (left) and day 84 (right). The mean change from baseline at FEV_1 in the salmeterol group (combined population) was significant (indicated by asterisk; $p < 0.001$) for each serial assessment at all visits. Within the ipratropium group, change from baseline was significant ($p < 0.026$) for all serial assessments except for hour 0 (predose) at day 84. Significant differences in serial FEV_1 between salmeterol and ipratropium treatment groups are indicated with a plus sign. (From Ref. 79.)

similar 1 hr after dosing; dyspnea ratings were similar with both broncho-dilators (108).

Significant data have been published defining the effect of long-acting beta agonists on HRQol in COPD patients, as enumerated in Table 6. Instruments utilized to assess HRQol have included a multidimensional general health questionnaire (SF-36) (109–111) and disease-specific instruments. The latter include the Chronic Respiratory Disease Questionnaire (CRDQ) (79,80,112,113) and the St. George's Respiratory Questionnaire (SGRQ) (81,106,111,112). Representative results are illustrated in Figure 8, which confirms a clinically significant change in the SGRQ with salmeterol 50 µg bid compared with salmeterol 100 µg bid or placebo (111). Similar, clinically important improvement has been confirmed when formoterol 12 µg bid was compared with placebo but not with 24 µg bid. Given the important relationship between HRQol and exacerbations of disease in patients with COPD (48,49), several groups have examined the effect of long-acting beta agonists on exacerbations. As enumerated in Table 6, a consistent decrease in exacerbation percentage has not been documented in all studies. One group has demonstrated a statistically longer time to exacerbation when comparing salmeterol, ipratropium, and placebo (Fig. 9). Importantly, salmeterol has been demonstrated to result in a lesser decrease in Pa_{O_2} than albuterol (114). A large analysis involving three cohort studies (12,294 patients treated with nedocromil, 15,407 with salmeterol, and 8098 with bambuterol) suggested an increased risk of adverse cardiac side effects with an oral beta agonist (bambuterol) but not with inhaled salmeterol (115). A smaller study of 12 COPD patients with pre-existing cardiac arrhythmias and hypoxemia ($Pa_{O_2} < 60$ mmHg) examined the effect of formoterol 12 µg bid, formoterol 24 µg bid, salmeterol 50 µg bid, and placebo (116). A higher heart rate and more frequent supraventricular or ventricular premature beats were noted with higher-dose formoterol than lower-dose formoterol or salmeterol. Therefore long-acting beta agonists seem to have favorable side-effect profiles.

D. Combination of Inhaled Bronchodilators

Given the different modes of action of anticholinergic and beta agonist agents, it is logical to consider their combination in the management of symptomatic

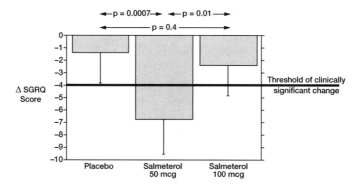

Figure 8 Change in St. George's Respiratory Questionnaire (SGRQ) total score over 16 weeks. Error bars are 95% confidence intervals. A reduction in score indicated improved health. (From Ref. 20.)

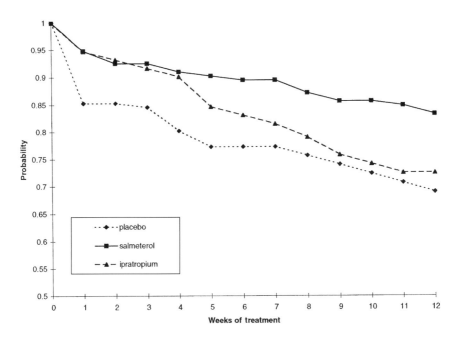

Figure 9 Kaplan-Meier survival analysis of time to first exacerbation. A significantly higher percentage of salmeterol-treated patients completed the study without experiencing a COPD exacerbation than did either ipratropium-treated ($p = 0.0411$) or placebo-treated ($p = 0.0052$) patients. (From Ref. 79.)

COPD. Indeed, many have examined the clinical and physiological effects of such combinations. Several studies have confirmed that the combination of ipratropium and short-acting beta agonists results in a greater physiological response than either agent administered separately (117–129). Other investigators have not confirmed these findings (130–132); some have suggested that the combination does not provide benefit over maximal doses of either agent alone (130), particularly higher doses of beta agonists (133). In a retrospective study of two randomized, double-blind, parallel, multicenter trials, Dorinsky and colleagues examined spirometric responses to the MDI administration of ipratropium bromide (36 µg qid), albuterol base (180 µg qid), or an equivalent combination of both drugs (120). Defining spirometric responses as increases in FEV_1 of 12 and 15%, the combination of bronchodilators proved more effective than either agent alone. A similar improvement has been demonstrated when nebulized (versus MDI) bronchodilators were compared (95). Interestingly, some investigators have suggested that beneficial effects of combination therapy are realized when the antimuscarinic therapy is administered before the beta agonist (134–136).

Some investigators have examined the combination of anticholinergic agents and long-acting beta agonists. The results have been contradictory. One group has suggested that the combination of salmeterol and ipratropium was not more effective than salmeterol alone (137), while another group has suggested that the combination of formoterol plus ipratropium was more effective than ipratropium alone but did not provide additional bronchodilation to formoterol alone (138). Similarly, the combination of oxitropium bromide and formoterol yielded additional bronchodilation (139), although this effect may depend on the dose of bronchodilator administered (140) and the timing of bronchodilator administration (139). Most recently, the combination of ipratropium (40 mg qid) and formoterol (12 µg bid) has resulted in a greater improvement in spirometry compared with salbutamol (200 µg qid) plus ipratropium (40 µg qid) (141). Long-term studies of these combinations are scarce. Van Noord et al. examined the effects of 12 weeks of salmeterol (50 µg bid) alone, salmeterol (50 µg bid) in combination with ipratropium (40 µg qid), and placebo (142). Interestingly, the combination produced a greater peak increase in FEV_1 (12%) compared to salmeterol alone (7%). A similar, albeit of lesser magnitude, advantage to the combination was noted after 12 weeks of treatment (5% increase in FEV_1 for salmeterol compared to 8% for salmeterol plus ipratropium).

Limited data have been published examining the effect of combined bronchodilator therapy on exercise capacity (74). Unfortunately the results on submaximal and maximal testing have been inconsistent. Additional improvement in symptoms with combination therapy have been marginal in some (95) but significant in other studies (119,141). During short-term treatment, the combination of formoterol/ipratropium provided better symptomatic relief than salbutamol/ipratropium (141); symptom scores using the SGRQ followed a similar improvement. Interestingly, a differential improvement in symptoms was not consistently seen during 12 weeks of therapy with salmeterol alone versus salmeterol plus ipratropium (142). These investigators noted a decrease in exacerbation rate between the groups treated with placebo (36%), salmeterol (23%), and salmeterol plus ipratropium (13%). The differences proved significant only in the patients treated with combination bronchodilation. In a separate publication, these investigators noted a clinically significant difference in mean symptom scores of the SGRQ with salmeterol and combination therapy compared with placebo (112). Similarly, the proportion of patients experiencing a clinically meaningful improvement in the Chronic Respiratory Questionnaire was greater with combination bronchodilation (40%) than with salmeterol monotherapy or placebo (112). An improved pharmacoeconomic picture has been suggested for the combination of an anticholinergic agent and beta agonists as described above. In fact, a recent analysis of a computerized prescription and hospitalization database in Saskatchewan, Canada, has confirmed a decrease in overall costs of therapy with a combination product of ipratropium and a beta agonist (RR 0.83, 95% CI 0.76 to 0.92) (143). These data support the use of combinations of bronchodilators in symptomatic patients with COPD. The ideal sequence of short-acting beta agonists, long-acting beta agonists, anticholinergic agents, and their combination remains controversial. Further prospective studies are required to better define the optimal sequence of inhaled bronchodilator therapy in symptomatic patients with COPD.

Methylxanthines

Methylxanthines such as caffeine and theophylline have been used to treat respiratory disorders for many decades (54), although the use of theophylline has decreased over the past decade; a recent summary of 10 bronchodilator trials performed between 1987 and 1995 identified a decrease in theophylline use from 63.4 to 29.0% (144). This change in practice pattern reflects the controversy regarding theophylline's benefits (67,145), the availability of alternative bronchodilator regimens (see above) (85), and theophylline's narrow therapeutic spectrum (67). Investigators over the past several decades have confirmed that theophylline is a weak bronchodilator in patients with COPD. In reviewing 15 studies involving COPD patients, vas Fragoso and Miller reported an improvement in FEV_1 ranging from 10 to 21% (145); the variability in results was felt to reflect differences in study format, patient characteristics, and treatment duration. Investigators have attempted to identify those patients more likely to experience spirometric improvements with theophylline therapy. Some have felt that patients experiencing an acute bronchodilator response to a short-acting beta agonist would be more likely to benefit from theophylline (146). Others have not confirmed these results (147,148). For example, Thomas et al. showed no significant correlation between acute FEV_1 bronchoreversibility and improvement after theophylline therapy (149). Similarly, Murciano et al. noted significant bronchodilation in 60 patients with "irreversible" airflow obstruction (150). A limited number of studies have compared various beta/agonists and theophylline administered alone or in combination. In general the mean increase in FEV_1 has been similar; when administered in combination, statistically significant additive effects have been observed (145,151). Data comparing theophylline and long-acting beta agonists are scarce. In general, the beta agonists seem to be more active in the short term, although the difference becomes less marked with prolonged therapy (85). In fact, the bronchodilatory effect of theophylline is most often achieved with prolonged administration (145). Salmeterol and theophylline have been demonstrated to result in similar spirometric improvements by several groups (152,153); the combination has been demonstrated to result in additional bronchodilation (153). Importantly, in this latter study, 150 of 1185 screened patients were unable to tolerate theophylline during a wash-in period and 30 additional patients were unable to achieve therapeutic theophylline levels (153). One may conclude, therefore, that theophylline may provide additional bronchodilation but is unlikely to be an effective initial bronchodilator.

Theophylline has been demonstrated to have additional beneficial effects, including improving mucociliary clearance, respiratory muscle function, cardiovascular function, and respiratory drive (67,145). Two of three studies have demonstrated improvements in mucociliary clearance (145). Similar controversy has been noted in studies examining the effect of theophylline on respiratory muscle function. For example, two of four studies examining transdiaphragmatic pressures have demonstrated a beneficial effect with methylthanxine therapy (67,145). Similarly, contradictory data have been presented suggesting that theophylline improves diaphragmatic fatigue resistance (67,145). Theophylline has been demonstrated in several studies to decrease pulmonary artery pressures, increase cardiac output, and improve right and left ventricular ejection fracture (145); the effects were more evident in patients without cor pulmonale (154,155), although this has not been confirmed by all (156). These additional effects may aid in explaining benefits in addition to spirometric changes that have been described with theophylline. For example, although theophylline provided only a small degree of bronchodilation compared to high-dose inhaled salbutamol and ipratropium, one-third of patients treated with additional theophylline experienced improved symptoms in one trial (157). Similarly, some but not all studies have suggested an improved exercise tolerance in patients treated with theophylline (74). In addition, a large study of salmeterol, theophylline, or the combination of the two confirmed additional improvement in dyspnea, symptom-free days and HRQol in patients treated with the combination of bronchodilators (153). Importantly, exacerbations were experienced by fewer patients treated with combined therapy (48 in 40 patients) than in those treated with theophylline alone (96 exacerbations in 62 patients) or salmeterol alone (71 exacerbations in 56 patients; $p = 0, 02$). It should be noted that theophylline therapy may not improve the cost-effectiveness of care. In a pharmacoeconomic analysis, Hilleman and colleagues noted that theophylline therapy alone was associated with greater treatment costs ($1946) in patients with milder COPD than ipratropium alone ($1362) or beta agonists alone ($1542) (8). Thus theophylline therapy is probably not the ideal bronchodilator, particularly in patients with milder disease.

The role of methylxanthines in COPD will likely be expanded by the new generation of phosphodiesterase receptor inhibitors. These enzymes have direct bronchodilating effects; similarly, PDE 4 receptors are present on inflammatory cells (54). Therefore inhibition of PDE 4, one of ten isoenzyme families, would be expected to result in an anti-inflammatory effect (158). One such agent, cilomilast, has been extensively studied (159). In a recent 6-week trial, 424 patients with severe COPD (FEV_1 46.8% predicted) were randomized to two doses of cilomilast or placebo (160). Cilomilast 15 mg demonstrated the maximal improvement in FEV_1 compared with placebo; this effect was most evident in the sixth week of treatment. Modest improvements were noted in HRQol. Thus, given the potential anti-inflammatory effect of methylxanthines, a potential beneficial effect would be expected in reducing exacerbation rate.

E. Corticosteroids

The role of corticosteroid therapy in COPD remains a highly controversial issue (161,162). The role of inflammation has been accepted and described by numerous authors (33). As recently reviewed, neutrophilic and lymphocytic inflammation have been described in the central airways of COPD patients, while a more intense lymphocytic inflammatory process (particularly $CD8 +$ lymphocytes) is present in the peripheral airways and parenchyma (33). Given the presence of inflammation in COPD patients and the known benefit of steroids in asthmatics (163), inhaled corticosteroids have frequently been used in clinical practice to treat patients with COPD. In fact, approximately 40% of COPD patients were receiving inhaled corticosteroids in recent analyses (144,164,165), rising from 13.2% in 1985 to 41.4% in 1995 in one study (144). The role of steroids in stable COPD has been reviewed by numerous authors in recent years (161,166–168).

As there is an active inflammatory process in patients with COPD, it is reasonable to expect an anti-inflammatory effect of corticosteroids, as noted in asthma (163). Unfortunately the inflammatory process in COPD patients differs from that of asthmatics, with a preponderance of neutrophils; this process may be less susceptible to the anti-inflammatory effect of corticosteroids (163,169). Numerous recent studies have examined the biological effect of inhaled steroids in patients with COPD (see Table 7). It is evident that some investigators have suggested little effect in COPD patients inhaling corticosteroids (169–173), while others have noted favorable effects on neutrophilic inflammation (174–176). This variability may reflect differences in patient selection, potency and dosage of inhaled steroids, duration of therapy, and endpoints reflecting inflammation. The importance of patient selection is highlighted by recent studies examining the effects of short-course oral steroid therapy in COPD patients. Several groups have suggested that an objective physiological response to oral steroid therapy is more likely to be seen in patients with eosinophilic airway inflammation (177–180). Some have suggested that this reflects patients with a similarity to asthmatics (168). Not all investigators have confirmed these findings (169). Importantly, some investigators have suggested that steroid responsiveness occurs as frequently in patients with physiological features of emphysema as in those without such features (181). Shedding light on this controversy, Fujimoto et al. examined steroid responsiveness in 24 patients with COPD with severe airflow obstruction (FEV_1 40.5% predicted) as well as anatomical emphysema documented by computed tomography (182). After 2 weeks of 20 mg prednisone daily, 12 patients experienced a greater than 12% increase in FEV_1; a significant relationship was noted between the percentage increase in FEV_1 and sputum eosinophil number.

Physiological endpoints after short-term steroid therapy have been examined by numerous groups. Reports regarding oral steroid therapy have been conflicting. A metanalysis of controlled trials performed through 1989 was reported by Callahan et al. (183). Response was defined as an increase in FEV_1 of 20%, and subjects in these trials achieved this level of change 10% more frequently after taking oral steroids than after placebo. As mentioned earlier, numerous groups have suggested that a subset of patients may be more susceptible to the beneficial effects of oral steroids (177–179,182). Interestingly, one group has suggested that these beneficial effects may continue past 14 days of steroid therapy (184). Long-term data with oral steroids are scarce. Two such retrospective studies noted a favorable effect of prednisolone on FEV_1 over a 20-year period (185). Interestingly, in a randomized study of elderly patients with "steroid-dependent" COPD, discontinuation of oral steroids did not result in a significant change in spirometric or other functional indices (186). Given the potential risks of oral steroid therapy (187), further data are required to adequately assess the risks and benefits of such therapy.

In an effort to improve the risk profile, multiple investigators have examined the role of inhaled steroids in COPD patients, as recently reviewed by several groups (161,163,167,168). Table 8 enumerates recent randomized, placebo-controlled studies in COPD patients. It is evident that physiological response is unusual, although some studies have suggested a significant response in some patients. Clear conclusions are limited by the varying study formats, different steroids and dosages, as well as a wide range of treatment durations. A clear definition of which patients are most likely to benefit remains unclear. Several large, randomized studies of inhaled steroids with long duration of follow-up have been published in the last several years; the majority of these studies emphasized long-term change in pulmonary function, as described in Tables 9 and 10. The patients enrolled varied widely between the trials, with two enrolling patients with milder disease (188,189) while the others included patients with more severely impaired lung function (190–192). The majority of the studies excluded patients with reversibility to beta agonists (188,190,191) and to oral steroids (189). Similarly, most studies included predominantly active smokers (188,189,192), while the others included predominantly ex-smokers (190,191). A wide range of equivalent steroid doses were employed (161), with the highest being utilized in the ISOLDE (191) and the International COPD Study Group (190). None of the studies demonstrated a consistent change in the rate of decline in FEV_1 over the course of follow-up (see Table 10), although different statistical models were used in these trials. Interestingly, the International COPD Study Group demonstrated a mild improvement in FEV_1 in patients treated with fluticasone for 6 months. Similarly, the EUROSCOP investigators demonstrated a change in FEV_1 favoring the budesonide group ($+17$ mL/year versus -81 mL/year) over the first 6 months of the trial, although the subsequent decline was similar between the two groups. Interestingly, the subsequent slopes differed based on the number of pack years smoked, with a more favorable effect of steroids in those patients who had smoked the least (< 35 pack years). The ISOLDE trial demonstrated the largest initial effect, which was significantly greater in ex-smokers, although the subsequent decline was similar between the treatment

Table 7 Recent Studies of Inhaled Corticosteroids and Inflammatory Markers in Patients with COPD

Reference	Treatment	Duration	N	Age	FEV$_1$	Smoking habit	Outcome
Thompson et al. (170)	BCM 2000 µg/day	6 weeks	20	50.6	72.6% pred	current	↓ Bronchial cellularity and albumin with ICS
	Placebo		10	47.0	72.0% pred		↑ Lysozyme and lactoferrin with placebo
Llewellyn-Jones et al. (174)	FP 1500 µg/day	8 weeks	8	65	0.73 L	4 ex/4 current	↓ Chemotactic activity of sputum sol phase
	Placebo		8	64	0.70 L	6 ex/3 current	↑ Sputum elastase inhibitory activity with ICS
Keatings et al. (169)	BUD 1600 µg/day	2 weeks	13	NR	35.1% pred	7 ex-smokers	No change in sputum cellularity, ECP, EPO, MPO, HNL or TNF-α
	Prednisolone 30 mg/day					6 current	
Confalonieri et al. (175)	BCM 1500 µg/day	8 weeks	17	58	60.2% pred	current	↓ Sputum total cells and neutrophils with ICS
			17	57	59.1% pred		↑ Macrophages with ICS
Cox et al. (171)	None BCM 1000 µg/day	28 days	30	33.7	3.91 L	current	No change in sputum cellularity

Culpitt et al. (172)	FP 1000 mg/day	4 weeks	13	62	49.5% pred	4 ex-smokers 9 current	No effect on sputum cellularity, IL-8, MMP-1, MMP-9, TIMP-1, elastase or SLPI
Balbi et al. (176)	BCM 1500 µg/day	6 weeks	8	61.1	69.8% pred	current	↓ BAL total cells and neutrophils, IL-8, MPO ↑ BAL macrophages and lymphocytes
Loppow et al. (173)	FP 1000 µg/day Placebo	4 weeks 4 weeks	19	55	83.4% pred	ex-smokers and current	No change in sputum cellularity, LDH, ECP, elastase, IL-8, iNOS
Ferreira et al. (271)	BCM 1000 µg/day Placebo	2 weeks	19	69.1	55% pred	ex-smokers	↓ Exhaled NO with ICS

Key: BCM, beclomethasone; BAL, bronchoalveolar lavage; ICS, inhaled corticosteroids; BUD, budesonide; NR, not reported; ECP, eosinophilic cationic protein; EPO, eosinophil peroxidase; MPO, myeloperoxidase; HNL, human neutrophil lipocalin; TNF-α, tumor necrosis factor α; L, liters; FP, fluticasone propionate; IL-8, interleukin 8; MMP, metalloproteinase; TIMP, tissue inhibitor of metalloproteinases; SLPI, antiproteases secretory leukoprotease inhibitor; LDH, lactate dehydrogenase; iNOS, inducible nitric oxide synthase; NO, nitric oxide.

Table 8 Recent Randomized, Placebo-Controlled, Short-Term Studies of Inhaled Corticosteroids in Patients with COPD

Reference	N	ICS dose (μg/day)	Follow-up (weeks)	Results FEV$_1$	Results Bronchial responsiveness	Results Symptoms
Weir et al. (272)	127	BCM 1500	2	Improved	NR	NR
Weir et al. (273)	105	BCM 1500 or 3000	3	Improved	No change	Improved
Wempe et al. (274)	10	BUD 1600	3	No change	No change	NR
Nishimura et al. (275)	30	BCM 3000	4	Improved	NR	Improved
Rutgers et al. (276)	44	BUD 1600	6	No change	No change	NR
Thompson et al. (170)	30	BCM 2000	6	Improved	NR	NR
Auffarth et al. (277)	24	BUD 1600	8	No change	No change	Improved
Watson et al. (278)	14	BUD 1200	12	No change	No change	No change

Study	N	Drug	Duration			
Cox et al. (171)	60	BCM 1000	4	No change	No change	NR
Culpitt et al. (172)	13	FP 1000	4	No change	NR	No change
Keatings et al. (169)	13	BUD 1600	2	PEFR No change	NR	No change
Loppow et al. (173)	19	FP 1000	4	No change	NR	NR
Ferreira et al. (271)	19	BCM 1000	2	No change	NR	NR
Bourbeau et al. (279)	79	BUD 1600	24	No change	NR	No change
Senderovitz et al. (280)	35	BUD 800	24	No change	NR	No change

NR, not reported; BCM, beclomethasone; BUD, budesonide; FP, fluticasone propionate; PEFR, peak expiratory flow rate.

Table 9 Descriptive Characteristics of Large, Placebo-Controlled Studies of Long-Term Therapy with Inhaled Steroids

Reference	N	Bronchoreversibility inclusion criteria	Treatment (µg/day)	Follow-Up time (months)	Patient characteristics			
					Age	FEV$_1$ (%pred)	Smoker (%)	Ex-smoker (%)
International COPD Study Group (190)	142	FEV$_1$ < 15% postsalbutamol	FP 1000	6	62	59	49	51
	139		Placebo		64	55	49	50
EUROSCOP (188)	634	FEV$_1$ < 10% postterbutaline	BUD 800	36	52.5	76.8	100	—
	643		Placebo		52.4	76.9	100	
Copenhagen City Lung	145	FEV$_1$ < 15% postprednisone	BUD 1200 for 6 months, then 800 for 30 months	36	59	86.2	75.9	—
Study (189)	145		Placebo		59.1	86.9	77.2	—
ISOLDE (191)	376	FEV$_1$ < 10% postsalbutamol	FP 1000 after 2 weeks prednisone	36	63.7	50.3	36.4	46.8
	375		Placebo		63.8	50.0	39.2	45.9
Lung Health Study II (192)	559	—	TA 1200	40	56.2	68.5	90.5	—
	537		Placebo		56.4	67.2	89.8	

Key: FP, fluticasone propionate; BUD, budesonide; TA, triamcinolone.

Table 10 Results of Large, Placebo-Controlled Studies of Long-Term Therapy with Inhaled Steroids

Reference	Treatment	Δ FEV₁ (mL/year)	Exacerbation (number per year)	Exacerbation (%reduction)	Change in symptoms	HRQol
International COPD Study Group (190)	FP Placebo	+0.11[a] −0.04	1.07 1.60	49%	Lower cough scores and sputum volume with FP; no difference in breathlessness.	NR
EUROSCOP (188)	BUD 800 Placebo	−57 −69	2.2 3.1	29%	NR	NR
Copenhagen City Lung Study (189)	BUD Placebo	−53.2 −49.6	0.36 0.38	2%	No difference in change in symptoms.	NR
ISOLDE (191)	FP Placebo	−50 −59	1.43 1.9	25%	NR	Less deterioration in FP group.
Lung Health Study II (192)	TRI	−44.2	0.35	44%	Dyspnea, unscheduled physician visits, and respiratory hospitalizations lessened in steroid group.	Mildly worsened mental health subscale of SF-36 in steroid group.

[a] 6-month study.
Key: HRQol, health-related quality of life; FP, fluticasone propionate; NR, not reported; BUD, budesonide; TRI, triamcinolone.

groups (Fig. 10). The differences between the studies likely reflect differences in study designs, patients enrolled, steroid dose used, or the statistical analyses employed (161). Minor improvements in selected patient populations cannot be excluded. O'Brien et al. recently demonstrated a mild decrement in pulmonary function in an elderly group of patients in whom long-term beclomethasone therapy was discontinued (193). Nevertheless, it is unlikely that inhaled corticosteroids alter deterioration in pulmonary function to any great extent.

As described earlier in the discussion of bronchodilators, spirometric results are imperfect measures of treatment response in COPD. Hence several groups have examined additional endpoints in the investigation of steroid therapy. A borderline survival advantage with fluticasone therapy was suggested by the ISOLDE investigators (Fig. 11), and an improvement in respiratory symptoms was reported by two groups (190,192). A greater degree of deterioration in HRQol has been noted with placebo therapy compared to fluticasone therapy using the St. George's Respiratory Questionnaire (Fig. 12) (194). Using the SF-36, one group noted little change with inhaled triamcinolone (192), although the ISOLDE investigators demonstrated significant differences in the rate of decline in 4 of the 8 domains with fluticasone (Fig. 12) (194).

An important potential benefit of steroid therapy is a modulation of exacerbation frequency (see Table 10). The International COPD Study Group, which was powered to detect differences in exacerbation frequency, noted no difference in the overall incidence of exacerbations; importantly, more patients treated with placebo experienced moderate or severe exacerbations (those requiring physician visits or hospitalizations) (86 versus 60%, $p < 0.001$) (190). The ISOLDE study, which included exacerbations as a secondary endpoint, demonstrated a decrease in the rate of exacerbations from 1.32 per year with placebo to 0.99 per year with fluticasone therapy; similarly, the rate of withdrawals secondary to respiratory disease was lowered by fluticasone (19 versus 25%, $p = 0.034$) (191). Interestingly, the studies that enrolled mildly affected patients demonstrated less impressive results, although exacerbations were imprecisely defined in these trials. An additional interesting insight is provided by a recent observational study utilizing the Ontario version of the Canadian Institute for Health Information hospital discharge database (195). These investigators examined outcome in all 22,260 patients above 65 years of age who were discharged from the hospital with a principal diagnosis of COPD between 1992 and 1996. Admission data were linked to subsequent inhaled steroid prescriptions and subsequent death or rehospitalization for COPD during year after the index hospitalization. Of the patients studied 11,481 received at least one inhaled steroid prescription within 3 months of discharge, compared to 11,139 who did not. After adjustment for age, gender, other medications, and comorbidity, the group receiving inhaled steroids after hospital discharge experienced an improved COPD hospitalization-free survival (Fig. 13). Similarly, an analysis of newly physician-diagnosed COPD

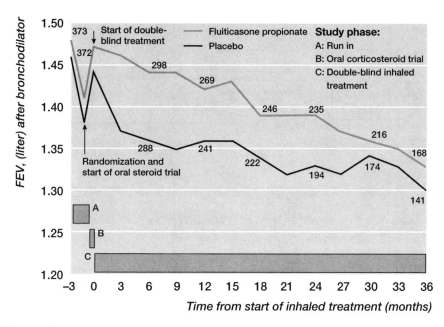

Figure 10 Mean FEV$_1$ (liters) after bronchodilator by time from start of double-blind treatment. Numbers reflect patients with valid reading at each time point. Measurements within 4 weeks of exacerbation are excluded. Direct comparisons of FEV$_1$ means at each time point are not possible because fewer patients remained in the study as it progressed. (From Ref. 191.)

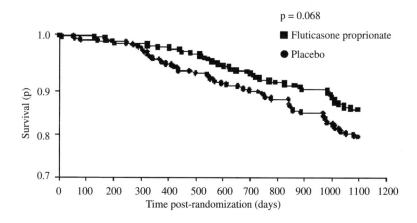

Figure 11 Survival of patients in the Inhaled Steroids in Obstructive Lung Disease (ISOLDE) trial, using an intention to treat population and Kaplan-Meier statistics. Fluticasone propionate dosage was 500 µg twice daily. (From Ref. 161.)

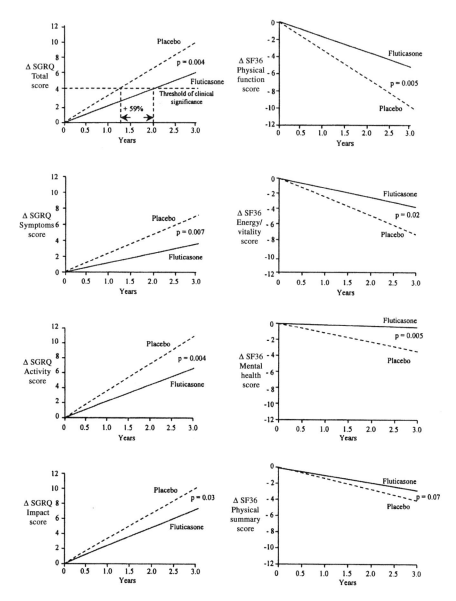

Figure 12 Slope of deterioration in health status calculated using estimates from a random coefficients hierachical model. The regression estimates are weighted by the number of observations and the variance contributed by each patient. A higher SGRQ score or a lower SF-36 score indicates worse health status. All SGRQ component scores are shown, together with selected SF-36 scores. (From Ref. 194.)

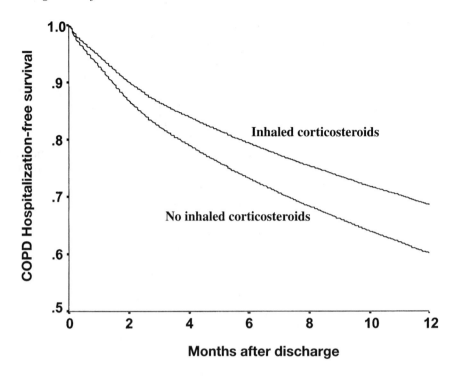

Figure 13 Adjusted probability of hospitalization-free survival in patients with chronic obstructive pulmonary disease who did and did not receive inhaled corticosteroids postdischarge (within 90 days of discharge). (From Ref. 11.)

patients in the U.K. General Practice Research Database suggested a survival advantage in patients treated with fluticasone propionate (FP) plus salmeterol (hazard ratio, HR 0.48, 95% CI 0.31–0.73) or FP alone (HR 0.62, 95% CI 0.45–0.85) compared to a reference group treated with other bronchodilators but not inhaled corticosteroids or long-acting β_2-agonists (195a). The totality of these data suggests that inhaled steroids may have a role in the treatment of patients with more severe disease as judged by more severely impaired pulmonary function, frequent exacerbations, or COPD-related hospitalization.

It should be noted that steroids have well-defined side effects, which may be more problematic in an elderly COPD patient. The potential side effects of systemic and topical steroids have been ably reviewed by several groups (166,167,187,196,197). Numerous potential side effects have been described with chronic steroid use, including topical effects, adrenal suppression, effects on bone, gastrointestinal toxicity, psychiatric effects, infectious complications, glucose intolerance, myopathic changes, cutaneous effects, cardiovascular effects, and ocular toxicity (166,167,187).

   The most feared adverse reactions have been the bone side effects
(197,198). It has been estimated that between 30 and 50% of patients receiving
long-term steroids will experience fractures and that the risk of fracture
increases to 50 to 100% for those taking oral steroids (198). Patients with
COPD are particulary susceptible to osteoporosis, given their age, inactivity,
comorbidity, and potentially medication use (197). Although some studies have
suggested that patients with mild COPD are not at increased risk of bone
abnormalities with ICS (196), others have suggested that worsening respiratory
disease increases the potential risks of steroids (199). A recent cross-sectional
study has shed light on these questions. McEvoy and colleagues evaluated the
association between steroid use and vertebral fractures in 312 patients, 50 years
of age or older, with COPD (200). Patients were categorized as those who never
used steroids ($n = 117$), those who used only inhaled steroids ($n = 70$) and those
who were administered systemic steroids for at least 2 weeks (at least 5 mg/day
or 10 mg as needed) during their lifetime ($n = 125$). Importantly, the prevalence
of one or more vertebral fractures was 48.7% in those patients who were never
administered steroids, 57.1% in the inhaled steroid users, and 63.3% in those
who were administered systemic steroids. Compared with never steroid users,
those who used systemic steroids were approximately two times more likely to
have vertebral fractures (OR 1.80, 95% CI 1.08–3.07); this association was
particularly strong in those on continuous systemic steroids (prednisone daily
or as needed for at least 6 consecutive months) (OR 2.36, 95% CI 1.26–4.38).
The relationship of steroid use was weaker for inhaled steroids; those patients
using inhaled steroid only were slightly more likely to have experienced a
vertebral fracture (OR 1.35, 95% CI 0.77–2.56). The recent data from long-
term studies of ICS in COPD have provided additional data. The EUROSCOP
investigators examined bone density in 102 patients in the budesonide group
and 92 patients in the placebo group (188); no difference was noted during
follow-up in bone density nor on the frequency of fractures (based on two sets
of spine radiographs obtained in 653 subjects). The ISOLDE investigators
noted no difference in new vertebral fractures (2.4% in fluticasone recipients
versus 4.6% in placebo recipients) (191). Importantly, the Lung Health Study II
investigators examined bone density in 412 patients; a significant decrease in
bone mineral density was confirmed with triamcinolone therapy in both men
and women (192). Therefore, although there may be benefits to steroid therapy
in COPD patients, it must be carefully weighed against the real risk of potential
toxicity.

F. Mucolytics

Mucus production is a frequent symptom in patients with COPD. Moreover,
increasing or a change in the character of sputum production is frequently seen
during an exacerbation of disease activity (201). Mucolytic drugs increase the
expectoration of sputum by reducing hypersecretion or the viscosity of the
secretions (202); hence these drugs would be expected to have a beneficial

impact on exacerbations in patients with COPD. A recent detailed, systematic review examining the role of oral mucolytic drugs in these patients has been published (203). These authors culled 23 randomized, placebo-controlled trials of oral mucolytic drugs taken for at least 2 months. In these studies, regular use of these agents was associated with a reduction of 0.07 exacerbations per patient month (95% CI -0.08 to -0.05). Therefore the odds ratio for having no exacerbation in the study period with mucolytic drug therapy compared with placebo was 2.22 (95% CI 1.93 to 2.54). The reduction in the exacerbation rate was greater in the two studies with patients with an FEV_1 <50% predicted (reduction of 0.13 per patient month). In addition, the reduction was greater for studies that lasted 3 months or less (0.13 per subject) than for those that lasted over three months (0.06 per subject) suggesting that the benefit was seen early in the course of therapy. In addition, mucolytic therapy was associated with a reduced number of days of illness and days that subjects took antibiotics. Interestingly, changes in spirometric indices were minor. Thus a wider role for these agents may be appropriate in selected patients, including those with greater airflow obstruction and/or more frequent exacerbations.

G. Long-Term Oxygen Therapy

One of the few therapeutic interventions that can positively affect survival in patients with COPD is the appropriate delivery of long-term oxygen therapy (204). Several randomized trials have consistently documented an improved survival in patients so treated as recently reviewed in a systematic Cochrane review (205). The five trials are summarized in Table 11. It is evident that oxygen therapy has improved survival in patients with more severe hypoxemia (206,207). The Medical Research Council (MRC) trial confirmed improved survival with O_2 administered for at least 15 hrs/day (206) while the Nocturnal Oxygen Therapy Trial (NOTT) trial confirmed a survival advantage for oxygen therapy continuously throughout the day compared to nocturnal administration (207). It therefore appears that continuous therapy is appropriate in patients that meet criteria for advanced hypoxemia (see Table 12), although a plausible mechanism for the improvement in survival is not clear (205). The role of oxygen therapy in patients with less severe hypoxemia remains unclear. In studies of patients with milder daytime hypoxemia (208–210), oxygen therapy did not result in significant benefits, although all studies were limited by low power. Two of these studies included patients with documented nocturnal desaturation (208,210). Further data from one of these groups defined the serial changes noted in patients with mild resting hypoxemia (Pa_{O_2} 63.4 mmHg) who exhibited nocturnal hypoxemia ($n = 35$) or no nocturnal desaturation ($n = 29$) (211). Although the number of patients available for follow-up after 2 years was limited, there was no difference in survival or right-heart function in either group; this suggests that nocturnal desaturation may not be a transitional state before worsening daytime hypoxemia. The effect of oxygen therapy on quality of life in these trials is difficult to ascertain. The

Table 11 Randomized Controlled Trial of Oxygen Therapy in COPD Patients

Trial	N	Age	FEV$_1$	PaO$_2$ (mmHg)	Treatment	Duration (months)	Outcomes
NOTT (207)	101 102	65.2 65.7	29.5% pred 29.9% pred	50.8 51.4	Continuous O$_2$ 1–4 L/min Nocturnal O$_2$ 1–4 L/min	26	Improved survival and right heart function with continuous O$_2$ at 24 months
MRC (206)	42	58.8	0.67 L	49.9	Continuous O$_2$ 15 hr/day	60	Improved survival in O$_2$ therapy group after 5 years
	45	57.8	0.64 L	51.2	No O$_2$		
Fletcher et al. (208)	19	62.1	—	73.7	Nocturnal O$_2$ 3 L/min	36	No difference in survival
	19	61.2	—	76.7	No O$_2$		
Gorecka et al. (209)	68	60.1	29.7% pred	59.5	O$_2$ adjusted to PaO$_2$ > 65 mmHg	36	No difference in survival
	67	62.4	29.8% pred	61.3	No O$_2$		
Chaouat et al. (210)	41	63	39% pred	62.6	Nocturnal O$_2$	24	No difference in survival or right heart function

MRC investigators noted general improvement in the sense of well-being, appetite, and general alertness with oxygen therapy (206). The NOTT trial reported small improvements in neuropsychological function and quality of life with continuous oxygen therapy (207,212). Further data are required to better define the role of O_2 therapy with milder hypoxemia, including exercise induced desaturation.

H. Pulmonary Rehabilitation

Pulmonary rehabilitation is a therapeutic intervention for COPD that has become more widely used, although it remains a method that is hotly debated in some circles. In part, this debate has risen from questions regarding the pathophysiology of improvement in COPD patients, questions regarding its overall utility and efficacy in all levels of COPD severity, and questions regarding the appropriate method that the therapy is delivered. The goals of pulmonary rehabilitation are to reduce symptoms, decrease disability, increase participation in physical and social activities, and improve overall quality of life in patients with COPD (213,214). These benefits occur in the face of irreversible lung architectural abnormalities because pulmonary rehabilitation addresses the presence of secondary comorbidities such as muscular deconditioning (215). Since pulmonary rehabilitation addresses "nonpulmonary" comorbidity, pulmonary function measurements such as FEV_1, FVC, and bronchial reversibility typically do not show significant changes and should not be used as outcome measures for improvement with pulmonary rehabilitation. The physiological rationale for the benefits seen remains an area of active

Table 12 Potential Indications for Long-Term Oxygen Therapy in COPD

O_2 therapy	Indications
Continuous	Resting $Pa_{O_2} \leqslant 55$ mmHg or O_2 saturation $\leqslant 88\%$
	Resting Pa_{O_2} of 56–59 mmHg or O_2 saturation of 89% with any of the following:
	Dependent edema
	P pulmonale on the electrocardiogram
	Erythocythemia (hematocrit > 56%)
	Resting $Pa_{O_2} > 59$ mmHg or O_2 saturation > 89%
	Reimbursable only with additional documentation justifying O_2 prescription
Noncontinuous	O_2 flow rate and number of hours per day must be specified
	During exercise, $Pa_{O_2} \leqslant 55$ mmHg or O_2 saturation $\leqslant 88\%$ with low-level exercise
	During sleep, $Pa_{O_2} \leqslant 55$ mmHg or O_2 saturation $\leqslant 88\%$ with associated complications, including pulmonary hypertension, daytime hypersomnolence, and cardiac arrhythmia

Source: Adapted from Ref. 204.

research. A reduction in ventilatory demand for similar activities appears to be a principal effect of physiological training (216–221). In addition, there is significant improvement in peripheral and ventilatory muscle function (218,219,222–225), although this has not been a consistent finding (226).

Clear benefits of pulmonary rehabilitation have been seen in improving exercise capacity and decreasing levels of breathlessness with exercise. A metanalysis of 14 randomized trials has been reported (227). In the 11 trials that measured maximal exercise capacity, the pooled effect size achieved significance, corresponding to an improvement of 8.3 W (95% CI 2.8–16.5). In addition, an improvement in 6-min walk distance of 55.7 m (95% CI 27.8–92.8) was noted in these studies. More consistent beneficial effects were seen in improving HRQol. A second, more recent systematic review has reached similar conclusions (228). The improvement in perceptions of dyspnea and in 6-min walk distance from an outpatient trial of pulmonary rehabilitation have been found to diminish but persist up to 2 years following a comprehensive 6-month program of pulmonary rehabilitation followed by maintenance rehabilitation of 6 months duration. The maintenance program did not have prescribed exercise targets, nor did the patients participate in controlled exercise regimens. The patients in the pulmonary rehabilitation arm of the study were found to have statistically significant lower frequency of exacerbations (3.7 ± 2.2) as compared to controls (6.9 ± 3.9) (229). Other recent studies have confirmed the benefit of similar long-term maintenance from pulmonary rehabilitation programs (229–232).

Patients with COPD who are candidates for pulmonary rehabilitation include those with chronic respiratory impairment who, despite optimal medical management, are persistently symptomatic, have reduced exercise tolerance, or experience a restriction in activities (214). Severity of symptoms, disability, and handicap—not the severity of the physiological impairment—should be the primary characteristics that determine the need for pulmonary rehabilitation (233). In a study of 38 men with a mean FEV_1 of $55.1 \pm 19.8\%$ predicted, all patients along the spectrum of severity of disease demonstrated increases in peak values for work rate and oxygen uptake (220). Less severe stages of COPD as defined by ATS criteria were found to respond to a trial of pulmonary rehabilitation in a similar fashion to their more severe counterparts. In a study of 151 patients with stages I, II, or III of COPD based on ATS criteria, all three groups increased their 6-min walk distance from baseline to follow-up after a 12-week trial of exercise rehabilitation. There was a trend for the mild and moderate groups to have greater increases in distance than the severe group (stage III). All three groups also showed significant improvements in their dyspnea and fatigue scores by disease-specific quality-of-life measures (234). Similarly, one group has demonstrated functional benefits in patients independent of age (235). Exclusion criteria for a rehabilitation program should be limited to (1) conditions that might interfere with the patient undergoing the rehabilitative process and (2) conditions that might place the patient at undue risk during exercise training (215).

Pulmonary rehabilitation should be a multimodal therapeutic intervention. Elements of a comprehensive program should include education, psychosocial/behavioral intervention, exercise training, ventilatory muscle training in selected patients, and clear outcome assessment (214,215,221,236,237). A clear delineation of improved clinical efficacy between inpatient, outpatient, and home rehabilitation has not been clearly made. Each program format has shown some therapeutic benefit (238–245). The important element is the comprehensive nature of the program, with incorporation of all of the elements described above. Guidelines for exercise prescription have been recently published (246,247).

Clearly, comprehensive pulmonary rehabilitation is a useful adjunctive therapy in situations where medical therapy for COPD has been maximized. COPD of all levels of clinical severity can benefit with improved exercise tolerance, perceived improvement in quality of life, and, likely, a reduction in health care utilization. Significant improvement or change in routine pulmonary function parameters is not expected, nor are they routinely found. Pulmonary rehabilitation should be a routine part of the overall comprehensive care of patients with COPD.

IV. Medical Management of the COPD Patient During an Exacerbation

As detailed above, COPD is associated with a significant economic burden. The majority of the cost attributed to COPD is associated with hospitalizations (9,248). Therefore the effective prevention or at least the effective outpatient management of COPD exacerbations has the potential to significantly decrease the economic burden of COPD by decreasing the number of hospitalizations. Furthermore, exacerbations of COPD significantly worsen individual patients' quality of life (QOL). In a recent study by Seemungal et al., patients having more that two exacerbations during a 1-year period had a significantly worse QOL as measured by the SGRQ compared to patients with two or fewer exacerbations per year (48). Other studies have also identified the number of exacerbations (49) and readmission for COPD as factors associated with decreased QOL (249). Finally Seemungal et al. evaluated the time course to recovery for patients with a COPD exacerbation (47). The median time for symptomatic recovery was 7 days (range 4–14 days); however, nearly 5% of patients failed to recover after a 3-month period and 3.4% of patients had another exacerbation prior to completely resolving their first exacerbation. In the following sections we briefly outline information regarding the treatment of COPD exacerbations. Several excellent recent reviews (2,250,251) have addressed this topic; their conclusions, in conjunction with supporting data, are presented in this chapter.

A. Bronchodilators

Both inhaled beta agonists and anticholinergic agents can decrease obstruction during COPD exacerbations. The magnitude of improvement varies between studies but was recently summarized as between 15 and 29% for FEV_1 and FVC over a period of 60 to 90 min (250). A recent evidence-based review concluded that short-acting beta agonists and anticholinergic inhaled bronchodilators have comparable effects on spirometry and a greater effect than parenterally administered bronchodilators (251). The combination of an anticholinergic agent with a beta agonist has the potential for increased therapeutic benefit by combining agents with different mechanisms of action. Studies evaluating the combination of these agents have shown varied results but on average do not seem to support the routine use of multiple agents for COPD exacerbations (251). It has been suggested that factors such as onset of action (more rapid with beta agonists) and the propensity for side effects (which may be lower with ipratropium bromide) be considered for initial therapy for patients having an exacerbation (250). It also seems reasonable to add a second agent to patients' medications if they are having exacerbations through their current home regimens. The evidence for and against the utility of adding a methylxanthine to inhaled bronchodilators is also conflicting (250,251), and the high incidence of adverse reactions makes it difficult to recommend their routine use for COPD exacerbations.

B. Corticosteroids

Several studies have evaluated the effect of corticosteroid therapy for the treatment of hospitalized patients with COPD exacerbations. The largest study evaluated 271 patients from 25 Veterans Affairs medical centers (252). Patients were randomized to placebo or one of two steroid treatment arms (SoluMedrol 125 mg/day for 3 days followed by either a 15-day or 8-week taper). Both corticosteroid groups were associated with a faster improvement in FEV_1, a lower number of treatment failures (Fig. 14) (252), and a shorter length of hospital stay. Patients in the corticosteroid groups were also more likely to experience complications of treatment; hyperglycemia was the most common. In a more recent study, investigators randomized patients hospitalized with a COPD exacerbation to methylprednisolone, 0.5 mg/kg every 6 hr for 3 days, followed by either no further steroids or a taper completed on day 10 (253). Patients treated with a longer course of corticosteroids experienced a greater improvement in FEV_1. Investigators from the United Kingdom randomized 56 patients admitted with a COPD exacerbation to a smaller dose of prednisone (30 mg daily for 14 days) versus placebo (254). Patients treated with prednisone had a faster and greater improvement in FEV_1 (26% predicted to 32% predicted for placebo versus 28% predicted to 42% predicted for prednisone; $p < 0.0001$). The median length of stay was also shorter in the steroid treated group (7 days versus 9 days; $p = 0.027$). Interestingly, there was no difference in percent predicted FEV_1 at the 6-week follow-up between the two groups. In a study of 27 outpatients with COPD exacerbations presenting to either clinic or emergency department, Thompson et al. randomized patients to treatment with 9 days of prednisone (60 mg for 3 days, 40 mg for 3 days, and 20 mg for 3 days) or placebo (254a). Patients treated with prednisone had a faster and greater improvement in oxygenation and FEV_1 while experiencing fewer treatment failures (0 versus 57%; $p = 0.002$).

Inhaled corticosteroids may be an alternative to oral corticosteroids for the treatment of COPD exacerbations. Maltais et al. randomized 199 patients to either placebo, nebulized budesonide (2 mg every 6 hr), or oral prednisone (30 mg every 12 hr) (255). Both active treatment arms had a greater improvement in FEV_1 compared to placebo, although there was no difference between budesonide and oral prednisone. The incidence of serious adverse events was similar in all groups, although the patients in the oral prednisone group experienced a higher incidence of hyperglycemia.

These studies suggest that corticosteroids are beneficial for the treatment of patients with COPD exacerbations. Although the best dose and duration of therapy are not known, it appears that for inpatients a moderate dose (approximately 30 mg/day) for a period of approximately 2 weeks seems reasonable. Fewer data are available for outpatients, although a taper over an approximate 10-day period seems reasonable. Further studies are required to

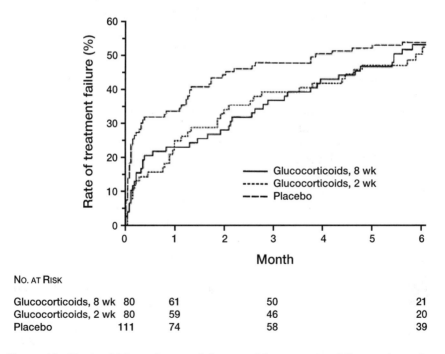

No. at Risk			
Glucocorticoids, 8 wk	80	61	50	21
Glucocorticoids, 2 wk	80	59	46	20
Placebo	111	74	58	39

Figure 14 Kaplan-Meier estimates of the rate of first treatment failure at 6 months, according to treatment group. (From Ref. 252.)

better define the role of inhaled corticosteroids for the management of inpatients and outpatients with COPD exacerbations.

C. Antibiotics

Bacteria are thought to be at least a contributing factor in 50 to 70% of COPD exacerbations (256); for these exacerbations, antibiotics should have a beneficial effect. The metanalysis by Saint et al. evaluated nine placebo-controlled trials for the treatment of COPD exacerbations (257) and identified a modest improvement in peak flow for the patients treated with antibiotics. A more recent placebo-controlled trial (258) for mechanically ventilated patients with a COPD exacerbation compared treatment with an antibiotic to placebo and found a marked decrease in mortality (4 versus 22% $p = 0.01$), days on ventilator (6.4 versus 10.6; $p = 0.04$), and length of stay (14.9 versus 24.5 days; $p = 0.01$) for patients who received an antibiotic. The differential magnitude of benefit between these studies is striking and likely relates to different patient populations and potentially to the prevalence of causal bacteria. One of the best studies evaluating which patients benefit from antibiotic therapy was performed by Anthonisen et al., who looked at 362 exacerbations in 173 patients (201). Patients with at least two symptoms (more dyspnea, more sputum volume, increased sputum purulence) were more likely to benefit from treatment with antibiotics compared to placebo. A more recent study evaluated the impact of sputum purulence and found that 32 of 34 patients with an exacerbation and mucoid sputum resolved their exacerbation without antibiotic therapy (259). Patients with purulent sputum were treated with antibiotics, and 77 or 87 resolved their exacerbation. These data suggest that multisymptom COPD exacerbations, or at least patients with new purulent sputum, are more likely to benefit from antibiotic therapy. The optimal choice of antibiotic remains controversial. The most likely pathogens are *Haemophilus influenzae*, *Moraxella catarrhalis*, and *Streptococcus pneumoniae*; patients with more severe obstruction (FEV_1 <50% predicted) are more likely to have infection with *H. influenzae* and *Pseudomonas aeruginosa* (260). This has led some (261–263) to advocate the use of broader-spectrum antibiotics for patients with more severe obstruction or other factors associated with a higher risk of relapse, such as more than four exacerbations in the previous year, home oxygen therapy, history of pneumonia/sinusitis, comorbid cardiopulmonary disease, and chronic steroid use (264–266). Although limited data suggest that treatment with initial broader-spectrum antibiotics may be associated with a lower total cost (267,268), this has not been confirmed in other trials (264), and further studies looking at antibiotic stratification schemes for the treatment of COPD exacerbations are needed.

D. Mucolytics

A recent analysis of five randomized controlled trials concluded that pharmacological mucus-clearance strategies do not shorten the course of treatment, although they may improve symptoms (251). The agents evaluated in these trials included domiodol, bromhexine, ambroxol, S-carboxymethyl-cysteine, and potassium chloride.

E. Oxygen Therapy

Oxygen therapy has been described as a cornerstone of hospital treatment for COPD exacerbations (2). The benefits include decreasing pulmonary vasocon-striction, decreasing right-heart strain and possible ischemia and improving cardiac output as well as subsequent oxygen delivery to the central nervous system and other vital organs (251). The concern regarding oxygen use is that it may lead to hypercarbia and subsequent respiratory failure. A recent review found that the administration of supplemental oxygen was associated with an increase in pa_{CO_2} in most patients; however, most patients did not require subsequent mechanical ventilation (251). Patients with combined baseline hypercarbia and more severe hypoxemia had the highest risk of requiring mechanical ventilation following the administration of supplemental oxygen (251). Therefore oxygen should be administered for patients with a COPD exacerbation, with a goal oxygen saturation of 90 to 92% (Pa_{O_2} 60–65 mmHg) (250).

F. Noninvasive Positive-Pressure Ventilation

Noninvasive positive-pressure ventilation (NPPV) has the potential benefit of resting fatigued muscles and subsequently preventing the need for endotracheal intubation and mechanical ventilation. The decreased need for mechanical ventilation and a potential survival advantage has been seen in several studies, which were recently reviewed (251). Patients suggested to benefit include those with worsened dyspnea with use of accessory muscles and paradoxical abdominal motion, acute respiratory acidosis and hypercarbia (pH 7.30–7.35, pa_{CO_2} 45–60 mmHg), worsening oxygenation, and tachypnea (respiratory rate >25 breaths per minute) (2,250). Patients not likely to benefit or excluded from trials include those with respiratory failure, cardiovascular instability, impaired mental status, agitation/uncooperative state, high aspiration risk, recent facial or gastroesophageal surgery, craniofacial trauma, and extreme obesity (2,250).

V. Conclusion

COPD is a common health problem with major repercussions on patient quality of life and survival. Furthermore, these patients utilize a large proportion of health care resources worldwide. Unfortunately, the impact of this disease is expected to worsen as the population ages and smoking continues. A comprehensive approach to medical management can improve physiology, quality of life, and, hopefully, long-term survival.

References

1. American Thoracic Society. ATS Statement. Standards for the diagnosis and care of patients with chronic obstructive pulmonary disease. Am J Respir Crit Care Med 1995; 152(suppl):S77–S120.
2. Pauwels RA, Buist AS, Calverley PMA, Jenkins CR, Hurd SS, GOLD Scientific Committee. Global strategy for the diagnosis, management, and prevention of chronic obstructive pulmonary disease. NHLBI/WHO Global Initiative for Chronic Obstructive Lung Disease (GOLD) Workshop Summary. Am J Respir Crit Care Med 2001; 163:1256–1276.
3. Flaherty KR, Kazerooni EA, Martinez FJ. Differential diagnosis of chronic airflow obstruction. J Asthma 2000; 37:201–223.
4. Barnes PJ. Chronic obstructive pulmonary disease. N Engl J Med 2000; 343:269–280.
5. Jeffery PK. Remodeling in asthma and chronic obstructive lung disease. Am J Respir Crit Care Med 2001; 164:S28–S38.
6. Friedman M, Hilleman DE. Economic burden of chronic obstructive pulmonary disease. Impact of new treatment options. Pharmacoeconomics 2001; 19:245–254.
7. Singh GK, Matthews TJ, Clarke SC, et al. Annual Summary of Births, Marriages, Divorces and Deaths: United States, 1994: Monthly Vital Statistics Report. Vol 43, No 13. Hyattsville, MD: National Center for Health Statistics, 1994.
8. Hilleman DE, Dewan N, Malesker M, Friedman M. Pharmacoeconomic evaluation of COPD. Chest 2000; 118:1278–1285.
9. Grasso ME, Weller WE, Shaffer TJ, Diette GB, Anderson GF. Capitation, managed care, and chronic obstructive pulmonary disease. Am J Respir Crit Care Med 1998; 158:133–138.
10. Ward MM, Javitz HS, Smith WM, Bakst A. Direct medical cost of chronic obstructive pulmonary disease in the USA. Respir Med 2000; 94:1123–1129.
11. Sin DD, Stafinski T, Ng YC, Bell NR, Jacobs P. The impact of chronic obstructive pulmonary disease on work loss in the United States. Am J Respir Crit Care Med 2002; 165:704–707.
12. Murray CJ, Lopez AD. Evidence-based health policy—lessons from the Global Burden of Disease Study. Science 1996; 274:740–743.
13. Murray CJL, Lopez AD, eds. The Global Burden of Disease: A Comprehensive Assessment of Mortality and Disability from Diseases, Injuries and Risk Factors in 1990 and Projected to 2020. Cambridge, MA: Harvard University Press, 1996.
14. Pearson MG, Bellamy D, Calverley PMA, Honeybourne D, MacNee W, Rudolf M, Wedzicha JA, Williams JP. BTS guidelines for the management of chronic obstructive pulmonary disease. Thorax 1997; 52(suppl 5):S1–S28.
15. Georgopoulas D, Anthonisen NR. Symptoms and signs of COPD. In: Cherniack N, ed. Chronic Obstructive Pulmonary Disease. Philadelphia: Saunders, 1991:357–363.
16. Calverley P, Bellamy D. The challenge of providing better care for patients with chronic obstructive pulmonary disease: the poor relation of airways obstruction? Thorax 2000; 55:78–82.

17. Vestbo J, Prescott E, Lange L, Copenhagen City Heart Study Group. Association of chronic mucous hypersecretion with FEV_1 decline and chronic obstructive pulmonary disease morbidity. Am J Respir Crit Care Med 1996; 153:1530–1535.

18. Wijnhoven HAH, Kriegsman DMW, Hesselink AE, Penninx BWJH, de Haan M. Determinants of different dimensions of disease severity in asthma and COPD. Pulmonary function and health-related quality of life. Chest 2001; 119:1034–1042.

19. Ferguson GT, Enright PL, Buist AS, Higgins MW. Office spirometry for Lung Health Assessment in Adults. A consensus statement from the National Lung Health Education Program. Chest 2000; 117:1146–1161.

20. Jones PW. Health status measurement in chronic obstructive pulmonary disease. Thorax 2001; 56:880–887.

21. Mahler DA, Mackowiak JI. Evaluation of the short-form 36-item questionnaire to measure health-related quality of life in patients with COPD. Chest 1995; 107:1585–1589.

22. Holleman DR, Simel DL, Goldberg JS. Diagnosis of obstructive airways disease from the clinical examination. J Gen Intern Med 1993; 8:63–68.

23. McIvor A, Chapman KR. Diagnosis of chronic obstructive pulmonary disease and differentiation from asthma. Curr Opin Pulm Med 1996; 2:148–154.

24. Holleman DR Jr, Simel DL. Does the clinical examination predict airflow limitation? JAMA 1995; 273:313–319.

25. Emerman CL, Lukens TW, Effron D. Physician estimation of FEV_1 in acute exacerbation of COPD. Chest 1994; 105:1709–1712.

26. Badgett RG, Tanaka DJ. Is screening for COPD justified? Prev Med 1997; 26:466–472.

27. Dow L. Asthma versus chronic obstructive pulmonary disease—exploring why "reversibility versus irreversibility" is no longer an appropriate approach. Clin Exp Allergy 1999; 29:739–743.

28. Papi A, Romagnoli M, Baraldo S, Braccioni F, Guzzinati I, Saetta M, Ciaccia A, Fabbri LM. Partial reversibility of airflow limitation and increased exhaled NO and sputum eosinophilia in chronic obstructive pulmonary disease. Am J Respir Crit Care Med 2000; 162:1773–1777.

29. Hajiro T, Nishimura K, Tsukino M, Ikeda A, Oga T. Stages of disease severity and factors that affect the health status of patients with chronic obstructive pulmonary disease. Respir Med 2000; 94:841–846.

30. Jeffery PK. Structural and inflammatory changes in COPD: a comparison with asthma. Thorax 1998; 53:129–136.

31. Piqueras MGC, Cosio MG. Disease of the airways in chronic obstructive pulmonary disease. Eur Respir J 2001; 18(suppl 34):41s–49s.

32. Chung KF. Cytokines in chronic obstructive pulmonary disease. Eur Respir J 2001; 18(suppl 34):50s–59s.

33. Saetta MP, Turato G, Maestrelli P, Mapp CE, Fabbri LM. Cellular and structural bases of chronic obstructive pulmonary disease. Am J Respir Crit Care Med 2001; 163:1304–1309.

34. Burrows B, Bloom JW, Traver GA, Cline MG. The course and prognosis of different forms of chronic airways obstruction in a sample from the general population. N Engl J Med 1987; 317:1309–1314.

35. Kazerooni EA, Whyte RI, Flint A, Martinez FJ. Imaging of emphysema and lung volume reduction surgery. Radiographics 1997; 17:1023–1036.

36. Kazerooni EA. Radiologic evaluation of emphysema for lung volume reduction surgery. Clin Chest Med 1999; 20:845–861.
37. Bergin CJ, Müller NL, Miller RR. CT in the qualitative assessment of emphysema. J Thorac Imaging 1986; 1:94–103.
38. Miller RR, Muller N, Vedal S, Morrison NJ, Staples CA. Limitations of computed tomography in the assessment of emphysema. Am Rev Respir Dis 1989; 139:980–983.
39. Müller NL, Staples CA, Miller RR, Abboud RT. "Density mask." An objective method to quantitate emphysema using computed tomography. Chest 1988; 94:782–787.
40. Gevenois PA, Yernault JC. Can computed tomography quantify pulmonary emphysema? Eur Respir J 1995; 8:843–848.
41. Gevenois PA, De Vuyst P, Sy M, Scillia P, Chaminade L, de Maertelaer V, Zanen J, Yernault JC. Pulmonary emphysema: quantitative CT during expiration. Radiology 1996; 199:825–829.
42. Kuwano K, Matsuba K, Ikeda T, Murakami J, Araki A, Nishitani H, Ishida T, Yasumoto K, Shigematsu N. The diagnosis of mild emphysema. Correlation of computed tomography and pathology scores. Am Rev Respir Dis 1990; 141:169–178.
43. Baldi S, Miniati M, Bellina CR, Battolla L, Catapano G, Begliomini E, Giustini D, Giuntini C. Relationship between extent of pulmonary emphysema by high-resolution computed tomography and lung elastic recoil in patients with chronic obstructive pulmonary disease. Am J Respir Crit Care Med 2001; 164:585–589.
44. Klein JS, Gamsu G, Webb WR, Golden JA, Muller NL. High-resolution CT diagnosis of emphysema in symptomatic patients with normal chest radiographs and isolated low diffusing capacity. Radiology 1992; 182:817–821.
45. O'Brien C, Guest PJ, Hill SL, Stockley RA. Physiological and radiological characterisation of patients diagnosed with chronic obstructive pulmonary disease in primary care. Thorax 2000; 55:635–642.
46. Celli BR. The importance of spirometry in COPD and asthma. Effect on approach to management. Chest 2000; 117:15S–19S.
47. Seemungal TAR, Donaldson GC, Bhowmik A, Jeffries DJ, Wedzicha JA. Time course and recovery of exacerbations in patients with chronic obstructive pulmonary disease. Am J Respir Crit Care Med 2000; 161:1608–1613.
48. Seemungal TAR, Donaldson GC, Paul EA, Bestall JC, Jeffries DJ, Wedzicha JA. Effect of exacerbation on quality of life in patients with chronic obstructive pulmonary disease. Am J Respir Crit Care Med 1998; 157:1418–122.
49. Doll H, Grey-Amante P, Duprat-Lomon I, Sagnier PP, Thate-Waschke I, Lorenz J, Rychlik R, Pfeil T. Quality of life in acute exacerbation of chronic bronchitis: results from a German population study. Respir Med 2002; 96:39–51.
50. Hankinson JL, Wagner GR. Medical screening using periodic spirometry for detection of chronic lung disease. Occup Med 1993; 8:353–361.
51. Smoking Cessation Clinical Practice Guideline Panel and Staff: The Agency for Health Care Policy and Research. Smoking cessation clinical practice guidelines. JAMA 1996; 275:1270–1280.
52. The Tobacco Use and Dependence Clinical Practice Guideline Panel Staff and Consortium Representatives. A clinical practice guideline for treating tobacco use and dependence. JAMA 2000; 282:3244–3254.

53. Lancaster T, Stead L, Silagy C, Sowden A. Effectiveness of interventions to help people stop smoking: findings from the Cochrane Library. Br Med J 2000; 321:355–358.

54. Ferguson GT. Update on pharmacologic therapy for chronic obstructive pulmonary disease. Clin Chest Med 2000; 21:723–738.

55. Fiore MC, Smith SS, Jorenby DE, Baker TB. The effectiveness of the nicotine patch for smoking cessation: a meta-analysis. JAMA 1994; 271:1940–1947.

56. Henningfield JE. Nicotine medications for smoking cessation. N Engl J Med 1995; 333:1196–1203.

57. Jorenby DE, Leischow SJ, Nides MA, Rennard SI, Johnston JA, Hughes AR, Smith SS, Muramoto ML, Daughton DM, Doan K, Fiore MC, Baker TB. A controlled trial of sustained-release bupropion, a nicotine patch, or both for smoking cessation. N Engl J Med 1999; 340:685–691.

58. Anthonisen NR, Connett JE, Kiley JP, Altose MD, Bailey WC, Buist AS, Conway WA, Enright PL, Kanner RE, O'Hara P, Scanlon PO, Tashkin DP, Wise RA, for the Lung Health Study Group. The effects of smoking intervention and the use of an inhaled anticholinergic bronchodilator on the rate of decline in FEV_1: the Lung Health Study. JAMA 1994; 272:1497–1505.

59. O'Donnell DE. Assessment of bronchodilator efficacy in symptomatic COPD. Is spirometry useful? Chest 2000; 117:42S–47S.

60. O'Donnell DE. Dyspnea in advanced chronic obstructive pulmonary disease. J Heart Lung Transplant 1998; 17:544–554.

61. O'Donnell DE, Revill SM, Webb KA. Dynamic hyperinflation and exercise intolerance in chronic obstructive pulmonary disease. Am J Respir Crit Care Med 2001; 164:770–777.

62. O'Donnell DE, Lam M, Webb KA. Measurement of symptoms, lung hyperinflation, and endurance during exercise in chronic obstructive pulmonary disease. Am J Respir Crit Care Med 1998; 158:1557–1565.

63. Diaz O, Villafranca C, Ghezzo H, Borzone G, Leiva A, Milic-Emili J, Lisboa C. Role of inspiratory capacity on exercise tolerance in COPD patients with and without tidal expiratory flow limitation at rest. Eur Respir J 2000; 16:269–275.

64. Gross NJ. Ipratropium bromide. N Engl J Med 1988; 319:486–494.

65. Disse B. Antimuscarinic treatment for lung diseases. From research to clinical practice. Life Sci 2001; 68:257–264.

66. On LS, Boonyongsunchai P, Webb S, Davies L, Calverley PMA, Costello RW. Function of pulmonary neuronal M_2 muscarinic receptors in stable chronic obstructive pulmonary disease. Am J Respir Crit Care Med 2001; 163:1320–1325.

67. Cazzola M, Spina D, Matera MG. The use of bronchodilators in stable chronic obstructive pulmonary disease. Pulm Pharmacol Ther 1997; 10:129–144.

68. Chapman KR. Clinical implications of anticholinergic bronchodilator therapy in COPD. Res Clin Forums 1991; 13:43–50.

69. Klock LE, Miller TD, Morris AH, Watanabe S, Dickman M. A comparative study of atropine sulfate and isoproterenol hydrochloride in chronic bronchitis. Am Rev Respir Dis 1975; 112:371–376.

70. Marini JJ, Lakshminarayan S. The effect of atropine inhalation in "irreversible" chronic bronchitis. Chest 1980; 77:591–596.

71. Braun SR, McKenzie WN, Copeland C, Knight L, Ellersieck M. A comparison of the effect of ipratropium and albuterol in the treatment of chronic obstructive pulmonary disease. Arch Intern Med 1989; 149:544–547.

72. Rennard SI, Serby CW, Ghafouri M, Johnson PA, Friedman M. Extended therapy with ipratropium is associated with improved lung function in patients with COPD. A retrospective analysis of data from seven clinical trials. Chest 1996; 110:62–70.

73. Littner MR, Ilowite JS, Tashkin DP, Friedman M, Serby CW, Menjoge SS, Witek TJ Jr. Long-acting bronchodilation with once-daily dosing of tiotropium (Spiriva) in stable chronic obstructive pulmonary disease. Am J Respir Crit Care Med 2000; 161:1136–1142.

74. Liesker JJW, Wijkstra PJ, Hacken NHTT, Koeter GH, Postma DS, Kerstjens HAM. A systematic review of the effects of bronchodilators on exercise capacity in patients with COPD. Chest 2002; 121:597–608.

75. Ikeda A, Nishimura K, Koyama H, Tsukino M, Mishima M, Izumi T. Dose response study of ipratropium bromide aerosol on maximum exercise performance in stable patients with chronic obstructive pulmonary disease. Thorax 1996; 51:48–53.

76. Tsukino M, Nishimura K, Ikeda A, Hajiro T, Koyama H, Izumi T. Effects of theophylline and ipratropium bromide on exercise performance in patients with stable chronic obstructive pulmonary disease. Thorax 1998; 53:269–273.

77. Oga T, Nishimura K, Tsukino M, Hajiro T, Ikeda A, Izumi T. The effects of oxitropium bromide on exercise performance in patients with stable chronic obstructive pulmonary disease. A comparison of three different exercise tests. Am J Respir Crit Care Med 2001; 161:1897–1901.

78. O'Donnell DE, Lam M, Webb KA. Spirometric correlates of improvement in exercise performance after anticholinergic therapy in chronic obstructive pulmonary disease. Am J Respir Crit Care Med 1999; 160:542–549.

79. Mahler DA, Donohue JF, Barbee RA, Goldman MD, Gross NJ, Wisniewski ME, Yancey SW, Zakes BA, Rickard KA, Anderson WH. Efficacy of salmeterol xinafoate in the treatment of COPD. Chest 1999; 115:957–965.

80. Rennard SI, Anderson W, ZuWallack R, Broughton J, Bailey W, Friedman M, Wiesniewski M, Rickard K. Use of a long-acting inhaled β_2-adrenergic agonist, salmeterol xinafoate, in patients with chronic obstructive pulmonary disease. Am J Respir Crit Care Med 2001; 163:1087–1092.

81. Dahl R, Greefhorst LAPM, Nowak D, Nonikov V, Byrne AM, Thomson MH, Till D, Della Cioppa G. Inhaled formoterol dry powder versus ipratropium bromide in chronic obstructive pulmonary disease. Am J Respir Crit Care Med 2001; 164:778–784.

82. Casaburi R, Mahler DA, Jones PW, Wanner A, San Pedro G, ZuWallack RL, Menjoge SS, Serby CW, Witek TJ Jr. A long-term evaluation of once-daily tiotropium in chronic obstructive pulmonary disease. Eur Respir J 2002; 19:217–224.

83. Vincken W, Van Noord JA, Greefhorst APM, Bantje ThA, Kesten S, Korducki L, Cornelissen PJG, Dutch/Belgian Tiotropium Study Group. Improved health outcomes in patients with COPD during 1 year's treatment with tiotropium. Eur Respir J 2002; 19:209–216.

84. Friedman M, Serby CW, Menjoge SS, Wilson JD, Hilleman DE, Witek TJ Jr. Pharmacoeconomic evaluation of a combination of ipratropium plus albuterol compared with ipratropium alone and albuterol alone in COPD. Chest 1999; 115:635–641.

85. Cazzola M, Donner CF. Long-acting β_2 agonists in the management of stable chronic obstructive pulmonary disease. Drugs 2000; 60:307–320.
86. Jarvis B, Markham A. Inhaled salmeterol. A review of its efficacy in chronic obstructive pulmonary disease. Drugs Aging 2001; 18:441–472.
87. Bartow RA, Brogden RN. Formoterol. An update of its pharmacological properties and therapeutic efficacy in the management of asthma. Drugs 1998; 55:303–322.
88. Johnson M, Rennard SI. Alternative mechanisms for long-acting β_2-adrenergic agonists in COPD. Chest 2001; 120:258–270.
89. Anthonisen NR, Wright EC, IPPB Trial Group. Bronchodilator response in chronic obstructive pulmonary disease. Am Rev Respir Dis 1986; 133:814–819.
90. Jaeschke R, Guyatt GH, Cook D, Morris J, Willan A, McIlroy W, Harper S, Ramsdale H, Haddon R, Fitzgerald MJ. The effect of increasing doses of beta agonists on airflow in patients with chronic airflow limitation. Respir Med 1993; 87:433–438.
91. Cook D, Guyatt GH, Wong E, Goldstein R, Bedard M, Austin P, Ramsdale H, Jaeschke R, Sears M. Regular versus as-needed short-acting inhaled β-agonist therapy for chronic obstructive pulmonary disease. Am J Respir Crit Care Med 2001; 163:85–90.
92. Belman MJ, Botnick WC, Shin JW. Inhaled bronchodilators reduce dynamic hyperinflation during exercise in patients with chronic obstructive pulmonary disease. Am J Respir Crit Care Med 1996; 153:967–975.
93. Saito S, Miyamoto K, Nishimura M, Aida A, Saito H, Tsujino I, Kawakami Y. Effects of inhaled bronchodilators on pulmonary hemodynamics at rest and during exercise in patients with COPD. Chest 1999; 115:376–382.
94. Guyatt GH, Townsend ER, Pugsley SO, Keller JL, Short HD, Taylor DW, Newhouse MT. Bronchodilators in chronic air-flow limitation. Effects on airway function, exercise capacity, and quality of life. Am Rev Respir Dis 1987; 135:1069–1074.
95. The COMBIVENT Inhalation Solution Study Group. Routine nebulized ipratropium and albuterol together are better than either alone in COPD. Chest 1997; 112:1514–1521.
96. Cazzola M, Santangelo G, Piccolo A, Salzillo A, Matera MG, D'Amato G, Rossi F. Effect of salmeterol and formoterol in patients with chronic obstructive pulmonary disease. Pulm Pharmacol 1994; 7:103–107.
97. Benhamou D, Cuvelier A, Muir JF, Leclerc V, Le Gros V, Kottakis J, Bourdeix I. Rapid onset of bronchodilation in COPD: a placebo-controlled study comparing formoterol (Foradil Aerolizer) with salbutamol (Ventodisk). Respir Med 2001; 95:817–821.
98. Cazzola M, Centanni S, Regorda C, di Marco F, Di Perna F, Carlucci P, Boveri B, Santus P. Onset of action of single doses of formoterol administered via Turbuhaler in patients with stable COPD. Pulm Pharmacol Ther 2001; 14:41–45.
99. Cazzola M, Matera MG, Santangelo G, Vinciguerra A, Rossi F, D'Amato G. Salmeterol and formoterol in partially reversible severe chronic obstructive pulmonary disease: a dose-response study. Respir Med 1995; 89:357–362.
100. Celik G, Kayacan O, Beder S, Durmaz G. Formoterol and salmeterol in partially reversible chronic obstructive pulmonary disease: a crossover, placebo-controlled comparison of onset and duration of action. Respiration 1999; 66:434–439.

101. Cazzola M, Di Perna F, Noschese P, Vinciguerra A, Calderaro F, Girbino G, Matera MG. Effects of formoterol, salmeterol or oxitropium bromide on airway responses to salbutamol in COPD. Eur Respir J 1998; 11:1337–1341.

102. Cazzola M, Di Lorenzo G, Di Perna F, Calderaro F, Testi R, Centanni S. Additive effects of salmeterol and fluticasone or theophylline in COPD. Chest 2000; 118:1576–1581.

103. Cazzola M, Vinciguerra A, Di Perna F, Matera MG. Early reversibility to salbutamol does not always predict bronchodilation after salmeterol in stable chronic obstructive pulmonary disease. Respir Med 1998; 92:1012–1016.

104. Ramirez-Venegas A, Ward J, Lentine T, Mahler DA. Salmeterol reduces dyspnea and improves lung function in patients with COPD. Chest 1997; 112:336–340.

105. Grove A, Lipworth BJ, Reid P, Smith RP, Ramage L, Ingram CG, Jenkins RJ, Winter JH, Dhillon DP. Effects of regular salmeterol on lung function and exercise capacity in patients with chronic obstructive airways disease. Thorax 1996; 51:689–693.

106. Boyd G, Morice AH, Pounsfod JC, Siebert M, Peslis N, Crawford C. An evaluation of salmeterol in the treatment of chronic obstructive pulmonary disease (COPD). Eur Respir J 1997; 10:815–821.

107. Patakas D, Andreadis D, Mavrofridis E, Argyropoulou P. Comparison of the effects of salmeterol and ipratropium on exercise performance and breathlessness in patients with stable chronic obstructive pulmonary disease. Respir Med 1998; 92:1116–1121.

108. Ayers ML, Mejia R, Ward J, Lentine T, Mahler DA. Effectiveness of salmeterol versus ipratropium bromide on exertional dyspnea in COPD. Eur Respir J 2001; 17:1132–1137.

109. Di Lorenzo G, Morici G, Drago A, Pellitteri ME, Mansueto P, Melluso M, Norrito F, Squassante L, Fasolo A. Efficacy, tolerability, and effects on quality of life of inhaled salmeterol and oral theophylline in patients with mild-to-moderate chronic obstructive pulmonary disease. SLMT02 Italian Study Group. Clin Ther 1998; 20:1130–1148.

110. Taccola M, Bancalari L, Ghignoni G, Paggiaro PL. Salmeterol versus slow-release theophylline in patients with reversible obstructive pulmonary disease. Monaldi Arch Chest Dis 1999; 54:302–306.

111. Jones PW, Bosh TK. Quality of life in COPD patients treated with salmeterol. Am J Respir Crit Care Med 1997; 155:1283–1289.

112. Rutten-van Molken M, Roos B, Van Noord J. A. An empirical comparison of the St George's Respiratory Questionnaire (SGRQ) and the Chronic Respiratory Disease Questionnaire (CRQ) in a clinical trial setting. Thorax 1999; 54:995–1003.

113. Cox F, Godwin B, Stanford R, et al. Using simple and relative difference to interpret changes in health-related quality-of-life scores for salmeterol, ipratropium, and placebo. J Managed Care Pharm 2000; 6:483–487.

114. Khoukaz G, Gross NJ. Effects of salmeterol on arterial blood gases in patients with stable chronic obstructive pulmonary disease. Comparison with albuterol and ipratropium. Am J Respir Crit Care Med 1999; 160:1028–1030.

115. Martin RM, Dunn NR, Freemantle SN, Mann RD. Risk of non-fatal cardiac failure and ischaemic heart disease with long acting b_2 agonists. Thorax 1998; 53:558–562.

116. Cazzola M, Imperatore F, Salzillo A, Di Perna F, Calderaro F, Imperatore A, Matera MG. Cardiac effects of formoterol and salmeterol in patients suffering from COPD with preexisting cardiac arrhythmias and hypoxemia. Chest 1998; 114:411–415.

117. COMBIVENT Inhalation Aerosol Study Group. In chronic obstructive pulmonary disease, a combination of ipratropium and albuterol is more effective than either agent alone: an 85-day multicenter trial. Chest 1994; 105:1411–1419.

118. Ikeda A, Nishimura K, Koyama H, Izumi T. Bronchodilating effects of combined therapy with clinical dosages of ipratropium bromide and salbutamol for stable COPD: comparison with ipratropium bromide alone. Chest 1995; 107:401–405.

119. Campbell S. For COPD a combination of ipratropium bromide and albuterol sulfate is more effective than albuterol base. Arch Intern Med 1999; 159:156–160.

120. Dorinsky PM, Reisner C, Ferguson GT, Menjoge SS, Serby CW, Witek TJ Jr. The combination of ipratropium and albuterol optimizes pulmonary function reversibility testing in patients with COPD. Chest 1999; 115:966–971.

121. Casali L, Grassi C, Rampulla C, et al. Clinical pharmacology of a combination of a bronchodilators. Int J Clin Pharmacol Biopharm 1979; 7:277–280.

122. Lees AW, Allan GW, Smith J. Nebulised ipratropium bromide and salbutamol in chronic bronchitis. Br J Clin Pract 1980; 3:240–242.

123. Leitch AG, Hopkin JM, Ellis DA, et al. The effect of aerosol ipratropium bromide and salbutamol on exercise tolerance in chronic bronchitis. Thorax 1978; 33:711–713.

124. Petrie GR, Palmer KNV. Comparison of aerosol ipratropium bromide and salbutamol in chronic bronchitis and asthma. Br Med J 1975; 1:430–432.

125. Lightbody IM, Ingram CG, Legge JS, Johnston RN. Ipratropium bromide, salbutamol and prednisolone in bronchial asthma and chronic bronchitis. Br J Dis Chest 1978; 72:181–186.

126. Wesseling G, Mostert R, Wouters EFM. A comparison of effects of anti-cholinergic and β_2-agonist and combination therapy on respiratory impedance in COPD. Chest 1992; 101:166–173.

127. Marlin GE. Studies of ipratopium bromide and fenoterol administered by metered-dose inhaler and aerosolized solution. Respiration 1986; 50(suppl 2):290–293.

128. Serra G, Giacopelli A. Controlled clinical study of a long-term treatment of chronic obstructive lung disease using a combination of fenoterol and ipratropium bromide in aerosol form. Respiration 1986; 50(suppl 2):249–253.

129. Morton O. Response to Duovent of chronic reversible airways obstruction—a controlled trial in general practice. Postgrad Med J 1984; 60(suppl 1):32–35.

130. Easton PA, Jadue C, Dhingra S, Anthonisen NR. A comparison of the bronchodilating effects of a beta-2 adrenergic agent (albuterol) and an anticholinergic agent (ipratropium bromide), given by aerosol alone or in sequence. N Engl J Med 1986; 315:735–739.

131. Lloberes P, Ramis L, Montserrat JM, Serra J, Campistol J, Picado C, Agusti-Vidal A. Effect of three different bronchodilators during an exacerbation of chronic obstructive pulmonary disease. Eur Respir J 1988; 1:536–539.

132. Le Doux EJ, Morris JF, Temple WP, Duncan C. Standard and double dose ipratropium bromide and combined ipratropium bromide and inhaled metapro-terenol in COPD. Chest 1989; 95:1013–1016.

133. Ullah MI, Newman GB, Saunders KB. Influence of age on response to ipratropium and salbutamol in asthma. Thorax 1981; 36:523–529.
134. Rebuck AS, Chapman KR, Abboud RT, Pare PD, Kreisman H, Wolkove N, Vickerson F. Nebulized anticholinergic and sympathomimetic treatment of asthma and chronic obstructive airway disease in the emergency room. Am J Med 1987; 82:59–64.
135. Lakshminarayan S. Iprartopium bromide in chronic bronchitis/emphysema: a review of the literature. Am J Med 1986; 81(Suppl 5A):76–80.
136. Newnham DM, Dhillon DP, Winter JH, et al. Bronchodilator reversibility to low and high doses of terbutaline and ipratropium bromide in patients with chronic obstructive pulmonary disease. Thorax 1993; 48:1151–1155.
137. Matera MG, Caputi M, Cazzola M. A combination with clinical recommended dosages of salmeterol and ipratropium is not more effecive than salmeterol alone in patients with chronic obstructive pulmonary disease. Respir Med 1996; 90:497–499.
138. Sichletidis L, Kottakis J, Marcou S, Constantinidis TC, Antoniades A. Bronchodilatory responses to formoterol, ipratropium, and their combination in patients with stable COPD. Int J Clin Pract 1999; 53:185–188.
139. Cazzola M, Di Perna F, Califano C, Vinciguerra A, D'Amato M. Incremental benefit of adding oxitropium bromide to formoterol in patients with stable COPD. Pulm Pharmacol Ther 1999; 12:267–271.
140. Cazzola M, Di Perna F, Centanni S, Califano C, D'Amato M, Mazzarella G. Influence of higher than conventional doses of oxitropium bromide on formoterol-induced bronchodilation in COPD. Respir Med 1999; 93:909–911.
141. D'Urzo AD, De Salvo MC, Ramirez-Rivera A, Almeida J, Sichletidis L, Rapatz G, Kottakis J. In patients with COPD, treatment with a combination of formoterol and ipratropium is more effective than a combination of salbutamol and ipratropium: a 3-week, randomized, double-blind, within-patient, multi-center study. Chest 2001; 119:1347–1356.
142. Van Noord JA, de Munck DRAJ, Bantje ThA, Hop WCJ, Akveld MLM, Bommer AM. Long-term treatment of chronic obstructive pulmonary disease with salmeterol and the additive effect of ipratropium. Eur Respir J 2000; 15:878–885.
143. Benayoun S, Ernst P, Suissa S. The impact of combined inhaled bronchodilator therapy in the treatment of COPD. Chest 2001; 119:85–92.
144. Van Andel AE, Reisner C, Menjoge SS, Witek TJ. Analysis of inhaled corticosteroid and oral theophylline use among patients with stable COPD from 1987 to 1995. Chest 1999; 115:703–707.
145. vas Fragoso CA, Miller MA. Review of the clinical efficacy of theophylline in the treatment of chronic obstructive pulmonary disease. Am Rev Respir Dis 1993; 147:S40–S47.
146. Dull WL, Alexander MB, Sadoul P, Woolson RF. The efficacy of isoproterenol inhalation for predicting the response to orally administered theophylline in chronic obstructive pulmonary disease. Am Rev Respir Dis 1982; 126:656–659.
147. Guyatt GH, Townsend M, Pugsley SO, Keller JL, Short HD, Taylor DW, Newhouse MT. Bronchodilators in chronic air-flow limitation. Effects on airway function, exercise capacity and quality of life. Am Rev Respir Dis 1987; 135:1069–1074.

148. Taylor DB, Buick B, Kinney C, Lowry RC, McDevitt DG. The efficacy of orally administered theophylline, inhaled salbutamol and a combination of the two as chronic therapy in the management of chronic bronchitis with reversible air-flow obstruction. Am Rev Respir Dis 1985; 131:747–751.

149. Thomas P, Pugsley JA, Stewart JH. Theophylline and salbutamol improve pulmonary function in patients with irreversible chronic obstructive pulmonary disease. Chest 1992; 101:160–165.

150. Murciano D, Auclair MH, Pariente R, Aubier M. A randomized, controlled trial of theophylline in patients with severe chronic obstructive pulmonary disease. N Engl J Med 1989; 320:1521–1525.

151. Nishimura K, Koyama H, Ikeda A, Izumi T. Is oral theophylline effective in combination with both inhaled anticholinergic agent and inhaled beta-2-agonist in the treatment of stable COPD. Chest 1993; 104:179–184.

152. Taccola M, Bancalari L, Ghignoni G, Paggiaro PL. Salmeterol versus slow-release theophylline in patients with reversible obstructive pulmonary disease. Monaldi Arch Chest Dis 1999; 54:302–306.

153. ZuWallack RL, Mahler DA, Reilly D, Church N, Emmett A, Rickard K, Knobil K. Salmeterol plus theophylline combination therapy in the treatment of COPD. Chest 2001; 119:1661–1670.

154. Parker JO, Ashekian PB, Di Giorgi S, West RO. Hemodynamic effects of aminophylline in chronic obstructive pulmonary disease. Circulation 1967; 35:365–372.

155. Parker JO, Kelkar K, West RO. Hemodynamic effects of aminophylline in cor pulmonale. Circulation 1966; 33:17–25.

156. Matthay MA, Berger HJ, Davies R, Loke J, Gottschalk A, Zaret BL. Improvement in cardiac performance by oral long-acting theophylline in chronic obstructive pulmonary disease. Am Heart J 1982; 104:1022–1026.

157. Nishimura K, Koyama H, Ikeda A, Suguira N, Kawakatsu K, Izumi T. The additive effect of theophylline on a high-dose combination of inhaled salbutamol and ipratropium in stable COPD. Chest 1995; 107:718–723.

158. Torphy TJ, Barnette MS, Underwood DC, Griswold DE, Christensen SB, Murdoch RD, Nieman RB, Compton CH. Ariflo TM (SB 207499), a second generation phosphodiesterase 4 inhibitor for the treatment of asthma and COPD: from concept to clinic. Pulm Pharmacol Ther 1999; 12:131–135.

159. Giembycz MA. Cilomilast: a second generation phosphodiesterase 4 inhibitor for asthma and chronic obstructive pulmonary disease. Exp Opin Invest Drugs 2001; 10:1361–1379.

160. Compton CH, Gubb J, Nieman R, Edelson J, Amit O, Bakst A, Ayres JG, Creemers JPHM, Schultze-Werninghaus G, Brambilla C, Barnes NC. Cilomilast, a selective phosphodiesterase-4 inhibitor for treatment of patients with chronic obstructive pulmonary disease: a randomised, dose-ranging study. Lancet 2001; 358:265–270.

161. Burge S. Should inhaled corticosteroids be used in the long term treatment of chronic obstructive pulmonary disease. Drugs 2001; 61:1535–1544.

162. Borron W, deBoisblanc BP. Steroid therapy for chronic obstructive pulmonary disease. Curr Opin Pulm Med 1998; 4:61–65.

163. Barnes PJ, Pederson S, Busse WW. Efficacy and safety of inhaled corticosteroids. New developments. Am J Respir Crit Care Med 1998; 157:1S–53S.

164. Jackevicius CA, Chapman KR. Prevalence of inhaled corticosteroid use among patients with chronic obstructive pulmonary disease: a survey. Annu Pharmacother 1997; 31:160–164.

165. Jackevicius C, Joyce DP, Kesten S, Chapman KR. Prehospitalization inhaled corticosteroid use in patients with COPD or asthma. Chest 1997; 111:296–302.

166. McEvoy CE, Niewoehner DE. Corticosteroids in chronic obstructive pulmonary disease. Clinical benefits and risks. Clin Chest Med 2000; 21:739–752.

167. Bonay M, Bancal C, Crestani B. Benefits and risks of inhaled corticosteroids in chronic obstructive pulmonary disease. Drug Saf 2002; 25:57–71.

168. Postma DS, Kerstjens HAM. Are inhaled glucocorticosteroids effective in chronic obstructive pulmonary disease? Am J Respir Crit Care Med 1999; 160:66S–71S.

169. Keatings VM, Jatakanon A, Worsdell YM, Barnes PJ. Effects of inhaled and oral corticosteroids on inflammatory indices in asthma and COPD. Am J Respir Crit Care Med 1997; 155:542–548.

170. Thompson AB, Mueller MB, Heires AJ, Bohling TL, Daughton D, Yancey SW, Sykes RS, Rennard SI. Aerosolized beclomethasone in chronic bronchitis. Improved pulmonary function and diminished airway inflammation. Am Rev Respir Dis 1992; 146:389–395.

171. Cox G, Whitehead L, Dolovich M, Jordana M, Gauldie J, Newhouse MT. A randomized controlled trial on the effect of inhaled corticosteroids on airways inflammation in adult cigarette smokers. Chest 1999; 115:1271–1277.

172. Culpitt SV, Maziak W, Loukidis S, Nightingale JA, Matthes JL, Barnes PJ. Effect of high dose inhaled steroid on cells, cytokines, and proteases in induced sputum in chronic obstructive pulmonary disease. Am J Respir Crit Care Med 1999; 160:1635–1639.

173. Loppow D, Schleiss MB, Kanniess F, Taube C, Jorres RA, Magnusson H. In patients with chronic bronchitis a four week trial with inhaled steroids does not attenuate airway inflammation. Respir Med 2001; 95:115–121.

174. Llewellyn-Jones CG, Harris TA, Stockley RA. Effect of fluticasone propionate on sputum of patients with chronic bronchitis and emphysema. Am J Respir Crit Care Med 1996; 153:616–621.

175. Confalonieri M, Mainardi E, Della Porta R, Bernorio S, Gandola L, Beghe B, Spanevello A. Inhaled corticosteroids reduce neutrophilic bronchial inflammation in patients with chronic obstructive pulmonary disease. Thorax 1998; 53:583–585.

176. Balbi B, Majori M, Bertacco S, Convertino G, Cuomo A, Donner CF, Pesci A. Inhaled corticosteroids in stable COPD patients. Do they have effects on cells and molecular mediators of airways inflammation? Chest 2000; 117:1633–1637.

177. Chanez P, Vignola AM, O'Shaugnessy T, Enander I, Li D, Jeffery PK, Bousquet J. Corticosteroid reversibility in COPD is related to features of asthma. Am Rev Respir Crit Care Med 1997; 155:1529–1534.

178. Pizzichini E, Pizzichini M, Gibson P, Parameswaran K, Gleich GJ, Berman L, Dolovich J, Hargreave FE. Sputum eosinophilia predicts benefit from prednisone in smokers with chronic obstructive bronchitis. Am J Respir Crit Care Med 1998; 158:1511–1517.

179. Brightling CE, Monteiro W, Ward R, Parker D, Morgan MDL, Wardlaw AJ, Pavord ID. Sputum eosinophilia and short-term response to prednisolone in

chronic obstructive pulmonary disease: a randomised controlled trial. Lancet 2000; 356:1480–1485.

180. Davies L, Nisar M, Pearson MG, Costello RW, Earis JE, Calverley PMA. Oral corticosteroid trials in the management of stable chronic obstructive pulmonary disease. QJ Med 1999; 92:395–400.

181. Weir DC, Gove RI, Robertson AS, Burge PS. Response to corticosteroids in chronic airflow obstruction: relationship to emphysema and airway collapse. Eur Respir J 1991; 4:1185–1190.

182. Fujimoto K, Kubo K, Yamamoto H, Yamaguchi S, Matsuzawa Y. Eosinophilic inflammation in the airway is related to glucocorticoid reversibility in patients with pulmonary emphysema. Chest 1999; 115:697–702.

183. Callahan CM, Dittus RS, Katz BP. Oral corticsteroid therapy for patients with stable chronic obstructive pulmonary disease: A meta-analysis. Ann Intern Med 1991; 114:216–223.

184. Weir DC, Gove RI, Roberts RS, Burge PS, Robertson AS. Time course of response to oral and inhaled corticosteroids in non-asthmatic chronic airflow obstruction. Thorax 1990; 45:118–121.

185. Postma DS, Steenhuis EJ, van der Weele LT, Sluiter HJ. Severe chronic airflow obstruction: can corticosteroids slow down obstruction? Eur J Respir Dis 1985; 67:56–64.

186. Rice KL, Rubins JB, Lebahn F, Parenti CM, Duane PG, Kuskowski M, Joseph AM, Niewoehner DE. Withdrawal of chronic systemic corticosteroids in patients with COPD. A randomized trial. Am J Respir Crit Care Med 2000; 162:174–178.

187. McEvoy CE, Niewoehner DE. Adverse effects of corticosteroid therapy for COPD. A critical review. Chest 1997; 111:732–743.

188. Pauwels RA, Lofdahl CS, Laitinen LA, Schouten JP, Postma DS, Pride NB, Ohlson LO, European Respiratory Society Study on Chronic Obstructive Pulmonary Disease. Long-term treatment with inhaled budesonide in persons with mild chronic obstructive pulmonary disease who continue smoking. N Engl J Med 1999; 340:1948–1953.

189. Vestbo J, Sorensen T, Lange P, Brix A, Torre P, Viskum K. Long-term effect of inhaled budesonide in mild and moderate chronic obstructive pulmonary disease: a randomized controlled trial. Lancet 1999; 353:1819–1823.

190. Paggiaro PL, Dahle R, Bakran I, Frith L, Hollingworth K, Efthimiou J. International COPD Study Group. Multicentre randomised placebo-controlled trial of inhaled fluticasone propionate in patients with chronic obstructive pulmonary disease. Lancet 1998; 351:773–780.

191. Burge PS, Calverley PMA, Jones PW, Spencer S, Anderson JA, Maslen TK. Randomised, double blind, placebo controlled study of fluticasone propionate in patients with moderate to severe chronic obstructive pulmonary disease: the ISOLDE trial. Br Med J 2000; 320:1297–1303.

192. The Lung Health Study Research Group. Effect of inhaled triamcinolone on the decline in pulmonary function in chronic obstructive pulmonary disease. N Engl J Med 2000; 343:1902–1909.

193. O'Brien A, Russo-Magno P, Karki A, Hiranniramol S, Hardin M, Kaszuba M, Sherman C, Rounds S. Effects of withdrawal of inhaled steroids in men with severe irreversible airflow obstruction. Am J Respir Crit Care Med 2001; 164:365–371.

194. Spencer S, Calverly PMA, Burge PS, Jones PW. Health status deterioration in patients with chronic obstructive pulmonary disease. Am J Respir Crit Care Med 2001; 163:122–128.

195. Sin DD, Tu JV. Inhaled corticosteroids and the risk of mortality and readmission in elderly patients with chronic obstructive pulmonary disease. Am J Respir Crit Care Med 2001; 164:580–584.

195a. Soriano JB, Vestbo J, Pride NB, Kiri V, Maden C, Maier WC. Survival in COPD patients after regular use of fluticasone propionate and salmeterol in general practice. Eur Respir J 2002; 20:819–825.

196. Jones A, Fay JK, Burr M, Stone M, Hood K, Roberts G. Inhaled corticosteroid effect on bone metabolism in asthma and mild chronic obstructive pulmonary disease. Cochrane Database Syst Rev 2002.

197. Biskobing DM. COPD and osteoporosis. Chest 2002; 121:609–620.

198. Adachi JD, Papaionnaou A. Corticosteroid-induced osteoporosis. Detection and management. Drug Saf 2001; 24:607–624.

199. van Staa TP, Leufkens HGM, Cooper C. Use of inhaled corticosteroids and risk of fractures. J Bone Miner Res 2001; 16:581–588.

200. McEvoy CE, Ensrud KE, Bender E, Genant HK, Yu W, Griffith JM, Niewoehner DE. Association between corticosteroid use and vertebral fractures in older men with chronic obstructive pulmonary disease. Am J Respir Crit Care Med 1998; 157:704–709.

201. Anthonisen N, Manfreda J, Warren C, Hersfield E, Harding G, Nelson N. Antibiotic therapy in exacerbations of chronic obstructive pulmonary disease. Ann Intern Med 1987; 106:196–204.

202. Del Donno M, Olivieri D. Mucoactive drugs in the management of chronic obstructive pulmonary disease. Monaldi Arch Chest Dis 1998; 53:714–719.

203. Poole PJ, Black PN. Oral mucolytic drugs for exacerbations of chronic obstructive pulmonary disease: systematic review. Br Med J 2001; 322:1–6.

204. Tarpy SP, Celli BR. Long-term oxygen therapy. N Engl J Med 1995; 333:710–714.

205. Crockett AJ, Cranston JM, Moss JR, Alpers JH. A review of long-term oxygen therapy for chronic obstructive pulmonary disease. Respir Med 2001; 95:437–443.

206. Medical Research Council Working Party. Long-term domiciliary oxygen therapy in chronic hypoxic cor pulmonale complicating chronic bronchitis and emphysema. Lancet 1981; 1:681–686.

207. Nocturnal Oxygen Therapy Trial Group. Continuous or nocturnal oxygen therapy in hypoxemic chronic obstructive lung disease. A clinical trial. Ann Intern Med 1980; 93:391–398.

208. Fletcher EC, Lukett RA, Goodnight-White S, Miller CC, Qian W, Costarangos-Galarza C. A double-blind trial of nocturnal supplemental oxygen for sleep desaturation in patients with chronic obstructive pulmonary disease and a daytime Pa_{O_2} above 60 mm Hg. Am Rev Respir Dis 1992; 145:1070–1076.

209. Gorecka D, Gorzelak K, Sliwinski P, Tobiasz M, Zielinski J. Effect of long term oxygen therapy on survival in patients with chronic obstructive pulmonary disease with moderate hypoxemia. Thorax 1997; 52:674–679.

210. Chaouat A, Weitzenblum E, Kessler R, Charpentier C, Ehrhart M, Schott R, Levi-Valensi P, Zielinski J, Delaunois L, Cornudella R, Moutinho dos Santos J.

A randomized trial of nocturnal oxygen therapy in chronic obstructive pulmonary disease patients. Eur Respir J 1999; 14:1002–1008.

211. Chaouat A, Weitzenblum E, Kessler R, Schott R, Charpentier C, Levi-Valensi P, Zielinski J, Delaunois L, Comudella R, Moutinho dos Santos J. Outcome of COPD patients with mild daytime hypoxaemia with or without sleep-related oxygen desaturation. Eur Respir J 2001; 17:848–855.

212. Grant I, Heaton RK, McSweeney AJ, Adams KM, Timms RM. Neuropsychologic findings in hypoxemic chronic obstructive pulmonary disease. Arch Intern Med 1982; 142:1470–1476.

213. Ries AL. Position paper of the American Assocciation of Cardiovascular and Pulmonary Rehabilitation: scientific basis of pulmonary rehabilitation. J Cardiopulm Rehabil 1990; 10:418–441.

214. Morgan MDL, Calverley PMA, Clark CJ, Davidson AC, Garrod R, Goldman JM, Griffiths TL, Roberts E, Sawicka E, Singh SJ, Wallace L, White R. Pulmonary rehabilitation. Thorax 2001; 56:827–834.

215. American Thoracic Society. Pulmonary rehabilitation—1999. Am J Respir Crit Care Med 1999; 159:1666–1682.

216. O'Donnell DE, McGuire M, Samis L, Webb KA. The impact of exercise reconditioning on breathlessness in severe chronic airflow limitation. Am J Respir Crit Care Med 1995; 152:2005–2013.

217. Casaburi R, Porszasz J, Burns MR, Carithers ER, Change RSY, Cooper CB. Physiologic benefits of exercise training in rehabilitation of patients with severe chronic obstructive pulmonary disease. Am J Respir Crit Care Med 1997; 155:1541–1551.

218. O'Donnell CR, McGuire M, Samis L, Webb KA. General exercise training improves ventilatory and peripheral muscle strength and endurance in chronic airflow limitation. Am J Respir Crit Care Med 1998; 157:1489–1497.

219. Maltais F, LeBlanc P, Simard C, Jobin J, Berube C, Bruneau J, Carrier L, Belleau R. Skeletal muscle adaptation to endurance training in patients with chronic obstructive pulmonary disease. Am J Respir Crit Care Med 1996; 154:442–447.

220. Vogiatzis I, Williamson AF, Miles J, Taylor IK. Physiological response to moderate exercise workloads in a pulmonary rehabilitation in patients with varying degrees of airflow obstruction. Chest 1999; 116:1200–1207.

221. Larson JL, Covey MK, Wirtz SE, Berry JK, Alex CG, Langbein WE, Edwards L. Cycle ergometer and inspiratory muscle training in chronic obstructive pulmonary disease. Am J Respir Crit Care Med 1999; 160:500–507.

222. Sala E, Roca J, Marrades RM, Alonso J, Gonzales de Suso JM, Moreno A, Barbera JA, Nadal J, de Jover L, Rodrigues-Roisin R, Wagner PD. Effects of endurance training on skeletal muscle bioenergetics in chronic obstructive pulmonary disease. Am J Respir Crit Care Med 1999; 159:1726–1734.

223. Serres I, Varray A, Vallet G, Micallef JP, Prefaut C. Improved skeletal muscle performance after individualized exercise training in patients with chronic obstructive pulmonary disease. J Cardiopulm Rehabil 1997; 17:232–238.

224. Mador MJ, Kufel TJ, Pineda LA, Steinwald A, Aggarwal A, Upadhyay AM, Khan MA. Effect of pulmonary rehabilitation on quadriceps fatigability during exercise. Am J Respir Crit Care Med 2001; 163:930–935.

225. Engelen MP, Wouters EF, Deutz NE, Does JD, Schols AM. Effects of exercise on amino acid metabolism in patients with chronic obstructive pulmonary disease. Am J Respir Crit Care Med 2001; 163:859–864.

226. Belman MJ, Kendregan BA. Exercise training fails to increase skeletal muscle enzymes in patients with chronic obstructive lung disease. Am Rev Respir Dis 1981; 123:256–261.

227. Lacasse Y, Wong E, Guyatt GH, King D, Cook DJ, Goldstein RS. Meta-analysis of respiratory rehabilitation in chronic obstructive pulmonary disease. Lancet 1996; 348:1115–1119.

228. Cambach W, Wagenaar R, Koelman T, van Keimpema A, Kemper H. The long-term effects of pulmonary rehabilitation in patients with asthma and chronic obstructive pulmonary disease: a research synthesis. Arch Phys Med Rehabil 1999; 80:103–111.

229. Guell R, Casan P, Belda J, Sangenis M, Morante F, Guyatt GH, Sanchis J. Long-term effects of outpatient rehabilitation of COPD. A randomized trial. Chest 2000; 117:976–983.

230. Griffiths TL, Campbell IA, Lewis-Jenkins V, Mullins J, Shiels K, Turner-Lawlor PJ, Newcombe RG, Lonescu AA, Thomas J, Tunbridge J. Results at 1 year of outpatient multidisciplinary pulmonary rehabilitation: a randomised controlled trial. Lancet 2000; 355:362–368.

231. Troosters T, Gosselink R, Decramer M. Short- and long-term effects of outpatient rehabilitation in patients with chronic obstructive pulmonary disease: a randomized trial. Am J Med 2000; 109:207–212.

232. Foglio K, Bianchi L, Bruletti G, Battista L, Pagani M, Ambrosino N. Long-term effectiveness of pulmonary rehabilitation in patients with chronic airway obstruction. Eur Respir J 1999; 13:125–132.

233. Bourjeily G, Rochester CL. Exercise training in chronic obstructive pulmonary disease. Clin Chest Med 2000; 214.

234. Berry MJ, Rejeski WJ, Adair NE, Zaccaro D. Exercise rehabilitation and chronic obstructive pulmonary disease stage. Am J Respir Crit Care Med 1999; 160:1248–1253.

235. Couser JI Jr, Guthman R, Hamadeh MA, Kane CS. Pulmonary rehabilitation improves exercise capacity in older elderly patients with COPD. Chest 1995; 107:730–734.

236. Scherer TA, Spengler CM, Owassapian D, Imhof E, Boutellier U. Respiratory muscle endurance training in chronic obstructive pulmonary disease. Impact on exercise capacity, dyspnea, and quality of life. Am J Respir Crit Care Med 2000; 162:1709–1712.

237. Riera HS, Rubio TM, Ruiz FO, Ramos PC, Otero DDC, Hernandez TE, Gomez JC. Effect on dyspnea, exercise performance, and quality of life. Chest 2001; 120:748–756.

238. Rochester CL. Which pulmonary rehabilitation program is best for your patient? J Respir Dis 2000; 21:539–546.

239. Goldstein RS, Gort EH, Stubbing D, Avendano MA, Guyatt GH. Randomised controlled trial of respiratory rehabilitation. Lancet 1994; 344:1394–1397.

240. Reardon J, Awad E, Normandin E, Vale F, Clark B, ZuWallack RL. The effect of comprehensive outpatient pulmonary rehabilitation on dyspnea. Chest 1994; 105:1046–1052.

241. Ries AL, Kaplan RM, Limberg TM, Prewitt LM. Effects of pulmonary rehabilitation on physiologic and psychosocial outcomes in patients with chronic obstructive pulmonary disease. Ann Intern Med 1995; 122:823–832.

242. Wijkstra PJ, van der Mark TW, Kraan J, van Altena R, Koeter GH, Postma DS. Long-term effects of home rehabilitation on physical performance in chronic obstructive pulmonary disease. Am J Respir Crit Care Med 1996; 153:1234–1241.

243. Strijbos JH, Postma DS, van Altena R, Gimeno F, Koeter GH. A comparison between an outpatient hospital-based pulmonary rehabilitation program and a home-care pulmonary rehabilitation program in patients with COPD. A follow-up of 18 months. Chest 1996; 109:366–372.

244. Ringbaek TJ, Broendum E, Hemmingsen L, Lybeck K, Nielsen D, Andersen C, Plange P. Rehabilitation of patients with chronic obstructive pulmonary disease. Exercise twice a week is not sufficient! Respir Med 2000; 94:150–154.

245. Green RH, Singh SJ, Williams J, Morgan MDL. A randomised controlled trial of four weeks versus seven weeks of pulmonary rehabilitation in chronic obstructive pulmonary disease. Thorax 2001; 56:143–145.

246. Cooper CB. Exercise in chronic pulmonary disease: aerobic exercise prescription. Med Sci Sports Exerc 2001; 33:S671–S679.

247. Storer TW. Exercise in chronic pulmonary disease: resistance exercise prescription. Med Sci Sports Exerc 2001; 33:S680–S686.

248. Wilson L, Devine EB, So K. Direct medical costs of chronic obstructive pulmonary disease: chronic bronchitis and emphysema. Respir Med 2000; 94:204–213.

249. Osman LM, Godden DJ, Friend JAR, Legge JS, Douglas JG. Quality of life and hospital re-admission in patients with chronic obstructive pulmonary disease. Thorax 1997; 52:67–71.

250. Stoller JK. Acute exacerbations of chronic obstructive pulmonary disease. N Engl J Med 2002; 346:988–988.

251. McCrory DC, Brown C, Gelfand SE, Bach PB. Management of acute exacerbations of COPD: A summary and appraisal of published evidence. Chest 2001; 119:1190–1209.

252. Niewoehner DE, Erbland ML, Deupree RH, Collins D, Gross NJ, Light RW, Anderson P, Morgan NA. Effect of systemic glucocorticoids on exacerbations of chronic obstructive pulmonary disease. N Engl J Med 1999; 340:1941–1947.

253. Sayner A, Aytemur ZA, Cirit M, Unsal I. Systemic glucocorticoids in severe exacerbations of COPD. Chest 2001; 119:726–730.

254. Davies L, Angus RM, Calverley PMA. Oral corticosteroids in patients admitted to hospital with exacerbations of chronic obstructive pulmonary disease: a prospective randomised controlled trial. Lancet 1999; 354:456–460.

254a. Thompson WH, Nielson CP, Carvalho P, Charan NB, Crowley JJ. Controlled trial of oral prednisone in outpatients with acute COPD exacerbation. Am J Respir Crit Care Med 1996; 154:407–412.

255. Maltais F, Ostinelli J, Bourbeau J, Tonnel AB, Jacquemet N, Haddon J, Rouleau M, Boukhana M, Martinot JB, Duroux P. Comparison of nebulized budesonide and oral prednisolone with placebo in the treatment of acute exacerbations of chronic obstructive pulmonary disease: a randomized controlled trial. Am J Respir Crit Care Med 2002; 165:698–703.

256. Sherk PA, Grossman RF. The chronic obstructive pulmonary disease exacerbation. Clin Chest Med 2000; 21:705–721.

257. Saint S, Bent S, Bittinghoff E, Grady D. Antibiotics in chronic obstructive pulmonary disease exacerbations: A meta-analysis. JAMA 1995; 273:957–960.

258. Nouira S, Marghli S, Belghith M, Besbes L, Elantrous S, Abroug F. Once daily oral ofloxacin in chronic obstructive pulmonary disease exacerbation requiring mechanical ventilation: a randomised placebo-controlled trial. Lancet 2001; 358:2020–2025.
259. Stockley RA, O'Brien A, Pye A, Hill SL. Relationship of sputum color to nature and outpatient management of acute exacerbations of COPD. Chest 2000; 117:1638–1645.
260. Miravitlles M, Espinosa C, Fernandez-Laso E, Martos JA, Maldonado JA, Gallego M, Study Group of Bacterial Infection in COPD. Relationship between bacterial flora in sputum and functional impairment in patients with acute exacerbations of COPD. Chest 1999; 116:40–46.
261. Wilson R. Outcome predictors in bronchitis. Chest 1995; 106 (suppl):53S–57S.
262. Grossman R. Guidelines for the treatment of acute exacerbations of chronic bronchitis. Chest 1997; 112 (suppl 6):311S–313S.
263. Flaherty KR, Saint S, Fendrick AM, Martinez FJ. The spectrum of acute bronchitis: using baseline factors to guide empirical therapy. Postgrad Med 2001; 109:39–47.
264. Dewan NA, Rafique S, Kanwar B, Satpathy H, Ryschon K, Tillotson GS, Niederman MS. Acute exacerbation of COPD: factors associated with poor treatment outcome. Chest 2000; 117:662–671.
265. Ball P, Harris J, Lowson D, Tillotson G, Wilson R. Acute infective exacerbations of chronic bronchitis. Q J Med 1995; 88:61–68.
266. Miravitlles M., Murio C., Guerrero T. Factors associated with relapse after ambulatory treatment of acute exacerbations of chronic bronchitis. DAFNE Study Group. Eur Respir J 2001; 17:928–933.
267. Destache CJ, Dewan N, O'Donohue WJ, Campbell JC, Angelillo VA. Clinical and economic considerations in the treatment of acute exacerbations of chronic bronchitis. J Antimicrob Chemother 1999; 43 (suppl A): 107–113.
268. Grossman R, Mukherjee J, Vaughan D, Eastwood C, Cook R, LaForge J, Lampron N. A 1-year community-based health economic study of ciprofloxacin vs usual antibiotic treatment in acute exacerbations of chronic bronchitis. The Canadian Ciprofloxacin Health Economic Study Group. Chest 1998; 113:131–141.
269. Casaburi R, Briggs DD Jr, Donohue JF, Serby CW, Menjoge SS, Witek TJ Jr. Group US Tiotropium Study. The spirometric efficacy of once-daily dosing with tiotropium in stable COPD. A 13-week multicenter trial. Chest 2000; 118:1294–1302.
270. Van Noord JA, Bantje ThA, Eland MA, Korducki L, Cornelissen PJG, Dutch Tiotropium Study Group. A randomised controlled comparison of tiotropium and ipratropium in the treatment of chronic obstructive pulmonary disease. Thorax 2000; 55:289–294.
271. Ferreira IM, Hazari MS, Gutierrez C, Zamel N, Chapman KR. Exhaled nitric oxide and hydrogen peroxide in patients with chronic obstructive pulmonary disease. Effects of inhaled beclomethasone. Am J Respir Crit Care Med 2001; 164:1012–1015.
272. Weir DC, Gove RI, Robertson AS, Burge PS. Corticosteroid trials in non-asthmatic chronic airflow obstruction: a comparison of oral prednisolone and inhaled beclomethasone dipropionate. Thorax 1990; 45:112–117.

273. Weir DC, Burge PS. Effects of high dose inhaled beclomethasone dipropionate, 750 micrograms and 1500 micrograms twice daily, and 40 mg per day prednisolone on lung function, symptoms, and bronchial hyperresponsiveness in patients with non-asthmatic chronic airflow obstruction. Thorax 1993; 48:309–316.

274. Wempe JB, Postma DS, Breederveld N, Kort E, van der Mark TW, Koeter GH. Effects of corticosteroids on bronchodilator action in chronic obstructive lung disease. Thorax 1992; 47:616–621.

275. Nishimura K, Koyama H, Ikeda A, Tsukino M, Hajiro T, Mishima M, Izumi T. The effect of high dose inhaled beclomethasone dipropionate in patients with stable COPD. Chest 1999; 115:31–37.

276. Rutgers SR, Koeter GH, van der Mark TW, Postma DS. Short-term treatment with budesonide does not improve hyperresponsiveness to adenosine 5'-monophosphate in COPD. Am J Respir Crit Care Med 1998; 157:880–886.

277. Auffarth BK, Postma DS, De Monchy JGR, van der Mark TW, Boorsma M, Koeter GH. Effects of inhaled budesonide on spirometric values, reversibility, airway responsiveness, and cough threshold in smokers with chronic obstructive lung disease. Thorax 1991; 46:472–477.

278. Watson A, Lim TK, Joyce H, Pride NB. Failure of inhaled corticosteroids to modify bronchochostrictor or bronchodilator responsiveness in middle-aged smokers with mild airflow obstruction. Chest 1992; 101:350–355.

279. Bourbeau J, Rouleau MY, Boucher S. Randomised controlled trial of inhaled corticosteroids in patients with chronic obstructive pulmonary disease. Thorax 1998; 53:477–482.

280. Senderovitz T, Vestbo J, Frandsen J, Maltbaek N, Noorgaard M, Nielsen C, Kampmann JP. Steroid reversibility test followed by inhaled budesonide or placebo in outpatients with stable chronic obstructive pulmonary disease. Respir Med 1999; 93:715–718.

8

Management of Bronchiectasis and Cystic Fibrosis

**VIVEK N. AHYA and
GREGORY TINO**

University of Pennsylvania
  School of Medicine and
University of Pennsylvania Medical Center
Philadelphia, Pennsylvania, U.S.A.

STANLEY B. FIEL

Drexel University College of Medicine
Philadelphia, Pennsylvania, U.S.A.

I. Overview

The true incidence of bronchiectasis is unknown because many patients are asymptomatic in early stages of the disease. Cystic fibrosis (CF) is the best understood of the bronchiectatic diseases; it is the most common cause of diffuse bronchiectasis in the United States and Europe. While many of the disease management modalities initially developed for the treatment of bronchiectasis have been applicable in CF, a growing number of clinical trials in CF have resulted in new treatment approaches that have also proven useful in bronchiectasis. This chapter provides a review of the pathogenesis, diagnosis, and management of bronchiectasis unrelated to CF. We then turn to the pathophysiology of CF, presenting the current tools and theoretical constructs in the medical management of CF. Due to space limitations, many of the related medical conditions and psychosocial issues—such as diabetes mellitus, sinusitis, nasal polyps, osteoporosis, and reproductive health in cystic fibrosis—are not covered.

II. Bronchiectasis: An Introduction

Bronchiectasis remains an important cause of advanced lung disease. If unrecognized, it may lead to progressive deterioration in lung function and cor pulmonale. Although this disease has been recognized for many years and was first described by Laennec in his classic monograph in 1819, bronchiectasis remains a difficult diagnostic and management problem for today's physicians (1).

Bronchiectasis is characterized pathologically by marked irreversible bronchial dilatation caused by recurrent inflammation and infection. Historically, the predominant causes of bronchiectasis were viral and severe necrotizing bacterial pneumonias. Modern medical interventions—powerful antibiotics and routine immunizations—have significantly reduced the incidence of this disease and changed the spectrum of likely etiologies.

III. Pathology

Over the years there have been a number of attempts to classify the pathological patterns of bronchiectasis. The most widely used classification system was established in 1950 by Reid, who compared the pathological abnormalities in surgically resected lobes to those seen by bronchography. Although these patterns of bronchiectasis—cylindrical, varicose, and saccular—have been useful for correlating anatomical findings with radiographic abnormalities, they do not impact the clinical management of the patient. Many of the diseases which cause bronchiectasis can produce any or all of the patterns described by Reid.

Permanent changes in bronchial anatomy result from inflammatory destruction of the elastic and muscular components of the airway wall. In general, the macroscopic findings of bronchiectasis include abnormally dilated airways with or without mucous plugs extending to the pleural surface, dilated bronchial arteries, edematous and inflamed bronchial mucosa, and numerous abscesses. Microscopic findings include thickened, dilated bronchial walls with inflammatory infiltrate, replacement of the ciliated airway epithelium with squamous or columnar epithelial cells, mucous gland hypertrophy, and formation of extensive anastomotic networks between the bronchial and pulmonary circulation. In advanced cases, there is loss of the elastin layer and destruction of bronchial muscle and cartilage (2).

IV. Pathophysiology

Regardless of etiology, an initial inflammatory insult damages the bronchial wall to a sufficient degree to predispose the patient to recurrent bacterial infections. This then perpetuates the vicious cycle of additional inflammation and bronchial destruction.

The severe bronchial inflammation is easily visible in pathological specimens. Several studies have also demonstrated elevations in surrogate markers of inflammation in patients with bronchiectasis. For example, it has been shown that the exhaled breath of patients with bronchiectasis has significantly elevated levels of hydrogen peroxide (a product of activated neutrophils) when compared to that of age-matched normal controls (3).

The sputum from patients with bronchiectasis is of three types: mucoid, mucopurulent, and purulent (4). The degree of sputum purulence has been directly correlated with the severity of bronchial inflammation. Purulent sputum contains increased numbers of neutrophils and neutrophil products, such as myeloperoxidase and neutrophil elastase (5). Interestingly, bronchial biopsy specimens from stable patients with only mucoid sputum also demonstrate increased numbers of neutrophils. This suggests that a stimulus for neutrophil recruitment persists even after resolution of the acute inflammatory event (6,7). Airway secretions from patients with bronchiectasis have recently been shown to have increased levels of proinflammatory cytokines, such as interleukin-8 (IL-8), interleukin-1 (IL-1), and tumor necrosis factor alpha (TNF-α). In addition, the inflammatory cells in the airway release toxic substances, such as collagenases and proteolytic enzymes, that can promote airway damage (8–11).

Investigations into discovering novel ways to reduce airway inflammation are in progress. Recently an in vitro study demonstrated that blocking neutrophil chemotactants such as IL-8 and leukotriene B4 reduced the ability of sputum from patients with bronchiectasis to attract neutrophils (12). Hopefully, these types of studies will lead to a better understanding of the destructive inflammatory stimulus and lead to new therapeutic options.

V. Etiology

Bronchiectasis is the end result of numerous pathogenic processes that predispose the patient to recurrent bronchial inflammation and infection (13). Historically, severe bacterial infections in childhood with *Staphylococcus aureus*, *Streptococcus pneumoniae*, *Bordetella pertussis*, and *Mycobacterium tuberculosis* were most commonly associated with bronchiectasis (14). Disease could be focal or multifocal, depending on the anatomical distribution of the infection. Viral infections with influenza or measles virus also caused bronchiectasis, either by inflicting direct bronchial damage or by permitting superinfections with bacterial pathogens. In the modern era, immunizations and early treatment with broad-spectrum antibiotics have significantly reduced acute primary respiratory infections as common causes of bronchiectasis. One notable exception has been the emergence of pulmonary infections with atypical mycobacterial organisms, especially *Mycobacterium avium-intracellulare* (MAI). These granulomatous infections, once presumed to represent benign colonization in the healthy host, have now been clearly implicated in the development of focal or multifocal bronchiectasis (15). Numerous genetic, immunological, and environmental conditions have also been associated with the development of bronchiectasis. Some of these conditions are discussed below.

VI. Focal Bronchiectasis

The primary cause of focal bronchiectasis in developing countries is severe childhood infection (Table 1). In developed countries, endobronchial narrowing or obstruction with resultant postobstructive infection is probably the most important cause of focal bronchiectasis. Endobronchial obstruction can be caused by aspiration of a foreign object, endobronchial tumors, amyloidosis, external compression from enlarged lymph nodes, vascular structures, mediastinal fibrosis or malignancy, and by inflammatory disorders of the airway such as relapsing polychondritis or ischemic injury. Although further discussion of these entities is beyond the scope of this article, it is important to consider them in the differential diagnosis (16).

VII. Diffuse Bronchiectasis

Diffuse bronchiectasis, because it is the result of widespread injury to the airways, is more likely to be progressive and to cause respiratory insufficiency (Table 2). Many causes of diffuse bronchiectasis have been described; they can be categorized into several general groups, including genetic disorders, immunodeficiency states, conditions characterized by an exaggerated immune response, toxic inhalation, diffuse infection, and miscellaneous disorders (17). These conditions are discussed in further detail below.

Table 1   Causes of Focal Bronchiectasis

Bronchial obstruction
  Tumor
  Foreign body
  Inspissated secretions
  Lymphadenopathy
Infection
  Bacterial pneumonia
  Childhood infection (pertussis, measles)
  Mycobacterial
Miscellaneous
  Bronchopulmonary sequestration
  Allergic bronchopulmonary aspergillosis (ABPA)

Table 2 Causes of Diffuse Bronchiectasis

Infectious
  Bacterial
  Mycobacterial
  Bordetella pertussis
  Viral (measles, influenza)
Genetic
  Cystic fibrosis
  Dyskinetic cilia syndrome
  α_1-Antitrypsin deficiency
Immunodeficiency states
  Chronic granulomatous disease
  Common variable immunodeficiency
  X-linked agammaglobulinemia
  HIV infection
Immune-mediated
  Allergic bronchopulmonary aspergillosis
  Rheumatoid arthritis
  Sjögren syndrome
  Inflammatory bowel disease
  Systemic lupus erythematosus
  Chronic lung allograft rejection
Anatomical abnormalities
  Swyer-James syndrome
  Williams-Campbell syndrome
  Mounier-Kuhn syndrome
  Traction bronchiectasis
Miscellaneous
  Yellow-nail syndrome
  Toxic fume inhalation

A. Genetic Predisposition

As mentioned earlier, the most common genetic predisposition to bronchiectasis is CF. Another autosomal recessive disorder that can cause diffuse bronchiectasis is primary ciliary dyskinesia. Normal ciliary function is critical for clearing airways of bacteria and other proinflammatory particles. Structural ciliary abnormalities such as absence of the dynein arms (a large, multisubunit ATPase that interacts with microtubules to generate force) renders airway cilia immotile, and predisposes the patient to frequent infections of the airways and sinuses. Male patients are often infertile, since dyskinetic or immotile cilia also impair sperm motility. Recently, several genes encoding various subunits of dynein arms have been identified, and further study should provide new insight into structural and functional ciliary abnormalities (18).

B. Immunodeficiency States

Patients with immune system impairments, especially humoral immunodeficiency states, have a predilection for developing recurrent respiratory infections with encapsulated micro-organisms. Patients with both primary and secondary hypogammaglobulinemias have been reported to have an increased incidence of bronchiectasis (19,20).

Defects in cell-mediated immunity may also contribute to bronchiectasis by impairing optimal development of a humoral response to bacterial infection or by predisposing the patient to recurrent viral infections. Recently, HIV-infected patients have been described to have progressive pulmonary disease from bronchiectasis (21).

C. Excessive Immune Responses

An exuberant or inappropriate immune response may also cause bronchiectasis. For example, bronchiectasis from allergic bronchopulmonary aspergillosis (ABPA) is caused by severe airway inflammation from an exaggerated host response to colonizing *Aspergillus* organisms (22). Several autoimmune diseases—such as rheumatoid arthritis, Sjögren's syndrome, and inflammatory bowel disease—have also been associated with bronchiectasis (23). A unique example of immune-mediated bronchial injury occurs in the setting of lung transplantation. The alloimmune response leads to bronchiolar inflammation and eventually fibrosis and obliteration. These obstructed airways hinder clearance of airway secretions; thus patients are likely to have recurrent airway infections and to develop bronchiectasis (24).

D. Anatomical Abnormalities

Certain anatomical abnormalities can also predispose the patient to diffuse bronchiectasis. Traction applied to the airway from parenchymal recoil in patients with pulmonary fibrosis can cause bronchial dilatation and subsequent pooling of airway secretions. This may lead to recurrent infection and bronchiectasis (25).

Another disorder, known as the Mounier-Kuhn syndrome, is defined by diffuse abnormal dilatation and atrophy of muscular and elastic tissues of the trachea and bronchi (26). These large floppy airways can result in pulmonary obstruction, impaired cough mechanics, and retention of mucus, which can lead to frequent pneumonias and bronchiectasis. Bronchiectasis has also been associated with a rare congenital disorder known as the Williams-Campbell syndrome, which is characterized by a deficiency of cartilage in subsegmental bronchi, and results in collapse of distal airways during expiration and airway obstruction (27).

E. Atypical Mycobacterial Infection

Although infections are less likely to cause bronchiectasis in this era, an important exception is infection due to atypical mycobacterial organisms. In the United States, there has been an increase in the prevalence of patients with chronic infection from atypical mycobacterial organisms (28). The most common respiratory pathogens are *Mycobacterium avium-intracellulare* (MAI) and *Mycobacterium kansasii*. Traditionally, nontuberculous mycobacterial pulmonary infections were thought to have a predilection for patients with an underlying chronic lung disease or defects in cell-mediated immunity. Often, these patients presented with an upper lobe fibrocavitary disease that mimicked tuberculosis. Positive cultures from otherwise healthy patients were felt to simply represent benign colonization. Recently, however, it has become clear that these organisms are pathogenic in healthy hosts and can cause progressive pulmonary disease, which may ultimately lead to bronchiectasis (15,29,30). A recent autopsy study of several patients with MAI infection and bronchiectasis demonstrated extensive granulomatous inflammation in association with bronchiectatic airways. Immunohistochemical techniques and pathological evaluation indicated that MAI infection was likely the cause of the destructive changes (31).

Unfortunately, it has been difficult to predict which patients will develop progressive disease. Many reports have described the occurrence of MAI infection and bronchiectasis, especially in the right middle lobe or lingula, in thin, healthy elderly women without underlying parenchymal disease or history of tobacco smoking. The term *Lady Windermere syndrome* was subsequently coined to describe this unusual pattern of infection and lung disease (32). Why these patients are particularly prone to develop infection and disease is unclear. Attempts to more specifically identify which patients are most likely to develop progressive lung disease from atypical mycobacterial infection have been disappointing so far. In a small study, 57 patients with previously diagnosed MAI were followed for more than 12 months without treatment. This study suggested that certain characteristics—such as an elevated erythrocyte sedimentation rate (ESR), C-reactive protein (CRP), and serum carbohydrate antigen 19-9 (CA19-9), as well as increased neutrophils in the bronchoalveolar lavage—might predict a group of patients with a high risk of developing progressive disease in the absence of treatment (33,34).

F. Toxic Substances

Inhalation or ingestion of numerous substances has been reported to be associated with bronchiectasis. Some of these toxins include smoke, anhydrous ammonia, mustard gas, gastric acid, mineral oil, and paraquat (35–39). Almost any substances that can acutely damage bronchiolar epithelium can initiate a process leading to irreversible bronchiolar damage and bronchiectasis.

G. Miscellaneous

As mentioned above, any process that initiates bronchial inflammation and damage can trigger a vicious cycle of infection, additional inflammation, and increased airway damage. Occasionally, however, the mechanism of bronchiectasis development cannot be readily explained. One such example is the yellow-nail syndrome, a rare disorder in which patients develop yellow nails, pleural effusions, lymphedema, and bronchiectasis. Although the lymphedema and pleural effusions are though to arise from hypoplasia or atresia of the lymphatic system, the etiology of the bronchiectasis remains a mystery. Some have hypothesized that bronchiectasis may be secondary to hypoplasia of the bronchial lymphatics or due to immunodeficiency from the loss of immunoglobulin loss (40).

VIII. Clinical Features

A. Symptoms

The hallmark of the disease is persistent or recurrent cough with production of purulent sputum, typically greater than 20 mL per day. Many patients have systemic symptoms such as fever, anorexia, and weight loss. Sinusitis is often present as well. Hemoptysis is usually scant but occasionally can be life-threatening. In the later stages of disease, patients develop progressively increasing dyspnea and symptoms of cor pulmonale.

B. Physical Examination

Physical examination, although often normal, may reveal clues to suggest bronchiectasis. Fetid breath is a classic but now rarely seen sign. Auscultation of the chest reveals diffuse or focal rales and rhonchi. Signs of airway obstruction such as wheezing, a prolonged expiratory phase, or a midinspiratory squeak may be present. Digital clubbing can be seen, as can evidence of cor pulmonale.

Physical findings can also suggest a more specific etiology. For example, vasculitic skin lesions or joint deformities may indicate that a collagen vascular disease is present. Nasal polyposis should alert the clinician to the possibility of CF.

C. Radiology

The plain chest radiograph may be normal in up to 20% of cases. When present, findings include "tram tracks" representing thickened bronchial walls, cystic spaces with or without air-fluid levels, nonspecific increase in bronchovascular markings, atelectasis, and hyperinflation (14). High-resolution computed tomography (HRCT) scan of the chest, on the other hand, has excellent sensitivity for detecting bronchiectasis and is now considered to be the diagnostic imaging tool of choice. HRCT findings include mucoid impaction; cystic airways with air-fluid levels; the "signet ring" sign, which occurs when the internal bronchial diameter is larger than its adjacent pulmonary artery (Fig. 1), and tram tracks, or dilated airways extending to mediastinal pleura or within 1 cm of the costal pleura, reflecting the lack of normal tapering of bronchi (Fig. 2) (41).

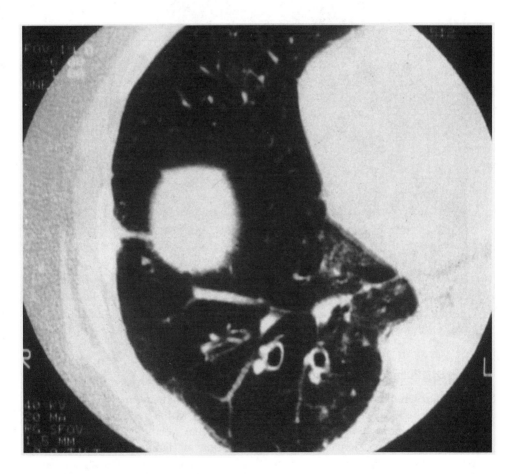

Figure 1 "Signet rings" of a bronchiectatic lung. Two signet rings comprising a pulmonary vessel adjacent to dilated bronchi are identified.

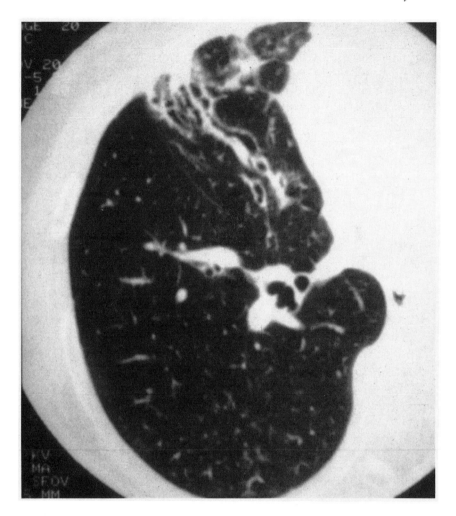

Figure 2 "Tram tracks" of a bronchiectatic lung. Tram tracks, representing dilated airways with thickened bronchial walls extending into the periphery, are clearly visible.

D. Pulmonary Function Testing

Pulmonary function testing (PFT) can also be normal in early or localized disease. The most common pattern is obstruction with a reduced FEV_1 and FEV_1/FVC ratio and hyperinflation. PFT may demonstrate a mixed obstructive and restrictive pattern in the setting of significant atelectasis or parenchymal fibrosis from chronic inflammation. In advanced disease, arterial hypoxemia and hypercapnia may be present and the diffusion capacity is reduced. In addition, patients with bronchiectasis often have abnormal airway hyperreactivity (42).

E. Diagnostic Approach

Once the diagnosis of bronchiectasis is entertained, an organized diagnostic plan should be employed. An important distinction should be made between focal and diffuse bronchiectasis, as the differential diagnosis and diagnostic approach diverge. Figure 3 outlines our approach.

Historically, bronchography was considered the "gold standard" for the diagnosis of bronchiectasis. This test required deposition of contrast material within the airways and was associated with significant risks such as

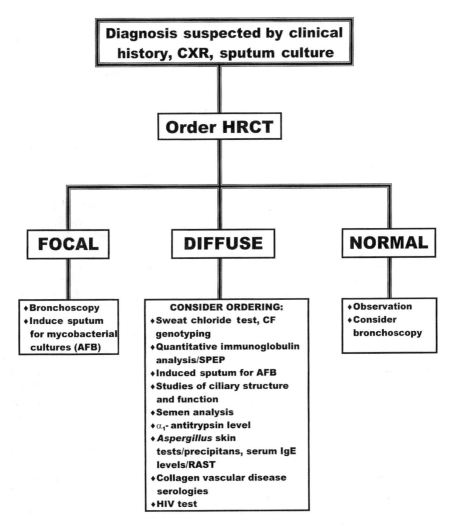

Figure 3 Diagnostic algorithm for bronchiectasis. CXR, chest x-ray; HRCT, high-resolution computed tomography; AFB, acid fast bacilli; SPEP, serum protein electrophoresis; RAST, radioallergosorbent test.

bronchospasm, increased ventilation/perfusion $(\dot{V}/\dot{Q})$ mismatching, and anaphylaxis. Currently, this test has been largely replaced by HRCT. With its 1.5-to 5.0-mm cuts, HRCT has a greater than 90% sensitivity and specificity for diagnosing bronchiectasis (14,42a).

F.   Specific Diagnostic Tests

Patients who have diffuse bronchiectasis warrant additional testing to identify a primary etiology. Some of these studies include the following:

>Sweat chloride and DNA testing for CF (43)
>Sputum culture to evaluate for atypical mycobacterial infections
>Quantification of immunoglobulins and HIV testing to evaluate for immunodeficiency states
>Ciliary studies and semen analysis to determine if a ciliary disorder is present (44)
>*Aspergillus* skin testing and serum IgE levels to identify patients with possible ABPA (22)

G.   Bronchoscopy

Fiberoptic bronchoscopy generally does not have a diagnostic role in patients with diffuse bronchiectasis unless it is used to obtain adequate microbiological samples for mycobacterial, fungal, or other unusual organisms. Patients with focal bronchiectasis, on the other hand, should undergo bronchoscopic inspection of the airways to exclude endobronchial obstruction as a nidus for recurrent infection. Bronchoscopy can be useful in patients with significant hemoptysis to localize an area of bleeding or to tamponade a bleeding segment until an appropriate therapeutic intervention can be performed (45).

H.   Sputum Analysis

Sputum culture may be helpful in guiding therapy and predicting prognosis in patients with bronchiectasis. The organisms most commonly isolated from the sputum of patients with bronchiectasis include *Staphylococcus aureus*, *Streptococcus pneumoniae*, *Haemophilus influenzae*, *Moraxella catarrhalis*, and mucoid and nonmucoid *Pseudomonas aeruginosa*. Numerous studies have demonstrated that patients with CF who are colonized with *P. aeruginosa* have more severe bronchiectasis and a more rapid decline in lung function. Recent studies in patients with bronchiectasis unrelated to CF reveal similar findings (46). Currently, it is not clear whether *P. aeruginosa* colonization is a cause or simply a marker of rapidly declining lung function. It has been clearly shown, however, that patients colonized by *P. aeruginosa* have a poorer quality of life than patients with similar lung function but colonized by other organisms (47).

I. Medical Treatment: Supportive

Since bronchiectasis is defined by irreversible damage to the bronchi, supportive therapy is aimed at treating acute flares and slowing the decline in lung function. Treatment can be general and applied to all patients with bronchiectasis or specific to the underlying cause of bronchiectasis.

J. Antibiotics

Antibiotics remain the most important therapeutic option for treating and preventing acute exacerbations of bronchiectasis. Surprisingly few data exist on the optimal duration, route of administration, and choice of antibiotics. The complex bacteriology of sputum in patients with bronchiectasis makes the selection of a narrow-spectrum antimicrobial agent based on sputum analysis difficult. In fact, a recent retrospective study of 123 patients with bronchiectasis, revealed that greater than 47.5% of patients demonstrated two or more organisms in the sputum, and 8.5% had four or more pathogens (48). It is clear that the antibiotic chosen should provide superior coverage for *S. pneumoniae* and *H. influenza*. Particular attention must be paid to the presence of *S. aureus* and *P. aeruginosa*, especially in patients with CF. Mild flareups may be treated with oral antibiotics.

Intravenous Antibiotics—Acute Flare

Patients who fail oral therapy often require intravenous antibiotics, administered on either an inpatient or outpatient basis. Treatment of patients with *Pseudomonas* infections should generally be with two sensitive antibiotics to reduce the risk of developing antibiotic resistance. Important antipseudomonal antibiotics include the fluoroquinolones, ureidopenicillins, carbapenems, some third- and fourth-generation cephalosporins, and aminoglycosides (1,49,50). Optimal duration of treatment has not yet been determined, but most clinicians generally recommend a prolonged course of antibiotics, often up to several weeks.

Chronic Antibiotic Therapy

As mentioned earlier, patients with both CF and non-CF bronchiectasis who are colonized with *P. aeruginose* have a more rapid decline in lung function than patients colonized with other organisms (46,51). This evidence has prompted many clinicians to chronically treat infected patients with antipseudomonal antibiotics to prevent acute exacerbations and reduce bacterial load. The development of oral antipseudomonal agents such as the quinolones has made this an even more attractive therapeutic option. However, few data exist to support a beneficial role of chronic therapy, even with rotating antibiotics. In addition, the risk of developing strains of highly resistant organisms precludes recommending this mode of therapy routinely.

Aerosolized Antibiotics

Another form of treatment that is gaining increasing popularity is the use of aerosolized antibiotics. This form of drug delivery has important theoretical advantages. The drug can be delivered at very high concentrations directly into the airways without significant systemic absorption, thus reducing the risk of antibiotic resistance and systemic toxicity (52). Although aerosolized anti-biotics were first developed in the 1950s, side effects such as bronchospasm prevented their widespread utilization. Improvements in antibiotic preparation and delivery as well as coadministration with a beta agonist to prevent bronchospasm have made aerosolized antibiotics an important therapeutic option. Recently, studies in patients with CF have demonstrated that aerosolized tobramycin resulted in improved lung function, decreased *Pseudomonas* sputum density, decreased use of systemic antipseudomonal antibiotics, and decreased number of days spent in the hospital (53). Smaller studies have suggested a similar benefit in patients with bronchiectasis from other causes (54–56). The largest study was a randomized, placebo-controlled multicenter study of 74 adult patients with bronchiectasis unrelated to CF or allergic bronchopulmonary aspergillosis and high-density *P. aeruginosa* cultured from the sputum. The study divided the 74 patients into two treatment groups, one receiving 300 mg of inhaled tobramycin twice a day for 4 weeks and another receiving placebo. After a 2-week observation period, the patients in the treatment group reported greater improvements in their general health status (62 versus 38%) and a 4.8 $\log_{10}$ reduction in sputum *P. aeruginosa* density. However, the patients in the treatment group did not demonstrate an improvement in lung function (60). Further study is required to see whether inhaled antibiotics will play an important role in the treatment of non-CF bronchiectasis. In the future, newer delivery systems such as dry-powder metered-dose inhalers may make the administration of inhaled antibiotics less cumbersome, less costly, and less time-consuming than with current nebulized techniques (58).

Other Antibiotics

Investigations into the treatment of diffuse panbronchiolitis—another disorder characterized by progressive decline in lung function, copious sputum production, and colonization with *P. aeruginosa*—indicate that long-term macrolide therapy can stabilize disease progression and reduce the incidence of acute exacerbations (59,60). These studies prompted a small, double-blind, placebo-controlled pilot investigation into the role of low-dose erythromycin in patients with bronchiectasis. Ten control patients received placebo tablets and 14 patients with idiopathic bronchiectasis received 500 mg of erythromycin twice a day for 8 weeks. At the end of the study period, the treatment group had better forced expiratory volume in 1 sec (FEV_1), forced vital capacity (FVC), and 24-hr sputum volume (61). The mechanism behind this improvement in both diseases remains unclear. It is certainly not due simply to its antimicrobial effect, since most of the study patients were heavily colonized with *P. aeruginosa*, a pathogen that is not susceptible to macrolide antibiotics. Laboratory studies suggest that the beneficial effect may be due to immunomodulatory properties such as inhibition of neutrophil chemotaxis (62). If these results confirmed by larger studies, macrolide therapy may become an important, relatively nontoxic option for chronic suppressive therapy.

K. Airway Clearance

Since airway secretions obstruct airflow and promote respiratory infections, it seems logical that methods to promote airway clearance would be beneficial. These measures called are called *bronchopulmonary hygiene physical therapy*. They include chest percussion, postural drainage, humidification, and special coughing and forced exhalation techniques with or without the use of flutter valves or vibrating vests. Although studies demonstrating benefit have been conducted primarily in patients with CF, it is reasonable to extend these observations to patients with bronchiectasis unrelated to CF (63).

L. Bronchodilators

Since many patients with bronchiectasis develop obstructive lung disease, bronchodilator therapy has been advocated for treatment; however, the mechanisms of airway obstruction in bronchiectasis are not well understood. It is likely that multiple factors such as mucosal edema, plugging of small airways with purulent secretions, glandular hyperplasia, peribronchiolar fibrosis, and bronchiolar collapse during expiration—in addition to bronchial hyperresponsive—play a role in the development of airway obstruction (64). In addition, these drugs may be beneficial because of their theoretical ability to enhance mucociliary clearance. Unfortunately but not unexpectedly, small observational studies have demonstrated only marginal improvement in lung function. Thus, bronchodilator administration should be reserved only for patients who demonstrate increased airway hyperreactivity and a response to therapy (65). Clinicians have also used long-acting beta$_2$ agonists. Further research is necessary to determine whether these drugs have a therapeutic role.

M. Anti-inflammatory Agents

Anti-inflammatory therapy with systemic steroids is not recommended for most patients with bronchiectasis because of numerous side effects of therapy and the potential for increased risk of infection secondary to immunosuppressive properties. Bronchiectasis patients with immune-mediated disorders may require steroid therapy to control disease activity, although the benefit of long-term inhaled steroids remains to be demonstrated. A recent preliminary investigation reported that a short course of inhaled steroids did not significantly change lung function measured by spirometry despite reduction in certain inflammatory mediators in the sputum (66,67). Further investigation is needed to determine whether longer courses of inhaled steroids will improve lung function and delay disease progression.

Inhaled indomethacin has been reported to diminish bronchorrhea in patients with bronchiectasis unrelated to CF. Unfortunately this small study did not report a benefit in other objective measures (68).

N. Mucolytics

Mucolytic therapy to thin respiratory secretions and facilitate their clearance has been advocated by some experts in the management of bronchiectasis. In 1994, an aerosolized recombinant human DNase (rhDNase) was approved as a mucolytic agent for the management of CF exacerbations after a large phase III multicenter trial investigating this agent revealed a modest (5%) improvement in FEV_1 as well as a slight reduction in disease exacerbations after 6 months of therapy (69). Whether the cost of therapy and its modest benefit justifies its use in CF remains controversial. A recently completed trial in patients with idiopathic bronchiectasis revealed that rhDNase was not effective and perhaps even harmful (70). Another mucolytic agent, bromhexine, was evaluated in a small study. At high doses, patients demonstrated reductions in sputum production and cough. Unfortunately, these patients did not show improvements in lung function (71). Thus, at this time, there is little evidence to recommend widespread use of mucolytics in patients with bronchiectasis.

O. Inhaled Hyperosmolar Agents

In experimental studies, hypertonic saline has been demonstrated to improve tracheobronchial clearance, probably by osmotically inducing liquid to move onto the airway surface and hydrating dry inspissated secretions (72). Inhaled dry-powder mannitol has been reported to have similar effects on tracheobronchial clearance. Two small studies by the same group investigated the effect of inhaled dry-powder mannitol in patients with bronchiectasis and reported that dry-powder mannitol increases short-term tracheobronchial clearance and reduces mucus retention. No adverse side effects were noted (73,74). Future investigation will determine if hyperosmolar agents will result in clinically meaningful improvements.

P. Miscellaneous

All patients with bronchiectasis should receive routine immunizations. These immunizations should include an annual influenza vaccine and a pneumococcal vaccine, administered every 5 to 10 years. Other measures to consider include supplemental oxygen therapy for hypoxemic patients either at rest or on exertion, optimization of nutritional status, pulmonary rehabilitation, and noninvasive positive-pressure ventilation for associated hypercapnia.

Q. Medical Treatment: Specific

Patients who develop bronchiectasis related to underlying primary diseases should be treated with appropriate specific therapy. For example, infections with MAI should be treated with clarithromycin or azithromycin with rifabutin and ethambutol. Patients with allergic bronchopulmonary aspergillosis or collagen vascular disease often require treatment with corticosteroids to control disease activity and patients with hypogammaglobulinemia may benefit from immunoglobulin replacement therapy.

R. Surgical Therapy

The first surgical resection of bronchiectasis was performed in 1901; since that time, a variety of operations including segmentectomy, lobectomy, and pneumonectomy have been utilized for treatment of this disease. With improvements in medical therapy, the role of surgical therapy has become increasingly controversial. However, patients should be considered for surgical resection if they have localized disease that is refractory to medical management or if they are unwilling to undergo chronic medical therapy. Preoperative management typically involves aggressive chest physiotherapy and a 2-week course of appropriate antibiotic therapy. During anesthesia, an epidural catheter is placed for regional anesthesia and continued for several post-operative days. The patient is then intubated with a double-lumen tube to avoid spillage of purulent secretions into the contralateral lung. In the present era, mortality for surgery in appropriate patients is about 2%, with most deaths occurring in patients undergoing complete pneumonectomy. In a recent retrospective review of the surgical experience with bronchiectasis at the Mayo Clinic, over 80% of the patients reported complete relief or significant improvement in their preoperative symptoms. However, complications from surgery occurred in over 24% of patients and included atelectasis requiring bronchoscopy, prolonged air leak (over 10 days), empyema, pneumonia, postoperative hemorrhage requiring reexploration, arrhythmias, postpneumonectomy pulmonary edema, respiratory failure, and bronchopulmonary fistula formation (75).

An absolute indication for surgery is the presence of massive hemoptysis, especially if adequate control cannot be achieved by interventional techniques such as bronchial artery embolization (76,77). Some have argued that because of the low surgical mortality and high chance of curing or significantly improving patients' symptoms, surgery should be performed earlier in the disease course (78). In the absence of randomized or controlled clinical trials comparing medical therapy to surgical intervention, it is not possible to make a general recommendation for earlier intervention.

Patients with severe end-stage lung disease from generalized bronchiectasis should be referred to a specialized center for consideration of bilateral or heart-lung transplantation (79,80).

S. Prognosis

As mentioned previously, the prognosis for patients with bronchiectasis has improved dramatically with vaccinations and powerful medications. Nevertheless, bronchiectasis and its related complications continue to provide a significant challenge for afflicted patients and their physicians. Prognosis depends primarily on the underlying etiology of bronchiectasis as well as local factors such as airway colonization by resistant virulent organisms. Overall, patients with CF appear to have the poorest prognosis, with mean survival into the fourth decade, while patients with bronchiectasis from other causes tend to have a better but more varied prognosis.

Patients with bronchiectasis continue to pose new diagnostic and management challenges. However, with a thorough, well-conceived evaluation, the disease can be suspected, diagnosed, and treated, with resulting improved survival and quality of life for the patient (2).

IX. Cystic Fibrosis: An Introduction

Cystic fibrosis (CF) is the most common inherited autosomal recessive genetic disease among Caucasians. There are approximately 30,000 children and adults in the United States with CF, and the frequency of this disorder among North American Caucasians is about 1 per 2500 live births (81). CF is a disorder of the exocrine glands characterized by thick viscous mucous secretions that lead to dysfunction in several organ systems, including the airways, pancreas, hepatobiliary, and reproductive systems. CF pathology alters the chemical properties of mucus so that it obstructs airways and exocrine ducts. In the lungs, the thickened mucus fosters bacterial growth leading to frequent pulmonary infections and a chronic inflammatory state. CF lung disease is characterized by thick occlusive mucus, recurrent infection, and inflammation that impair local host defense mechanisms and lead to progressive bronchiectasis (Fig. 4). This vicious disease cycle repeats throughout the patient's lifetime, eventually leading to respiratory failure, which is the principal cause of death in CF patients. The most common clinical manifestations of CF include endobronchial inflammation (i.e., chronic recurrent airways obstruction), pancreatic insufficiency with intestinal malabsorption, meconium ileus, fatty infiltration of the liver, focal biliary cirrhosis, glucose intolerance, and an increased risk of heat prostration arising from severe salt depletion. Improved medical management—particularly of CF pulmonary disease, which accounts for approximately 98% of CF mortality—has transformed CF from a fatal disease where patients rarely reach adulthood to a chronic illness with most patients attaining adulthood. Because of these improvements in disease management, the average life expectancy in CF is into the fourth decade of life.

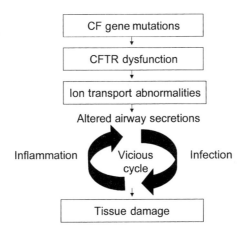

Figure 4 Vicious cycle of CF pathophysiology.

X. Pathogenesis

A. Cystic Fibrosis Transmembrane Conductance Regulator

The most important advancement in elucidating the pathogenesis of CF came in 1989, with the identification and cloning of the gene on the long arm of chromosome 7, which encodes the cystic fibrosis transmembrane conductance regulator (CFTR) (82). CFTR is found on the apical cell membrane of secretory epithelial cells. In normal individuals, this protein regulates the exchange of sodium and chloride across epithelial cells. Thus, CFTR has a significant role in controlling the volume and electrolyte composition of airway secretions. Absence or dysfunction of CFTR results in dysfunctional or altered chloride channels. While the clinical manifestations of CF appear to result from defective transepithelial ion transport, scientific controversy remains regarding the underlying mechanism of this effect. A number of theories— some conflicting—have been suggested. They include defective intracellular vesicular function, leading to abnormal protein processing, loss of the ability to regulate other membrane transporting proteins, defective airway submucosal gland secretion, abnormal composition of airway surface liquid (ASL), a reduction in intrinsic antimicrobial action, and hyperabsorption of airway fluid (83).

One hypothesis proposes that defective or absent CFTR affects chloride retention at the cell membrane, causing dehydration of the ASL. This alteration in ASL causes an increased uptake of sodium and water at the cellular membrane. Some researchers believe that this series of osmotic compensations facilitates the production of abnormally viscous mucus and greatly contributes to—if not causes—impaired ciliary clearance, fostering a bacterial breeding ground in the CF airways (84,85).

An alternate hypothesis suggests that chloride and sodium are not absorbed by airway epithelia, which leads to ASL that is normally hydrated but with a significantly increased chloride concentration (86). This hypothesis is bolstered by studies suggesting that beta defensins, antimicrobial peptides found in the normal lung, become inactive in high chloride concentrations, thus facilitating survival of lung pathogens (86a). If the ASL contains too much salt for normal antimicrobial action, the addition of a hypotonic solution to dilute ASL will ameliorate the condition. If the ASL is underhydrated, the addition of hypertonic solution to draw water into the airway could be efficacious. Several drugs aimed at treating ion imbalances are currently under investigation.

Final resolution of the pathophysiology of CF will significantly enhance opportunities for the development of new therapeutic agents and improve the medical management of declining pulmonary function in CF patients. Bolstered in the interim by new findings such as these, researchers continue to investigate mechanisms, techniques, and agents to ameliorate the ion imbalance present in the CF airways.

B. CFTR Class Mutations

To date, more than 1000 CFTR mutations have been identified. Five classifications have been designated to describe functional differences at the cellular level and identify mechanisms of CFTR dysfunction (Table 3) (87). Class I mutations result in defective CFTR synthesis, leading to a defect in protein production and a loss of function. Class II mutations cause defective processing of the CFTR protein. Class III mutations affect the regulation and activation of CFTR at the cell surface, and class IV mutations interfere with chloride channel conductance. Class V mutations result in reduced CFTR synthesis.

The class II delta F508 mutation—a phenylalanine deletion on the gene— is the most prevalent of the CF mutations. Individuals with this delta F508 mutation make up $\sim 70\%$ to 75% of the North American CF population. The delta F508 mutation produces defects in folding of the CFTR protein; thus the defective protein is rejected and degraded prematurely. A small amount of defective CFTR is incorporated into the cell membrane and results in abnormal functioning of the chloride channel. Delta F508 is usually accompanied by pancreatic insufficiency.

Genotype-phenotype relationships in CF are not predictable. The correlation between genotype and severity of airways disease is low, but the relationship between genotype and pancreatic insufficiency is robust. Genotype also influences the presence of meconium ileus, age at diagnosis, sweat chloride concentrations, and male infertility.

Table 3 Examples of CFTR Mutations Organized by Classification of the Defect in CFTR Biosynthesis

Type	Genotype	Phenotype	Defect	Drugs that may improve phenotype
Class I (64)	G542X 621 + 1 G→T 3905insT W1282X R553X 1717-1 G→A	PI	No CFTR protein No cell surface chloride transport	Gentamicin G418
Class II (64)	ΔF508 N10303K (P574H)[a] (Δ455E)[a]	PI	Defective CFTR processing Defective CFTR trafficking No cell surface chloride transport	Chemical chaperones CPX Phenylbutyrate Deoxyspergualin
Class III (64)	G551D G551S	PI	Defective chloride channel Regulation Reduced or absent cell surface Chloride transport	Genistein Pyrophosphate
Class IV (64,66)	R117H R334W G314E R347P (ΔF508)[a] P574H	PS	Reduced chloride conductance Reduced levels of cell surface Chloride transport	Genistein Milrinone Phenylbutyrate
Class V (64)	3849 + 10kb C→T 2789 + 5 G→A 3272 − 26 A→G A455E 3120 + 1 G→A 1811 + 1.6kb A→G 5T[b]	PS	Normal CFTR channels Reduced numbers of normal CFTR Reduced cell surface chloride Transport	Genistein Milrinone Phenylbutyrate

[a]Some mutants have features of more than one class of defect.
[b]5T is an intron variant that is not considered a bonafide mutation but renders different levels of expression of a normal CFTR.
Source: Ref. 87.

XI. Current Medical Management of CF

At present, there is no definitive treatment or cure for CF. Medical management of airways disease is based on three principles: airway clearance, management of infection, and management of inflammation. Recent improvements in median survival (almost 40 years) reflect more aggressive medical management tactics, which are sometimes accompanied by complementary and alternative medicine (i.e., meditation and relaxation techniques, chiropractic) to combat the clinical consequences of the basic CF defect.

A. Airway Clearance Techniques

Thick neutrophil-derived mucous secretions retained in the airways are a hallmark of CF. They contribute to its pathophysiology in three ways: (1) mechanical obstruction of airways with viscous secretions, leading to a ventilation/perfusion regulatory defect and overinflation of the lungs; (2) exacerbation of infection due to decreased clearance and stagnation of mucus; and (3) exposure to inflammatory mediators, such as cytokines and leukotrienes, as well as increased levels of elastase, which result in bronchospasm and eventually progressive parenchymal injury and fibrosis.

Mobilization of secretions by means of percussion and postural drainage is the cornerstone intervention in CF. Removal of secretions helps preserve lung function where peak expiratory flow rates are too low to clear mucus even with coughing. Airway clearance is still an essential part of daily CF care. In mild to moderate CF, it may be required only once a day, while patients with severe airways disease may need to undergo physical clearance of airways several times a day. It may be performed in conjunction with aerosolized bronchodilators or mucolytics to aid in mobilization and expectoration of secretions.

In a study of older children with mild to moderate CF airways obstruction, patients receiving regular chest physiotherapy (CPT) showed an increase in peak expiratory flow rate (PEFR) 30 min after therapy. When CPT was discontinued for 3 weeks, both FVC and peak flow rates were reduced. This decrement was reversible with resumption of CPT (88).

Postural drainage uses gravity-assisted positions to aid in clearance; it can be performed alone by the patient or with assistance. Postural drainage with percussion is the only airways mobilization technique available for use in infants and small children, and it is frequently effective in older CF patients as well. The major drawback of this technique is that if the patient requires assistance, issues of autonomy and quality of life may be negatively affected. In addition, some patients experience symptoms of gastroesophageal reflux following postural drainage. A variety of forced expiratory maneuvers such as "huff and cough" also have been introduced and can be performed in conjunction with postural drainage or percussion. Autogenic breathing (self-drainage) uses controlled breathing techniques to optimize airflow in the bronchi and mobilize secretions. Although autogenic breathing can be time-consuming, it is easy to learn and can be practiced anywhere without assistance. In addition, some patients find autogenic breathing to be relaxing.

Several devices including the Flutter (VarioRaw SA), the Positive Expiratory Pressure (PEP) mask (Astra Meditech), the Vibracare percussor (General Physiotherapy), and the Vest Airway Clearance System (Advanced Respiratory Inc.; a product formerly marketed as the THAIRapy® vest) are also available. The Flutter is a small handheld device that resembles a pipe. When patients exhale into it, rapid air pressure fluctuations are induced in the airways, helping to vibrate secretions loose. PEP masks may help prevent airways closure during expiration and increase collateral ventilation. The mask may also be adapted to deliver bronchodilators prior to postural drainage. The Vest Airway Clearance System is a chest wall oscillator, worn as a vest, which is coupled to a compressor. The vest is expensive and not portable; some patients find it uncomfortable or restrictive.

Personal characteristics—such as activity level, lifestyle, age, and psychosocial issues—may play a role in determining the selection of one or more therapeutic techniques. Different types of airway clearance techniques may be needed for each patient. Carefully matching patient and airway clearance techniques will enhance adherence.

B. Exercise

The role of exercise in CF care cannot be overemphasized. As with any individual, it enhances cardiovascular fitness and functional capacity, helps manage mood, and improves quality of life. In CF patients, exercise has been shown to slow the decline in lung function (89), and it is considered an essential adjunct to airway clearance techniques. Patients should be encouraged to participate in aerobic exercise such as walking, cycling, or swimming three to four times per week.

C. Nutrition

Chronic undernutrition is a serious and common problem in CF patients. In children, undernutrition may lead to growth failure and pubertal delay. Undernutrition in CF results from the increased energy expenditures created by the extra effort required to breathe, the battle against chronic infection, and abnormalities in digestion and nutrient absorption. While pancreatic exocrine insufficiency is probably the leading cause of impaired nutrient absorption, reduced bile salts and increased intestinal mucus may also contribute.

Pancreatic insufficiency in CF results in intestinal malabsorption of fats, proteins, and, to some degree, carbohydrates. Mean fecal fat excretion is high, resulting in poor weight gain, chronic abdominal discomfort, deficiency of subcutaneous fat and muscle tissue, and deficiencies of fat-soluble vitamins (A, D, E, K), essential fatty acids, and albumin. Patients with pancreatic insufficiency require lifelong lipase replacement therapy. Close monitoring is important due to the increased risk of fibrosing colonopathy that has been associated with high-dose lipase therapy (90). A recent CF Adult Care Consensus Report (91) recommends the prescription of proprietary brands of pancreatic enzyme products, since generic products may not dissolve in an equivalent manner and could be less effective.

CF patients should eat a high-calorie diet that is unrestricted in fat, with liberal salt intake and vitamin-plus-mineral supplementation. It is generally recommended that CF patients receive 120 to 150% of the recommended daily allowance for caloric intake (92,93) to counter the unfavorable energy balance. Children experiencing growth problems may benefit from supplemental nighttime enteral feedings. The importance of maintaining body weight has been demonstrated in several studies. Body wasting has been shown to be a significant predictor of survival independent of pulmonary function, arterial blood oxygen, or carbon dioxide tensions (94). The same study found that as nutritional status worsens, the probability of death for any percent predicted FEV_1 increased significantly. Patients who were >110% over their ideal body weight had a better prognosis than those whose weight was normal. This supports findings from an earlier study in which better median survival rates were associated with better nutrition in one center when compared to another (95).

D. Complementary and Alternative Medicine in CF

Complementary and alternative medicine (CAM)—such as acupuncture, massage, various forms of energetic medicine and hypnosis—may have a place in CF palliative care. These therapies may provide relief for some of the symptoms that accompany CF, such as pain, anxiety, and moodiness or depression. However, these therapies must be considered as *complements* rather than alternatives to standard medical therapy.

Few controlled studies of CAM have been carried out in CF, but trials of acupuncture, chiropractic, and massage have shown these approaches to be beneficial in asthma, which shares some characteristics with CF, including airways inflammation, bronchial obstruction, increased airways secretions, dyspnea, and wheezing.

E. Acupuncture

Acupuncture is one of the more accepted and regulated forms of CAM available in the United States. Along with other eastern medical approaches, acupuncture aims to correct the flow of vital energy, or *qi* in Chinese medicine, throughout the body. According to this system, diseases arise from blockages or weakness in *qi*. *Qi* can be unblocked by inserting fine needles or deeply pressing (acupressure) on active points along energy lines known as meridians. Acupuncture may reduce pain by enhancing the flow of endorphins or by modifying efferent pain signals.

A 1997 National Institutes of Health (NIH) Consensus Report (96) concluded that acupuncture was safe and effective in treating several conditions, including pain and asthma, where it can be used as part of a comprehensive management program or as an acceptable alternative capable of reducing the need for inhaled corticosteroids. Acupuncture may be helpful in managing some common CF symptoms, including gastrointestinal problems, sinusitis, pain, and anxiety.

F. Massage

Massage has been used successfully to improve lung function, reduce anxiety, and to improve mood in asthma. In one study (97), children with asthma received either 30 min of massage by parents over three areas of the body or standard relaxation exercises. In the massage group, children aged 4 to 8 years of age showed improvements in peak flow rates (PFR), FVC, and FEV_1. Both parents and children were found to have reduced levels of anxiety. In 9- to 14-year-olds, salivary cortisol levels were lower. Stress reduction may play an important role in CF as well and may be reflected by improved immune and nutritional status and reduced dyspnea (97).

G. Self-Hypnosis

A trained physician or an accredited hypnotherapist can teach self-hypnosis in several sessions. This technique appears to be beneficial in reducing anxiety and controlling the discomforts of the disease and may enhance patients' feelings of self-control. In a study of CF patients ≥ 7 years of age, 49 subjects agreed to be taught self-hypnosis by their pulmonologists (98). The study subjects used the technique for relaxation, relief of pain associated with headache and medical procedures, to improve the palatability of medications, and for control of other CF symptoms.

H. Herbal Remedies and Nutritional Supplements

Herbal remedies and nutritional supplements are used by many patients with chronic diseases such as CF. Informal investigations done at Boston Children's Hospital suggested that pediatric and adult CF patients use herbal remedies and nutritional supplements often. Such products could include herbal teas and remedies; vitamin, mineral, and nutritional supplements; homeopathic remedies; and probiotics (to restore intestinal function while receiving antibiotics). Importantly, the unsupervised use of high-dose vitamins and herbs is most likely to cause harm. Throughout the literature, herbal remedies have been reported to be associated with untoward side effects, herb–drug interactions and, in some cases, serious medical conditions (99,100). For example, Gingko biloba inhibits platelet aggregation and has been associated with cases of spontaneous bleeding. In CF patients, use of Ginkgo biloba may contribute to hemoptysis. St John's wort, widely promoted as an antidepressant, also may produce dry mouth, dizziness, confusion, gastrointestinal symptoms, allergic reactions, and fatigue. Patients need to be informed of possible risks when choosing these products and of the importance of consulting with their physicians before initiating any changes to their established routine of care.

A variety of nontraditional therapies may be helpful to some CF patients. Although the medical benefits are presently controversial, not objectively measurable, and have yet to be determined, the majority of herbal and nutritional supplements do no harm and patients may experience a strong placebo effect. The simple act of making choices about complementary therapies may enhance a patient's feelings of being in control, which can be therapeutic. Data have demonstrated that reductions in anxiety and depression, as well as increases in physical and psychological comfort, may be attained through alternative therapies, including therapeutic touch, reiki (a Japanese form of healing), and aromatherapy. Physical movement and positioning techniques—such as the Feldenkrais method, the Alexander technique, and yoga—may improve breath control, strength, and flexibility.

XII.   Medical Management of CF Airways Disease

Increasingly, data suggest that early and aggressive treatment of CF airways disease is important to preserve lung function, improve health status, and enhance patients' quality of life. Chronic infection and pulmonary exacerbations (PEs) contribute to CF morbidity and mortality both directly and indirectly.

A.   Treatment of Infection

Improvements in antibiotic therapy represent the single most important contribution to increased longevity and improved quality of life that is now attainable for CF patients. Antibiotics are employed to reduce bacterial load, decrease airways inflammation, and reduce airways obstruction. In the management of PEs, antibiotics improve the CF patient's clinical status and may be used as prophylactic maintenance therapy to suppress chronic infection and slow disease progression. In very young or newly colonized CF patients, it may be possible to achieve bacterial eradication with early, aggressive antibiotic intervention.

The predominant organisms found in CF airways evolve based on age and health status of the patient. At birth, *S. aureus* predominates, however, by the onset of the second decade of life, *P. aeruginosa* becomes more prevalent. *H. influenzae*, *Stentotrophomonas maltophilia*, and *Burkholderia cepacia* are less prevalent. Colonization by *Pseudomonas* is significant because, once established in the airways, it evolves to the "mucoid" form. Mucoid strains produce a thick layer of biofilm composed of alginate, an exopolysaccharide. The mucoid biofilm confers several survival advantages that render the organism difficult to control. It is believed to be important in aiding bacterial adherence to epithelial cells and in making the organisms resistant to mucociliary

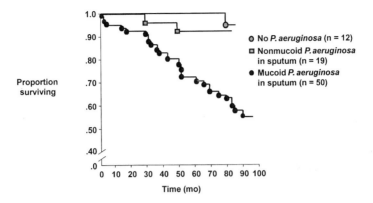

Figure 5 Presence of mucoid *Pseudomonas aeruginosa* in cystic fibrosis patients. (From Ref. 103.)

clearance. It may protect against destruction by antibacterials as well as by leukocytes and phagocytes (101,102). Figure 5 shows the significant survival differences according to the presence or absence of mucoid strains of *P. aeruginosa* (103).

The presence of mucoid strains of *P. aeruginosa* is virtually pathognomonic of CF; mucoid *Pseudomonas* is rarely observed in the airways infection of any non-CF patient.

B. Bacterial Eradication

One of the most aggressive approaches in the management of CF airways disease today is bacterial eradication. At the initial detection of infection, aggressive targeted intervention offers clinicians the best chance to eradicate the organism(s). Successful eradication is more likely to be achieved in very young or newly colonized CF patients and in CF patients colonized with nonmucoid strains of *P. aeruginosa*. Eradication may require an extended period of antibiotic therapy. In a study (104) of 15 newly colonized CF patients receiving 80 mg tobramycin formulated for inhalation twice daily for 12 months, *P. aeruginosa* eradication was achieved in 14 of 15 subjects. Eradication was maintained in most patients after the termination of therapy.

A sputum culture can provide valuable treatment information to optimize the impact of antibiotic therapy. Annual or more frequent culture intervals in CF patients can provide clinicians with an accurate assessment of the airways bacterial status and facilitate the choice of appropriate antibiotic therapy to minimize loss of lung function and disease progression.

C. Treatment of Pulmonary Exacerbations

Antimicrobial therapy is universally employed for the treatment of Pulmonary exacerbations (PEs) characterized by acute, subacute, or gradual worsening in pulmonary symptoms. PEs may be due to viral infection, bacterial colonization, or allergic reactions, or they may be idiopathic. Recent data from the *Epidemiologic Study of Cystic Fibrosis* indicate that the correlation between the initiation of antibiotic therapy and slowing the decline in lung function in patients with PEs is highly inconsistent (105). On closer examination, researchers recognized that the inconsistent finding might reflect the absence of definitive clinical criteria for diagnosis of a PE. This led the group to establish a consensus panel and to develop a list of common signs and symptoms associated with PEs (Table 4) (106).

Acute or subacute PEs can be treated with intravenous, oral, or inhaled antibiotics. The goal of parenteral therapy in treating a severe PE is to return the patient to his or her baseline pulmonary status and level of sputum production. Intravenous treatment is generally reserved for patients with severe PEs, and treatment duration of 2 to 3 weeks is usually sufficient. In selecting an antibiotic regimen, it is important to select appropriate antibiotics on the basis of sputum cultures and bacterial sensitivity testing and to administer the agents at sufficient dosages. Antibiotic combination therapy is less apt to lead to the emergence of drug-resistant bacterial strains. This is likely due to the potential synergy of the combined agents against *P. aeruginosa*. Drug synergy testing also is available to aid in harnessing this effect. In addition, clinicians must be aware that differences in the volume of distribution and rate of elimination in CF patients require higher doses and shorter dosing intervals for many antibiotics (107).

Table 4 Signs and Symptoms of Pulmonary Exacerbation

Increased cough

Increased sputum production and/or a change in appearance of expectorated sputum

Fever ($\geqslant 100.5\,°F$ ($\leqslant 38\,°C$) for at least 4 hr in a 24-hr period) or more than one occasion in the previous week

Weight loss $\geqslant 1\,kg$ or 5% of body weight associated with anorexia and decreased dietary intake or growth failure in an infant or child

School or work absenteeism (because of illness) in the previous week

Increased respiratory rate and/or rate of breathing

New findings on chest examination (e.g., rales, wheezing, crackles)

Decreased exercise tolerance

Decreased FEV_1 of $\geqslant 10\%$ from previous baselines study within past 3 months

Decreased hemoglobin saturation (as measured by oximetry) of $\geqslant 10\%$ from baseline value within past 3 months

New finding(s) on chest radiograph

Source: Adapted from Ref. 106.

Although the choice of specific agents depends on susceptibility testing and local resistance patterns, combinations such as an aminoglycoside (e.g., gentamicin or tobramycin) plus a beta lactam (including the semisynthetic penicillins and cephalosporins such as ceftazidime) are frequently employed in this setting. If *S. aureus* is isolated in sufficient concentrations to require treatment, a penicillin/sulbactam combination may be used. However, increasing resistance may mandate the use of vancomycin or clindamycin. Because of the potential complexity of such therapy, clinicians need to routinely review all aspects of a medical regimen to assess patient adherence and response to treatment as well as the potential side effects of medications.

Home intravenous therapy, which is less costly and less disruptive of the patient's life, may be appropriate for those who do not require hospitalization otherwise; however, close monitoring of the patient's status and progress is critical. For patients with frequent PEs or those who require long-term home care, a central intravenous line may be placed. A professional home care company may be able to provide valuable support and to permit the use of home care during parenteral therapy.

Oral antibiotic therapy is useful only in mild or moderate PEs and to reduce the use of IV antibiotics. Oral therapy is limited by the small number of drugs that remain effective against *P. aeruginosa*. Oral ciprofloxacin is frequently used and is efficacious in patients who have not received many courses of it for prior exacerbations. However, resistance is a problem with ciprofloxacin monotherapy; it is best reserved for brief, intermittent courses. Aerosolized antibiotics may be given in place of oral antibiotics for mild to moderate exacerbations, but there is a paucity of data supporting their use.

While PEs are clearly an important contributor to the loss of lung function in CF patients, spirometry measurements continue to decline even in the absence of an acute exacerbation in patients without severe pulmonary disease (Fig. 6) (108). Therefore, the assumption supporting symptom-guided treatment, such that the majority of tissue damage leading to decreased pulmonary function largely results from PEs, may be erroneous. This finding would suggest the need for intermittent chronic therapy rather that symptom-guided treatment. Several approaches to prophylactic maintenance therapy have been developed.

D. Chronic Suppressive Antibiotic Therapy

Some centers—notably in Denmark—have employed scheduled parenteral antibiotic therapy several times per year for suppressive therapy. Retrospective and uncontrolled studies have suggested that scheduled therapy with 2-week courses of parenteral antibiotics four times per year, regardless of symptoms, may improve survival (109). However, a recent randomized trial comparing

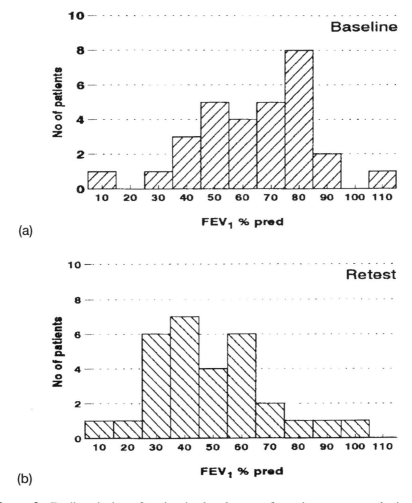

Figure 6 Declines in lung function in the absence of a pulmonary exacerbation in cystic fibrosis patients without severe disease. Distribution of FEV_1 at (a) baseline testing (mean 69% predicted) and (b) repeat testing (mean 54% predicted) in 30 subjects, showing significant decline in FEV_1 in the period between assessments (mean time interval, 6.3 years). (From Ref. 108.)

scheduled prophylactic maintenance therapy versus standard therapy for exacerbations showed no difference in outcome between groups (110). Inhaled antibiotic therapy using tobramycin for inhalation (TOBI) represents the most widely studied form of chronic prophylaxis in CF patients.

E. Inhalational Therapy in Cystic Fibrosis

Nebulized Antibiotics

Systemic antibiotic therapy via the oral or parenteral route is often associated with systemic toxicity (e.g., the hearing loss and kidney damage seen with systemic aminoglycosides). In addition, respiratory tract infection often shows a poor response to systemic antimicrobial therapy due to low drug penetration into bronchial secretions and the altered pharmacokinetic disposition of certain classes of antimicrobials. These drawbacks have led to experimentation with the direct application of antimicrobials into the respiratory tract to maximize therapeutic effect by delivering higher concentrations of the drug directly to the site of infection. Direct application may also reduce dosages necessary for therapeutic effect.

Over the past 50 years, antibiotic inhalational therapy using gentamicin, tobramycin, colistin, carbenicillin, ticarcillin, neomycin, polymixin, amphotericin B, and ceftazidime have been used with some success in patients with CF. However, these drugs, which were formulated for intravenous use, presented significant drawbacks, including bronchospasm, coughing, irritation, bad taste, foaming when aerosolized, and incompatibility with normal saline. Many of these side effects were related to preservatives and other additives found in the intravenous solutions that were nebulized.

The formulation of antibiotics for aerosol delivery is significantly different from that for intravenously delivered drugs. Tolerability, effectiveness of therapy, and drug delivery depend on osmolality, pH, and antibiotic concentration. The solution should be free of any preservatives (e.g., such as phenol—a neurotoxin, and bisulfites) that may cause bronchospasm when administered by inhalational therapy. Preservatives may also have a bad taste or may slow nebulization rates. The addition of detergents, such as methylparaben, can affect particle size and drug dispersal in situ. Osmolality affects cough and bronchoconstriction. The osmolality of inhaled solutions should be >150 and $<550 \, \text{mOsm/kg}$ (111). It has been shown in asthma patients that acidic aerosols can cause bronchoconstriction in direct proportion to pH. Airway resistance may increase significantly if the pH is $\leqslant 2$ (112,113).

It is challenging to deliver consistent levels of drug by inhalation because of anatomical differences and variations in breathing patterns and coughing. Certain drugs—including antibiotics, recombinant products, and other large peptides—must be delivered via nebulizer. Agents to be nebulized should not foam or precipitate. Nebulizers are intrinsically inefficient, delivering only part of the dosage to the lungs. Factors that can influence pulmonary drug distribution include aerosol particle size, aerosol velocity, inspiratory flow rate, lung volume, and airway caliber. When particles are too small in size, they are deposited mainly in the alveoli. This can increase systemic absorption and the antibiotic may fail to reach the site of infection. Particles that are too large are deposited more proximally in the oropharynx and the central airways. The choice of nebulizer/compressor system has an important impact on the pharmacodynamic results for all inhaled therapeutics. Not all aerosol delivery systems are recommended for all inhaled drugs.

A metanalysis of the use of continuous nebulized gentamicin, tobramycin, colistin, and ceftazidime prepared from intravenous formulations in the treatment of chronic *Pseudomonas* infections concluded that they decreased bacterial load, decreased the frequency of PEs requiring supplemental antibiotic therapy, and decreased the decline in pulmonary function (114). However, because of the adverse effects associated with the use of "home brews" based on intravenous formulations of antibiotics, tobramycin formulated for inhalation (TOBI) is the most commonly used. Inhaled colistin is widely used in Europe. However, bronchospasm is a common problem. Controlled trials are required to establish its benefits relative to other inhaled drugs.

In a multicenter, double blind, placebo-controlled study of intermittent high-dose tobramycin for inhalation, 520 patients were randomized to receive either 300 mg nebulized tobramycin twice daily in 28-day on/off cycles for 6 months or placebo (53). At 24 weeks, the TOBI group showed a 10% increase in FEV_1 versus a 2% decrease in controls ($p < 0.001$). The tobramycin group also showed decreased significant reduction in *Pseudomonas* density in sputum and was less likely than placebo-treated patients to be admitted to hospital or to require intravenous antibiotics.

An open-label extension study (115) demonstrated continued safety and maintenance of pulmonary function above normal for up to 96 weeks. These findings suggest that the reduction of *Pseudomonas* density by chronic intermittent suppressive therapy helps preserve lung function in CF.

The Microbiology of Nebulized Antipseudomonal Therapy

The long-term microbiological consequences of chronic antipseudomonal therapy are still unclear, and there is concern over the emergence of resistant *Pseudomonas* strains as well as the level of intrinsically aminoglycoside-resistant strains of *B. cepacia* and *S. maltophilia*, the possible decreases in tobramycin susceptibility and deleterious effects on the microbiology of the CF airway. Several studies (116–118) showed the emergence of tobramycin-resistant strains within 3 to 6 months of continuous therapy and an increase in tobramycin minimum inhibitory concentration (MIC). The resistant *Pseudomonas* strains regained sensitivity after the discontinuation of aerosol therapy. These data suggest that parenteral antibiotic breakpoints may not predict response to combination intravenous therapy in CF patients (119).

While antimicrobial susceptibility testing is recommended to optimize the management of PEs and for surveillance, further studies are needed to elucidate the significance of bacterial resistance in the management of CF airways disease.

Inhaled Mucolytic Therapy

Tenacious mucus plugs are virtually universal in CF. The viscosity of CF airway mucus is partly due to the breakdown products of bacteria, neutrophils, and other cellular debris. DNase cleaves DNA found in this debris, decreasing its viscosity and facilitating expulsion of mucus.

In the 1990s, an aerosolized recombinant human DNase (rhDNase) became available as a mucolytic. In a recent study of 474 young CF patients with mild to moderate airways disease (mean FVC 102% predicted, mean FEV_1 95–96% predicted), patients receiving rhDNase showed an early improvement in FEV_1, which was maintained for the course of the study (Fig. 7) (120). At week 96, the difference in FEV_1 between active treatment and placebo was about 3%. FEF_{25-75}, which was 85% predicted at the start of the study, was increased nearly 4% in the treatment group and declined by approximately 4% from baseline in the placebo group. By the end of the study, 24% of the placebo group and 17% of the treatment group had had at least one PE. It was calculated that the risk of a first PE was reduced by about 34% in the rhDNase group (119). The authors concluded that early intervention with rhDNase [Pulmozyme (dornase alfa recombinant) Inhalation Solution,

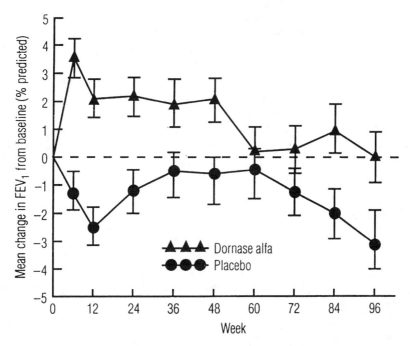

Figure 7   Mean change in FEV_1 from baseline—a 2-year trial of dornase alfa. Vertical bars represent $\pm$ standard error of the mean. (From Ref. 120.)

manufactured by Genentech, Inc., South San Francisco, CA] results in a substantial reduction in exacerbations and a sustained benefit in lung function. These finding clearly demonstrate the importance of early initiation of therapy to prevent loss of lung function, even in young patients who initially present with mild lung disease. It has been suggested that aggressive treatment in young or newly diagnosed patients may be more beneficial to long-term health and maintenance of pulmonary function than later aggressive therapy, when lung function has already shown a significant decline.

In a large phase III randomized, double-blind placebo-controlled trial, patients treated with DNase 2.5 mg daily or twice daily for 24 weeks showed reductions in PEs (28 and 37% in the once- and twice-daily groups, respectively). Time spent in the hospital (~ 1.2 fewer days over 6 months) and on intravenous antibiotics (~ 2.5 fewer days) was not substantially different between the two treatment groups and the placebo group. Nevertheless, even those patients who did not show improvements in spirometry showed decreased *P. aeruginosa* density (69). Postmarketing surveillance data has confirmed the safety of Pulmozyme, and it is appropriate to administer the drug during either a stable period or during a PE. Hoarseness, voice alteration, and chest pain were occasionally seen.

Currently 49% of CF patients in the United States use rhDNase (121). It is unclear at present which patients benefit from this therapy, as some individuals show very little clinical response. However, many clinicians believe that its impact on the frequency of respiratory tract infections is significant enough to support therapeutic trials in many patients. Some studies suggest that results after 3 months of rhDNase therapy predict response at 12 months (122).

Inhaled hypertonic saline has been suggested as a mucolytic. It appears to improve mucociliary clearance and increases coughing. In a short trial of 6% hypertonic saline in patients with mild to moderate disease, patients reported improvements in the feeling of chest clearance. FEV_1 was improved 15% compared to results obtained with isotonic saline inhalation (123). Longer studies will be required before this therapy can be widely recommended for routine use.

Inhaled Bronchodilator Therapy

Bronchodilators may be of value in CF patients with airway hyperreactivity or those who have concomitant asthma. Nebulized beta-adrenergic agonists are the agents most commonly prescribed in this setting. Two studies (124,125) indicated that patients treated with albuterol showed a sustained reversal of the decline in lung function. Beta agonists are generally well tolerated by CF patients, although some show paradoxical decreases in flow rates after inhalation. Some patients may show greater improvement on the anticholinergic ipratropium bromide. This is particularly true of adults, who may have greater bronchoreactivity and secretions than younger CF patients.

Others may do best on a combination of a beta agonist and an anticholinergic agent. A therapeutic trial is warranted for patients whose bronchospasm is not sufficiently controlled by either therapy alone.

F. Treatment of Inflammation

It is clear that airways infection and inflammation account for most CF morbidity and mortality, but there is a continuing controversy as to which comes first. The traditional view has been that inflammation resulted from repeated bacterial infections in an environment of reduced mucociliary clearance and mucous stasis. However, later studies (126) suggested that airway inflammation is already present in the early neonatal period and may exist independently of infection. Several groups reported increased levels of the proinflammatory cytokine, interleukin-8 (IL-8) and of neutrophils and neutrophil-derived elastase in the bronchoalveolar lavage fluid of children as young as 4 weeks of age, even in the absence of infection (127,128). At this point, there is still controversy as to whether the regulation of the inflammatory response is abnormal in CF airways from birth or whether inflammation is secondary to infection.

While this question remains unresolved, several approaches currently exist to manage inflammation with the goal of reducing the rate of decline in lung function, slowing the progression of airways disease, and contributing to quality of life. The most frequently used at present are oral and inhaled corticosteroids and ibuprofen.

One study of alternate-day or daily prednisolone (2 mg/kg/day for 2 weeks followed by an additional 10 weeks at 1 mg/kg qod) showed improvements in lung function and decreased markers of inflammation (129). However, a large, randomized, multicenter trial compared alternate-day prednisone at either 1 or 2 mg/kg to placebo and found an increased incidence of cataracts, glucose intolerance and growth deficits (130). Although steroids were beneficial to long-term pulmonary function in patients infected with *P. aeruginosa*, the adverse effects are considered to be too great for routine use, particularly in growing children.

Inhaled corticosteroids have been proposed as a way of avoiding the systemic adverse events that occur with oral dosing. Studies using beclomethasone 400 µg/day (131) and budesonide (800 µg bid) (132) have failed to show a demonstrable benefit on markers in inflammation. Higher doses of inhaled corticosteroids may to be promising, but further study is needed before this approach can be safely recommended.

In another approach designed to manage inflammation, high-dose ibuprofen (20–30 mg/kg up to 1600 mg bid) was shown to slow the progression of lung disease in patients with mild CF ($FEV_1 > 60\%$), particularly in patients 5 to 12 years of age (133). In this 4-year double blind, placebo-controlled trial, patients were randomized to receive ibuprofen or placebo in addition to standard CF care. Intent-to-treat analysis after 4 years showed a 40% relative reduction in the annual rate of pulmonary decline in ibuprofen-treated patients. This group also gained 0.2% of ideal body weight while the placebo group lost nearly 4%.

Later analysis of these data showed the greatest benefit in patients aged 5 to 12 years who were adherent to therapy. These patients showed a decline in FEV_1 of approximately 1.5% per year compared to approximately 4.2% per year in placebo-treated patients.

While the use of anti-inflammatories is theoretically of benefit, the only agents available at present have drawbacks or limited applicability. The search for effective anti-inflammatory therapy with fewer side effects continues.

G. Lung Transplantation

Despite advances in all areas of CF care, 85% of patients die of lung disease. At present, bilateral lung transplantation is the only alternative to the treatment of end-stage CF airways disease. The first lung transplant in a CF patient was performed in 1983. Table 5 lists indications and contraindications for lung transplantation, although there is some variability by center.

Although these criteria may appear quite straightforward, in fact the decision to pursue lung transplantation is extremely complicated. Emotional and physical strength as well as significant psychosocial and financial resources are required to make the decision to undergo the procedure and to endure the long wait for an organ, which can be 18 to 24 months. The stresses on both patient and family are significant. Recovery can be debilitating and the requirement for lifelong immunosuppression adds to the stresses associated with transplantation.

The earliest lung transplants in CF patients consisted of en bloc heart and lung grafts from cadaver donors. However, this operation has been replaced by bilateral single-lung transplants with bibronchial anastomoses. Although some lung diseases can be treated with single-lung transplantation, this is not possible in CF patients because of the likelihood of transmission of infection

Table 5   Potential Contraindications for Lung Transplantation in Cystic Fibrosis[a]

Liver disease with significant hepatocellular dysfunction or portal hypertension
Severe malnutrition (<80% of ideal body weight)
Extensive pleural scarring from prior thoracic surgery
Ventilator dependence (excluding noninvasive ventilation)
Airway colonization with *Burkholderia cepacia*
Aspergilloma with extensive pleural reaction
Severe osteoporosis with history of vertebral compression fractures

[a]Policies regarding transplantation of patients with the above features vary among centers and none should be viewed as an absolute contraindication.
Source: Ref. 152.

from the remaining lung into the immunocompromised donor lung and the effect of rejection prophylaxis and treatment on the remaining native lung.

Recently, the technique of living-related lobar transplantation has been introduced, whereby a single lobe is transplanted from each of two donors. This approach appears to be as successful as cadaveric transplantation and potentially offers the advantages of scheduling the procedure, less stress on patient and family, the opportunity to better screen donors for infectious diseases, and less ischemia time for the donor organ.

The posttransplant prognosis is variable. One large series (134) is reporting 1- and 3-year survival rates of 84 and 61%, respectively. Most recipients of successful transplants have improved lung function, exercise tolerance, and quality of life.

XIII. The Future

At the beginning of the twenty-first century, we are entering what might be termed the "golden age" of CF therapeutics. With the data from the Human Genome Project and the new understanding of CF provided by the cloning of CFTR, we are closer than ever before to understanding the pathogenesis of this complex disease and to developing novel therapeutic strategies, like developing gene therapy to replace the mutated CFTR with wild-type CFTR in an effort to correct the underlying genetic defect. Pharmacological interventions include new approaches to the management of airway infection and inflammation, methods of improving the function of mutant CFTR, and ways of modifying airway ion transport. Another promising outgrowth of our deepened understanding of the genetic basis of CF is the burgeoning science of pharmacogenetics—genetics in the service of pharmacotherapy to elucidate how genes influence individual responses to treatment. This new science will expand our ability to tailor treatment based on microgenetic differences rather than employing the current "one size fits all" therapeutic paradigm.

The Cystic Fibrosis Foundation's Therapeutic Development Grants Program and its phase I and II clinical trials network, the Therapeutics Development Network, have been developed to aid in the advancement of promising therapies.

Two new strategies, high-throughput screening and DNA microarrays, have contributed significantly to drug discovery and overall understanding of CF therapeutics. High-throughput screening relies on robotic equipment to screen thousands of compounds per day based on lead compounds with some known activity against CF. At present, this technique is being used to screen for compounds that affect normal processing and functioning of CFTR mutants. The use of DNA microarrays is central to the translation of data generated by the Human Genome Project and other initiatives such as the *Pseudomonas* Genome Project. This technology involves the hybridization of fluorescent-labeled DNA/cDNA probes made from total cellular mRNA to an array of DNA representing human genes. This enables measurement of cellular levels of mRNA (135) and thus the simultaneous monitoring of the gene expression of thousands of genes. Microarray technology in conjunction with information about the genomic sequence of *P. aeruginosa* is presently being employed to put all of the *Pseudomonas* genes onto microchips that can be used to compare drug-resistant and drug-sensitive *P. aeruginosa*.

A. Gene Therapy

While all of the therapies discussed here are capable of ameliorating symptoms, preserving lung function, and improving quality of life, none is capable of reversing the underlying defect in CFTR.

Since the 1989 cloning of CFTR, hopes for an eventual cure have been pinned upon the development of gene therapy to replace the mutated CFTR gene with normal copies. At present, gene therapy is being targeted to CF airways disease. The therapy would likely be delivered during the neonatal period before the development of CF lung disease. Unfortunately, there is a wide divergence between what can be executed in vitro and what can be accomplished in a living system. Although in vivo gene transfer has been accomplished in CF, many barriers to successful gene therapy in CF remain (136–140).

Choice of Vector

Several different types of vectors, both viral and nonviral, have been developed and subjected to clinical testing in CF patients. For gene therapy to be effective, the normal gene must reach the cell and result in long-term expression of normal CFTR. Most groups have used viral vectors made from adenovirus (Ad) and adenovirus-associated viruses (AAV) for gene transduction into the cell. Drawbacks to these vectors include concerns about host safety and the immunological disposition of the viral vectors. Adenoviruses, which are naturally efficient at infecting the airways, have been used most often in human studies. Although efficient for gene transfer, these vectors had dose-limiting side effects arising from innate host immune responses to the viral proteins (140–142). Later generations of Ad vectors were manufactured with fewer or no viral genes, resulting in less destruction via cell-mediated immunity and prolonged expression in some animal models (143). Unfortunately, it has been shown that neutralizing antibodies to these vectors develop following repeated administration. At present, based on airway epithelial cell turnover rates, it is thought that successful gene therapy will rely on repeated administration at approximately monthly intervals.

Several strategies—including encasing the vector in a nonimmunogenic coating, modifying immunogenic epitopes or inducing tolerance to wild-type adenoviruses—have been proposed to circumvent this problem (144).

Adenovirus-associated vectors (AAVs) are also being developed. These vectors can enter the host cell genome and become latent, affording the possibility of long-duration gene transfer. So far, animal studies have not revealed immunogenic or inflammatory responses to these vectors.

Retroviruses, with some structural genes deleted to permit insertion of normal CFTR genes, integrate into the host cell genome and may be capable of long-duration expression. A modified Sendai virus vector, which may be capable of efficient gene transfer following only brief contact with host receptors, is also promising.

Cationic liposomes are lipid-DNA complexes that usually have a positive-charged cationic end, which enhances interaction with DNA, and a hydrophobic lipophilic end that promotes cellular uptake and membrane fusion (137,144,145). They enter the cell by endocytosis. These vectors appear to be less efficient than viral vectors, with a shorter duration of gene transfer, because they do not incorporate into the host cell genome and may not continue to be expressed with cell division. However, they appear not to stimulate immune and inflammatory responses, thus permitting repeat dosing.

Other hindrances that remain to be overcome before correction of the genetic defect can become a reality include how to penetrate the characteristic thick mucus and how to avoid mucociliary clearance systems. If this can be reliably effected, which airways cells will be the most appropriate targets for gene transfer, and do they have receptors for gene transfer at their apical surface? The highest levels of CFTR are expressed in the serous cells of the submucosal glands. Nebulized delivery of vectors is most apt to reach the surface epithelial cells that express much lower levels of CFTR. Is delivery to these cells sufficient to effect long-term expression of CFTR? Although it has been shown that 5% of normal CFTR function results in about 50% normal chloride transport (146), no clinical trials have reported correction of sodium ion transport. Will incomplete gene transfer be capable of restoring other functions of normal CFTR? These and other questions remain to be answered before the goal of gene therapy in CF can be reached.

B. Future Pharmacotherapy

While gene replacement therapy is the long-term hope of CF therapy, there are other avenues for correcting the underlying defect. One approach is to improve the function of CFTR, since it is estimated that as little as 10% of normal CFTR function is sufficient for the correction of chloride—though not sodium—channels (147). Although it has been shown that cooling CF cells or treating them with glycerol improved delta F508 folding and increased its delivery to its correct position on the apical cell membrane, at present neither method is practical for clinical use. High-throughput screening is being employed to search for compounds capable of promoting normal folding. Several compounds in the flavinoid and benzoquinoliziniums have shown promise in vitro.

In another approach, the aminoglycoside gentamicin has been shown to be capable of partially correcting stop mutations that result in the absence of functional CFTR. The application of gentamicin 0.3% nasal drops resulted in beneficial changes in nasal potential difference in patients who were homozygous for stop mutations (148).

Several xanthines, particularly 8-cyclopentyl-1,3-dipropylxanthine (CPX) and 4-phenylbutyrate, a drug used to treat Hansen's disease, appear capable of increasing chloride efflux in vitro (149,150), though neither has yet shown clinical efficacy. The isoflavone genistein, which can activate both mutant and normal CFTR, may be capable of potentiating drugs that increase CFTR on cell surfaces (150).

Another approach involves the development of synthetic cationic peptides that could act synergistically with antibiotics to replace normal lung antimicrobial peptides (defensins), which may be inactivated by high salt concentrations in the ASL of CF patients. However, the success of this approach will depend on the final verdict regarding the salt concentration of ASL in this disease (151). One new antibiotic based on the hypothesis that lung defensins function is compromised in CF, IB367, is presently in clinical trials.

XIV. Summary

The twentieth century witnessed a revolution in the diagnosis, understanding, and treatment of CF. It can no longer be considered a childhood disease whose victims rarely survive into adulthood, but rather as a disease of childhood onset with 37% of patients currently 18 years of age and older (121). It is now clear that the three-tiered approach to CF therapy—management of secretions, infection, and inflammation—is theoretically correct. The contributions of the gene revolution and related new drug development techniques will continue to add new therapies to the existing armamentarium. The highest hopes lie farther in the future, when gene therapy may well be capable of correcting the defect in CFTR early in life, before its absence or malfunction leads to the full cascade of clinical disease events.

References

1. Laennec RTH. De l'auscultation medicale, un traite di diagnostic des maladies des poumons et du coeur. Paris: Brossonet Chaude, 1819.
2. Swartz M. Bronchiectasis. In: Fishman A, ed. Fishman's Pulmonary Diseases and Disorders. New York: McGraw Hill, 1998:2045–2070.
3. Loukides S, Horvath I, Wodehouse T, et al. Elevated levels of expired breath hydrogen peroxide in bronchiectasis. Am J Respir Crit Care Med 1998; 158:991–994.
4. Stockley RA, Hill SL, Morrison HM, Starkie CM. Elastinolytic activity in sputum and its relation to purulence and lung function in patients with bronchiectasis. Thorax 1984; 39:408–413.
5. Stockley RA, Hill SL, Burnett D. Proteinases in chronic lung infection. Ann NY Acad Sci 1991; 624:257–266.

6. DiStefano A, Maestrelli P, Roggeri A. Up-regulation of adhesion molecules in the bronchial mucosa of subjects with chronic obstructive bronchitis. Am J Respir Crit Care Med 1995; 149:803–810.

7. Stockley RA, Shaw J, Hill SL, Burnett D. Neutrophil chemotaxis in bronchiectasis: a study of peripheral cells and lung secretions. Clin Sci (Colch) 1988; 74:645–650.

8. Fahy JV, Schuster A, Ueki I, et al. Mucus hypersecretion in bronchiectasis: the role of neutrophil proteases. Am Rev Respir Dis 1992; 146:1430.

9. Lloberes P, Montserrat E, Montserrat JM, et al. Sputum sol phase proteins and elastase activity in patients with clinically stable bronchiectasis. Thorax 1992; 47:88.

10. Sepper R, Konttinen YT, Ingman T, et al. Presence, activities, and molecular forms of cathespin G, elastase, alpha 1-antitrypsin and alpha 1-antichymotrypsin in bronchiectasis. J Clin Immunol 1995; 15:27.

11. Shum DK, Chan SC, Ip MS. Neutrophil-mediated degradation of lung proteoglycans: stimulation by tumor necrosis factor-alpha in sputum of patients with bronchiectasis. Am J Respir Crit Care Med 2000; 162:1925–1931.

12. Mikami M, Llewellyn-Jones CG, Bayley D, et al. The chemotactic activity of sputum from patients with bronchiectasis. Am J Respir Crit Care Med 1998; 157:723–728.

13. Cole PJ. Inflammation: a two edged sword—the model of bronchiectasis. Eur Respir J 1986; 69:6–15.

14. Fraser R, Colman N, Muller N, Pare P. Bronchiectasis and other bronchial abnormalities. In: Fraser and Pare Diagnosis of Diseases of the Chest, Vol 4 Philadelphia: Saunders, 1999:2265–2297.

15. Prince DS, Peterson DD, Steiner RM, et al. Infection with *Mycobacterium avium* complex in patients without predisposing conditions. N Engl J Med 1989; 321:863–868.

16. Liaw YS, Yang PC, Wu ZG, et al. The bacteriology of obstructive pneumonitis. Am J Respir Crit Care Med 1994; 149:1648–1653.

17. Pasteur MC, Helliwell SM, Houghton SJ, et al. An investigation into causative factors in patients with bronchiectasis. Am J Respir Crit Care Med 2000; 162:1277–1284.

18. Milisav I. Dynein and dynein-related genes. Cell Motil Cystoskel 1998; 39:261–272.

19. Kainulainen L, Varpula M, Liippo K, et al. Pulmonary abnormalities in patients with primary hypogammaglobulinemia. J Allergy Clin Immunol 1999; 104(5):1031–1036.

20. De Gracia J, Rodrigo MJ, Morell R, et al. IgG subclass deficiencies associated with bronchiectasis. Am J Respir Crit Care Med 1996; 153:650.

21. Bard M, Couderc L, Saimot A, et al. Accelerated obstructive pulmonary disease in HIV-infected patients with bronchiectasis. Eur Respir J 1998; 11:771–775.

22. Cockrill B, Hales C. Allergic bronchopulmonary aspergillosis. Annu Rev Med 1999; 50:303–316.

23. Cohen M, Sahn S. Bronchiectasis in systemic disease. Chest 1999; 116:1063–1074.

24. Boehler A, Kesten S, Weder W, Speich R. Bronchiolitis obliterans after lung transplantation: a review. Chest 1998; 114:1411–1426.

25. Westcott JL, Cole SR. Traction bronchiectasis in end-stage pulmonary fibrosis. Radiology 1986; 161:665–669.

26. Al-mallah Z, Quantock OP. Tracheobronchomegaly. Thorax 1968; 23:230–234.

27. Palmer SM Jr, Layish DT, Kussin PS, et al. Lung transplantation for Williams-Campbell syndrome. Chest 1998; 113:534–537.

28. Kennedy TP, Weber DJ. Nontuberculous mycobacteria: an under-appreciated cause of geriatric lung disease. Am J Respir Crit Care Med 1994; 149:1654–1658.

29. Huang JH, Kao PN, Adi V, Ruoss SJ. *Mycobacterium avium-intracellulare* pulmonary infection in HIV-negative patients without pre-existing lung disease: diagnostic and management limitations. Chest 1999; 115:1044–1040.

30. Rossman M. Colonization with *Mycobacterium avium* complex—an outdated concept. Eur Respir J 1999; 13:479.

31. Fujita J, Ohtsuki Y, Suemitsu I, et al. Pathological and radiological changes in resected lung specimens in *Mycobacterium avium intracellulare* complex disease. Eur Respir J 1999; 13:535–540.

32. Reich JM, Johnson RE. *Mycobacterium avium* complex pulmonary infection presenting as isolated lingular or middle lobe pattern: the Lady Windermere syndrome. Chest 1992; 101:1605–1609.

33. Kubo K, Yamazaki Y, Hanaoka M, et al. Analysis of HLA antigens in *Mycobacterium avium-intracellulare* pulmonary infection. Am J Respir Crit Care Med 2000; 161:1368–1371.

34. Yamazaki Y, Kubo K, Takamizawa A, et al. Markers indicating deterioration of pulmonary *Mycobacterium avium-intracellulare* infection. Am J Respir Crit Care Med 1999; 160:1851–1855.

35. Emad A, Rezaian GR. The diversity of the effects of sulfur mustard gas inhalation on respiratory system 10 years after a single, heavy exposure: analysis of 197 cases. Chest 1997; 112:734–738.

36. Amshel CE, Fealk MH, Phillips BJ, Caruso DM. Anhydrous ammonia burns case report and review of the literature. Burns 2000; 26:493–497.

37. Annobil SH, Morad NA, Kameswaran M, et al. Bronchiectasis due to lipid aspiration in childhood: clinical and pathological correlates. Ann Trop Paediatr 1996; 16:19–25.

38. Lee SH, Lee KS, Ahn JM, et al. Paraquat poisoning of the lung: thin-section CT findings. Radiology 1995; 195:271–274.

39. Tasaka S, Kanazawa M, Mori M, et al. Long-term course of bronchiectasis and bronchiolitis obliterans as late complication of smoke inhalation. Respiration 1995; 62:40–42.

40. Hiller E, Rosenow EC III, Olsen AM. Pulmonary manifestations of the yellow nail syndrome. Chest 1972; 61:452–458.

41. Hansell D. Bronchiectasis. Radiol Clin North Am 1998; 36:107–128.

42. Luce J. Bronchiectasis. In: Murray J, Nadel J, eds. Textbook of Respiratory Medicine. Philadelphia: Saunders, 1994: 1398–1416.

42a. Young K, Aspestrand F, Kolbenstredt A. High resolution CT and bronchography in the assessment of bronchiectasis. Acta Radiol 1991; 32:439–441.

43. Rosenstein, BJ. Making and confirming the diagnosis. In: Orenstein DM, Stern RC, eds. Treatment of the Hospitalized Cystic Fibrosis Patient. New York: Marcel Dekker, 1998:1–35.

44. Tsang KWT, Zheng L, Tipoe G. Ciliary Assessment in bronchiectasis. Respirology 2000; 5:91–98.

45. Cahill B, Ingbar D. Massive hemoptysis. Clin Chest Med 1994; 15:147–168.

46. Evans S, Turner S, Bosch B, et al. Lung function in bronchiectasis: the influence of *Pseudomonas aeruginosa*. Eur Respir J 1996; 9:1601–1604.
47. Wilson C, Jones P, O'Leary C, et al. Effect of sputum bacteriology on the quality of life of patients with bronchiectasis. Eur Respir J 1997; 10:1754–1760.
48. Nicotra BM, Rivera M, Dale A, et al. Clinical, pathophysiologic, and microbiologic characterization of bronchiectasis in an aging cohort. Chest 1995; 108:955–961.
49. Darley ER, Bowker KE, Lovering AM, et al. Use of meropenem 3 g once daily for outpatient treatment of infective exacerbations of bronchiectasis. J Antimicrob Chemother 2000; 45:247–250.
50. Tsang KW, Chan WM, Ho PI, et al. A comparative study on levofloxacin and ceftazadime in acute exacerbation of bronchiectasis. Eur Respir J 1999; 14:1206–1209.
51. Packe GE, Hodson ME. Changes in spirometry during consecutive admissions for infective pulmonary exacerbations in adolescent and adult cystic fibrosis. Respir Med 1992; 86:45–48.
52. Kuhn R. Formulation of aerosolized therapeutics. Chest 2001; 120:94S–98S.
53. Ramsey BW, Pepe MS, Quan JM, et al. Intermittent administration of inhaled tobramycin in patients with cystic fibrosis. N Engl J Med 1999; 340:23–30.
54. Barker AF, Couch L, Fiel SB, et al. Tobramycin solution for inhalation reduces sputum *Pseudomonas aeruginosa* density in bronchiectasis. Am J Respir Crit Care Med 2000; 162:481–485.
55. Orriols R, Roig J, Ferrer J, et al. Inhaled antibiotic therapy in non-cystic fibrosis patients with bronchiectasis and chronic bronchial infection by *Pseudomonas aeruginosa*. Respir Med 1999; 93:476–480.
56. Lin H, Cheng H, Wang C, et al. Inhaled gentamycin reduces airway neutrophil activity and mucus secretion in bronchiectasis. Am J Respir Crit Care Med 1997; 155:2024–2029.
57. Couch LA. Treatment with tobramycin solution for inhalation in bronchiectasis patients with *Pseudomonas aeruginosa*. Chest 2001; 120:114s–117s.
58. Crowther-Labiris NR, Holbrook AM, Chrystyn H, et al. Dry powder versus intravenous and nebulized gentamycin in cystic fibrosis and bronchiectasis. *Am J Respir Crit Care Med* 1999; 160:1711–1716.
59. Kudoh S, Uetake T, Hagiwara K, et al. Clinical effect of low-dose long-term erythromycin chemotherapy of diffuse panbronchiolitis. Jpn J Thorac Dis 1987; 25:632–642.
60. Nagai H, Shishido H, Yoneda R, et al. Long-term low-dose administration of erythromycin to patients with diffuse panbronchiolitis. Respiration 1991; 58:145–149.
61. Tsang KWT, Ho Pl, Chan KN, et al. A pilot study of low-dose erythromycin in bronchiectasis. Eur Respir J 1999; 13:361–364.
62. Nakamura H, Fujishima S, Inoue T, et al. Clinical and immunoregulatory effects of roxithromycin therapy in chronic respiratory tract infection. Eur Resp J 1999; 13:1371–1379.
63. Hardy KA. A review of airway clearance: new techniques, indications, and recommendations. Respir Care 1994; 39:440–452.
64. Roberts HR, Wells AU, Milne DG, et al. Airflow obstruction in bronchiectasis: correlation between computed tomography features and pulmonary function tests. Thorax 2000; 55:198–204.

65. Hassan JA, Saadiah S, Roslan H, Zainudin B. Bronchodilator response to inhaled beta-2 agonist and anticholinergic drugs in patients with bronchiectasis. Respirology 1999; 4:423–426.

66. Tsang K, Ho P, Iam W, et al. Inhaled fluticasone reduces sputum inflammatory indices in severe bronchiectasis. Am J Respir Crit Care Med 1998; 158:723–727.

67. Elborn JS, Johnston B, Allen F, et al. Inhaled steroids in patients with bronchiectasis. Respir Med 1992; 86:121–124.

68. Tamaoki J, Chiyotani A, Kobayashi K, et al. Effect of indomethacin on bronchorrhea in patients with chronic bronchitis, diffuse panbronchiolitis, or bronchiectasis. Am Rev Respir Dis 1992; 145:548–552.

69. Fuchs H, Borowitz D, Christiansen D, et al. Effect of aerosolized recombinant human DNase on exacerbation of respiratory symptoms and on pulmonary function in patients with cystic fibrosis. N Engl J Med 1994; 331:637–642.

70. O'Donnell AE, Barker A, Ilowite J, Fick R. Treatment of idiopathic bronchiectasis with aerosolized recombinant human DNase I. Chest 1998; 113:1329–1334.

71. Olivieri D, Ciaccia A, Marangio E, et al. Role of bromhexine in exacerbations of bronchiectasis. Respiration 1991; 58:117–121.

72. Daviskas E, Anderson SD, Gonda I, et al. Inhalation of hypertonic saline aerosol enhances mucociliary clearance in asthmatic and healthy subjects. Eur Respir J 1996; 9:725–732.

73. Daviskas E, Anderson SD, Eberl S, et al. Inhalation of dry powder mannitol improves clearance of mucus in patients with bronchiectasis. Am J Respir Crit Care Med 1999; 159:1843–1848.

74. Daviskas E, Anderson SD, Eberl S, et al. The 24-h affect of mannitol on the clearance of mucus in patients with bronchiectasis. Chest 2001; 119:414–421.

75. Agasthian T, Deschamps C, Tratek V, et al. Surgical management of bronchiectasis. Ann Surg 1996; 62:976–980.

76. Osaki S, Nakanishi Y, Wataya H, et al. Prognosis of bronchial artery embolization in the management of hemoptysis. Respiration 2000; 67:412–416.

77. Jean-Baptiste E. Clinical assessment and management of massive hemoptysis. Crit Care Med 2000; 5:1642–1647.

78. Prieto D, Bernardo J, Matos M, et al. Surgery for bronchiectasis. Eur J Cardiothorac Surg 2001; 20:19–24.

79. Arcasoy S, Kotloff R. Lung transplantation. N Engl J Med 1999; 340:1081–1091.

80. Rao JN, Forty J, Hasan A, et al. Bilateral lung transplant: the procedure of choice for end-stage septic lung disease. Transplant Proc 2001; 33:1622–1623.

81. Fitzsimmons SC. Cystic Fibrosis Foundation 1995 Annual Patient Registry Data Report. Bethesda, MD: Cystic Fibrosis Foundation, 1996.

82. Riordan JR, Rommens JM, Kerem B, et al. Identification of the cystic fibrosis gene: cloning and characterization of complementary DNA. Science 1989; 245:1066–1073.

83. Verkman AS. Lung disease in cystic fibrosis: is airway surface liquid composition abnormal? Am J Physiol Lung Cell Mol Physiol 2001; 281:L306–L308.

84. Boucher RC. Human airway ion transport, part one. Am J Respir Crit Care Med 1994; 150(1):271–281.

85. Boucher RC. Human airway ion transport, part two. Am J Respir Crit Care Med 1994; 150(2):581–593.

86. Zabner J, Smith JJ, Karp PH, et al. Loss of CFTR chloride channels alters salt absorption by cystic fibrosis airway epithelia in vitro. Mol Cell 1998; 2:229–236.

86a. Goldman MJ, Anderson GM, Stolzenberg ED, et al. Human β-defensin-1 is a salt-sensitive antibiotic in lung that is inactivated in cystic fibrosis. Cell 1997; 88:553-560.

87. Zeitlin PL. Future pharmacological treatment of cystic fibrosis. Respiration 2000; 67:351–357.

88. Desmond KJ, Schwenk WF, Thomas E, et al. Immediate and long-term effects of chest physiotherapy in patients with cystic fibrosis. J Pediatr 1983; 103:224–225.

89. Schneiderman-Walker JSL, Pollock M, Corey DD, et al. A randomized, controlled trial of a 3-year home exercise program in cystic fibrosis. J Pediatr 2000; 136:304–310.

90. Borowitz DS, Grand RJ, Durie PR. Use of pancreatic enzyme supplements for patients with cystic fibrosis in the context of fibrosing colonopathy. J Pediatr 1995; 127:681–684.

91. Sokol RJ, Durie PR. Recommendations for management of liver and biliary tract disease in cystic fibrosis. Cystic Fibrosis Foundation Hepatobiliary Disease Consensus Group. J Pediatr Gastroenterol Nutr 1999; 28(suppl 1):S1–S13.

92. Ramsey BW, Rannell PM, Pencharz P. Nutritional assessment and management in cystic fibrosis: a consensus report. Am J Clin Nutr 1992; 55:108–116.

93. Daniels LA, Davidson GP. Current issues in the nutritional management of children with cystic fibrosis. Aust Paediatr J 1989; 25(5):261–266.

94. Sharma R, Florea VG, Bolger AP, et al. Wasting as an independent predictor of mortality in patients with cystic fibrosis. Thorax 2001; 56:746–750.

95. Corey M, McLaughlin FJ, Williams M, et al. A comparison of survival, growth and pulmonary function in patients with cystic fibrosis in Boston and Toronto. J Clin Epidemiol 1988; 41:583–591.

96. Acupuncture. NIH Consensus Statement Online. November 3–5, 1997; 15(5):1–34.

97. Hernandez-Reif M, Field T, Krasnegor J, et al. Children with cystic fibrosis benefit from massage therapy. J Pediatr Psychol 1999; 24:175–181.

98. Anbar RD. Self-hypnosis for children with cystic fibrosis. Pediatr Pulmonol 2000; 30:461–465.

99. Cupp MJ. Herbal remedies: adverse effects and drug interactions. Am Fam Physician 1999; 59(5):1239–1245.

100. Shaw D, Leon C, Kolev S, Murray V. Traditional remedies and food supplements: a 5-year toxicological study (1991–1995). Drug Saf 1997; 17(5):342–356.

101. Gilligan PH. Microbiology of cystic fibrosis lung disease. In: Yankaskas JR, Knowles MR, eds. Cystic Fibrosis in Adults. Philadelphia: Lippincott-Raven, 1999:97.

102. Lam J, Chan R, Lam K, et al. Production of mucoid microcolonies by *Pseudomonas aeruginosa* within infected lungs in cystic fibrosis. Infect Immunol 1980; 28:546–556.

103. Henry RL, Mellis CM, Petrovic L. Mucoid *Pseudomonas aeruginosa* is a marker of poor survival in cystic fibrosis. Pediatr Pulmonol 1992; 12:158–161.

104. Ratjen F, Doring G, Nikolaizik WH. Effect of inhaled tobramycin on early Pseudomonas aeruginosa colonisation in patients with cystic fibrosis. Lancet 2001; 358:983–984.

105. Konstan MW, Butler SM, Schidlow DV, et al for the Investigators and Coordinators of the Epidemiologic Study of Cystic Fibrosis. Patterns of medical practice in cystic fibrosis. Part II—Use of therapies. Pediatr Pulmonol 1999; 28(4):248–254.

106. Cystic Fibrosis Foundation. Microbiology and infectious disease in cystic fibrosis. Clinical Practice Guidelines for Cystic Fibrosis. Vol. 1. Bethesda, MD: Cystic Fibrosis Foundation, 1997:25.

107. Moutin JW, Kerrebijn KF. Antibacterial therapy in cystic fibrosis. Med Clin North Am 1990; 74:837–850.

108. Moorcroft AJ, Dodd ME, Webb AK. Long-term change in exercise capacity, body mass, and pulmonary function in adults with cystic fibrosis. Chest 1997; 1111(2):338–343.

109. Szaff M, Hoiby N, Flensborg EW. Frequent antibiotic therapy improves survival of cystic fibrosis patients with chronic *Pseudomonas aeruginosa* infection. Acta Paediatr Scand 1983; 72:651–657.

110. Elborn JS, Prescott RJ, Stack BHR, et al. Elective versus symptomatic treatment in cystic fibrosis patients with chronic *Pseudomonas* infection of the lungs. Thorax 2000; 55:355–358.

111. Weber A, Morlin G, Cohen M, et al. Safety of aerosol tobramycin administration for 3 months to patients with cystic fibrosis. Pediatr Pulmonol 1997; 23:249–260.

112. Pai V, Nahata MC. Efficacy and safety of aerosolized tobramycin in cystic fibrosis. Pediatr Pulmonol 2001; 32:314–327.

113. Utell MJ, Marrow PE, Speers DM, et al. Airway responses to sulfate and sulfuric acid aerosols in asthmatics: an exposure-response relationship. Am Rev Respir Dis 1983; 128:444–450.

114. Mukhopadhyay S, Singh M, Carter JL, et al. Nebulised anti-pseudomonal antibiotic therapy in cystic fibrosis: a meta-analysis of benefits and the risks. Thorax 1996; 551:364–368.

115. Nickerson B, Montgomery AB, Kylstra JW, Ramsey BW. Safety and effectiveness of 2 years of treatment with TOBI (tobramycin solution for inhalation) in CF patients (abstr). Pediatr Pulmonol 1999; 19(suppl): 243.

116. Steinkamp G, Tummler B, Gappa M, et al. Long-term tobramycin aerosol therapy in cystic fibrosis. Pediatr Pulmonol 1989; 6:91–98.

117. MacLusky IB, Gold R, Corey M, Levison H. Long-term effects of inhaled tobramycin in patients with cystic fibrosis colonized with *Pseudomonas aeruginosa*. Pediatr Pulmonol 1989; 7(1):42–48.

118. Smith AL, Ramsey BW, Hedges DL, et al. Safety of aerosol tobramycin administration for 3 months to patients with cystic fibrosis. Pediatr Pulmonol 1989; 7:265–271.

119. Burns JL, Ramsey BW, Fiel SB. In vitro antibiotic susceptibility testing of CF *Pseudomonas* isolates does not predict FEV_1 response to combination intravenous antibiotic therapy. Presented at European Cystic Fibrosis Conference, June 4–8, 2000, Stockholm Sweden.

120. Quan JM, Tiddens HAWM, Sy JP, et al. A two-year randomized placebo-controlled trial of dornase alfa in young cystic fibrosis patients with mild lung function abnormalities. J Pediatr 2001; 139:813–820.

121. Cystic Fibrosis Foundation. 1999 Annual Patient Registry Data Report. Bethesda; MD: Cystic Fibrosis Foundation, 1999.

122. Thomson AH. Human recombinant DNase in cystic fibrosis. J R Med Soc 1995; 88:24–29.

123. Eng PA, Morton J, Douglas JA, et al. Short-term efficacy of ultrasonically nebulized hypertonic saline in cystic fibrosis. Pediatr Pulmonol 1996; 21:77–83.

124. Konig PD, Gayer G, Barbero J, Shaffer J. Short-term and long-term effects of albuterol aerosol therapy in cystic fibrosis: a preliminary report. Pediatr Pulmonol 1995; 20:205–214.

125. Konig P, Poehler J, Barbero G. A placebo-controlled, double blind trial of the long-term effects of albuterol administration in patients with cystic fibrosis. Pediatr Pulmonol 1998; 25:32–36.

126. Kahn TZ, Wagener JS, Bost T, et al. Early pulmonary inflammation in infants with cystic fibrosis. Am J Respir Crit Care Med 1995; 151:1075–1082.

127. Armstrong DS, Grimwood K, Carzino R, et al. Lower respiratory tract infection and inflammation in infants with newly diagnosed cystic fibrosis. Br Med J 1995; 310:1571–1572.

128. Balough K, Mc Cubbin M, Weinberger M, et al. The relationship between infection and inflammation in the early stages of lung disease from cystic fibrosis. Pediatr Pulmonol 1995; 20:63–70.

129. Greally P, Hussain MJ, Vergani D, Price JF. Interleukin-1 alpha, soluble interleukin-2 receptor and IgG concentrations in cystic fibrosis treated with prednisolone. Arch Dis Child 1994; 71:35–39.

130. Eigen H, Rosenstein BJ, FitzSimmons S, Schidlow DV for the Cystic Fibrosis Foundation Prednisone Trial Group. A multicenter study of alternate-day prednisone therapy in patients with cystic fibrosis. J Pediatr 1995; 126:515–523.

131. Schiotz PO, Jorgenson M, Flensborg EW, et al. Chronic *Pseudomonas* lung infection in cystic fibrosis: a longitudinal study of immune complex activity and inflammatory response in sputum sol-phase of cystic fibrosis patients with chronic *Pseudomonas aeruginosa* lung infections—influence of local steroid treatment. Acta Paediatr Scand 1983; 72:283–287.

132. Van Haren EHJ, Lammers JWJ, Heijerman HGM, et al. The effects of the inhaled corticosteroid budesonide on lung function and bronchial hyperrespon-siveness in patients with cystic fibrosis. Respir Med 1995; 89:209–214.

133. Konstan MW, Byard PJ, Hoppel CL, Davis PB. Effect of high-dose ibuprofen in patients with cystic fibrosis. N Engl J Med 1995; 332:848–854.

134. Mendeloff EN, et al. Pediatric and adult lung transplantation for cystic fibrosis. J Thorac Cardiovasc Surg 1998; 115:404–413.

135. Alam R, Gorska M. Genomic microarrays: arraying order in biological chaos? Am J Respir Crit Care Med 2001; 25:405–408.

136. Flotte TR, Laube BL. Gene therapy in cystic fibrosis. Chest 2001; 120:124s–131s.

137. Rosenfeld MA, Siegfried W, Yoshimura K, et al. Adenovirus-mediated transfer of a recombinant alpha-1-antitrypsin gene to the lung epithelium in vivo. Science 1991; 252:431–434.

138. Rosenfeld MA, Yoshimura K, Trapnell BC, et al. In vivo transfer of the human cystic fibrosis transmembrane conductance regulator gene to the airway epithelium. Cell 1992; 68:143–155.

139. Flotte TR, Afione SA, Conrad C, et al. Stable in vivo expression of the cystic fibrosis transmembrane conductance regulator with an adenovirus-associated vector. Proc Natl Acad Sci USA 1993; 90:10613–10617.

140. Crystal RG, McElvaney NG, Rosenfeld MA, et al. Administration of an adeno-associated virus CFTR gene vector in adult CF patients with mild lung disease. Hum Gene Ther 1996; 7:1145–1159.
141. Boucher RC, Knowles MR, Johnson LG, et al. Gene therapy for cystic fibrosis using E1-deleted adenovirus: a phase I trial in the nasal cavity. The University of North Carolina at Chapel Hill. Hum Gene Ther 1994; 5:615–639.
142. Harvey BG, Hackett NR, Ely S, et al. Host responses and persistence of vector genome following intrabronchial administration of an E1(-) and E3(-) adenovirus gene transfer vector to normal individuals. Mol Ther 2001; 3:206–215.
143. Fisher KJ, Choi H, Burda J, et al. Recombinant adenovirus deleted of all viral genes for gene therapy of cystic fibrosis. Virology 1996; 217:11–22.
144. Knowles MR, Hohneker KW, Zhou Z, et al. A controlled study of adenoviral-mediated gene transfer in the nasal epithelium of patients with cystic fibrosis. N Engl J Med 1995; 333:823–831.
145. Flotte TR. Recent advances in gene transfer methods for the treatment of cystic fibrosis. Curn Res Ion Channel Mod 1998; 3:41–50.
146. Dorin JR, Farley R, Webb S, et al. A demonstration using mouse models that successful gene therapy for cystic fibrosis requires only partial gene correction. Gene Ther 1996; 3:797–801.
147. Johnson LG, Olson JC, Sarkadi B, et al. Efficiency of gene transfer for restoration of normal airway function in cystic fibrosis. Nat Genet 1992; 2:21–25.
148. Wilschanski M, Famini C, Blau H, et al. A pilot study of the effect of gentamicin on nasal potential difference measurements in cystic fibrosis patients carrying stop mutations. Am J Respir Crit Care Med 2000; 16:860–865.
149. Tonelli MR, Aitken ML. New and emerging therapies for pulmonary complications of cystic fibrosis. Drugs 2001; 61:1379–1385.
150. Andersson C, Roomans G. Activation of delta F508 CFTR in a cystic fibrosis respiratory epithelial cell line by 4-phenylbutyrate, genisten and CPX. Eur Respir J 2000; 15:937–941.
151. Cantin AM. Novel approaches to inflammation and infection in the cystic fibrosis lung. Pediatr Pulmonol 2001; 23:94–96.
152. Zuckerman JB, Kotloff RM. Lung transplantation for cystic fibrosis. Clin Chest Med 1998; 19(3): 8.1–8.20.

9

Pulmonary Interstitial Disease
Idiopathic, Autoimmune, and Drug-Related

EDWARD MOLONEY

Imperial College School of Medicine
National Heart and Lung Institute
and Royal Brompton Hospital
London, England

JIM J. EGAN

Mater Misericordiae Hospital and
St. Vincent's University Hospitals
Dublin, Ireland

I. Introduction

The idiopathic interstitial pneumonias (IIPs) are a heterogeneous group of nonneoplastic disorders resulting from injury to the lung parenchyma. They comprise a number of clinicopathological syndromes that are sufficiently different from one another to be designated as separate disease entities (1). Idiopathic pulmonary fibrosis (IPF) is the commonest subgroup in patients with suspected IIP and is a fatal condition (2). The prevalence of IPF has been estimated to be between 20 and 30 per 100,000 of the general population (3). Most patients are between 40 and 80 years old, with a mean age of 65 years. Men are affected more commonly than women by a ratio of 2 to 1. The natural history of IPF appears to be progressive in all cases, with a mean survival of 2.9 years (4). A number of possible factors involved in the pathogenesis of IPF have been described, including genetic factors (5,6), autoimmune responses (5,6), infection (7,8), cigarette smoking (5), and environmental injury (9). In particular, exposure to wood dust or metal dust (9), acid reflux (10), and Epstein-Barr virus coinfection (11) may lead to repeated injury, resulting in progressive tissue remodeling. This chapter deals with 1) the classification of idiopathic interstitial pneumonias (IIPs), 2) connective tissue disorders and IIP, 3) drug-induced pulmonary disease, 4) drug therapy for IPF, and 5) the management of patients with advanced pulmonary fibrosis.

Table 1 Histological Classification in Idiopathic Interstitial Pneumonias (IIP)

Idiopathic pulmonary fibrosis (IPF)/usual interstitial pneumonia (UIP)
Nonspecific interstitial pneumonia (NSIP)
Desquamative interstitial pneumonia (DIP)
Respiratory bronchiolitis–associated interstitial lung disease (RBILD)
Acute interstitial pneumonia (AIP)

A. Usual Interstitial Pneumonia

Usual interstitial pneumonia (UIP) is the histopathological pattern that is synonymous with the clinical syndrome of IPF and accounts for 65% of IIP cases (1). UIP reduces the surface area of the lung and obliterates pulmonary vessels, resulting in ventilation perfusion mismatch, hypoxemia, and breathlessness. The histological features show fibrotic areas of varying age and activity (2). Typically, honeycombing is interspersed with areas of relatively normal lung tissue. Interstitial inflammation is mild, and fibroblastic foci are a major characteristic feature (2). The clinical diagnosis of IPF is based upon three criteria: (1) exclusion of other causes of interstitial lung disease (ILD); (2) abnormal pulmonary function tests (PFTs), showing a restrictive pattern and/or decreased diffusing lung capacity (DL_{CO}); and (3) a radiological pattern on high-resolution computed tomography (HRCT) showing bibasilar reticular abnormalities and minimal "ground glass" attenuation (1). A clinical diagnosis is usually adequate for diagnostic purposes (12). Therefore surgical biopsy is generally considered unnecessary, particularly in light of a significant risk associated with it. Utz et al., in a study of 60 UIP patients undergoing surgical lung biopsy, demonstrated a mortality of 17% within 30 days of the procedure (13). However, if there are atypical features on HRCT—including nodules or predominant ground glass attenuation or consolidation, particularly in a younger patient—consideration should be given to surgical biopsy. As

Table 2 Diagnostic Criteria for UIP/IPF

Major criteria
    Exclusion of other causes of interstitial lung disease
    Abnormal pulmonary function tests—restrictive pattern and/or reduced DL_{CO}
    Typical bibasilar reticular abnormalities with minimal ground-glass opacities on HRCT scans
Minor criteria
    Age > 50 years
    Insidious onset of otherwise unexplained dyspnea on exertion
    Duration of illness less than or equal to 3 months
    Bibasilar, inspiratory crackles (dry or "Velcro" type in quality)

indicated above, UIP has a poor prognosis, with a median survival of 2.9 years (4).

B. Nonspecific Interstitial Pneumonia (NSIP)

Surgical lung biopsies of patients with IIP occasionally reveal a chronic interstitial pneumonia that lacks the characteristic variegate pattern of UIP. This is referred to as NSIP (14). These lesions are characterized by a relatively uniform appearance at low magnification due to a cellular interstitial infiltrate of mononuclear inflammatory cells associated with varying degrees of interstitial fibrosis. Introduction of the term *NSIP* by Katzenstein et al. led to a reappraisal of the classification of IIP (14). However, NSIP is likely to have been formerly described by Scadding et al. as "cellular" cryptogenic fibrosing alveolitis (CFA) (6). Within the group of patients described as having CFA, it was recognized that a subgroup of patients had a favorable prognosis associated with a uniformly cellular change on biopsy in a manner comparable to NSIP (4). NSIP is the commonest histological pattern of IIP associated with systemic sclerosis (15). The clinical presentation of NSIP is similar to that of UIP but affects younger patients, mean age 57 years. HRCT shows bilateral symmetrical ground-glass opacities or mixed bilateral airspace consolidation and interstitial thickening, but the specificity of HRCT based diagnosis of NSIP is unknown (16). NSIP patients have a good prognosis with a median survival of greater than 10 years (17).

C. Desquamative Interstitial Pneumonia (DIP)

DIP is a distinct clinicopathological entity that differs substantially from UIP (2). It is rare, with an incidence <3%, and it typically affects cigarette smokers in their fourth or fifth decade of life. Most patients present with a subacute (weeks to months) illness characterized by dyspnea and cough. HRCT shows ground-glass attenuation. Lung biopsy reveals uniform, diffuse intra-alveolar macrophage accumulation (1). As a consequence, it has been suggested that DIP should be renamed as "acute macrophage pneumonia." Clinical recognition of DIP is important because the prognosis is excellent, and it responds to corticosteroid treatment. It rarely progresses to advanced pulmonary fibrosis and is associated with an overall survival of about 70% after 10 years (4).

D. Respiratory Bronchiolitis–Associated Interstitial Lung Disease (RBILD)

Like DIP, RBILD is a rare condition found in current or former cigarette smokers, typically during their fourth or fifth decades of life (18). The clinical presentation resembles that of patients with other IIP, including cough, breathlessness, and sparse crackles on auscultation. HRCT scanning shows

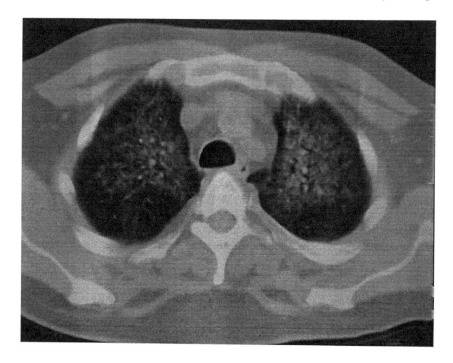

Figure 1 HRCT of a patient with acute interstitial pneumonia. There is bilateral symmetrical ground-glass attenuation interspersed with areas of consolidation.

mild, diffuse, fine reticulonodular opacities in a bibasilar distribution. RBILD is characterized histologically by the presence of pigmented intraluminal macrophages within first- and second-order respiratory bronchioles. The changes are patchy at low magnification and have a bronchiolocentric distribution, accompanied by a patchy submucosal and peribronchiolar infiltrate of lymphocytes and histiocytes. RBILD appears to be a relatively benign and self-limited condition (19).

E.   Acute Interstitial Pneumonia (Hamman-Rich Syndrome)

Acute interstitial pneumonia (AIP) is a rare, fulminant form of lung injury that presents acutely, usually in a previously healthy individual (20). Symptoms include fever, shortness of breath, and cough. This acute presentation is comparable to acute respiratory distress syndrome (ARDS), differing only in that it is not preceded by a catastrophic event (i.e., the condition is idiopathic). Ventilatory support is invariably required. AIP has a poor prognosis, with a mortality of up to 70% (20). Diffuse bilateral airspace opacification is seen on chest radiograph, and HRCT scans show bilateral, patchy, symmetrical areas of ground-glass attenuation (Fig. 1). Bilateral areas of airspace consolidation may also be present (21). The lung biopsy typically shows diffuse involvement, although there may be variation in the severity of the changes among different histological fields. Features typical of diffuse alveolar damage (DAD)—including edema, hyaline membranes, and interstitial acute inflammation—are characteristically seen (22). Loose organizing fibrosis is mostly seen within alveolar septa, but it may also be observed within airspaces. The latter pattern may be a prominent feature in more than one-third of cases. If the patient survives, complete recovery is possible. However in approximately 25% of cases, the process can recur, progressing to chronic interstitial fibrosis potentially requiring lung transplantation (20).

II. Interstitial Lung Disease in Connective Tissue Disorders

A. Interstitial Lung Disease in Rheumatoid Arthritis

Ellman and Ball first observed an association between interstitial lung disease (ILD) and rheumatoid arthritis (RA) in 1948 (23). ILD associated with RA is most common in men (M:F = 3:1) between 50 to 60 years of age and is most frequently associated with seropositive and erosive joint disease (28). A study of 36 patients with recent-onset rheumatoid disease (joint symptoms <2 years) demonstrated that 58% of patients had evidence of ILD on either chest x-ray, HRCT, bronchial lavage, or lung physiology (24). However, pulmonary involvement was clinically apparent in only 14% of patients (24). The onset of pulmonary symptoms usually postdates the onset of joint symptoms by up to 5 years. In a HRCT surveillance study of 84 RA patients, heterogeneous changes were identified. Bronchiectasis in the absence of fibrosis occurred in 30% of patients, pulmonary nodules in 22%, subpleural micronodules in 17%, ground-glass attenuation in 14%, nonseptal linear attenuation in 18%, and honeycombing in 10% (25). In another HRCT study, bullous emphysema was an additional common finding, occurring in 66% of patients (26). This emphasizes that smoking is an important risk factor for ILD in RA. In a study of 336 RA patients, it was observed that in those with a >25 pack-year smoking history, there was a significant association with radiographic evidence of ILD (27). If surgical lung biopsy is completed, a spectrum of findings may be present, including inflammatory disease, a mixed pattern, or more commonly UIP (29). The prognosis and natural history of IIP associated with RA is not precisely defined, but in general it appears to be better than IPF. However, when hospital admission for pulmonary disease is required, the median survival is limited. In a study of 49 RA patients who required hospitalization for ILD, the median survival was only 3.5 years (30).

B. Systemic Sclerosis and Interstitial Lung Disease

Pulmonary disease is the second most common visceral complication after esophageal involvement in patients with systemic sclerosis (31). The two main pulmonary manifestations are interstitial lung disease (ILD) and pulmonary vascular disease. ILD occurs in more than 75% of patients with systemic sclerosis and vascular disease in approximately 10% (32). ILD is seen in both diffuse and limited cutaneous scleroderma, although it usually occurs at an earlier stage and may progress more rapidly in diffuse sclerosis. The most common symptoms of ILD are fatigue, breathlessness on exertion, and a dry cough. A pronounced reduction in DL_{CO} is usually associated with a restrictive pattern on pulmonary function testing (33). The presence of reduced DL_{CO} and normal lung volumes may suggest isolated vascular disease. ILD is a significant determinant of outcome in systemic sclerosis and is now the most common disease-related cause of death. In patients with diffuse cutaneous systemic sclerosis and pulmonary disease, the median survival is 78 months (34). Although ILD in systemic sclerosis is associated with a reduced survival among patients with systemic sclerosis, the survival is more favorable than in patients with isolated IPF. This may be explained by the fact that up to 50% of patients with IIP associated with systemic sclerosis have a histological diagnosis of NSIP (14). In systemic sclerosis patients with isolated pulmonary hypertension, the prognosis may be poor. Systemic sclerosis patients with pulmonary hypertension and a DL_{CO} of less than 25% of predicted have a median survival of less than 1 year (34).

C. Systemic Lupus Erythematosus (SLE) and Interstitial Lung Disease

Acute lupus pneumonitis—presenting as cough, dyspnea, pleuritic pain, hypoxemia, and fever—has been reported to occur in 1 to 4% of patients with SLE (35). However, controversy exists as to whether acute lupus pneumonitis is a unique entity. In a large autopsy study, every case of clinically diagnosed lupus pneumonitis could be explained by other factors such as infection, aspiration, cardiac dysfunction, or uremia (36). Chronic interstitial pneumonitis has been reported to occur in 3 to 13% of SLE patients (37). Asymptomatic pulmonary disease is thought to be relatively common, as abnormalities in pulmonary function tests have been documented in up to two-thirds of SLE patients (38,39). Fenlon et al. (38) assessed chest radiographs, pulmonary function tests, and HRCT scans in 34 SLE patients. Eleven patients were judged to have interstitial lung disease on HRCT scanning, nine of whom were asymptomatic. Therefore symptomatic chronic interstitial peumonitis is rarely a dominant feature of SLE and severe pulmonary fibrosis is very uncommon (35). Forinstance in an autopsy based study moderate or severe pulmonary fibrosis was documented in only four of 120 SLE patients (36). Histological features of chronic interstitial pneumonitis complicating SLE are of the nonspecific pneumonia pattern including varying degrees of chronic inflammatory cell infiltrates, peribronchial lymphoid hyperplasia, interstitial fibrosis, and hyperplasia of type 2 pneumocytes (35). Data relating to the specific treatment of interstitial pneumonitis in SLE are scanty. Corticosteroids, and or immunosuppressive, agents would be the recommended treatment.

III. Drug-Induced Pulmonary Disease

A. Amiodarone Pulmonary Disease

The most serious adverse effect of amiodarone is interstitial pneumonitis, which occurs in 5 to 15% of patients (40). Although exceptions occur, pulmonary toxicity correlates more closely with the total cumulative dose rather than with serum drug levels (40). Interstitial pneumonitis is usually recognized after 2 months of therapy, especially in patients in whom the daily dose exceeds 400 mg (40). Amiodarone-induced interstitial pneumonitis is characterized by a nonspecific interstitial pneumonitis predominantly composed of mononuclear cells, type II cell hyperplasia, and fibrosis. A characteristic finding in all patients exposed to amiodarone is the presence of numerous foamy macrophages in the airspaces (41). An organizing pneumonia with or without bronchiolitis obliterans [cryptogenic organizing pneumonia (COP) pattern] is seen in approximately 25 percent of cases (42). Acute lung injury is a rare but potentially fatal form of pulmonary toxicity. It is characterized by a fulminant course in patients being treated with amiodarone who have undergone surgery (43) or pulmonary angiography (44). The diagnosis of amiodarone-induced pneumonitis can be difficult in certain circumstances, for instance, may mimic pulmonary edema in patients with left ventricular dysfunction, or elderly IPF patients may give a remote history of coincidental amiodarone exposure. These patients are usually unsuitable candidates for tissue biopsy. Therefore criteria have been devised to facilitate the diagnosis of amiodarone-induced pulmonary toxicity (Table 3), the treatment of which consists primarily of stopping amiodarone. Corticosteroid therapy is indicated in severe cases and for patients with mild disease in whom amiodarone withdrawal is not desirable. Due to its accumulation in fatty

Table 3 Criteria for Amiodarone-Induced Pulmonary Toxicity[a]

New or worsening signs or symptoms
New abnormalities on chest roentgenogram
A decline in total lung capacity (15%) or in DL_{CO} (>20%)
Presence of foamy macrophages in the airspaces
A CD8 + lymphocytosis in lavage fluid
Histological evidence showing diffuse alveolar damage, organizing pneumonia, interstitial pneumonitis, or fibrosis
Improvements in lung manifestations following withdrawal of the drug (with or without steroid therapy)

[a]Three or more of these criteria suggest the "clinical diagnosis" of amiodarone pulmonary toxicity.

tissues and long elimination half-life (approximately 45 days), pulmonary toxicity may initially progress despite amiodarone cessation and may recur upon premature steroid withdrawal. The prognosis of amiodarone lung disease is generally favorable. Three-quarters of patients may stabilize or improve after withdrawal of the drug with or without corticosteroid treatment (45). Death attributable to amiodarone pneumonitis is believed to occur in 10 percent of cases, although the actual mortality in clinical practice may be less (46).

B. Cyclophosphamide Pulmonary Disease

Cyclophosphamide-induced pulmonary injury is rare. There are two patterns of pulmonary toxicity: an acute pneumonitis that occurs early in the course of treatment and a chronic progressive fibrotic process that occurs after prolonged therapy (47). In the acute presentation, symptoms of dry cough and dyspnea occur 1 to 6 months following initiation of therapy. HRCT shows diffuse ground-glass attenuation. The diagnosis is difficult, as infection needs to be excluded. Discontinuation of the drug and institution of corticosteroid therapy may result in complete resolution (47). Late-onset pulmonary toxicity develops in patients who have received prolonged therapy. The disorder differs

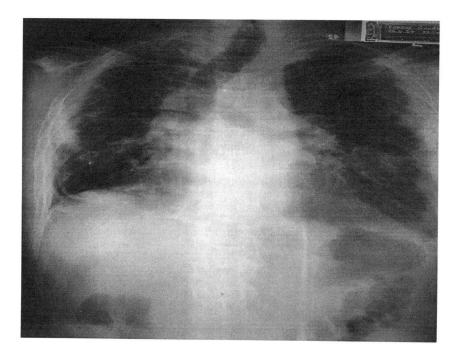

Figure 2   A chest x-ray of a patient exposed to cyclophosphamide for 5 years. There is bilateral pleural thickening and interstitial fibrosis as well as a small right basal pneumothorax. This is an example of cyclophosphamide-induced pulmonary fibrosis.

from UIP in that clubbing and inspiratory crackles are rare, and the reticular infiltrates on HRCT do not have the typical bibasilar predominance seen in UIP (47). Bilateral pleural thickening of the middle and upper zones is a common feature, allowing differentiation from UIP (Fig. 2) (48). Late-onset pulmonary toxicity appears not to respond to corticosteroids. Cyclophosphamide withdrawal is advised and treatment is largely supportive. Lung transplantation may be considered in selected cases remote from malignancy or in those patients with quiescent autoimmune disease (47).

C. Busulfan-Induced Pulmonary Disease

Busulfan was the first cytotoxic drug to be associated with pulmonary toxicity (49). Symptomatic pulmonary injury is estimated to occur in fewer than 5% of patients (50). Occult pulmonary injury may occur in many patients exposed to the drug (51). The mechanism of busulfan-induced lung injury is unknown. Direct toxicity of busulfan to epithelial lining cells is suggested, but cytological and histological findings are nonspecific. Lung biopsy specimens reveal pneumocyte dysplasia, atypical bronchial lining cells, mononuclear cell infiltration, and fibrosis (52). The risk of pulmonary toxicity due to busulfan appears to correlate with the cumulative dose. The threshold dose beyond which the risk of pulmonary toxicity may increase is 500 mg (53). The interval between initiation of therapy and onset of pulmonary symptoms is usually greater than 4 years. However, symptoms may occur early, after only 8 months, or late, up to 10 years following onset of busulfan exposure (50). The diagnosis of busulfan-induced pulmonary toxicity is usually established clinically and is a diagnosis of exclusion. Withdrawal of the drug is the initial step, but there are anecdotal reports of responses to corticosteroids (54).

D. Bleomycin-Induced Lung Disease

Bleomycin therapy may lead to a life-threatening pneumonitis that is dose- and time-dependent and progresses to interstitial pulmonary fibrosis in up to 10% of patients (55). Bleomycin is inactivated in vivo by bleomycin hydrolase, a cytosolic aminopeptidase. This hydrolase is active in all tissues with the exception of the skin and lungs, which accounts for the toxicity of the drug to these organs (55). High concentrations of oxygen are believed to increase the risk of bleomycin-induced lung injury (56). Oxygen therapy may result in oxygen radical formation, augmenting bleomycin lung injury. Symptoms of bleomycin-induced lung injury usually develop 1 to 6 months after treatment and include dyspnea, dry cough, and substernal chest pain. HRCT demonstrates a bilateral subpleural fibroproliferative infiltration (57). The mortality due to bleomycin pulmonary toxicity in a study of 180 patients treated for germ-cell tumors between 1991 and 1995 was 2.8% (58). Corticosteroids or other anti-inflammatory therapy would be the recommended treatment for bleomycin-induced fibrosis.

E. Carmustine (BCNU)–Induced Lung Disease

Carmustine was formerly a compound frequently used in the treatment of malignant brain tumors. Pulmonary fibrosis is a recognized complication occurring in 20 to 30% of patients (59). The total cumulative amount of administered carmustine and female gender are independent variables associated with the development of lung disease. Formerly, lung disease was reported as occurring within 3 years of exposure to the drug (59). However, it is now recognized that pulmonary fibrosis can occur up to 20 years after exposure to the compound following a prolonged symptom-free period (60). Carmustine-induced fibrosis is characterized by an upper lobe distribution (61). No specific treatment is recommended, but given a remote history of malignancy, lung transplantation can be considered.

IV. Drug Therapy for UIP/IPF

Historically, the concept that inflammation of the lower respiratory tract (alveolitis) leads to pulmonary fibrosis has resulted in the use of anti-inflammatory therapy for IPF. As a consequence, oral corticosteroids are considered to be the cornerstone of treatment, while other therapies—including immunosuppressive, cytotoxic, and antifibrotic agents—have also been utilized. To date, no pharmacological therapy has been proven to alter or reverse the clinical course of IPF (62). As a consequence, some authors have gone so far as to argue that current anti-inflammatory therapy for IPF provides no benefit and may even be detrimental (5,63).

A. Corticosteroids

Corticosteroids constitute the recommended therapy for UIP despite the absence of any randomized placebo-controlled trial. In initiating corticosteroid treatment in IPF, it is recommended to do so as early as possible with the hope of slowing progression of the disease. What constitutes the most effective dose and period of treatment is also unknown. A dose of 0.5 mg/kg/day for 4 weeks followed by does reduction to 0.25 mg/kg/day has been advocated (62). The application of corticosteroids is based on a variety of historical reports. In a retrospective analysis of 127 patients who received oral corticosteroid therapy with a follow-up of 4 years, 17% of patients demonstrated an objective response to treatment (64). In this study, corticosteroid therapy identified a subgroup with an improved survival who were younger and who had a more cellular lung biopsy. In retrospect, these patients may now be reclassified as suffering with NSIP. Carrington et al. (65) described 40 DIP patients and 53 UIP patients among whom 66% of the DIP patients responded to corticosteroid therapy compared to 11% of UIP patients. Therefore a trial of corticosteroids may have a role in selecting patients with suspected treatment-responsive disease (DIP, NSIP), particularly younger patients below 65 years of age (64). By implication, the majority of patients not responding to corticosteroid therapy may have UIP. These patients are commonly elderly (mean age 65 years), male, have a BAL characterized by an excess of neutrophils and HRCT with honeycombing, traction bronchiectasis, and no ground-glass attenuation. Flaherty et al. (66) have prospectively identified 30 side effects in UIP patients exposed to corticosteroid therapy in line with international guidelines. Of these patients, 76% complained of insomnia, 73% became cushingoid, and 61% suffered with irritability and blurred vision. In light of the significant side-effect profile of corticosteroids, and the lack of documented efficacy in UIP, IPF patients should be exposed to corticosteroids only after careful consideration.

B. Cytotoxic and Antifibrotic Agents

A number of alternative cytotoxic, immunomodulatory, and antifibrotic agents have been employed in the treatment of IPF, usually administered in conjunction with oral corticosteroid therapy. These agents include azathio prine, cyclophosphamide, colchicine, methotrexate, penicillamine, cyclosporine, and interferon gamma.

Azathioprine

Azathioprine, which is commonly used as a steroid-sparing agent in IPF, is a purine antagonist that inhibits DNA synthesis resulting in suppression of cellular and humoral immunity. Raghu et al. (67) suggested that the use of azathioprine at 3 mg/kg/day in conjunction with corticosteroids conferred a survival advantage over those patients receiving oral corticosteroids at 20 mg/day. In this study, age was identified as an important determinant of outcome. When the survival analysis was adjusted for age, there was a significantly better survival in those patients receiving azathioprine. However, 27% of patients died in the first year, and a difference in survival became apparent only after 4 years of follow-up. We now recognize that survival beyond 3 years is unusual in patients with UIP; therefore, inadvertently, the prolonged survival associated with azathioprine may reflect the fact that 63% of the azathioprine patients were female. Nevertheless, the trend toward improved survival from a prospective randomized study has resulted in azathioprine and corticosteroids being a recommended form of therapy. As a consequence, the American Thoracic Society (ATS) guidelines recommend a dose of 2 to 3 mg/kg/day to a maximum dose of 150 mg/kg/day (62). Gastrointestinal side effects—including nausea, vomiting, and diarrhea—are common. Patients exposed to azathioprine who are deficient in thiopurine methyltransferase are at increased risk of bone marrow suppression. Mild thiopurine methyltransferase deficiency occurs in 11% of the general population.

Cyclophosphamide

Cyclophosphamide has been administered widely as therapy for IPF because it impairs neutrophil activity. O'Donnell et al. (68) demonstrated a cyclophosphamide-induced reduction in bronchoalveolar lavage (BAL) neutrophil concentration. In this 6-month study, 14 patients receiving cyclophosphamide 1.5 mg/kg had a significant reduction in BAL neutrophil count in comparison to 14 patients receiving corticosteroid therapy. A randomized study of cyclophosphamide in patients with biopsy-proven IPF compared prednisolone, 60 mg/day tapering to 20 mg on alternate days, to cyclophosphamide 100 mg/day plus prednisolone 20 mg on alternate days (69). These data were widely interpreted as suggesting that cyclophosphamide conferred a significant survival advantage. However, the data were biased in favor of cyclophosphamide. More than 50% of patients receiving cyclosphosphamide had a total lung capacity of greater than 80% predicted, in contrast to greater than 50% of patients receiving prednisolone alone, who had a total lung capacity below 60% of predicted. In spite of this physiological advantage in favor of cyclophosphamide, there was still no significant difference in survival between the two groups. Intravenous cyclophosphamide is an alternative to oral cyclophosphamide and results in a lower total cumulative dose of cyclophosphamide being administered to patients. A patient being given 100 mg of oral cyclophosphamide per day for 3 weeks receives a total dose of 2.1 g. In contrast, pulse intravenous cyclophosphamide on a three-weekly basis results in a dose of between 800 and 1500 mg being administered episodically. As a result, intravenous cyclophosphamide is associated with less risk in terms of carcinogenesis, but it is labor-intensive and demands appropriate nursing infrastructures. There is no randomized study involving the use of intravenous cyclophosphamide, but an open, noncontrolled study (70) reported on 33 patients, 30% of whom died in the first 6 months of the study period. This study demonstrated that intravenous cyclophosphamide had little impact in patients with progressive disease but facilitated steroid tapering in patients who selected themselves out as having nonprogressive disease. Because cyclophosphamide has little effect on survival, the impact of potential side effects is of considerable importance. Nausea, alopecia, and bone marrow suppression are common reversible side effects. Infertility, hemorrhagic cystitis, and malignancy are particularly significant adverse effects. Patients with Wegener's granulomatosis receiving cyclophosphamide have a threefold increased risk of carcinoma (71). This is important to IPF patients, as they are inherently at a greater risk for the development of lung cancer (72). Patients with IPF are recognized as having increased p53 oncogene expression in pulmonary tissues (73). Late after lung transplantation, malignant disorders are the second commonest cause of death (15%) in IPF patients (Fig. 3) (74). This may reflect the use of cyclophosphamide in IPF patients prior to transplantation. These concerns argue for a critical review of the traditional role that cyclophosphamide therapy has in the treatment of UIP.

Cyclosporine

As many IPF patients are under the care of physicians with an interest in transplantation, increasing numbers of patients have been exposed to cyclosporine therapy. Cyclosporine is an immunophylin-binding drug that forms a complex with cyclophylin and inactivates calcineurin. Calcineurin is an enzyme critical to the transcription of cytokines, including IL-2, IL-3, IL-4, IL-5, interferon-γ, and tumor necrosis factor α. In IPF patients awaiting lung transplantation, cyclosporine has been advocated as an effective means of facilitating steroid withdrawal or reduction. In a study by Venuta et al. (75), 10 patients receiving high-dose prednisolone (>50 mg/day), were given cyclosporine (4–7 mg/kg/day). Achieving cyclosporine levels of 300 to 400 ng/mL, facilitated the reduction in dose of steroids, and this resulted in a mild improvement in the 6-min walk test in 5 of 10 patients. These were encouraging results, as inevitably patients awaiting transplantation have advanced disease, although these 10 patients were receiving questionably high doses of corticosteroids. The application of cyclosporine facilitating dose reduction of

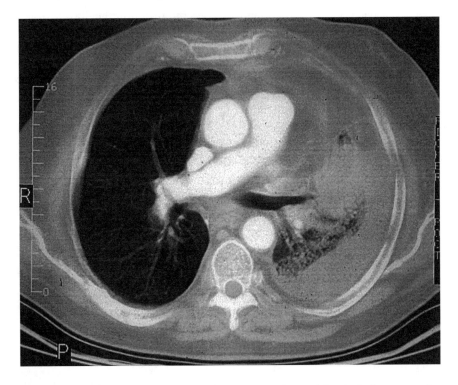

Figure 3 A thoracic CT scan of a patient 5 years after a right single-lung transplant for IPF. The transplanted lung is normal. In the left native lung there is an intrapulmonary mass and an associated pleural effusion. This is a non-small-cell lung cancer occurring in the native IPF lung.

corticosteroids and maximizing exercise capacity is an acceptable therapeutic goal. Two other open, nonrandomized studies have reported on the application of cyclosporine in IPF. Moolman et al. (76) described the impact of cyclosporine administered for 9 months in 10 patients, of whom 5 patients had IPF and 5 had histological features suggestive of NSIP. While receiving cyclosporine 3 mg/kg/day, all 5 patients with NSIP and 3 patients with UIP experienced an improvement in exercise capacity and vital capacity. Alton et al. (77) evaluated once-daily cyclosporine at a dose of 5 mg/kg/day in 10 patients in whom cyclophosphamide therapy had failed. Survival analysis suggested that there was an improvement in survival of 2.5 to 5 months in comparison to a matched historical control group of 7 patients receiving cyclosporine. Further studies are required before cyclosporine can be recommended as form of therapy, particularly as cyclosporine is a fibrogenic compound.

Colchicine

In vitro studies have demonstrated that colchicine is an inhibitor of fibroblast function, particularly fibroblast proliferation and collagen synthesis (78). However, it has little effect on other cytokines important in the fibrotic disease process, particularly transforming growth factor β (79). Colchicine has been advocated as a potential treatment of IPF following a study in which it was administered to 23 patients who had received previous corticosteroid therapy (80). While receiving colchicine 600 mg/day, 30% of patients improved, 30% remained stable, and 40% worsened. Douglas et al. (81) have subsequently emphasized the favorable outcome of IPF patients receiving colchicine in contrast to prednisolone. In a prospective, randomized study, 12 subjects treated with prednisolone experienced a higher incidence of serious side effects, a more rapid decline in pulmonary function, and reduced survival, compared to 14 patients treated with colchicine alone (81). These data emphasize that corticosteroid therapy had negligible efficacy and more side effects than colchicine, which had negligible efficacy but a favorable side-effect profile.

Methotrexate

Methotrexate is a folic acid analog that inhibits the enzyme dihydrofolate reductase. Its immunosuppressive properties can probably be attributed to inhibition of replication and function of T lymphocytes and possibly B lymphocytes. It may also interfere with neutrophil chemotaxis. There are very few published reports using methotrexate in IPF, probably because of its known pulmonary toxicity. At present there is no evidence to support its application in IPF.

Penicillamine

Several animal studies suggest a possible role for penicillamine in the treatment of fibrotic lung disorders. However, controlled trials of penicillamine therapy in IPF do not exist. There are a number of open-label, nonrandomized uncontrolled trials (82,83) and one case series in the literature (84) demonstrating that penicillamine has little or no benefit in IPF, and side effects appear to be frequent. If this drug is initiated, 125 or 250 mg is given orally as a single daily dose, with gradual increments to a final dose of 500 mg/ day. It is thought that a response to treatment requires 3 to 6 months of therapy.

Antioxidants

The antioxidant substance glutathione is deficient in the alveolar lining fluid of IPF patients (85). Therefore augmenting the availability of this substance may reduce the oxidative damage contributing to the pathogenesis of IPF. The administration of N-acetylcysteine (NAC) has been shown to elevate BAL glutathione levels in IPF patients (86). A single 12-week open-label study of oral NAC 600 mg 3 times per day in a group of 18 patients receiving maintenance immunosuppression has been undertaken (87). This study reported that NAC administration was associated with an improvement in lung function. These data are encouraging, and the low side-effect profile of this therapy suggest that this therapeutic approach deserves further study.

Perfenidone

Perfenidone is an agent that inhibits transforming growth factor beta ($TGF\text{-}\beta$) stimulated collagen synthesis, decreases the extracellular matrix, and blocks fibroblast proliferation in vitro. One open label phase II trial of the drug in 54 patients with IPF has suggested that it may result in the stabilization of lung function (88). Perfenidone appeared to facilitate the withdrawal of conventional therapy in 38 patients. One- and 2-year survival was 78 and 63% respectively (88). The drug administered to a maximum dose of 3600 mg/day was reasonably well tolerated, with nausea and photosensitivity as the most commonly reported adverse effects. Further studies are required of this potentially important compound.

Interferon Gamma 1b

Interferon gamma 1b is a potential therapeutic compound for the treatment of IPF. This is because in animal studies, interferon gamma has been shown to inhibit fibroblast and collagen synthesis. Furthermore, it is recognized that patients with IPF have reduced levels of interferon gamma in BAL compared to controls (89). Therefore it is believed that there may be an imbalance between interferon gamma and TGF-β in IPF patients. Ziesche et al. (90) have attempted to redress this imbalance by administering interferon gamma to UIP patients. In an open-label, randomized pilot study, they showed that patients receiving interferon gamma demonstrated a statistically significant 9% improvement in total lung capacity over 1 year and a reduction in TGF-β

expression in tissue obtained by serial transbronchial biopsy. In this study, IPF patients received interferon gamma 200 mg three times per week with 7.5 mg of oral corticosteroids per day, and the control patients received a symptom-driven schedule of oral corticosteroids. The IPF patients were carefully selected on the basis of two criteria: first, a failure to respond to steroids over 1 year and, second, histological evidence of UIP acquired by open-lung biopsy. This diligent selection process and efforts to exclude patients with potentially steroid-responsive disease (i.e., NSIP) may have introduced a selection bias inadvertently. To identify patients with progressive disease from whom a surgical biopsy and serial transbronchial lung biopsies can be obtained is unusual. Another important factor to be considered in interpreting the data is that the control group, who clearly had steroid unresponsive disease, were exposed to oral corticosteroids (25–50 mg), potentially worsening lung function. This decline in the control group may have been due to the promotion of Epstein-Barr virus replication within the pulmonary tissue or to the increase in body-mass index with corticosteroids. The deterioration in control patients receiving corticosteroids alone conferred an advantage on the group receiving interferon gamma, which highlights the necessity for novel therapies for UIP-pattern IPF to be compared with either placebo or no treatment. Nevertheless, this study represents an important step forward, and if these benefits are confirmed in other studies, the use of interferon gamma 1b could represent a significant advance in the treatment of IPF.

V. Management of Patients with Advanced Pulmonary Fibrosis

A. Oxygen Therapy

Historically, physicians have had some reluctance toward prescribing oxygen therapy, because of the hypothetical disadvantage of augmenting oxygen radical production. However this has not been substantiated. In a multivariate analysis of variables associated with disease progression (91), oxygen therapy was not associated with a decline in the clinical status of the patient. Indeed there are two complementary avenues of data demonstrating that oxygen therapy is beneficial. First, it has been shown that in patients with pulmonary fibrosis, an acute challenge of oxygen therapy significantly reduces the mean pulmonary artery pressure in those patients with secondary pulmonary hypertension. Second, it has been demonstrated that nocturnal hypoxemia is associated with daytime impairment of quality of life and that the administration of nocturnal oxygen therapy attenuates the daytime symptoms and improves quality of life (92). Patients should be warned of the side effects of oxygen therapy, which are predominantly local, in that the cold, dry oxygen can irritate the nose, causing dryness and epistaxis. An alternative method of oxygen delivery is the transtracheal route, but its application is often determined by local medical practice or physician interest. Briefly, a small stent is placed percutaneously under local anaesthetic, and following the development of a mature tract, a catheter is placed in the trachea. Complications include mucous plugging, local infection, and potentiation of the patient's existing cough. One theoretical advantage to transtracheal oxygen is that by reducing the upper airway dead space, there is less oxygen and air admixture, promoting oxygen delivery and reducing workload.

It should not be forgotten when prescribing oxygen therapy that both the concentration and flow should be considered. It is reasonable to titrate the oxygen therapy according to resting oxygen saturations, but it must be remembered that augmented flows of oxygen are required immediately following exercise and coughing in order to correct for oxygen deficit. It is difficult to administer greater more than 4L of oxygen per minute for patients while they are actively exercising; and therefore they should be advised to have additional supplemental oxygen supply available to them in circumstances where intense exercise is required. For instance, an additional cylinder delivering a higher flow of oxygen should be available at the top of the stairs. In this context, in order to prevent distressing breathlessness, early consideration should be given to altering the patient's environment. In particular a stair lift should be contemplated for a patient with a short life span, because bureaucratic delays may prevent the timely provision of a stair lift. Many IPF patients utilize portable breath-activated oxygen delivery systems in order to conserve oxygen, allowing prolonged mobilization from the patient's home. This is a useful strategy, but it must be remembered that if patients with advanced disease become extremely tachypnoeic, the breath-activated delivery system may not keep pace with the rate of breath. Paradoxically then, in advanced disease, the patient might be advised to use a continuous rather than intermittent supply when away from the home and to compensate the shorter supply time by bringing an additional cylinder.

B. Pulmonary Hypertension

An important but underemphasized feature of advanced IPF is secondary pulmonary hypertension. This results from (1) hypoxemia, (2) architectural disruption of the arterial bed by fibrosis, (3) in situ arteriolar thrombosis, and (4) imbalance of vasomotor tone. The management of hypoxemia is critical and has been dealt with above, while the cessation of the fibroproliferative process remains as the major challenge in the treatment of IPF. Anticoagulation potentially offers some protection against vascular thrombosis. There are no data to support the application of anticoagulation in IPF. Anticoagulation in IPF patients awaiting lung transplantation must be undertaken with care and judgment and specifically is ill advised in patients with marked pleural disease. However, it is the authors' practice to anticoagulate patients with advanced IPF and secondary pulmonary hypertension provided that they can easily be subjected to anticoagulation surveillance and have no contraindications. An imbalance of vasomotor tone is also believed to be an important factor in the development of secondary pulmonary hypertension in IPF. Endothelial-cell production of the vasodilators prostacyclin and nitric oxide (NO) is thought to be impaired in patients with secondary pulmonary hypertension. Correction of these deficiencies might thus be a therapeutic measure for IPF. Olschewski et al. (93) have demonstrated, in an acute challenge study, that nebulized iloprost significantly reduces pulmonary artery pressures without augmenting the pulmonary shunt. Although attractive, because nebulized therapy should target normal ventilated parts of the lung, nebulized iloprost is not without practical problems and has not been shown to be beneficial when administered chronically. Significantly, iloprost must be nebulized every 3 hr, and a specific ultrasonic nebulizer that achieves particles of less than 3 μm is recommended (94). Encouragingly, there is no evidence to suggest that the cessation of nebulized iloprost results in rebound pulmonary hypertension in a fashion similar to inhaled nitric oxide (NO). Inhaled NO has also been successfully applied in IPF and secondary pulmonary hypertension. Channick et al. (95) demonstrated that the inhalation of NO in IPF patients with secondary pulmonary hypertension led to a significant fall in pulmonary artery pressure. The therapeutic application of NO is potentially limited by the lack of availability of suitable delivery systems for outpatients, although a recent report describes the chronic application of NO to an IPF patient as a bridge to lung transplantation (96). In this study, using a pulsed delivery system, the patient continued to receive outpatient inhaled NO for 30 months while waiting for lung transplantation. Exercise and echocardiogram studies in this patient, after 3 months of inhaled NO, showed an improvement in arterial oxygenation, pulmonary hypertension, and exercise tolerance (96). With continuing advances in the treatment of primary pulmonary hypertension, novel strategies including oral sildenafil are emerging for the management of secondary pulmonary hypertension.

C. Reflux

Another important concomitant problem in IPF patients is oesophageal reflux. Tobin et al. (10) have demonstrated that IPF patients have a significantly increased incidence of acid reflux in comparison to control subjects. Utilizing ambulatory esophageal pH monitoring, 16 of 17 IPF patients, compared to 4 of 8 controls, had an increased incidence of acid reflux. Very importantly only 25% of these IPF patients actually had symptoms pertaining to reflux. Therefore it is advisable to treat all IPF patients with proton pump inhibitors.

D. Cough

Cough is a major problem in IPF patients. There are no data in the literature as to what is the best management strategy for this problem. The cough may be dry, but many patients may produce large amounts of mucoid sputum. Inhaled beclomethasone, which is administered using the HFA propellant in order to achieve small airway distribution, may offer relief to some individuals. Cough is frequently associated with reflux esophagitis; therefore, in patients complaining of cough, reflux therapy should be administered. In the authors' experience, nebulized lignocaine and nebulized narcotic therapy do not substantially ameliorate the symptoms.

In the advanced stages of pulmonary fibrosis, cough frequently precipitates profound hypoxemia. In this circumstance, it is important to administer high-flow oxygen, over and above what the patient normally uses, to ameliorate the hypoxemia.

E. Pneumothorax

Another problem that arises in patients with IPF is the development of a spontaneous pneumothorax. If this occurs early in the course of disease, it should be treated aggressively. Surgical pleurodesis should be considered in order to prevent profound respiratory failure should the pneumothorax recur. Alternatively, pneumothorax frequently signals a terminal phase of disease. In this circumstance, it should be acknowledged that palliative care is the key component of management, and surgical treatment or ventilation should be avoided.

F. Minimalism/Best Supportive Care

The majority of IPF patients are "nonresponders" to medical therapy. These patients are commonly elderly, male, have a BAL characterized by an excess of neutrophils, and a HRCT with honeycombing, traction bronchiectasis, and no ground-glass attenuation. In these patients, particularly those above 65 years of age, a strategy of minimalism should be considered (63). Minimalism involves avoiding immunosuppression, dose reduction, and drug withdrawal. There are little or no data to support chronic corticosteroid therapy or second-line therapy in patients with advanced disease. Indeed, much of the data support a strategy of minimalism. Johnson et al. (69) demonstrated that low-dose corticosteroid therapy was as effective as high-dose steroid therapy, and the addition of cyclophosphamide failed to improve survival. Douglas et al. (97) highlighted the concept of minimalism by demonstrating that in well-matched but clinically stable patients, corticosteroid therapy was associated with a decline in lung physiology. In contrast, colchicine was associated with preservation of lung function. Raghu et al. (67) and Lok et al. (98) have demonstrated that older patients in particular fail to benefit from intensive immunosuppression. Therefore minimalism/best supportive care should be acknowledged as a specific and important treatment strategy in patients with IPF, particularly elderly IPF patients and those awaiting lung transplantation.

G. Referral for Lung Transplantation

IPF has an extremely limited prognosis, with a median survival of 2.9 years (4). After the failure of medical treatment, single-lung transplantation results in an actuarial survival of 73% at 1 year and 57% at 3 years (99). In the United States, lung transplantation for IPF has been shown to confer an improved survival compared with patients remaining on the waiting list (74). A limited window of opportunity exists to refer IPF patients for lung transplantation. The short transplant window is reflected in the high mortality rate in IPF patients awaiting lung transplantation (74). Currently, the median waiting period for single-lung transplantation in the United Kingdom is 351 days [confidence interval (CI) 293 to 427 days]. Given an expected median survival of 34 months after the diagnosis of IPF and a mean waiting list for transplantation of 12 months, there is a window of just 22 months for referral for transplantation. It is because of this limited transplant window and the difficulty predicting survival that IPF patients in the United States are given a 3-month waiting advantage compared with patients with emphysema (100). Despite this, IPF patients still have the highest death rate while awaiting lung transplantation (74). International guidelines recommend that symptomatic patients with IPF below 65 years of age should be discussed with the transplant center after a failed trial of corticosteroid therapy and referred in any of the following circumstances: $DL_{CO} < 50$ to 60%, $FVC < 60$ to 70%, resting hypoxia or pulmonary hypertension (101). Since the publication of these guidelines, two important concepts have been developed. First, Gay et al. (102) have emphasized that lung function is a poor marker for survival. This corroborates previous data, which showed that there was no correlation between morphological fibrosis and lung function. Second, it has been demonstrated that HRCT quantification of the extent of fibrosis is superior to histological quantification of fibrosis in predicting survival (103). In light of these developments, recent data have shown that 2-year survival can be estimated in IPF patients, potentially optimizing the timing of transplantation. The model described utilizes simple criteria, including HRCT fibrosis score and DL_{CO}. In a study 136 IPF patients below 65 years of age, a DL_{CO} of less than 40% of predicted combined with a HRCT fibrosis score of greater than 2 has a sensitivity and specificity of 80% in predicting 2-year survival (104).

H. Organization of Care

To resolve the continuing difficulty in treating patients with IPF, there is an urgent need for ongoing randomized therapeutic trials. The absence of randomized studies facilitates the poor outcome experienced by IPF patients. The development of "shared care" specialist clinics should facilitate early referral and encourage the recruitment of adequate numbers of patients at an early stage of their disease to power randomized studies (105). Lok et al. have reported that IPF patients attending a specialist fibrosis clinic have a significantly better survival rate than those IPF patients who attend a general pulmonary service (105). Appropriately designed studies are needed at a time when a variety of agents—including perfenidone, antioxidants, interferon, and endothelin antagonists—have been shown to have potential as therapeutic agents in IPF. Therefore scientifically oriented pulmonologists need to dispense with the philosophy of patient ownership and collaborate with centers with a declared interest that also offer transplantation as an alternative to failed medical therapy. Encouragingly, this concept is being increasingly adopted, with practical examples including the Greater Manchester Lung Fibrosis Consortium, the Michigan Fibrotic Lung Disease Network, and the Mayo Clinic Fibrosis Network.

References

1. American Thoracic Society/European Respiratory Society: International Multi-disciplinary Consensus Classification of the Idiopathic Interstitial Pneumonias. Am J Respir Crit Care Med 2002; 165:277–304.
2. Katzenstein AA, Myers JL. Idiopathic pulmonary fibrosis, clinical relevance of pathologic classification. Am J Respir Crit Care Med 1998; 157:1301–1315.
3. Coultas DB, Zumwalt ZE, Black WC, Sobonya RE. The epidemiology of interstitial lung diseases. Am J Respir Crit Care Med 1994; 150:967–972.
4. Bjoraker JA, Ryu J, Edwin MK, Myers JL, Tazelaar HD, Schroeder DR, Offord KP. Prognostic significance of histologic subsets in idiopathic pulmonary fibrosis. Am J Respir Crit Care Med 1998; 157:199–203.
5. Gross TJ, Hunninghake GW. Idiopathic pulmonary fibrosis. N Engl J Med 2001; 345(7):517–525.
6. Scadding JG, Hinson KFW. Diffuse fibrosing alveolitis (diffuse interstitial fibrosis of the lungs): correlation with histology of biopsy with prognosis. Thorax 1967; 22:291–304.
7. Egan JJ, Stewart JP, Haselton PS, Arrand JR, Carroll KB, Woodcock AA. Epstein-Barr virus replication with pulmonary epithelial cells in cryptogenic fibrosing alveolitis. Thorax 1995; 50:1234–1239.
8. Egan JJ, Woodcock AA, Stewart JP. Viruses and idiopathic pulmonary fibrosis. Eur Respir J 1997; 10:1433–1437.
9. Hubbard R, Lewis S, Richards K, Johnston I, Britton J. Occupational exposure to metal or wood dust and etiology of cryptogenic fibrosing alveolitis. Lancet 1996; 347:284–289.
10. Tobin RW, Pope CE, Pellefrini CA, Emond MJ, Sillery J, Raghu G. Increased prevalence of gastroesophageal reflux in patients with idiopathic pulmonary fibrosis. Am J Respir Crit Care Med 1998; 158:1804–1808.
11. Stewart JP, Egan JJ, Haselton PS, Lok S, Nash AA, Woodcock AA. The detection of EBV DNA in lung biopsy specimens from patients with idiopathic pulmonary fibrosis. Am J Respir Crit Care Med 1999; 159:1336–1341.
12. Raghu G, Mageto YN, Lockhart D, Schmidt RA, Wood DE, Godwin JD. The accuracy of the clinical diagnosis of new-onset idiopathic pulmonary fibrosis and other interstitial lung disease: a prospective study. Chest 1999; 116(5):1168–1174.

13. Utz JP, Ryu JH, Douglas WW, Hartman TE, Tazelaar HD, Myers JL, Allen MS, Schroder DR. High short-term mortality following lung biopsy for usual interstitial pneumonia. Eur Respir J 2001; 17(2):175–179.
14. Katzenstein AL, Fiorelli RF. Nonspecific interstitial pneumonia/fibrosis: histologic features and clinical significance. Am J Surg Pathol 1994; 18:136–147.
15. Fugita J, Yoshinouchi T, Ohtsuki Y, Tokuda M, Yang Y, Yamadori I, Bandoh S, Ishida T, Takahara J, Ueda R. Non-specific interstitial pneumonia as pulmonary involvement of systemic sclerosis. Ann Rheum Dis 2001; 60:281–283.
16. Park JS, Lee KS, Kim JS, Park CS, Suh YL, Choi DL, Kim KJ. Nonspecific interstitial pneumonia with fibrosis: radiographic and CT findings in seven patients. Radiology 1995; 195:645–648.
17. Daniil ZD, Gilchrist FC, Nicholson AG, Hansell DM, Harris J, Colby TV, du Bois RM. A histologic pattern of nonspecific interstitial pneumonia is associated with a better prognosis than usual interstitial pneumonia in patients with cryptogenic fibrosing alveolitis. Am J Respir Crit Care Med 1999; 160:899–905.
18. Myers JL. Respiratory bronchiolitis associated interstitial lung disease. In: Epler GR, ed. Diseases of the Bronchioles. New York: Raven Press, 1994:297.
19. Nicholson AG, Colby TV, du Bois RM, Hansell DM, Wells AU. The prognostic significance of the histologic pattern of interstitial pneumonia in patients presenting with the clinical entity of cryptogenic fibrosing alveolitis. Am J Respir Crit Care Med 2000; 162:2213–2217.
20. Olsen J, Colby T, Elliott C. Hamman-Rich syndrome revisited. Mayo Clin Proc 1990; 65:1538–1548.
21. Katzenstein AL, Myers JL, Mazur MT. Acute interstitial pneumonia. A clinicopathologic, ultrastructural, and cell kinetic study. Am J Surg Pathol 1986; 10:256–267.
22. Vourlekis JS, Brown KK, Cool CD, Young DA, Cherniack RM, King TE, Schwarz MI. Acute interstitial pneumonitis. Case series and review of the literature. Medicine 2000; 79(6):369–378.
23. Ellman P, Ball RE. Rheumatoid disease with joint and pulmonary manifestations. Br Med J 1948; 2:816–820.
24. Gabbay E, Tarala R, Will R, Carroll G, Adler B, Cameron D, Lake FR. Interstitial lung disease in recent onset rheumatoid arthritis. Am J Respir Crit Care Med 1997; 156:528–535.
25. Remy-Jardin M, Remy J, Cortet B, Mauri F, Delcambre B. Lung changes in rheumatoid arthritis: CT findings. Radiology 1994; 193:375–382.
26. Dawson JK, Fewins HE, Desmond J, Lynch MP, Graham DR. Fibrosing alveolitis in patients with rheumatoid arthritis as assessed by high resolution computed tomography, chest radiography, and pulmonary function tests. Thorax 2001; 56(8):622–627.
27. Saag KG, Kolluri S, Koehnke RK, Georgou TA, Rachow JW, Hunninghake GW, Schwartz DA. Rheumatoid arthritis lung disease: determinants of radiographic and physiologic abnormalities. Arthritis Rheum 1996; 39:1711–1719.
28. Hunninghake GW, Fauci AS. Pulmonary involvement in collagen vascular diseases. Am Rev Respir Dis 1979; 119:471–503.
29. Yousem SA, Colby TV, Carrington CB. Lung biopsy in rheumatoid arthritis. Am Rev Respir Dis 1985; 131:770–777.
30. Hakala M. Poor prognosis in patients with rheumatoid arthritis hospitalized for interstitial lung fibrosis. Chest 1988; 93:114–118.

31. Wells AU, Hansell DM, Rubens MB, Cullinan P, Haslam PM, Black CM, du Bois RM. Fibrosing alveolitis in systemic sclerosis. Bronchoalveolar findings in relation to computed tomographic appearance. Am J Respir Crit Care Med 1994; 150:462–468.
32. Alton E, Turner-Warwick M. Lung involvement in scleroderma. In: Black CM, Jayson MIV, eds. Systemic Sclerosis (Scleroderma). Chichester, UK: Wiley, 1988.
33. Wells AU, Hansell DM, Rubens MB, King AD, Cramer D, Black CM, du Bois RM. Fibrosing alveolitis in systemic sclerosis. Indices of lung function in relation to extent of disease on computed tomography. Arthritis Rheum 1997; 40:1229–1229.
34. Altman RD, Medsger TA Jr, Bloch DA, Michel BA. Predictors of survival in systemic sclerosis (scleroderma). Arthritis Rheum 1991; 34:403–413.
35. Orens JB, Martinez FJ, Lynch JP III. Pleuropulmonary manifestations of systemic lupus erythematosus. Rheum Dis Clin North Am 1994; 20:159–193.
36. Haupt HM, Moore GW, Hutchins GM. The lung in systemic lupus erythematosus. Analysis of the pathologic changes in 120 patients. Am J Med 1981; 71:791–798.
37. Todd NW, Wise RA. Respiratory complications in the collagen vascular diseases. Clin Pulm Med 1996; 3:101–112.
38. Fenlon HM, Doran M, Sant SM, Breatnach E. High resolution chest CT in systemic lupus erythematosus. Am J Roentgenol 1996; 166:301–307.
39. King TE, Jr. Connective tissue disease. In: Schwarz MI, King TE, Jr, eds. Interstitial Lung Disease. London: Decker, 1998:451–506.
40. Martin WJ, Rosenow EC. Amiodarone pulmonary toxicity. Recognition and pathogenesis. Chest 1988; 93:1067–1075.
41. Mason JW. Amiodarone. N Engl J Med 1987; 316:455–466.
42. Dean PJ, Groshart KD, Porterfield JG, Iansmith DH, Golden EB. Amiodarone associated pulmonary toxicity. A clinical and pathologic study of eleven cases. Am J Clin Pathol 1987; 87:7–13.
43. Van Mieghem W, Coolen L, Malysse I, Lacquet LM, Deneffe GJ, Demedts MG. Amiodarone and the development of ARDS after lung surgery. Chest 1994; 105:1642–1645.
44. Wood DL, Osborn MJ, Rooke J, Holmes DR Jr. Amiodarone pulmonary toxicity: report of two cases associated with rapidly progressive fatal respiratory distress syndrome after pulmonary angiography. Mayo Clin Proc 1985; 60:601–603.
45. Coudert B, Bailly F, Lombard JN, Andre F, Camus P. Amiodarone pneumonitis. Brochoalveolar lavage findings in 15 patients and review of the literature. Chest 1992; 102:1005–1012.
46. Myers JL, Kennedy JI, Plumb VJ. Amiodarone lung: pathologic findings in clinically toxic patients. Hum Pathol 1987; 18:349–354.
47. Malik SW, Myers JL, DeRemee RA, Specks U. Lung toxicity associated with cyclophosphamide use. Two distinct patterns. Am J Respir Crit Care Med 1996; 154:1851–1856.
48. Abdel Karim FW, Ayash RE, Allam C, Salem PA. Pulmonary fibrosis after prolonged treatment with low dose cyclophosphamide. Oncology 1983; 40:174–176.
49. Oliner H, Schwartz R, Rubio F, Dameshek W. Interstitial pulmonary fibrosis following busulphan therapy. Am J Med 1961; 31:134.

50. Cooper JAD, White DA, Mattay RA. Drug induced pulmonary disease. Part 1: Cytotoxic drugs. Am Rev Respir Dis 1986; 133:321–340.

51. Heard BE, Cooke RA. Busulphan lung. Thorax 1968; 23:187–193.

52. Vergnon J, Boucherons S, Riffart J, Guy C, Blanc P, Emonot A. Pneumopathies interstitielles au busulfan: analyse histologique, evolutive et par lavage broncho-alveolaire de trios observations. Rev Med Intern 1988; 9:377–383.

53. Ginsberg SS, Comis RL. The pulmonary toxicity of antineoplastic agents. Semin Oncol 1982; 9:34–51.

54. Podell LN, Winkler SS. Busulphan lung: report of two cases and review of the literature. Am J Roentgenol 1974; 120:151.

55. Jules-Elysee K, White DA. Bleomycin-induced pulmonary toxicity. Clin Chest Med 1990; 11:1.

56. Tryka AF, Skornic WA, Godleski JJ, Brain JD. Potentiation of bleomycin-induced lung injury by exposure to 70 percent oxygen. Am Rev Respir Dis 1982; 126:1074–1079.

57. Belamy E, Husband J, Blaquire R, Law M. Bleomycin-related lung damage: CT evidence. Radiology 1985; 156:155–158.

58. Simpson AB, Paul J, Graham J, Kaye SB. Fatal bleomycin pulmonary toxicity in the west of Scotland 1991–1995: a review of patients with germ cell tumours. Br J Cancer 1998; 78:1061–1066.

59. Reiss RB, Poster DS, Penta JS. The nitrosureas and pulmonary toxicity. Cancer Treat Rev 1981; 8:111–125.

60. O'Driscoll BR, Haselton PS, Taylor PM, Poulter LW, Gattamaneni HR, Woodcock AA. Active lung fibrosis up to 17 years after chemotherapy with carmustine (BCNU) in childhood. N Engl J Med 1990; 323:378–382.

61. Taylor PM, O'Driscoll BR, Gattamaneni HR, Woodcock AA. Chronic lung fibrosis following carmustine (BCNU) chemotherapy: radiological features. Clin Radiol 1991; 44:299–301.

62. American Thoracic Society. Idiopathic pulmonary fibrosis: diagnosis and treatment. International consensus statement. American Thoracic Society (ATS), and the European Respiratory Society (ERS). Am J Respir Crit Care Med 2000; 161:646.

63. Egan JJ. Pharmacologic therapy of idiopathic pulmonary fibrosis. J Heart Lung Transplant 1998; 17:1039–1044.

64. Turner-Warwick M, Burrows B, Johnson A. Cryptogenic fibrosing alveolitis: response to corticosteroid treatment and its effect on survival. Thorax 1980; 35:593–599.

65. Carrington CB, Gaensler EA, Coutu RE, Fitzgerald MX, Gupta RG. Natural history and treated course of usual and desquamative interstitial pneumonia. N Engl J Med 1978; 298:801–809.

66. Flaherty KR, Toews GB, Lynch JP, Kazerooni EA, Gross BH, Strawderman RL, Hariharan K, Flint A, Martinez FJ. Steroids in idiopathic pulmonary fibrosis: a prospective assessment of adverse reactions, response to therapy, and survival. Am J Med 2001; 110(4):278–282.

67. Raghu G, Depaso WJ, Cain K, Hammar SP, Wetzel CE, Dreis DF, Hutchinson J, Pardee NE, Winterbauer RH. Azathioprine combined with prednisolone in the treatment of idiopathic pulmonary fibrosis: a prospective, double-blind randomised, placebo-controlled clinical trial. Am Rev Respir Dis 1991; 144:291–296.

68. O'Donnell K, Keogh B, Cantin A, Crystal RG. Pharmacological suppression of the neutrophil component of the alveolitis in idiopathic pulmonary fibrosis. Am Rev Respir Dis 1987; 136:288–292.

69. Johnson MA, Kwan S, Snell NJC, Nunn AJ, Darbyshire JH, Turner-Warwick M. Randomised controlled trial comparing prednisolone alone with cyclophosphamide and low dose prednisolone in combination in cryptogenic fibrosing alveolitis. Thorax 1989; 44:280–288.

70. Baughman RP, Lower EE. Use of intermittent, intravenous cyclophosphamide for idiopathic pulmonary fibrosis. Chest 1992; 102:1090–1094.

71. Hoffman GS, Kerr GS, Leavitt RY, Hallahan CW, Lebovics RS, Travis WD, Rottem M, Fauci AS. Wegeners granulomatosis: an analysis of 158 patients. Ann Intern Med 1992; 116:488–498.

72. Turner-Warwick M, Lebowitz M, Burrows B, Johnson A. Cryptogenic fibrosing alveolitis and lung cancer. Thorax 1980; 35:496–499.

73. Kuwano K, Kunitake R, Kawasaki M, Nomoto Y, Hagimoto N, Nakanishi Y, Haru N. P21 WAFI/CIPI/SD11 and p53 expression in association with DNA strand breaks in idiopathic pulmonary fibrosis: a prospective double-blind, randomised, placebo controlled clinical trial. Am J Respir Crit Care Med 1996; 154:477–483.

74. Hosenpud JD, Bennett LE, Keck BM, Edwards EB, Novick RJ. Effect of diagnosis on survival benefit of lung transplantation for end-stage lung disease. Lancet 1998; 351:24–27.

75. Venuta F, Rendina EA, Ciriaco P, De Giacomo T, Pompeo E, Bachetoni A, Ricci C. Efficacy of cyclosporine to reduce steroids in patients with idiopathic pulmonary fibrosis before lung transplantation. J Heart Lung Transplant 1993; 12:909–914.

76. Moolman JA, Bardin PG, Roussouw DJ, Joubert JR. Cyclosporin as a treatment for interstitial lung disease of unknown etiology. Thorax 1991; 46:592–595.

77. Alton EWF, Johnson M, Turner-Warwick M. Advanced cryptogenic fibrosing alveolitis: preliminary report on treatment with cyclosporine A. Respir Med 1989; 83:277–279.

78. Rennard SI, Bitterman PB, Ozaki T, Rom WN, Crystal RG. Colchicine suppresses the release of fibroblast growth factors from alveolar macrophages in vitro. Am Rev Respir Dis 1988; 137:181–185.

79. Entzian P, Scklaak M, Seitzer U, Bufe A, Acil Y, Zabel P. Antiinflammatory and antifibrotic properties of colchicines: implications for idiopathic pulmonary fibrosis. Lung 1997; 175:41–51.

80. Peters SG, McDougall JC, Douglas WW, Coles DT, DeRemee RA. Colchicine in the treatment of pulmonary fibrosis. Chest 1993; 103:101–104.

81. Douglas WW, Ryu JH, Swensen SJ, Offord KP, Schroeder DR, Caron GM, DeRemee RA. Colchicine versus prednisolone in the treatment of idiopathic pulmonary fibrosis. Am J Respir Crit Care Med 1998; 158(1):220–225.

82. Goodman M, Turner-Warwick M. Pilot study of D-penicillamine therapy in corticosteroid failure patients with widespread pulmonary fibrosis. Chest 1978; 74(3):338.

83. Selman M, Carrillo G, Salas J, Padilla RP, Perez-Chavira R, Sansores R, Chapela R. Colchicine, D-penicillamine and prednisolone in the treatment of idiopathic pulmonary fibrosis. Chest 1998; 114(2):507–512.

84. Liebetrau G, Pielesch W, Ganguin HG, Jung A, Jung H. Die therapie der lungenfibrosen mit D-penizillamin. Z Ges Inn Med 1982; 37:263–266.
85. Cantin AM, Hubbard RC, Crystal RG. Glutathione deficiency in the epithelial lining fluid of the lower respiratory tract in idiopathic pulmonary fibrosis. Am Rev Respir Dis 1989; 139(2):370–372.
86. Meyer A, Buhl R, Kampf S, Magnussen H. Intravenous N-acetylcysteine and lung glutathione of patients with pulmonary fibrosis and normals. Am J Respir Crit Care Med 1995; 152(3):1055–1060.
87. Behr J, Maier K, Degenkolb B, Krombach F, Vogelmeier C. Antioxidative and clinical effects of high-dose N-acetylcysteine in fibrosing alveolitis. Adjunctive therapy to maintenance immunosuppression. Am J Respir Crit Care Med 1997; 156(6):1897–1901.
88. Raghu G, Johnson WC, Lockhart D, Mageto Y. Treatment of idiopathic pulmonary fibrosis with a new antifibrotic agent, perfenidone. Am J Respir Crit Care Med 1999; 159:1061–1069.
89. Prior C, Haslam CM. In vivo levels and in vitro production of interferon-gamma in fibrosing interstitial lung diseases. Clin Exp Immunol 1992; 88(2):280–287.
90. Ziesche R, Hofbauer E, Wittmann K, Petkov V, Block LH. A preliminary study of long-term treatment with interferon-gamma-lb and low dose prednisolone in patients with idiopathic pulmonary fibrosis. N Engl J Med 1999; 341:1246–1249.
91. Douglas WW, Ryu JH, Scroeder DR. Idiopathic pulmonary fibrosis: impact of oxygen and colchicine, prednisolone or no therapy on survival. Am J Respir Crit Care Med 2000; 161:1172–1178.
92. Clark M, Cooper B, Singh S, Cooper M, Carr N, Hubbard R. A survey of nocturnal hypoxaemia and health related quality of life in patients with cryptogenic fibrosing alveolitis. Thorax 2001; 56:482–486.
93. Olschewski H, Ghofrani HA, Walmrath D, Schermuly R, Temmesfeld-Wollbruck B, Grimminger F, Seeger W. Inhaled prostacyclin and ilioprost in severe pulmonary hypertension secondary to lung fibrosis. Am J Respir Crit Care Med 1999; 160(2):600–607.
94. Gessler T, Schmehl T, Hoeper MM, Rose F, Ghofrani HA, Olschewski H, Grimminger F, Seeger W. Ultrasonic versus jet nebulization of iloprost in severe pulmonary hypertension. Eur Respir J 2001; 17(1):14–19.
95. Channick RN, Hoch RC, Newhart JW, Johnson FW, Smith CM. Improvement in pulmonary hypertension and hypoxemia during nitric oxide inhalation in a patient with end-stage pulmonary fibrosis. Am J Respir Crit Care Med 1994; 149(3):811–814.
96. Yung GL, Kriett JM, Jamieson SW, Johnson FW, Newhart J, Kinninger K, Channick RN. Outpatient inhaled nitric oxide in a patient with idiopathic pulmonary fibrosis: a bridge to lung transplantation. J Heart Lung Transplant 2001; 20(11):1224–1227.
97. Douglas WW, Ryu JH, Bjoraker JA, et al. Colchicine versus prednisolone as treatment of usual interstitial pneumonia. Mayo Clin Proc 1997; 72:201–209.
98. Lok S, the Greater Manchester Lung Fibrosis Consortium. The survival of idiopathic pulmonary fibrosis patients treated with cyclosporine and cyclophosphamide. Am J Respir Crit Care Med 1998; 157:A278.
99. Egan JJ, Haselton PS. Cryptogenic fibrosing alveolitis: diagnosis and treatment. Hosp Med 1998; 59:364–368.
100. Dark JH. Priorities for lung transplantation. Lancet 1998; 351:4–5.

101. Maurer J, Frost A, Estenne M, Higenbottam T, Glanville AR. International guidelines for the selection of lung transplant candidates. Am J Respir Crit Care Med 1998; 158:335–339.

102. Gay SE, Kazerooni EA, Toews GB, Lynch JP, Gross BH, Cascade PN, Spizarny DL, Flint A, Schork MA, Whyte RI, Povich J, Hyzy R, Martinez FJ. Idiopathic pulmonary fibrosis: predicting response to therapy and survival. Am J Respir Crit Care Med 1998; 157:1063–1072.

103. Wells A. Clinical usefulness of HRCT in cryptogenic fibrosing alveolitis. Thorax 1998; 53:1080–1087.

104. Mogulkoc N, Brutsche MH, Bishop PW, Greaves MS, Horrocks AW, Egan JJ. Pulmonary function in idiopathic pulmonary fibrosis and referral for lung transplantation. Am J Respir Crit Care Med 2001; 164(1):103–108.

105. Lok S. Interstitial lung disease clinics for the management of idiopathic pulmonary fibrosis: a potential advantage to patients. J Heart Lung Transplant 1999; 18:884–890.

10

Sarcoidosis, Lymphangioleiomyomatosis, and Histiocytosis

FORTUNE O. ALABI

Henry Ford Hospital
Detroit, Michigan, U.S.A.

FRANCIS X. McCORMACK

University of Cincinnati School of
Medicine
Cincinnati, Ohio, U.S.A.

I. Sarcoidosis

A. Overview of Chronic Sarcoidosis

Sarcoidosis is a systemic disease of unknown etiology characterized by lymphocytic and granulomatous inflammation and organ dysfunction. It can produce a spectrum of pulmonary manifestations ranging from asymptomatic infiltrates on chest x-ray to end-stage fibrosis and respiratory failure and has a tendency to relapse and remit unpredictably. Although the lung and the intrathoracic lymph nodes are involved in over 90% of cases, virtually any organ can be affected (1), including the eye, skin, liver, brain, and peripheral lymph nodes. Some presentations of acute sarcoidosis, such as the combination of bilateral hilar adeonopathy and erythema nodosum, can be so unmistakable that the diagnosis can made on clinical grounds alone and managed by observation. In most cases of acute or chronic sarcoidosis, however, an insidious or protean presentation, an atypical feature, or progressive organ dysfunction compels the clinician to seek a definitive diagnosis based on the demonstration of noncaseating granulomata in tissue samples. Even with pathological confirmation of granulomatous change, the clinical context is also critical, since tuberculosis, histoplasmosis, berylliosis, lymphoma, and a host of other diseases can mimic sarcoidosis (2). The overall prognosis of sarcoidosis is excellent, with spontaneous resolution occurring in almost two-thirds of cases (3,4), but the remaining patients may develop persistent or progressive disease associated with significant morbidity and mortality (5). Of those with chronic disease, one-fourth will eventually die of respiratory failure (6).

The basic tenet in the treatment of chronic pulmonary sarcoidosis is that therapy has never been proven to alter the course of the disease, so that decisions to treat are based on alleviation of symptoms alone. This discussion focuses on difficult management issues in chronic sarcoidosis, including predicting which patients will develop persistent or progressive disease, deciding which symptoms warrant initiation of treatment, choosing the dose and duration of chronic corticosteroid therapy, and the selection and timing of alternative agent use. The elements of sarcoidosis pathophysiology that form the basis for various therapeutic strategies are also reviewed. Other sarcoidosis topics covered in this volume include pathology (Chap. 2), pulmonary physiology (Chap. 5), and extrapulmonary disease (Chaps. 15 and 16).

B. Pathogenesis of Chronic Sarcoidosis

The histological hallmark of sarcoidosis is the noncaseating granuloma (Fig. 1), composed of giant cells, epitheloid cells, and lymphocytes (7,8). The granuloma results from a response to an as yet undiscovered antigen that has

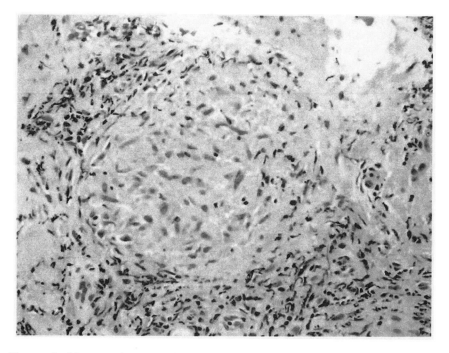

Figure 1 Noncaseating granuloma of sarcoidosis characterized by giant cells, palisading histiocytes, and lymphocytes.

been processed by the macrophage and then presented to antigen-specific T lymphocytes (9,10). Most of the T cells in sarcoid granulomas are CD4+, interspersed among the epitheloid cells and giant cells. At sites of active disease, striking increases in CD4+ lymphocytes and increased CD4+/CD8+ ratios are characteristic (11,12). The predominant T-lymphocyte populations in active lesions have been shown to express a Th1 cytokine pattern, although Th2 lymphocytes are also present (13–15). Th1 cytokine secretion likely contributes to the induction of the immune response, T-cell replication, and activation of monocytes. T lymphocytes are thought to be the key mediators of the alveolitis phase of sarcoidosis, and increased levels of CD4+ cells in bronchoalveolar lavage have been shown to correlate with disease activity (16) (Fig. 2). In general, chronic disease develops more commonly in patients who have persistent elevation in the CD4/CD8 ratios in bronchoalveolar lavage (BAL), while spontaneous remission is often heralded by a fall in the CD4/CD8 ratio into the normal range (17). Although Th2 lymphoctyes may contribute to disease resolution, the Th2 response may also lead to fibrosis (18). Interleukin-4 (IL-4), a signature Th2 cytokine, has been shown to augment fibroblast proliferation and collagen production (19). Furthermore,

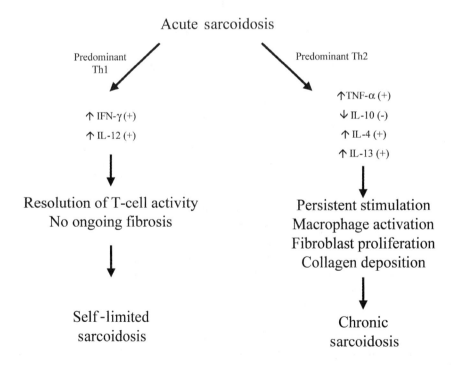

Figure 2 Hypothetical scheme of the cellular and molecular basis for persistence and progression of sarcoidosis. The (+) or (−) denotes pro- or anti-inflammatory effects of the cytokine, respectively.

IL-4 inhibits the expression of many interferon (IFN)-γ–inducible genes and the ability of IFN-γ to suppress fibroblast proliferation.

Lymphocytes are not the only activated cell type in sarcoidosis, however (9). Sarcoidosis macrophages spontaneously release proinflammatory cytokines, such as IL-1, IL-6, IL-12, tumor necrosis factor alpha (TNF-α), and granulocyte macrophage colony-stimulating factor (GM-CSF) (20–26). Fibroblasts deposit collagen at the periphery of the granuloma in the early phases of the disease, which matures and organizes in the chronic phase. Although fibroblasts have traditionally been regarded as effector cells that produce matrix components under the influence of T cells and macrophages, there is mounting evidence that fibroblasts play an important role in the perpetuation of chronic sarcoidosis (27). Alveolar fibroblasts have been shown to elaborate stem cell factors (SCF), which stimulate proliferation of hematopoietic progenitor cells involved in mast and stromal cell interaction (28). Alveolar fibroblasts also indirectly induce recruitment of eosinophils via the elaboration of IL-5 (28) and enhance capacity for IL-6 secretion in vitro (29,30).

Neutrophils may also contribute to the pathogenesis of chronic fibrotic sarcoidosis. IL-8 levels in BAL are elevated during the chronic phase (31,32), and Roth et al. found that patients with advanced disease including fibrosis or bullous changes on chest radiographs had increased BAL neutrophilia compared to those with early disease (33). Elevated plasma leukocyte elastase levels were demonstrated in patients with fibrotic radiological changes, which implies the presence of ongoing activation of neutrophils (34).

The events driving the transition from the inflammatory alveolitis phase of sarcoidosis to fibrosis are not fully understood, but increasing attention has been focused on TNF-α and other monocyte/macrophage derived chemokines (35). TNF-α signaling plays a role in the upregulation and secretion of profibrotic cytokines, including transforming growth factors alpha and beta (TGF-α, TGF-β) and platelet-derived growth factors (PDGFs) (36,37) and animal data suggests that TNF-α may be important for early activation of the fibrotic process. In a mouse model of asbestos-induced lung fibrosis, animals that are deficient in TNF-α receptors do not develop early fibroproliferative lesions (38). In patients with sarcoidosis, increased expression of members of the TNF receptor superfamily have been demonstrated on T lymphocytes (39). Subjects with stage 1 sarcoidosis have increased amounts of TNF-soluble receptors compared to stage 2 and 3 patients, perhaps representing a homeostatic mechanism that quenches chronic inflammation from excessive TNF-α stimulation. Polymorphisms of the TNF-α gene promoter and the TNF-β intron 1 have been described in sarcoidosis, but thus far they do not appear to correlate with the level of TNF production (40). The TNFB 1 allele was reported to be a marker of chronic disease (41), whereas the TNFA 2 allele was found more frequently in patients with Lofgren's syndrome, with a high rate of spontaneous resolution (42).

Several centers have presented provocative evidence that sarcoidosis may have an infectious or environmental etiology. The spatial clustering of cases in a study from the Isle of Man suggested possible person-to-person transmission or common exposure to an environmental agent (43,44). Clustering of disease has also been described among nurses (45,46), firefighters (47), and personnel on U.S. Navy aircraft carriers (48). Cell wall–deficient acid-fast bacilli have been grown from the blood of patients with sarcoidosis (49), and genetic evidence of the presence of mycobacteria has been detected in some studies (50), but not in others (51) using specific primers and the polymerase chain reaction. Furthermore, Ishige et al. reported the presence of *Propionibacterium acnes* or *granulosum* DNA in the lymph node biopsies of 15 patients with sarcoidosis (52).

C. Diagnosis

The differential diagnosis of chronic pulmonary sarcoidosis encompasses all fibrosing lung diseases, as well as a variety of infectious granulomatous disorders such as histoplasmosis and tuberculosis. There are few physical findings to assist the clinician in differentiating between the possibilities. Extrapulmonary manifestations of sarcoidosis such as acute arthritis, lupus pernio, or uveitis are obviously helpful diagnostically. Clubbing is frequent in patients with idiopathic pulmonary fibrosis and is uncommon in sarcoidosis, but it can occur with virtually any end-stage disease. Auscultation of the lung is remarkably uninformative in sarcoidosis and rarely reveals crackles except when there is superimposed pulmonary edema or pneumonia (53). Neurological manifestations, especially cranial neuropathies, occur in about 5% of patients with sarcoidosis. Pleural effusions, hemoptysis, and spontaneous pneumothorax are rare in sarcoidosis but do occur. Punched out bone lesions on radiographs of the hands and feet, hypercalcemia, and elevated liver enzymes are also found in patients with sarcoidosis. Restrictive ventilatory defects are observed on pulmonary function testing in virtually all patients with chronic pulmonary sarcoidosis, and obstructive lung disease is present in approximately 20% especially smokers with concomitant emphysema. Reduction in DL_{CO} is common in fibrotic sarcoidosis but are generally less severe than in patients with interstitial pulmonary fibrosis (IPF) (54). Chest x-ray and CT scanning of the chest (Fig. 3) identify characteristic features of chronic sarcoidosis, including nodular and fibrotic peribronchiolar changes, cystic destruction, and honeycombing; these modalities can help to exclude alternative diagnoses such as cancer (55,56) or myocobacterial or fungal infection (57). The diagnostic yield of transbronchial biopsy is reduced in chronic sarcoidosis (58) compared to acute sarcoidosis; rare patients may require larger tissue samples obtained by video-assisted thoracoscopic biopsy. Biopsy of alternative sites—such as the liver, peripheral lymph nodes, and skin—may also be considered in patients with extrapulmonary disease.

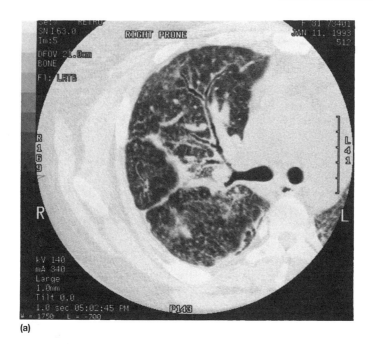

(a)

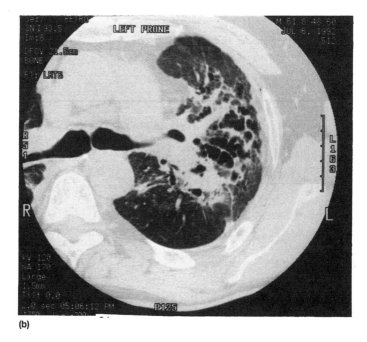

(b)

Figure 3 High-resolution CT scans of chronic pulmonary sarcoidosis revealing bronchostenosis (a) and fibrocystic change (b).

D. Clinical Features That Predict Persistence or Progression of Chronic Sarcoidosis

Geraint James defined chronic sarcoidosis as disease that is present for more than 2 years (59,60). He noted that some features of sarcoidosis, such as lupus pernio and neurological diseases, were associated with a low rate of remission, while others, such as erythema nodusum, were associated with a high rate of spontaneous resolution within 2 years. Other manifestations of sarcoidosis that have been associated with chronicity include age equal to or greater than 40 years, dyspneic presentation, splenomegaly, absence of erythema nodosum, and progressive parenchymal infiltrates on x-ray (61) (Table 1).

The percentage of patients with chronic disease varies between regions, perhaps reflecting different ethnic backgrounds among the studied populations. Race is one of several factors that predict chronicity, and, in general, black patients have a worse prognosis (62). For example, a patient population in Philadelphia (63) consisting predominantly of African Americans had a higher relapse rate than a Caucasian population treated in Iowa (64). The percentage of patients who required continued corticosteriod therapy varied widely, from 18% in a mostly Irish population in Iowa (64) to 4% in an Italian cohort (65) to 53% in predominantly African-American population (63,64).

E. Radiographic Features of Chronic Sarcoidosis That Predict Persistence or Progression

The hallmark of chronic pulmonary sarcoidosis is fibrosis (Fig. 3). The chest radiograph may demonstrate reticular pulmonary infiltrates, hilar retraction, cystic changes, and bullae. Parenchymal lesions in sarcoidosis are characteristically distributed along bronchovascular bundles and lymphatics, especially in the upper lobes, in contrast to IPF, which has a proclivity for subpleural and basilar regions of the lung. Septal lines and subpleural nodules may be present.

Table 1 Predicting Progression of Sarcoidosis

Markers associated with spontaneous remission	Markers associated with potential reversibility	Markers associated with persistence or progression
Erythema nodosum	Ground-glass appearance on high-resolution computed tomography of the chest	Neurosarcoidosis Lupus pernio Black race Splenomegally Age > 40 Absence of erythema nodosum Dyspneic presentation
Radiographic stage I		Radiographic stages II, III, IV

Cystic spaces may become colonized with *Aspergillus*, and intraluminal fungus balls and air-fluid levels may be seen. Pneumothoraces, pleural thickening, and pleural effusion (rarely) can occur (66,67).

Calcification of hilar or mediastinal nodes may be seen in long-standing sarcoidosis (68). The radiographic presentation of sarcoidosis may be difficult to distinguish from that of chronic fungal or tuberculosis infection (69). Computed tomography (CT) of the chest (especially using high-resolution algorithms) is more sensitive than conventional chest radiography for defining the extent of pulmonary involvement, but it is usually not required to diagnose or stage sarcoidosis (70).

Wurm (71) and Scadding (72) classified involvement on chest x-ray in sarcoidosis into five stages: stage 0, no abnormality; stage I, bilateral hilar or paratracheal adenopathy with clear chest x-ray; stage II, hilar adenopathy with pulmonary infiltration; stage III, pulmonary infiltration without hilar adenopathy; and stage IV, evidence of pulmonary fibrosis (Table 2). Although the Scadding roentgenographic classification was not designed for assessment of extent or activity of the disease, it correlates well with chronicity and the frequency of spontaneous resolution (72). Radiographic changes generally improve or stabilize in patients with hilar adenopathy alone (radiographic stage I), but tend to persist or progress in patients with parenchymal infiltrates (stages II and III). More recently, the chest CT scan has also been used to predict progression and guide therapy. For example, ground-glass changes, while uncommon in sarcoidosis, suggest active inflammation that may be amenable to therapy (73). In contrast, honeycombing, traction bronchiectasis, distortion of lung parenchyma, volume loss, linear bands, bronchiectasis, cystic radiolucencies, and bullae are characteristic of end-stage fibrosis that does not warrant aggressive therapies with substantial toxicities.

Table 2 Prognosis Based on Roentgenographic Classifications

Stage	Chest film findings	Prognosis
0	Normal	
I	BHL[a] only	Spontaneous remission in 70–85%
II	BHL with parenchymal infiltrates	Spontaneous remission in 30–60%
III	Parenchymal infiltrates without BHL	Spontaneous remission in <20%
IV	Pulmonary fibrosis	Persistent disease

[a]Bilateral hilar adenopathy.

F. Other predictors

The baseline level of angiotensin converting enzyme, which is elevated in 30 to 50% of patients with sarcoidosis, is not predictive of deterioration or improvement and should not be used as a basis for initiation of therapy. Gallium scanning is also unhelpful (74). The identities and amounts of various inflammatory cells and markers in BAL fluid have not proved to be reliable predictors of the course of disease in sarcoidosis.

G. Treatment

The universally accepted indication for initiating treatment in patients with pulmonary sarcoidosis is for the amelioration of symptoms. The most common symptoms prompting intervention are dyspnea, persistent disabling cough unresponsive to conservative measures, and bronchoscopic evidence of bronchostenosis (Table 3). Corticosteroids have been the mainstay of therapy for chronic sarcoidosis since the 1950s (75,76). Most patients with chronic sarcoidosis will require treatment for symptoms at some point during their clinical course, and some will require treatment indefinitely. Moderate to low initiating doses (0.5–0.7 mg/kg) produce symptomatic and limited radiographic improvement in most patients (17,77–79). Once initiated, the steroid trial should continue for at least 3 months and be tapered slowly to a maintenance level. Decisions to continue treatment should be based on objective responses such as improvement in pulmonary function tests, radiographic shadowing, or performance on the 6-min walk test.

   Predictable side effects—including weight gain, cataracts, fluid retention, glucose intolerance, bone loss, and susceptibility to infection—limit the dose and duration of prednisone use. Therefore diligent attempts to taper the drug to levels below 15 mg/day should be made. The efficacy of chronic corticosteroid therapy in sarcoidosis is not proven, and randomized trials have failed to demonstrate long-term benefit for the patients beyond the time on treatment. Patients with radiographic evidence of end-stage fibrosis—such as extensive honeycombing, bronchiectasis, or cystic changes—should not be

Table 3 Indications for Therapy of Chronic Sarcoidosis

Pulmonary	Extrapulmonary
Dyspnea	Chronic uveitis
Debilitating cough, refractory to	Iritis
conservative measures	Hypercalcemia
	Cardiac involvement
	Lupus pernio
	Neurosarcoidosis

subjected to prolonged steroid trials or toxic agents if their initial clinical response is poor; they should be considered for early transplant evaluation. Inhaled corticosteroids can be tried in patients with persistent cough, (80) and stenting can be considered for patients with bronchostenosis (81). Given the high frequency of relapses when therapy is discontinued, the relatively safety of low daily or every-other-day prednisone therapy—and anectodal evidence that chronic suppression may prevent fibrotic manifestations of the disease—some investigators favor long-term, low-dose therapy to control symptoms and sustain radiographic and pulmonary function stability (82). However, some patients progress to end-stage fibrosis even while being treated with corticosteroids (83), and recurrence of sarcoidosis in aggressively immunosuppresed transplant patients is well documented (84–87). All patients on chronic steroids should be evaluated for osteoporosis and treated appropriately to minimize bone loss.

H.   Alternative Agents—Overview

Corticosteroids are clearly the most efficacious available agents for the treatment of sarcoidosis. The use of alternative agents should be limited to patients who progress despite steroid therapy, those with intolerable side effects from steroids, or those who refuse to take them. Unfortunately, the benefits of all alternative agents used for the treatment of sarcoidosis are uncertain, there are few data on which to base informed decisions, and the toxicities for most of the drugs outlined below are substantial.

Antimalarials

Chloroquine and hydroxychloroquine were both initially developed for treating malaria but were subsequently found to have anti-inflammatory properties in rheumatoid arthritis (88,89). The efficacy of chloroquine in the treatment of cutaneous sarcoidosis has been well established (90,91), but the benefits of antimalarials for treatment of pulmonary sarcoidosis are less clear. In a double-blind trial involving 57 patients, the British Tuberculosis Association reported that chest radiographs improved in the chloroquine-treated sarcoidosis patients compared to those on placebo at 4 and 6 months but not at 12 months (92). In another study, Siltzbach and associates treated 43 patients with cutaneous and pulmonary sarcoidosis with chloroquine for a period of 8 months (range 4 to 17 months) (93). All patients had intrathoracic sarcoidosis, but some were asymptomatic and 14 had concomitant cutaneous involvement. None of the patients had received prior corticosteroid therapy. Chest radiographs improved in 11 of 14 patients with stage I disease; 14 of 18 patients with stage II disease; and 6 of 11 patients with stage III disease. Improvement in chest radiographs was generally apparent within 1 to 3 months, with maximal improvement by 3 to 6 months. The study was inconclusive, however, because of difficulty in differentiating the effects of chloroquine therapy from spontaneous improvement. Baltzan et al. conducted the first randomized trial of chloroquine in patients with biopsy-proven chronic sarcoidosis (94). In their study, 23 patients with symptomatic chronic sarcoidosis were treated with chloroquine for a period of 6 months. This initial treatment led to a significant improvement in symptoms, pulmonary function, angiotensin-converting enzyme (ACE) level, and extent of disease based on lung gallium scan. Patients were randomized to the maintenance chloroquine therapy group (250 mg/day) or to an observation group ($n = 8$ patients). The treated group showed a slower decline in pulmonary function and had fewer relapses than the observation group. This study suggested that chloroquine might be effective in patients with chronic sarcoidosis. The major complication of chloroquine treatment is ocular toxicity (95), which can be minimized by using lower dosages (96), treating with hydroxychloroquine rather than chloroquine (97), or discontinuing therapy at the first sign of visual impairment based on biannual funduscopic and visual field examinations (98).

Methotrexate

Methotrexate (MTX) is a folate antagonist with potent anti-inflammatory and immunosuppressive properties. The mechanism of action of MTX in sarcoidosis is unknown, but the effect does not appear to be T lymphocyte-dependent (97,99). Low-dose MTX suppressed alveolar macrophage cytokine release and lymphocytic alveolitis in a study of 12 patients with active pulmonary sarcoidosis (100,101). The use of MTX as a corticosteroid-sparing agent or alternative in patients who are intolerant of corticosteroid therapy has been reported, though many of the studies were conducted by a small number of investigators (102–104). Lower et al. reported favorable responses to MTX in 14 of 16 patients with chronic sarcoidosis (101), most of whom were unresponsive to treatment with corticosteroid therapy for at least 2 years. Symptomatic improvement on MTX therapy was noted within 4 to 6 months, but objective improvement was delayed for up to 6 months. The same investigators also reported the outcome of a long-term follow-up of 50 patients treated with oral MTX for at least 2 years (105). Most of the patients had received corticosteroids before the initiation of MTX. Overall, 33 (66%) patients had favorable responses, and a corticosteroid-sparing effect was noted in 25 of 30 patients. There is still no randomized study of the efficacy of MTX in chronic sarcoidosis, and the use of this agent is not without complications, including pulmonary, hematological, and hepatic toxicity (106–109). Routine hepatic enzyme studies have not been shown to be reliable for predicting drug-induced liver injury (110), and liver biopsy every 1 to 2 years is recommended (111). MTX may be considered for patients with chronic sarcoidosis who are intolerant of or unresponsive to corticosteroid therapy.

Azathioprine

Azathioprine is a purine analog that is metabolized intracellularly to 6-mercaptopurine, its active form. This compound inhibits DNA synthesis and has pronounced suppressive effects on T and B lymphocytes (112). The effectiveness of azathioprine as an immunosuppressive and anti-inflammatory agent has been well established in autoimmune disorders and inflammatory bowel diseases (113–115). However,there are only a handful of reports of the effect of azathioprine in chronic sarcoidosis. Although some centers have reported a favorable response (116–118), the trials have generally involved small numbers of patients and were not placebo-controlled. Azathioprine has been used as corticosteroid-sparing agent (116,119), as a second-line agent for patients unresponsive to corticosteroids (118), and for patients with chronic relapsing disease (116). Some investigators contend that azathioprine is effective for corticosteroid-sparing purposes but has limited activity in patients who do not respond to corticosteroids (120). Collectively, the available data suggests that azathioprine might be a reasonable alternative or adjunct to corticosteroids in some patients with chronic sarcoidosis, but additional studies will be needed to clarify its place in the treatment armamentarium.

Cyclosporin A

Cyclosporin A inhibits T-lymphocyte function by blocking interleukin 2 (IL-2). Although cyclosporin A has in vitro lympholytic properties suggesting that it may be an ideal agent in sarcoidosis, its in vivo efficacy has been disappointing (121). Wyser and associates found no significant differences in response between the treatment groups randomized to cyclosporin A alone or cyclosporin A with corticosteroids (122). Although some favorable responses had been reported in the treatment of cutaneous and neurosarcoidosis (123–125), available data do not support the use of cyclosporine A for treating patients with chronic pulmonary sarcoidosis.

Alkylating Agents

Chlorambucil has been studied as a potential alternative for patients with chronic pulmonary sarcoidosis who are not responding to or are intolerant of corticosteroids. Although two studies have reported some favorable responses (126,127), enthusiasm for this agent has been dampened by serious adverse side effects, including myelosuppression (128) and induction of secondary neoplasms (129,130).

Tumor Necrosis Factor Alpha (TNF-α) Antagonists

The inhibition of TNF-α function using soluble TNF receptors (Etanercept) or monoclonal antibodies to TNF-α (Infliximab) has been approved for the management of refractory Crohn's disease and rheumatoid arthritis (131–133), two chronic diseases where TNF-α plays a central role in the pathogenesis of tissue injury. The finding that TNF-α levels are high in the sputum, BAL fluid, and lymph nodes of patients with sarcoidosis has suggested the possible utility of anti-TNF agents in the chronic, refractory forms of the disease (134–136).

Recently, two groups reported their experiences with the use of anti-TNF antibodies in patients with chronic sarcoidosis (137,138). One of these, Baughman and associates, treated three patients with chronic pulmonary sarcoidosis that was refractory to corticosteroids and other immunosuppressive treatment with 5 mg/kg of anti-TNF-α IgG. There was objective improvement in the index organ function in all patients. A follow-up study by the same investigators involving 11 patients also showed significant improvement in 10 of 11 patients treated (139). Other drugs known to inhibit TNF-α activity have also been reported to have potential utility in the treatment of chronic pulmonary sarcoidosis, including pentoxyfylline (140) and thalidomide (141,142). In addition to inhibiting TNF-α release from alveolar macrophages (143,144), thalidomide had also been shown to inhibit IL-12 production from monocytes (145). IL-12 is an essential cytokine for Th1 differentiation (146). Firm conclusions and recommendations regarding anti-TNF-α strategies in sarcoidosis must await the results of randomized trials. The use of these agents can be complicated by reactivation of tuberculosis and dissemination of histoplasmosis (147,148).

I. Cytokine Modulation

Other key Th2 cytokines that have been reported to play important roles in the pathogenesis of pulmonary fibrosis—such as IL-4, IL-10, IL-5, and IL-13—are promising targets for monoclonal antibody-based treatments of sarcoidosis. Treatment with antifibrotic cytokines, such as gamma interferon 1b which has shown promise in patients with idiopathic pulmonary fibrosis, may also be considered (149). This approach has the theoretical potential to worsen granuloma formation and alveolitis in sarcoidosis, however.

J. Inhaled Corticosteroids

Inhaled corticosteroids may have utility in the treatment of sarcoidosis. At the cellular level, the use of inhaled corticosteroids was shown to decrease BAL T lymphocytosis and change the phenotype and functional characteristics of alveolar macrophages (150). Inhaled corticosteroids also decreased the ACE level and beta2 microglobulin level when compared to placebo (151). In several studies, treatment with inhaled steroids improved symptom scores without significant differences in pulmonary function studies or radiographic findings (152–154). However, other investigators have found no significant differences between inhaled corticosteroids and placebo (80,155). Although no aerosol studies have specifically targeted patients with chronic pulmonary sarcoidosis, we believe that an empiric trial of inhaled corticosteroids, given their favorable safety profile, is a reasonable approach to patients with endobronchial sarcoidosis who have increased airway reactivity and/or persistent cough.

K. Transplantation

Lung transplantation is the last resort for patients with end-stage lung disease (156,157). Patients with sarcoidosis are generally young and fit candidates for transplantation, but multiorgan involvement and multiorgan failure are relative and absolute contraindications, respectively (158). The 5-year survival of patients transplanted for chronic sarcoidosis is comparable to that for other lung diseases (87). Single-lung transplantation is the most common procedure, although double-lung and heart-and-lung transplantation have been success-fully performed (159–161). While clinically silent recurrence identified by tissue biopsy is not uncommon, organ failure or mortality due to recurrence is rare (84–87). The prevalence of acute rejection and obliterative bronchiolitis is not different from lung transplantation for other lung diseases (87,162). A recent study reported that nearly 50% of their listed sarcoidosis patients died while awaiting lung transplantation (163); this highlights the importance of early enrollment, especially in patients with elevated right atrial pressures (163).

L. Summary

The management of chronic sarcoidosis is challenging. For most patients, deciding when to initiate therapy with corticosteroids and how long to continue them is the major clinical issue. Minimizing steroid-induced side effects by titrating to the lowest effective dose, treatment with antiosteoporotic therapy, and vigilance for glucose intolerance, cataracts, and infection are critically important responsibilities for the clinician. In cases where steroids fail, alternative therapies with cytotoxic agents, antimalarials, and anticytokine agents are available, although data supporting their efficacy are inconclusive. There are several promising therapies on the horizon that have emerged from recent advances in our understanding of the pathogenesis of sarcoidosis (164).

II. Lymphangioleiomyomatosis

A. Overview

Lymphangioleiomyomatosis (LAM) is an uncommon, progressive, cystic lung disease of women that is characterized by diffuse infiltration of the pulmonary parenchyma with histologically benign smooth muscle-like cells (165). Extrapulmonary disease manifestations—including axial lymphadenopathy, abdominal lymphangiomyomas, and renal, hepatic or abdominal angiomyo-lipomas—also occur in LAM. LAM presents both sporadically (S-LAM), and in patients with tuberous sclerosis (TSC-LAM) (166), an autosomal dominant syndrome characterized by hamartomatous growths in multiple organs including skin, eye, kidney, and central nervous system. Although LAM occurs almost exclusively in women, radiographic cystic changes consistent with LAM (167) and biopsy-confirmed disease have also been reported in men with TSC (168). Registry-based efforts to locate LAM patients in the United

States (169), France (170), and the United Kingdom (171) have yielded a value for minimum prevalence of 2 to 6 per million women. Recent studies, however, indicate that LAM occurs in up to 26 to 39% of women with TSC, suggesting a total of over 100,000 LAM patients worldwide (172–174). The clinical course of LAM varies widely, from relatively stable disease over decades to relentlessly progressive dyspnea on exertion, recurrent pneumothoraces, and chylous pleural effusions. After an average age of onset of 35 years, the mean survival is frequently reported to be less than 10 years (170,175–178), but recent data suggest a more optimistic prognosis (179–181). LAM is often radiographically undetectable in the early stages, when the clinical presentation mimics asthma. For these reasons, the diagnosis is delayed for an average of 5 years or more, and most patients seen in practice and studied in clinical series present with advanced disease (170,175–178).

B. Genetics and Pathogenesis

Great strides in our understanding of the genetic basis of LAM have been made in the past few years. Clinicians have long suspected, based on nearly identical histopathological presentations, that the cystic lung disease familiar to neurologists who follow patients with TSC and the sporadic LAM seen by pulmonary physicians treating adults may have a common genetic basis (182,183). TSC is known to result from mutations in either of two tumor suppressor genes, the hamartin gene (TSC1) on chromosome 9 (9q34) (184) or the tuberin gene (TSC2) locus on chromosome 16 (16p13.3) (185,186). TSC is a tumor-suppressor syndrome, meaning that mutational events that cause complete loss of the growth-suppression function of hamartin or tuberin result in the formation of a tumor. Both the maternal and paternal alleles must be "hit" for unrestricted growth to occur. In most cases of TSC, the patient inherits a bad copy of a TSC gene from a parent, or develops a mutation during embryogenesis or development, and then suffers a second spontaneously occurring, inactivating mutation in a somatic organ or tissue. The mechanism by which hamartin and tuberin regulate cellular proliferation is not known, but coimmunoprecipitation experiments demonstrating that the two proteins interact intraceullularly suggest that their molecular pathways converge. Tuberin contains a Rap1-GAP homology domain near its COOH terminus (185) and has been shown to have Rap1-GAP activity (187) as well as Rab5 Gap activity (188). Tuberin has also been reported to bind to calmodulin via a specific COOH terminal domain and to be involved in cell cycle control and transcriptional events (189,190). Hamartin may play a role in cellular adhesion events and rho-dependent signaling for actin stress fiber formation through interactions with ezrin-radixin-moesin (ERM) proteins (191).

Over 600 mutations have been identified in TSC1 and TSC2, including protein truncating mutations, missense (TSC2 only) and nonsense mutations, splice mutations, and small and large deletions and insertions (192–194). Although familial TSC results from inheritance of germ line mutations, de novo mutations arising during embryogenesis account for two-thirds of TSC cases. TSC-LAM has been reported in patients with mutations in either TSC1 or TSC2 (194), but TSC2 related LAM appears to be much more common. Recent data suggest a reduced rate of germline and sporadic mutations in TSC1. Overall, the clinical presentation of patients with TSC1 and TSC2 disease are quite similar, although a recent detailed study has suggested that TSC1 mutations may produce somewhat milder disease (192).

The presence of TSC genetic abnormalities in sporadic LAM patients were independently identified and jointly reported by Smolarek and Henske in 1998. They found loss of heterozygosity (LOH) for TSC2 in AMLs and lymph nodes from patients with S-LAM (195), but TSC mutations were not found in the circulating blood cells from S-LAM patients (196). Carsillo et al. subsequently demonstrated the presence of missense and protein truncating TSC2 mutations associated with LOH in the lesional lung and kidney tissue of patients with S-LAM (197). Interestingly, the circulating lymphocytes and perilesional normal lung and kidney tissue in S-LAM patients were free of detectable TSC2 mutations. These data suggest that S-LAM may arise through two somatic mutations rather than the more typical tumor suppressor mechanism involving a combination of a germline mutation and a somatic mutation. The lack of any documented cases of mother-daughter transmission of S-LAM, which has been reported TSC-LAM (198), is also consistent with a somatic origin for biallelic mutations in patients with S-LAM. To date, only TSC2 mutations have been reported to cause S-LAM.

Additional genetic and clinical evidence suggests that the smooth muscle cell infiltration and cystic degeneration of lung tissue in LAM may be a consequence of seeding of the lung with "benign" angiomyolipoma cells. This hypothesis was original proposed by Carsillo et al., based on the finding of matching TSC2 mutations in the kidney and lung lesions of four LAM patients (199). The data are consistent with either a subdetectable level of mosaicism for TSC2 mutations or with benign metastasis of tumor forming cells from the kidney to the lung (or lung to kidney). The recurrence of LAM in the donor lung of LAM patients who have undergone lung transplant is also consistent with the metastatic theory, although in two studies the proliferating lesional cells appeared to be of donor origin (200–202). In a small prospective study of female TSC patients, lung cysts were more frequently associated with large or problematic angiomyolipomas, raising the possibility that more extensive kidney tumors may more readily seed the lung and cause cyst formation (173). This mechanism may not apply to all LAM cases, since only about 50% of S-LAM patients have radiographically apparent angiomyolipomas (203). It is possible, however, that the LAM cells that are deposited in the lung could originate from other sources, such as CT-invisible angiomyolipomas, axial lymph nodes, and lymphangiomyoma, which are present in at least an additional 25% of patients (204). The metastatic theory of LAM pathogenesis is provocative and controversial; if validated, it may provide new opportunities for early intervention in LAM.

Whether LAM cells have pulmonary or extrapulmonary origins, there is intense interest in the mechanism of accumulation of LAM cells in the lung and the relationship between smooth muscle cell infiltration and cystic change. LAM cells may accumulate because of a persistent proliferative stimulus, which may be extrinsic or intrinsic, or a failure of apoptosis. Two reports that the proliferating cells in recurrent LAM lesions posttransplant are donor derived suggest a circulating mitogenic stimulus (200–202). Recent data indicate that tuberin- and hamartin-deficient mesenchymal cells derived from angiofibromas secrete substances that stimulate the proliferation of tuberin- and hamartin-sufficient endothelial cells (205). In another study, LAM cells exhibited robust expression of Bcl-2, an antiapoptotic cell surface molecule, possibly contributing to an imbalance between proliferation and cell death in LAM (206). It is also possible that proliferating LAM cells are "bystanders" in a reactive response to an unknown lung injury. The finding that some early LAM lesions have pronounced cystic changes in the presence of only trivial smooth muscle cell infiltration is consistent with this notion. A more widely held hypothesis is that LAM cells express metalloproteinases and other matrix-degrading enzymes that produce cystic changes. Hayashi et al. described increased expression of MMP-2, MMP-9, and MMP-1 without an associated increase in immunostaining for tissue inhibitors of metalloproteinases (TIMPs) (207). The authors speculated that elastin degradation may play a role in cyst formation in LAM through an increase in MMP-2 and MMP-9 that is unbalanced by an increase TIMPs.

C. Epidemiology

The incidence of TSC-LAM has previously been estimated at 0.1 to 1% of TSC patients in a review of cases in the literature through 1971 and 2.3% of TSC patients that presented to the Mayo Clinic over a 43-year period (208). A recent retrospective analysis of abdominal and chest CT scans indicated that LAM may affect up to 26% of women with TSC, and two recent prospective series indicated that up to 34 to 39% of women with TSC have cystic changes consistent with LAM (172,173). The estimated incidence of tuberous sclerosis is 1 per 6000 to 11,000 births, and the estimated North American and worldwide prevalence of TSC is 40,000 and 1 million people, respectively (209). Based on these data, and the equal gender distribution of TSC, there may be as many as 10,000 patients with LAM in the North America and 200,000 LAM patients worldwide.

D. Clinical Presentation

The screening of female TSC patients for lung cysts identifies a LAM population with far fewer disease manifestations than are seen in the S-LAM patient population. The finding that up to 40% of women with TSC had cystic pulmonary changes was quite surprising, because based on the paucity of TSC-LAM reports in the literature, these patients come to medical attention relatively infrequently. There are several possible explanations for these discrepancies, including the fact that TSC-LAM may be a milder disease than S-LAM or that TSC comorbidities may limit life span or prevent TSC-LAM from becoming a health priority for TSC patients. Prior to 2001, there were only two series of TSC-LAM patients in the literature, both involving fewer than 10 patients (167,210). In the more recent Costello study, 7 of 9 patients had presenting pulmonary complaints of dyspnea or pneumothorax, and all of those had severe obstructive physiology and advanced cystic changes on HRCT of the chest (167,174). While 8 of 9 had renal AML, none had chylous complications. Franz et al. reported that 3 of 9 of the cyst-positive TSC patients identified by CT screening of currently asymptomatic patients had a remote history of pneumothorax. Most patients had mild to moderate cystic changes on HRCT of the chest, and there were no chylous complications (173). Although definitive conclusions must await a properly designed study, it seems likely that LAM manifestations will prove to be similar in TSC and non-TSC patients who present with breathlessness—with the possible exception of a reduced incidence of chylous effusions in TSC-LAM patients (174).

Symptomatic LAM patients may be identified very early or very late in their disease course, depending on the disease manifestations that bring them to medical attention. Acute or subacute shortness of breath or chest pain due to pneumothorax or chylous pleural effusion may be the presenting features of patients with a wide range of pulmonary involvement, including those with very few pulmonary cysts. Therapeutic intervention in these "early" patients may have the greatest potential impact. The most common presentation, however, is progressive breathlessness (170,171,176,177). LAM patients who present with chronic progressive dyspnea on exertion usually have advanced cystic changes on chest x-ray or HRCT scanning of the chest (Fig. 4). Additional atypical presentations of LAM include abdominal mass, flank pain due to hemorrhage into an angiomyolipoma, ascites, chyloptysis, chyluria, hemoptysis, or chylopericardium.

E. Diagnosis

The differential of the thin walled, cystic lung disease of the type seen in LAM includes emphysema or pulmonary Langerhans cell histiocytosis (PLCH), also known as pulmonary histiocytosis X or eosinophilic granuloma. Centrilobular emphysema and pulmonary histiocytosis X are very uncommon in nonsmoking patients, but genetic emphysema due to alpha$_1$-antitrypsin deficiency must be excluded. In the nonsmoker with normal alpha$_1$-antitrypsin levels, the diagnosis of pulmonary LAM can be made on clinical grounds on the basis of typical, diffuse, thin-walled cystic changes on HRCT scanning of the chest and at least one other associated feature, including known tuberous sclerosis, renal or lymphatic masses containing fat density on CT or ultrasound scanning of the abdomen, chylous ascites, chylous pleural effusion or other chylous collection, or aberrant drainage (e.g., chyluria). Recurrent pneumothoraces in

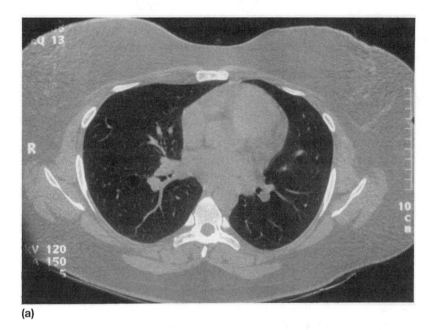

(a)

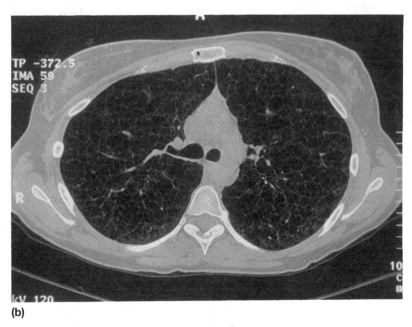

(b)

Figure 4 High resolution CT scans of early LAM in an asymptomatic TSC patient screened for cystic changes (a) and a sporadic LAM patient who presented with dyspnea (b).

a young nonsmoking female are suggestive of LAM, but even in the face of a consistent HRCT, they are not generally specific enough to obviate the need for tissue confirmation.

F. Treatment

LAM is empirically managed with antiestrogen therapies, based largely on the observed gender restriction and reports that birth control pills and pregnancy can worsen the disease (211,212). However, there is no convincing evidence that these strategies are effective. There have been no prospective randomized trials of hormonal therapy, and the available literature is limited to isolated case reports, metanalyses of compiled case reports, and retrospective case series that are inconclusive. The state of the science is such that "no pharmacologic treatment" for pulmonary LAM manifestations is generally accepted as a completely reasonable alternative for LAM patients at all disease stages.

Antiestrogen therapies were first suggested as a treatment for LAM in 1969 and first implemented by Shuman in 1979 (213). There are isolated reports of disease stabilization with oophorectomy (214–216), but Taylor et al. described no effect of castration on disease course in a series of 16 patients analyzed retrospectively (217), and there is currently little support for this aggressive therapy. Progesterone has been used as an empirical therapy for LAM for decades. The first reported use of medroxprogesterone acetate, by McCarthy et al. in a single LAM patient, was associated with resolution of her pleural effusion, cessation of hemoptysis, and improved gas exchange and exercise tolerance (218). Worsening of her clinical status with withdrawal of therapy and apparent remission upon reinstitution provided convincing evidence for efficacy. Unfortunately, such dramatic responses have not been realized for most of the hundreds of patients who have received the drug following that report, and the empirical suprapharmacological dose chosen, 400 mg IM, has become the standard of care for LAM (217). This dose, which is much higher than what is routinely used for birth control or suppression of menstruation (the typical medroxyprogesterone dose is 150 mg IM every 3 months), often results in significant side effects of mood swings, fluid retention, and fatigue. There is significant accumulation of this lipophilic drug in fat stores, and many LAM patients who are withdrawn from medroxyprogesterone 400 mg IM do not resume menstruation for up to 8 to 12 months. Because of these problems, some clinicians have chosen to use oral progestins at more conventional doses, such as those that are routinely used to suppress the growth of uterine fibroids [e.g., norethrindone acetate (Aygestin) at 10 to 20 mg/day PO], and to titrate to cessation of menstruation or to a targeted serum estrogen level. This modification of the most commonly used LAM therapy, while logical, is untested in the literature.

Whether progesterone has an effect on the progression of LAM has been debated. The proposed mechanism of action is that the drug downregulates estrogen receptor expression, antagonizes estrogen action, and suppresses estrogen levels, albeit less effectively than other agents, such as GnRH agonists. Four small case studies have suggested that progesterone may stabilize disease progression in some patients (170,177,178,219), especially those with chylous effusions and ascites. The latter result may contain inherent bias, since effusions are perhaps the most measurable manifestation of LAM. Improvements, based on outcomes of dyspnea or an increase in FEV_1, were uncommon but consistently reported in all four series. A retrospective study from the United Kingdom suggested that progesterone reduced the rate of decline in FEV_1 in premenopausal LAM patients from -170 to -47 ml/year, although the effect did not quite reach statistical significance ($p = 0.06$). Progesterone treatment did slow the decline in diffusion capacity for carbon monoxide (DL_{CO}) from -2.15 to -0.19 mL/min/mmHg per year ($p < 0.05$) (220). Although the available data concerning the clinical efficacy of progesterone are flawed by retrospective design, concomitant use of multiple treatments and heterogeneity in patient populations, the anecdotal reports of benefit, the reasonable safety profile, and the lack of any acceptable alternative will likely continue to perpetuate its use until a definitive clinical trial is performed.

G. Other Therapies

GnRH agonists such as goserelin and leuprolide have been used in a few patients, but these agents are expensive and there are not enough data concerning their effects on progression of LAM to formulate a recommendation (177,222,223).

Antiestrogen therapy with tamoxifen, a partial estrogen antagonist, is generally not recommended because of a low rate of clinical response and isolated case reports of clinical worsening (215). Aggressive therapies—including ovarian radiation and oophorectomy—are no longer used because of the lack of proof of efficacy and the often irreversible effects on bone mass. Similarly, there is no support for the use of corticosteroids, cytotoxic agents, or androgens (224,225).

Patients with LAM should been treated with supplemental oxygen to maintain saturations greater than 90% with rest, exercise, and sleep. Bone densitometry should be routinely obtained at baseline and, as part of routine follow-up, and bone loss aggressively treated. LAM patients on antiestrogen therapies are at increased risk for atherosclerotic cardiovascular disease, and should be screened for hyperlipidemia and counseled regarding diet and exercise.

Agents that have been discussed as potentially promising future therapies include Ak+ pathway inhibitors such as rapamycin, aromatase inhibitors, metalloproteinase inhibitors, cytokines that inhibit smooth muscle proliferation such as interferon-α, angiogenesis inhibitors, and the tyrosine kinase inhibitor imatinib mesylate (Gleevec).

H. Special Management Issues in LAM

Pulmonary Transplantation

The first successful LAM transplant procedure was a heart-lung transplant performed in 1983 (226,227), and the first reported single-lung transplant for LAM occurred in 1988. At the time of this writing, there have been well over 100 LAM transplants worldwide. A retrospective analysis of the outcome of lung transplantation for LAM was reported by Boehler et al. (228). They compiled questionnaire data on 34 LAM patients who were treated at 16 transplant centers from 1983 to 1995, including 3 patients with known TSC. The average ages of the patients at disease onset, diagnosis, and transplantation were 29 ± 8, 34 ± 10, and 40 ± 9 years, respectively. Almost all patients had chronic dyspnea; disease manifestations also included a history of pneumothorax in 25, chylothorax in 7, and chylous ascites in 1 patient. Of the total, 26 patients had severe obstructive physiology, 3 had restrictive defects, and 3 had a mixed picture. One patient with relatively well-preserved lung function was transplanted for recurrent and persistent pneumothoraces. The overall survivals after 1 and 2 years were 69 and 58%, figures not substantially different from the values for pulmonary transplantation performed for other lung diseases. Extensive pleural adhesions in more than half of the patients caused significant intraoperative problems, including moderate to severe hemorrhage in 4 patients, repeat thoracotomy in 2 patients, and 1 intraoperative death. There were 4 additional early deaths due to acute lung injury and anastomotic dehiscence and 11 deaths from 2 to 43 months posttransplant, including 8 due to infection, 2 due to bronchiolitis obliterans and 1 due to metastatic nephroblastoma transferred by the lung allograft. One year after surgery, the average FEV_1 of 25 patients was 49% percent of predicted. The postoperative course was complicated by 35 episodes of pneumonia and 37 episodes of acute rejection. There were also 6 episodes of pneumothorax in the native lung after single-lung transplantation in 5 patients and chylothorax in 3. There was one episode of recurrent LAM discovered at autopsy of a patient who died from disseminated aspergillosis. Of 26 patients with available follow-up, 8 were receiving continued hormonal therapy for LAM and 18 were on no LAM-specific therapy. The conclusion of the study was that, despite excessive LAM complications of intraoperative hemorrhage due to adhesions, pneumothorax in the native lung following single-lung transplant, and recurrence of LAM in the allograft, pulmonary transplantation is a valuable therapeutic alternative for patients with end-stage LAM.

Recurrence

The three case reports of recurrent LAM in the donor allograft of LAM patients who have undergone lung transplants are precious experiments of nature that have much to teach us about the pathogenesis of LAM (200–202). The transplant recipients in studies from Munich, St. Louis, and Pittsburgh were females 34 to 45 years of age and each received a lung from a male donor

(Table 4). All three women succumbed to infection or acute respiratory failure 20 to 30 months posttransplant. Progressive deterioration in lung function due a worsening obstructive defect and repeated episodes of rejection/bronchiolitis suggested chronic bronchiolitis obliterans (BO) in the Munich and St. Louis cases, but pathological confirmation of BO was present only in the Munich case. This led the authors to speculate that recurrent LAM may have contributed to airflow obstruction in the St. Louis patient. In the case from Pittsburgh, the patient presented with a pneumothorax in the grafted lung, which could have been due to recurrent LAM. Very few details of the terminal emergency room visit were available for that patient, however, and the evidence that LAM may have contributed to the deterioration in graft function

Table 4 Clinical Features of Posttransplant LAM Recurrences

Clinical feature	Munich	Pittsburgh	St. Louis
Age at transplant	34	45	41
Cause of death	Acute respiratory failure	Sepsis	ARDS/*Aspergillus* pneumonia
Transplant to death	24 months	30 months	20 months
Donor lung	Male	15-year-old male	16-year-old male
Angiomyolipoma	?	8 × 5 × 4 cm	Not present on CT
Lymphadenopathy	+	+	?
Hormonal agents posttransplant	?	?	−
Complications	Reject/ bronchiolitis	Reject/ bronchiolitis	Reject/ bronchiolitis
Posttransplant pneumonia	Pneumonia, graft	PE/pneumonia native lung	−
Physiology posttransplant	Progressive obstruction	?	Progressive obstruction
Bronchiolitis posttransplant	+	+	−
Stains and probes			
Desmin	+	?	+
smooth muscle actin	+++	?	+++
Vimentin	+++	?	+++
HMB-45	+++	?	?
Estrogen/ progesterone	+/+	?	?
FISH Y chromosome	+	+	?

Key: PE, pulmonary embolism; ARDS, acute respiratory distress syndrome; CT, computed tomography.

in either case must therefore be considered circumstantial. The pathology of the LAM lesion in all three patients revealed multifocal involvement of the walls of blood vessels and bronchioles by proliferation of spindle cells that generally mirrored the lymphatic investment of the structures. In at least two of the cases, the lesion did not appear to involve the alveolar septa extensively, which is an uncommon finding in more advanced LAM. These cases may represent our best opportunities to observe the development of a LAM lesion within a defined time frame. The immunohistochemical staining characteristics described in two studies were consistent with a smooth muscle lineage for the lesional cells. However, only the Munich case was stained with the HMB-45 antibody, which is relatively specific for LAM. It is important to note in this context that smooth muscle lesions have been described in the transplanted lung of an emphysema patient (229), suggesting caution in attributing the smooth muscle pathological changes to LAM in the St. Louis and Pittsburgh cases without corroborating HMB-45 antibody data. In the Pittsburgh and Munich patients, in situ hybridization with a Y-chromosome probe suggested that the proliferating cells in the LAM lesion were of male (donor) origin, but more recent FISH and genetic analysis of the recurrent lesion in the St. Louis patient indicated that the cells were from the recipient (229a). Candidate sites for the origin of a mitogenic stimulus or a metastatic cell may have been the angiomyolipoma, which was present in the Pittsburgh patient; lymphadeno-pathy, which was present in the Munich and St. Louis patients; or the native lung in all three patients. Since recurrent LAM has never been directly implicated in compromised graft function, recurrent disease should not be a factor in determining candidacy or single- versus double-lung transplant.

Pleural space Complications

Recurrent pneumothoraces and chylous pleural effusions are common in patients with LAM and present challenging management problems, because interventions have the potential to increase the risk of complications upon subsequent lung transplantation. Of 35 patients evaluated at the National Institutes of Health (NIH), 24 had at least one pneumothorax, and the average number of pneumothoraces per patient was 5 ± 6 (176). Small pneumothoraces occupying less than 15% of the hemothorax are occasionally detected on screening x-rays and CT scans of LAM patients and may be managed with observation in some cases, with careful follow-up. Conservative management with chest-tube drainage may be a reasonable approach for symptomatic first pneumothoraces, especially in patients who are candidates for lung transplant and who have had a sclerosis or pleurodesis procedure on the contralateral hemithorax. In a British study, however, 20 of 30 (66%) patients treated conservatively for a first pneumothorax had recurrences in the ipsilateral hemithorax (223). Approximately 60% of those treated conservatively for the second and third pneumothoraces also had recurrences. These data suggest that LAM patients who suffer a first pneumothorax are very likely to have recurrences and chemical pleurodesis with talc after a first event is our preferred approach, especially for patients who have limited access to health care, who fly frequently, or in those with life-threatening presentations such as tension or bilateral pneumothoraces. Pleural abrasion, talc poudrage or pleurectomy may be considered for patients with recurrent pneumothoraces following chemical pleurodesis (170).

Chylothorax occurs in 20 to 30% of LAM patients at some point in their disease course (230–232). Small to moderate-sized, stable, chronic chylous effusions are not inflammatory, do not cause plural fibrosis, and do not necessarily require intervention. Chylothoraces requiring repeated taps for alleviation of dyspnea or chronically draining chylothoraces in patients with indwelling chest tubes can cause severe protein and nutrient depletion. A retrospective analysis suggests that progesterone may reduce chylous pleural effusions, especially in combination with oophorectomy, but these data are not conclusive. Other medical interventions have included a medium-chain triglyceride diet and hyperalimentation (233). Octreotide, which has been used for the treatment of chylothorax in other conditions, is currently under evaluation for problematic chylous effusions in LAM. Surgical interventions that have been reported include chemical or surgical pleurodesis, ligation of the subdiaphragmatic thoracic duct, and pleuroperitoneal, pleurocutaneous, and pleurovenous shunts (234).

Other Chylous Complications

Other chylous complications—including chyloptysis, chylopericardium, ascites, chyluria—can be major management problems in patients with LAM (170,171,176,177). Somatostatin and the better-tolerated peptide analog octreotide, which have been successfully used for treatment of chylous ascites due to other conditions (235–237), are currently being evaluated for some of these in LAM manifestations but no data are yet available.

Pregnancy

There are several case reports of worsening of LAM during pregnancy (212,238–243). In a British study, 28 of 50 LAM patients had been pregnant (223). All but 7 had their children before the onset of symptoms, including 4 who had developed their first symptom with pregnancy and 3 who had become pregnant after symptoms had developed. Complications of chylous pleural effusions (2 patients), one or more pneumothoraces (3 patients), and requirement for lung surgery (3 patients) occurred in 5 of 7 patients, an incidence that was 11 times higher than the average 9-month complication rate for nonpregnant patients. In the French study, 9 of 46 patients with a history of pregnancy reported that the onset of LAM symptoms began during childbearing, but only 2 reported a marked exacerbation of LAM (170). Several LAM patients have borne children without obvious adverse consequences, but in most cases no objective baseline pulmonary were data available for comparison because the diagnosis of LAM followed the pregnancy (221). Only a carefully performed prospective study can definitively determine the safety of pregnancy in women with LAM.

Meningiomas

Of 250 female patients with LAM followed at a clinical protocol at the NIH, 8 were found to have meningiomas on screening CT and magnetic resonance imaging (MRI) of the brain (221). Three of the women had TSC, including one who had two meningiomas, and five of the women did not have TSC, including one with seven tumors. The rest of the women had only one meningioma. Five of the patients with meningiomas had been treated with progesterone. Size and clinical manifestations due to the tumor were not reported. Based on the 2:1 female-to-male prevalence of meningiomas, the presence of progesterone receptors on the surface of cells in LAM, evidence that progestins are mitogenic for meningioma cells, and the uncertain clinical efficacy of progestins in LAM patients, the authors recommended that LAM patients with documented meningiomas not be given progestins for LAM.

I. Summary

The current therapeutic options for LAM patients include watchful observation, progestin therapy at suprapharmacological or conventional doses, or GnRH agonist therapy. Given the bone and cardiovascular risks of antiestrogen therapies and the uncertain benefits of currently available therapies, we generally avoid treatment of asymptomatic patients. No therapy or progestins (usually low-dose) is considered for patients who have had an initial pneumothorax or who have stable symptomatic disease, and progestins (high- or low-dose) or GnRH agonists are recommended for patients who wish to try therapy for progressive disease, recurrent pneumothoraces, or chylothoraces.

III. Langerhans Cell Histocytosis

A. Overview

Pulmonary Langerhans cell histocytosis (PLCH), also referred to as pulmonary histiocytosis X or pulmonary eosinophilic granuloma, is an uncommon, smoking-related, diffuse interstitial lung disease that primarily affects young adults (244,245). While PLCH is most commonly isolated to the lungs, some patients may also present with pituitary and bone involvement. Langerhans cell (LC) infiltration of multiple organs—including lung bone, skin, pituitary gland, liver, lymph nodes, and thyroid—occurs in neoplastic disorders of children known as systemic histiocytosis X, Letterer-Siwe disease, or Hand-Schuller-Christian disease (246). Protean presentations of these diseases can mimic PLCH. This discussion is limited to PLCH, the form of LC infiltration that is most frequently encountered by specialists in adult pulmonary medicine.

Patients with PLCH are typically smokers who present with worsening dyspnea, cough, or spontaneous pneumothorax associated with reticular pulmonary infiltrates. The hallmark of LCH is a pulmonary parenchymal lesion containing an abundance of dendritic (Langerhans) cells in a bronchiolocentric pattern that mirrors the distribution of LC cells in the normal lung. The LCH lesion has a stellate appearance at low power under the microscope and a nodular appearance on HRCT scanning of the chest. Cystic degeneration of the lung parenchyma often coexists with nodular changes until the late stages of the disease, when cystic changes predominate. The natural history of LCH usually includes a favorable outcome but varies considerably, ranging from spontaneous remission to progressive respiratory deficiency and death.

B. Pathogenesis

LCs, the only cells of dendritic lineage in the lung, are normally present in the tracheobronchial epithelium, where their main function is to recognize and process inhaled antigens. The morphology of pulmonary LCs is similar to that of LCs in other tissues (247); the cells can be easily identified by their abundant eosinophilic cytoplasm, reniform nuclei, intracytoplasmic organelles (Birbeck bodies) seen on electron microscopy (248), and the universal expression of CD1a and S100 glycoproteins (249). LCs increase in number in the presence of damaged epithelium and with increases in the levels of GM-CSF (250), which is known to occur as a result of cigarrette smoking. LC-rich interstitial granulomatous inflammation in mice is induced by exposure to tobacco smoke (251). The prevailing theory is that factors in cigarette smoke—including particulates, P glycoprotein, and other molecules—promote the recruitment and activation of LCs within the lung. The finding that CD1 + and/or S100 cells isolated from patients with LCH are clonal has confirmed suspicions of the neoplastic basis of these diseases (252). A single study that analyzed the clonality of lesions in patients with PLCH found that most lesions (71%) were not clonal (253). In 5 of 13 patients, clonal nodules were found, but in 3 of those cases nonclonal lesion were also present. Given the mixed nature of these results, the fact that the HUMARA assay used to assess clonality can produce artifactual results, and that clonal proliferation can occasionally be seen with inflammatory disorders (253), these authors felt that the data were most consisent with a reactive rather than a neoplastic pathogenesis for PLCH. Patients with diffuse LCH in childhood may develop radiographic evidence of lung involvement with cystic and nodular changes years later, in some cases possibly precipitated by cigarette smoking (254,255).

C. Presentation

The prevalence of LCH is unknown, but the disease appears to affect young people more commonly. Early studies suggested a male predominance for PLCH (256), perhaps reflecting the demographics of smoking in the middle of the 20th century, but more recent series reveal an equal gender distribution (257) or a slight female predominance (258). The disease appears to be more prevalent in Caucasians, unusual in African Americans, and virtually nonexistent in Asians. Although almost all patients with isolated pulmonary LCH are smokers, only a tiny fraction of smokers develop LCH. There is no evidence for familial clustering to suggest an inheritable genetic basis for PLCH other than a single case report of father-to-son transmission in 1973 (259). PLCH occurs predominantly in young adults aged 20 to 40 years (259). Virtually all (90–100%) patients in recent series smoke cigarettes (245,260) and are frequently quite heavy tobacco users based on average daily tobacco consumption (261). Most patients with PLCH have symptoms (75%), usually cough and dyspnea, but fortuitous discovery on routine chest x-rays is the method of ascertainment in up to 36% of patients in some series (262). Although spontaneous pneumothorax is a commonly reported complication, it occurs during the course of illness in only about 25% of patients. About one-third of patients present with systemic symptoms of fever, malaise, or weight loss, which may stimulate a search for malignancy or chronic infection.

D. Diagnosis

Chest roentgenotgrams reveal reticulonodular changes in a diffuse bilateral and symmetrical pattern, often with an upper and middle lung zone predominance that spares the costophrenic angles (Fig. 5). The HRCT appearance may reveal multiple nodules associated with thin-walled cysts in the upper lung zones in the early stages, evolving into a predominant cystic and diffuse pattern as the disease progresses (263) (Fig. 5). In the most advanced cases, the lung parenchyma becomes almost completely replaced by reticular networks of interconnecting cysts. Pulmonary physiology may be normal in the face of radiographic changes in up to 10 to 15% of patients and obstructive, restrictive, or mixed patterns of airflow limitation have been reported. Lung volumes are often normal or even slightly increased, with a reduced vital capacity (VC) and normal or increased residual volume (RV). The presence of predominantly obstructive physiology with normal or increased lung volumes in the setting of diffuse interstitial changes on x-ray should suggest PLCH or LAM (264). Bronchoscopy with bronchoalveolar lavage can be quite useful in the evaluation of patients with PLCH (265). The presence of >5% LCs in the bronchoalveolar lavage fluid, identified by immunostaining for LC marker CD1a, is highly suggestive of PLCH (266,267). Unfortunately, the sensitivity for this threshold level is quite low (<25%), and lower levels of CD1a in BAL (2–3%) are diagnostically indeterminate, a picture also seen in heavy smokers

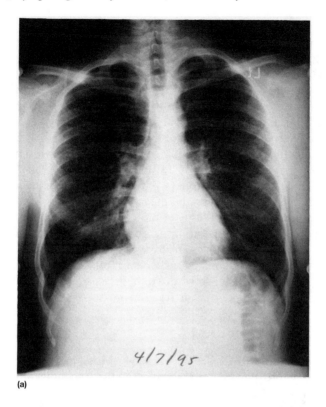

(a)

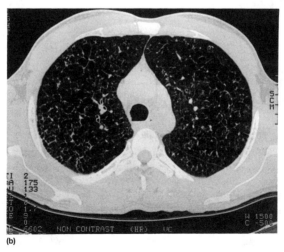

(b)

Figure 5 Radiographs from a patient with PLCH demonstrating reticular interstitial markings sparing the costophrenic angles on chest x-ray (a) and diffuse cystic change on HRCT (b).

and patients with other interstitial lung diseases. Transbronchial biopsy has a low diagnostic yield in PLCH because of the patchy nature of the disease, but it has been reported to produce useful information in 10 to 40% of cases (268). PLCH can be difficult to distinguish from emphysema, fibrocystic sarcoidosis, granulomatous infections such as tuberculosis and histoplasmosis, lymphangioleiomyomatosis, and several other disorders. In the appropriate clinical context, the clinical diagnosis of PLCH may be sufficiently certain to obviate the need for lung biopsy by thoracoscopy or thoracotomy. For instance, in smokers presenting with worsening dyspnea, cough, or pneumothorax associated with a compatible HRCT (upper and middle lobe–predominant cavitary nodules and cystic pulmonary parenchymal changes) and >5% LC in BAL, the diagnosis of LCH may be made without tissue biopsy. In atypical cases, wedge biopsy by thoracotomy or thoracoscopy is recommended, and CT should be used to identify regions which contain nodules for the surgeon to target. Since there are no known effective therapeutic interventions for other than smoking cessation, the major justification for biopsy may be to rule out other treatable illnesses (e.g., sarcoidosis, hypersensitivity pneumonitis) or to provide an incentive for the patient to quit smoking.

E. Prognosis

The natural history of PLCH is variable. Most patients do well, with stabilization, improvement, or remission either spontaneously or while receiving corticosteroids. About 10 to 20% of patients suffer a downhill course leading to respiratory insufficiency and cor pulmonale. Recurrent pneumothoraces, multisystem disease, extremes of age, systemic symptoms, major abnormalities in pulmonary function, and extensive cystic changes with a reduced diffusion capacity are associated with a poor prognosis (262,269). Pregnancy has been reported to exacerbate diabetes insipidus associated with PLCH but does not appear to cause deterioration in lung function (270,271). Lung carcinoma and lymphoma may occur with increased frequency in patients with PLCH, and PLCH has been reported in few patients after treatment with chemotherapy and radiation therapy for cancer (272–277).

F. The Recurrence of LCH in Lung Transplantation

To our knowledge, there have been four cases of recurrent LCH in lung-transplant patients reported in the English literature (278–280). The characteristics of the patients depicted in Table 5 suggest that LCH can recur in patients with multifocal disease as well as those with disease restricted to lung, even in patients that deny resumption of smoking after transplant. Although the number of cases is small, the fact that three of four recurrences were reported in patients with diffuse disease may suggest that this posttransplant complication is more likely in patients with multiorgan involvement. Recurrence despite the use of prednisone and other immunosup-

Table 5 Clinical Features of Posttransplant PLCH Recurrences

Clinical features	Burke	Corris	Mornex	Mornex
Age at diagnosis	27	32	19	27
Age at transplant	29	32	22	31
Original site of involvement	Lung	Lung, pituitary	Lung, bone	Lung, pituitary
Type of transplant	Single	Double	Single	Single
Time to recurrence (years)	2	2	1	1
Smoking posttransplant	No	No	Yes	Yes
Immunosuppression	Azathiorpine, cyclosporine, prednisone ?	Azathioprine, cyclosporine, prednisone		Azathioprine, cyclosporine, prednisone
Stain for S100	Yes	Yes	?	Yes
CD1	?	?	Yes	?
Clonality of lesion	?	?	?	?

pressive drugs in the posttransplant period challenges the rationale for the use of cytoxic and glucocorticoid therapy in the treatment of the histiocytoses.

G. Management of PLCH

Spontaneous resolution had been described in several patients after smoking cessation, and all patients should be encouraged to discontinue tobacco use (281–283). Persistent symptoms develop in only about 25% of patients (258), and 5 to 6% will develop progressive end-stage disease, in some cases culminating in death from respiratory failure. There is no proven pharmacological treatment for progressive PLCH, although steroids continue to be widely prescribed for progressive and symptomatic disease. A few success stories with the use of corticosteroid therapy continue to fuel this approach (258,284,285). In one series, corticosteroids were found to be associated with improvement in symptoms and radiographic infiltrates but not with improvement in pulmonary function (262). A trial of corticosteroids is appropriate in nonsmoking patients with nodular changes on HRCT or chest x-ray, systemic symptoms, and/or progressive disease. A tapering course of prednisone over 6 to 12 months beginning at 0.5 to 0.75 mg/kg is a typical regimen for these patients.

The use of cytotoxic therapy in LCH has also been reported, especially in patients with multisystemic involvement (286,287). Data to support the use of chemotherapeutic agents in PLCH are lacking; if these agents are used at all they should be restricted to salvage regimens for patients with progressive disease and who fail corticosteroids.

Pamidronate therapy is effective in the treatment of bone pain in patients with osteolytic lesions from LCH (288). Pamidronate was reported to reduce bone pain in a 14-year-old boy with with long-standing multisystemic LCH that had been refractory to treatment with corticosteroids and cytotoxic agents (289). Speculation that bisphosphonates may also be useful in the treatment of PLCH is supported by the antimacrophage properties of these agents (290).

H. Summary

PLCH is an uncommon smoking-related interstitial lung disease that is usually associated with a favorable outcome. Smoking cessation is the most important intervention, and corticosteroids may have utility in patients who progress after tobacco use is discontinued. The role of cytotoxic therapy is PLCH is unclear.

References

1. Lynch JP III, Sharma OP, Baughman RP. Extrapulmonary sarcoidosis. Semin Respir Infect 1998; 13:229–254.
2. Hunninghake GW, Costabel U, Ando M, et al. ATS/ERS/WASOG statement on sarcoidosis. American Thoracic Society/European Respiratory Society/World Association of Sarcoidosis and other Granulomatous Disorders. Sarcoidosis Vasc Diffuse Lung Dis 1999; 16:149–173.
3. Mana J, Salazar A, Manresa F. Clinical factors predicting persistence of activity in sarcoidosis: a multivariate analysis of 193 cases. Respiration 1994; 61:219–225.
4. Reich JM, Johnson RE. Course and prognosis of sarcoidosis in a nonreferral setting. Analysis of 86 patients observed for 10 years. Am J Med 1985; 78:61–67.
5. Siltzbach LE, James DG, Neville E, et al. Course and prognosis of sarcoidosis around the world. Am J Med 1974; 57:847–852.
6. Keller AZ. Hospital, age, racial, occupational, geographical, clinical and survivorship characteristics in the epidemiology of sarcoidosis. Am J Epidemiol 1971; 94:222–230.
7. Mitchell DN, Scadding JG, Heard BE, Hinson KF. Sarcoidosis: histopathological definition and clinical diagnosis. J Clin Pathol 1977; 30:395–398.
8. Soler P, Basset F. Morphology and distribution of the cells of a sarcoid granuloma: ultrastructural study of serial sections. Ann NY Acad Sci 1976; 278:147–160.
9. Thomas PD, Hunninghake GW. Current concepts of the pathogenesis of sarcoidosis. Am Rev Respir Dis 1987; 135:747–760.
10. Hunninghake GW, Kawanami O, Ferrans VJ, Young RC Jr, Roberts WC, Crystal RG. Characterization of the inflammatory and immune effector cells in the lung parenchyma of patients with interstitial lung disease. Am Rev Respir Dis 1981; 123:407–412.
11. Moller DR. Involvement of T cells and alterations in T cell receptors in sarcoidosis. Semin Respir Infect 1998; 13:174–183.

12. Agostini C, Basso U, Semenzato G. Cells and molecules involved in the development of sarcoid granuloma. J Clin Immunol 1998; 18:184–192.
13. Baumer I, Zissel G, Schlaak M, Muller-Quernheim J. Th1/Th2 cell distribution in pulmonary sarcoidosis. Am J Respir Cell Mol Biol 1997; 16:171–177.
14. Shigehara K, Shijubo N, Ohmichi M, et al. Enhanced mRNA expression of Th1 cytokines and IL-12 in active pulmonary sarcoidosis. Sarcoidosis Vasc Diffuse Lung Dis 2000; 17:151–157.
15. Prasse A, Georges CG, Biller H, et al. Th1 cytokine pattern in sarcoidosis is expressed by bronchoalveolar CD4 + and CD8 + T cells. Clin Exp Immunol 2000; 122:241–248.
16. Ward K, O'Connors C, Odlun C, Fitzgerald FX. Prognostic value of bronchoalveolar lavage in sarcoidosis: the critical influence of disease presentation. Thorax 1989; 44:6–12.
17. Ceuppens JL, Lacquet LM, Marien G, Demedts M, Van Den Eeckhout A, Stevens E. Alveolar T-cell subsets in pulmonary sarcoidosis: correlation with disease activity and effect of steroid treatment. Am Rev Respir Dis 1984; 129:563–568.
18. Romagnani S. T-cell subsets (Th1 versus Th2). Ann Allergy Asthma Immunol 2000; 85:9–18.
19. Kunkel SL, Lukacs NW, Strieter RM, Chensue SW. Th1 and Th2 responses regulate experimental lung granuloma development. Sarcoidosis Vasc Diffuse Lung Dis 1996; 13:120–128.
20. Bost TW, Riches DW, Schumacher B, et al. Alveolar macrophages from patients with beryllium disease and sarcoidosis express increased levels of mRNA for tumor necrosis factor-alpha and interleukin-6 but not interleukin-1 beta. Am J Respir Cell Mol Biol 1994; 10:506–513.
21. Foley NM, Millar AB, Meager A, Johnson NM, Rook GA. Tumour necrosis factor production by alveolar macrophages in pulmonary sarcoidosis and tuberculosis. Sarcoidosis 1992; 9:29–34.
22. Homolka J, Muller QJ. Increased interleukin 6 production by bronchoalveolar lavage cells in patients with active sarcoidosis. Lung 1993; 171:173–183.
23. Ishioka S, Saito T, Hiyama K, et al. Increased expression of tumor necrosis factor-alpha, interleukin-6, platelet-derived growth factor-B and granulocyte-macrophage colony-stimulating factor mRNA in cells of bronchoalveolar lavage fluids from patients with sarcoidosis. Sarcoidosis Vasc Diffuse Lung Dis 1996; 13:139–145.
24. Kim DS, Jeon YJ, Shim TS, et al. The value of interleukin-12 as an activity marker of pulmonary sarcoidosis. Sarcoidosis Vasc Diffuse Lung Dis 2000; 3:271–276.
25. Steffen M, Petersen J, Oldigs M, et al. Increased secretion of tumor necrosis factor-alpha, interleukin-1-beta, and interleukin-6 by alveolar macrophages from patients with sarcoidosis. J Allergy Clin Immunol 1993; 91:939–949.
26. Terao I, Hashimoto S, Horie T. Effect of GM-CSF on TNF-alpha and IL-1-beta production by alveolar macrophages and peripheral blood monocytes from patients with sarcoidosis. Int Arch Allergy Immunol 1993; 102:242–248.
27. Agelli M, Wahl SM. Cytokines and fibrosis. Clin Exp Rheumatol 1986; 4:379–388.

28. Fireman E, Kivity S, Shahar I, Reshef T, Mekori YA. Secretion of stem cell factor by alveolar fibroblasts in interstitial lung diseases. Immunol Lett 1999; 67:229–236.

29. Tamura R, Sato A, Chida K, Suganuma H. Fibroblasts as target and effector cells in Japanese patients with sarcoidosis. Lung 1998; 176:75–87.

30. Shahar I, Fireman E, Topilsky M, et al. Effect of IL-6 on alveolar fibroblast proliferation in interstitial lung diseases. Clin Immunol Immunopathol 1996; 79:244–251.

31. Car BD, Meloni F, Luisetti M, Semenzato G, Gialdroni-Grassi G, Walz A. Elevated IL-8 and MCP-1 in the bronchoalveolar lavage fluid of patients with idiopathic pulmonary fibrosis and pulmonary sarcoidosis. Am J Opthalmol 1994; 149:655–659.

32. Yokoyama T, Kanda T, Kobayashi I, Suzuki T. Serum levels of interleukin-8 as a marker of disease activity in patients with chronic sarcoidosis. J Med 1995; 26:209–219.

33. Roth C, Huchon GJ, Arnoux A, Stanislas-Leguern G, Marsac JH, Chretien J. Bronchoalveolar cells in advanced pulmonary sarcoidosis. Am Rev Respir Dis 1981; 124:9–12.

34. Hind CR, Latchman YE, Brostoff J. Circulating human leucocyte elastase levels in patients with pulmonary sarcoidosis. Sarcoidosis 1988; 5:38–42.

35. Losa Garcia JE, Rodriguez FM, Martin de Cabo MR, et al. Evaluation of inflammatory cytokine secretion by human alveolar macrophages. Mediators Inflamm 1999; 8:43–51.

36. Brass DM, Hoyle GW, Poovey HG, Liu JY, Brody AR. Reduced tumor necrosis factor-alpha and transforming growth factor-beta$_1$ expression in the lungs of inbred mice that fail to develop fibroproliferative lesions consequent to asbestos exposure. Am J Pathol 1999; 154:853–862.

37. Sime PJ, Marr RA, Gauldie D, et al. Transfer of tumor necrosis factor-alpha to rat lung induces severe pulmonary inflammation and patchy interstitial fibrogenesis with induction of transforming growth factor-beta$_1$ and myofibroblasts. Am J Pathol 1998; 153:825–832.

38. Liu JY, Brass DM, Hoyle GW, Brody AR. TNF-alpha receptor knockout mice are protected from the fibroproliferative effects of inhaled asbestos fibers. Am J Pathol 1998; 153:1839–1847.

39. Agostini C, Zambello R, Sancetta R, et al. Expression of tumor necrosis factor-receptor superfamily members by lung T lymphocytes in interstitial lung disease. Am J Respir Crit Care Med 1996; 153:1359–1367.

40. Somoskovi A, Zissel G, Seitzer U, Gerdes J, Schlaak M, Muller Q. Polymorphisms at position -308 in the promoter region of the TNF-alpha and in the first intron of the TNF-beta genes and spontaneous and lipopolysaccharide-induced TNF-alpha release in sarcoidosis. Cytokine 1999; 11:882–887.

41. Yamaguchi E, Itoh A, Hizawa N, Kawakami Y. The gene polymorphism of tumor necrosis factor-beta, but not that of tumor necrosis factor-alpha, is associated with the prognosis of sarcoidosis. Chest 2001; 119:753–761.

42. Seitzer U, Swider C, Stuber F, et al. Tumour necrosis factor alpha promoter gene polymorphism in sarcoidosis. Cytokine 1997; 9:787–790.

43. Parkes SA, Baker SB, Bourdillon RE, Murray CR, Rakshit M. Epidemiology of sarcoidosis in the Isle of Man—1: A case controlled study. Thorax 1987; 42:420–426.

44. Hills SE, Parkes SA, Baker SB. Epidemiology of sarcoidosis in the Isle of Man—2: Evidence for space-time clustering. Thorax 1987; 42:427–430.

45. Bresnitz EA, Stolley PD, Israel HL, Soper K. Possible risk factors for sarcoidosis. A case-control study. Ann NY Acad Sci 1986; 465:632–642.

46. Edmondstone WM. Sarcoidosis in nurses: is there an association? Thorax 1988; 43:342–343.

47. Kern DG, Neill MA, Wrenn DS, Varone JC. Investigation of a unique time-space cluster of sarcoidosis in firefighters. Am Rev Respir Dis 1993; 148:974–980.

48. Sarcoidosis among U.S. Navy enlisted men, 1965–1993. MMWR 1997; 46:539–543.

49. Almenoff PL, Johnson A, Lesser M, Mattman LH. Growth of acid fast L forms from the blood of patients with sarcoidosis. Thorax 1996; 51:530–533.

50. Fidler HM. Mycobacteria and sarcoidosis: recent advances. Sarcoidosis 1994; 11:66–68.

51. Bocart D, Lecossier D, De Lassence A, Valeyre D, Battesti JP, Hance AJ. A search for mycobacterial DNA in granulomatous tissues from patients with sarcoidosis using the polymerase chain reaction. Am Rev Respir Dis 1992; 145:1142–1148.

52. Ishige I, Usui Y, Takemura T, Eishi Y. Quantitative PCR of mycobacterial and propionibacterial DNA in lymph nodes of Japanese patients with sarcoidosis. Lancet 1999; 354:120–123.

53. Baughman RP, Shipley RT, Loudon RG, Lower EE. Crackles in interstitial lung disease. Comparison of sarcoidosis and fibrosing alveolitis. Chest 1991; 100:96–101.

54. Dunn TL, Watters LC, Hendrix C, Cherniack RM, Schwarz MI, King TE Jr. Gas exchange at a given degree of volume restriction is different in sarcoidosis and idiopathic pulmonary fibrosis. Am J Med 1988; 85:221–224.

55. Askling J, Grunewald J, Eklund A, Hillerdal G, Ekbom A. Increased risk for cancer following sarcoidosis. Am J Respir Crit Care Med 1999; 160:1668–1672.

56. Yamaguchi M, Odaka M, Hosoda Y, Iwai K, Tachibana T. Excess death of lung cancer among sarcoidosis patients. Sarcoidosis 1991; 8:51–55.

57. Winterbauer RH, Kraemer KG. The infectious complications of sarcoidosis: a current perspective. Arch Intern Med 1976; 136:1356–1362.

58. Teirstein AS, Chuang M, Miller A, Siltzbach LE. Flexible-bronchoscope biopsy of lung and bronchial wall in intrathoracic sarcoidosis. Ann NY Acad Sci 1976; 278:522–527.

59. Neville E, Walker AN, James DG. Prognostic factors predicting the outcome of sarcoidosis: an analysis of 818 patients. QJ Med 1983; 208:525–533.

60. James DG, Turiaf J, Hosoda Y, et al. Description of sarcoidosis: report of the Subcommittee on Classification and Definition. Ann NY Acad Sci 1976; 278:742.

61. Mana J, Badrinas F, Manresa F, Valverde J, Fernandez-Nogues F. Predictive factors of the persistence of sarcoidosis activity 2 years after diagnosis. Med Clin (Barc) 1991; 97:769–773.

62. Israel HL, Karlin P, Menduke H, DeLisser OG. Factors affecting outcome of sarcoidosis. Influence of race, extrathoracic involvement, and initial radiologic lung lesions. Ann NY Acad Sci 1986; 465:609–618.

63. Gottlieb JE, Israel HL, Steiner RM, Triolo J, Patrick H. Outcome in sarcoidosis. The relationship of relapse to corticosteroid therapy. Chest 1997; 111:623–631.

64. Hunninghake GW, Gilbert S, Pueringer R, et al. Outcome of the treatment for sarcoidosis. Am J Respir Crit Care Med 1994; 149:893–898.

65. Rizzato G, Montemurro L, Colombo P. The late follow-up of chronic sarcoid patients previously treated with corticosteroids. Sarcoidosis 1998; 15:52–58.

66. Soskel NT, Sharma OP. Pleural involvement in sarcoidosis. Curr Opin Pulm Med 2000; 6:455–468.

67. Chusid EL, Siltzbach LE. Sarcoidosis of the pleura. Ann Intern Med 1974; 81:190–194.

68. Israel HL, Lenchner G, Steiner RM. Late development of mediastinal calcification in sarcoidosis. Am Rev Respir Dis 1981; 124:302–305.

69. Teirstein AL, Siltzbach LE. Sarcoidosis of the upper lung fields simulating pulmonary tuberculosis. Chest 1973; 64:303–308.

70. Mana J, Teirstein AS, Mendelson DS, Padilla ML, DePalo LR. Excessive thoracic computed tomographic scanning in sarcoidosis. Thorax 1995; 50:1264–1266.

71. Wurm K, Rosner R. Prognosis of chronic sarcoidosis. Ann NY Acad Sci 1976; 278:732–735.

72. Scadding JG. Prognosis of intrathoracic sarcoidosis in England. Br Med J 1961; 4:1165–1172.

73. Tazi A, Desfemmes-Baleyte T, Soler P, Valeyre D, Hance AJ, Battesti JP. Pulmonary sarcoidosis with a diffuse ground glass pattern on the chest radiograph. Thorax 1994; 49:793–797.

74. Turner-Warwick M, McAllister W, Lawrence R, Britten A, Haslam PL. Corticosteroid treatment in pulmonary sarcoidosis: do serial lavage lymphocyte counts, serum angiotensin converting enzyme measurements, and gallium-67 scans help management? Thorax 1986; 41:903–913.

75. Siltzbach LE, Posner A, Medine MM. Cortisone therapy in sarcoidosis. JAMA 1951; 147:927–929.

76. Stone M, Israel HL, Dratman MB. Effect of cortisone in sarcoidosis. N Engl Med 951; 244:209–213.

77. Selroos O, Sellergren TL. Corticosteroid therapy of pulmonary sarcoidosis. Scand J Respir Dis 1979; 60:215–212.

78. Pinkston P, Saltini C, Muller-Quernheim J, Crystal RG. Corticosteroid therapy suppresses spontaneous interleukin 2 release and spontaneous proliferation of lung T lymphocytes of patients with active pulmonary sarcoidosis. J Immunol 1987; 139:755–760.

79. Young RL, Harkelroad LE, Lorden RE, Weg JG. Pulmonary sarcoidosis: a prospective evaluation of glucocorticoid therapy. Ann Intern Med 1970; 73:207–212.

80. du Bois RM, Greenhalgh PM, Southcott AM, Johnson NM, Harris TA. Randomized trial of inhaled fluticasone propionate in chronic stable pulmonary sarcoidosis: a pilot study. Eur Respir J 1999; 13:1345–1350.

81. Olsson T, Bjornstad-Pettersen H, Stjernberg NL. Bronchostenosis due to sarcoidosis: a cause of atelectasis and airway obstruction simulating pulmonary neoplasm and chronic obstructive pulmonary disease. Chest 1979; 75:663–666.

82. Johns CJ, Michele TM. The clinical management of sarcoidosis. A 50-year experience at the Johns Hopkins Hospital. Medicine (Baltimore) 1999; 78:65–111.

83. Eule H, Roth I, Ehrke I, Weinecke W. Corticosteroid therapy of intrathoracic sarcoidosis stages I and II—results of a controlled clinical trial. Z Erkr Atmungsorgane 1977; 149:142–147.

84. Johnson BA, Duncan SR, Ohori NP, et al. Recurrence of sarcoidosis in pulmonary allograft recipients. Am Rev Respir Dis 1993; 148:1373.

85. Kazerooni EA, Cascade PN. Recurrent miliary sarcoidosis after lung transplantation (letter). Radiology 1995; 194:913.

86. Muller C, Briegel J, Haller M, et al. Sarcoidosis recurrence following lung transplantation. Transplantation 1996; 61:1117–1119.

87. Nunley DR, Hattler B, Keenan RJ, et al. Lung transplantation for end-stage pulmonary sarcoidosis. Sarcoidosis Vasc Diffuse Lung Dis 1999; 16:93–100.

88. Seidel K. The immunopathogenesis of chronic rheumatoid polyarthritis and new ways of its treatment. Z Gesamte Inn Med 1968; 23:545–550.

89. Zvaifler NJ. Antimalarial treatment of rheumatoid arthritis. Med Clin North Am 1968; 52:759–764.

90. Jones E, Cagen JP. Hydroxychloroquine is effective therapy for control of cutaneous sarcoidal granulomas. Am Acad Dermatol 1990; 23:487–490.

91. Zie J, Horowitz D, Arzubiaga C, King L. Treatment of cutaneous sarcoidosis with chloroquine: review of the literature. Arch Dermatol 1991; 127:1034–1040.

92. Chloroquine in the treatment of sarcoidosis. A report from the Research Committee of the British Tuberculosis Association. Tubercle 1967; 48:257–272.

93. Siltzbach LE, Teirstein AS. Chloroquine therapy in 43 patients with intrathoracic and cutaneous sarcoidosis. Acta Med Scand 1964; 425:302S–308S.

94. Baltzan M, Mehta S, Kirkham TH, Cosio MG. Randomized trial of prolonged chloroquine therapy in advanced pulmonary sarcoidosis. Am J Respir Crit Care Med 1999; 160:192–197.

95. Easterbrook M. Chloroquine retinopathy. Arch Ophthalmol 1991; 109:1362.

96. Olansky AJ. Antimalarials and ophthalmologic safety. J Am Acad Dermatol 1982; 6:19–23.

97. Zic JA, Horowitz DH, Arzubiaga C, King LE, Jr. Treatment of cutaneous sarcoidosis with chloroquine. Review of the literature. Arch Dermatol 1991; 127:1034–1040.

98. Bartel PR, Roux P, Robinson E, Anderson IF. Visual function and long-term chloroquine treatment. S. Afr Med J 1994; 84:32–34.

99. Hu SK, Mitcho YL, Oronsky AL, Kerwar SS. Studies on the effect of methotrexate on macrophage function. J Rheumatol 1988; 15:206–209.

100. Baughman RP, Lower EE. The effect of corticosteroid or methotrexate therapy on lung lymphocytes and macrophages in sarcoidosis. Am Rev Respir Dis 1990; 142:1268–1271.

101. Lower EE, Baughman RP. The use of low dose methotrexate in refractory sarcoidosis. Arch Intern Med 1990; 299:153–157.

102. Albera C, Pozzi E, Palmulli P, Guerra S, Nicali R, Ghio P. Low dose steroid plus methotrexate in the treatment of pulmonary sarcoidosis. Eur Respir J 2000; 16:370s.

103. Baughman RP, Lower EE. Steroid-sparing alternative treatments for sarcoidosis. Clin Chest Med 1997; 18:853–864.

104. Lacher MJ. Spontaneous remission response to methotrexate in sarcoidosis. Ann Intern Med 1968; 69:1247–1248.

105. Lower EE, Baughman RP. Prolonged use of methotrexate for sarcoidosis. Arch Intern Med 1995; 155:846–851.

106. Sostman HD, Matthay RA, Putman GE. Methotrexate-induced pneumonitis. Medicine 1976; 55:371–388.

107. Hargreaves MR, Mowat AG, Benson MK. Acute pneumonitis associated with low dose methotrexate treatment for rheumatoid arthritis: report of five cases and review of published reports. Thorax 1992; 47:628–633.

108. Tolman KG, Clegg DO, Lee RG, Ward JR. Methotrexate and the liver. J Rheumatol 1985; 12:S29–S34.

109. Van de Kerkhof PCM, Hoefnagels WHL, van Haelst JGM, Mali JWH. Methotrexate maintenance therapy and liver damage in psoriasis. Clin Exp Dermatol 1985; 10:194–200.

110. Baughman RP. Methotrexate for sarcoidosis. Sarcoidosis Vasc Diffuse Lung Dis 1998; 15:147–149.

111. Baughman RP, Lower EE. A clinical approach to the use of methotrexate for sarcoidosis. Thorax 1999; 54:742–746.

112. Lynch JPI, McCune WJ. Immunosuppressive and cytotoxic pharmacotherapy for pulmonary disorders. Am J Respir Crit Care Med 1997; 155:395–420.

113. Present DH. 6-Mercaptopurine and other immunosuppressive agents in the treatment of Crohn's disease and ulcerative colitis. Ann Intern Med 1989; 18:57–71.

114. Sachar DB, Present DH. Immunotherapy in inflammatory bowel disease. Med Clin North Am 1978; 62:173–183.

115. Savolainen HA, Kautiainen H, Isomaki H, Aho K, Verronen P. Azathioprine in patients with juvenile chronic arthritis: a long-term follow-up study. J Rheumatol 1997; 24:2444–2450.

116. Muller-Quernheim J, Kienast K, Held M, Pfeifer S, Costabel U. Treatment of chronic sarcoidosis with an azathioprine/prednisolone regimen. Eur Respir 1999; 14:1117–1122.

117. Pacheo Y, Marechal C, Marechal F, Biot N, Perrin-Fayolle M. Azathioprine treatment of chronic pulmonary sarcoidosis. Sarcoidosis 1985; 2:107–113.

118. Sharma OP, Hughes DTD, James DG, Naish P. Immunosuppressive therapy with azathioprine in sarcoidosis. In: Levinsky L, Macholoa F, eds. Fifth International Conference on Sarcoidosis and Other Granulomatous Disorders. Prague: Universita Karlova, 1971:635–637.

119. Hof DG, Hof PC, Godfrey WA. Long-term use of azathioprine as a steroid-sparing treatment for chronic sarcoidosis. Am J Respir Crit Care Med 1996; 153:A870.

120. Lewis SJ, Ainslie GM, Bateman ED. Efficacy of azathioprine as second-line treatment in pulmonary sarcoidosis. Sarcoidosis Vasc Diffuse Lung Dis 1999; 16:87–92.

121. Martinet Y, Pinkston P, Saltini C, Spurzem J, Muller-Quernheim J, Crystal RG. Evaluation of the in vitro and in vivo effects of cyclosporine on the lung T-lymphocyte alveolitis of active pulmonary sarcoidosis. Am Rev Respir Dis 1996; 138:1242–1248.

122. Wyser CP, van Schalkwyk EM, Alheit B, Bardin PG, Joubert JR. Treatment of progressive pulmonary sarcoidosis with cyclosporin A: a randomized controlled trial. Am J Respir Crit Care Med 1997; 156:1571–1576.

123. Kavanaugh AF, Andrew SL, Cooper B, Lawrence EC, Huston DP. Cyclosporine therapy of central nervous system sarcoidosis. Am J Med 1987; 82:387.
124. Stern BJ, Krumholz A, Johns C, Scott P, Nissim J. Sarcoidosis and its neurological manifestations. Arch Neurol 1985; 42:909–917.
125. Bielory L, Holland C, Gascon P, Frohman L. Uveitis, cutaneous and neurosarcoid: treatment with low-dose cyclosporine A. Transplant Proc 1988; 20:144–148.
126. Kataria YP. Chlorambucil in sarcoidosis. Chest 1980; 78:36–42.
127. Israel HL, McComb BL. Chlorambucil treatment of sarcoidosis. Sarcoidosis 1991; 8:35–41.
128. Baughman RP, Lower EE. Use of intermittent, intravenous cyclophosphamide for idiopathic pulmonary fibrosis. Chest 1992; 102:1090–1094.
129. Baker GL, Kahl LE, Zee BC, Stolzer BL, Agarwal AK, Medsger TA. Malignancy following treatment of rheumatoid arthritis with cyclophosphamide. Am J Med 1987; 83:1–9.
130. Travis LB, Curtis RE, Glimelius B, et al. Bladder and kidney cancer following cyclophosphamide therapy for non-Hodgkin's lymphoma. J Natl Cancer Inst 1995; 87:524–530.
131. Bankhurst AD. Etanercept and methotrexate combination therapy. Clin Exp Rheum 1999; 17:S69–S72.
132. Hurd LB, Lichtenstein GR. Therapeutic potential of infliximab in inflammatory bowel disease. Gastroenterol Nurs 1999; 22:199–208.
133. Moreland LW, Schiff MH, Baumgartner SW, et al. Etanercept therapy in rheumatoid arthritis. A randomized, controlled trial. Ann Intern Med 1999; 130:478–486.
134. Spatafora M, Merendino A, Chiappara G, et al. Lung compartmentalization of increased TNF releasing ability by mononuclear phagocytes in pulmonary sarcoidosis. Chest 1989; 96:542–549.
135. Armstrong L, Foley NM, Millar AB. Inter-relationship between tumour necrosis factor-alpha (TNF-alpha) and TNF soluble receptors in pulmonary sarcoidosis. Thorax 1999; 54:524–530.
136. Moodley YP, Dorasamy T, Venketesamy S, Naicker V, Lalloo UG. Correlation of CD4:CD8 ratio and tumor necrosis factor (TNF) alpha levels in induced sputum with bronchoalveolar lavage fluid in pulmonary sarcoidosis. Thorax 2000; 55:696–699.
137. Yee AM, Pochapin MB. Treatment of complicated sarcoidosis with infliximab anti-tumor necrosis factor-alpha therapy. Ann Intern Med 2001; 135:27–31.
138. Baughman RP, Lower EE. Infliximab for refractory sarcoidosis. Sarcoidosis Vasc Diffuse Lung Dis 2001; 18:70–74.
139. Alabi OF, Lower EE, Baughman RP. Use of infliximab in refractory sarcoidosis. Am J Respir Crit Care Med 2001; 163:A557.
140. Zabel P, Entzian P, Dalhoff K, Schlaak M. Pentoxifylline in treatment of sarcoidosis. Am J Respir Crit Care Med 1997; 155:1665–1669.
141. Lee JB, Koblenzer PS. Disfiguring cutaneous manifestation of sarcoidosis treated with thalidomide: a case report. J Am Acad Dermatol 1998; 39:835–838.
142. Carlesimo M, Giustini S, Rossi A, Bonaccorsi P, Calvieri S. Treatment of cutaneous and pulmonary sarcoidosis with thalidomide. J Am Acad Dermatol 1995; 32:866.

143. Moreira AL, Tsenova Berkova L, Wang J, et al. Effect of cytokine modulation by thalidomide on the granulomatous response in murine tuberculosis. Tuber Lung Dis 1997; 78:47–55.

144. Tavares JL, Wangoo A, Dilworth P, Marshall B, Kotecha S, Shaw RJ. Thalidomide reduces tumour necrosis factor-alpha production by human alveolar macrophages. Respir Med 1997; 91:31–39.

145. Moller DR, Wysocka M, Greenlee BM, Ma X, Wahl L, Flockhart DA. Inhibition of IL-12 production by thalidomide. J Immunol 1997; 159:5157–5161.

146. Moller DR, Forman JD, Liu MC, et al. Enhanced expression of IL-12 associated with Th 1 cytokine profiles in active pulmonary sarcoidosis. J Immunol 1996; 156:4952–4960.

147. Keane J, Gershon S, Wise RP, et al. Tuberculosis associated with infliximab, a tumor necrosis factor alpha-neutralizing agent. N Engl J Med 2001; 345:1098–1104.

148. Bean AG, Roach DR, Briscoe H, et al. Structural deficiencies in granuloma formation in TNF gene-targeted mice underlie the heightened susceptibility to aerosol *Mycobacterium tuberculosis* infection, which is not compensated for by lymphotoxin. J Immunol 1999; 162:3504–3511.

149. Ziesche R, Hofbauer E, Wittmann K, Petkov V, Block LH. A preliminary study of long-term treatment with interferon gamma-1b and low-dose prednisolone in patients with idiopathic pulmonary fibrosis (see comments). N Engl J Med 1999; 341:1264–1269.

150. Spiteri MA, Clarke SW. The nature of latent pulmonary involvement in primary biliary cirrhosis. Sarcoidosis 1989; 6:107–110.

151. Erkkila S, Froseth B, Hellstrom PE, et al. Inhaled budesonide influences cellular and biochemical abnormalities in pulmonary sarcoidosis. Sarcoidosis 1988; 5:106–110.

152. Alberts C, van der Mark TW, Jansen HM. Inhaled budesonide in pulmonary sarcoidosis: a double-blind, placebo-controlled study. Dutch Study Group on Pulmonary Sarcoidosis. Eur Respir J 1995; 8:682–688.

153. Zych D, Pawlicka L, Zielinski J. Inhaled budesonide vs prednisone in the maintenance treatment of pulmonary sarcoidosis. Sarcoidosis 1993; 10:56–61.

154. Pietinalho A, Tukiainen P, Haahtela T, Persson T, Selroos O, Group FPSS. Oral prednisolone followed by inhaled budesonide in newly diagnosed pulmonary sarcoidosis: a double-blind, placebo-controlled, multicenter study. Chest 1999; 116:424–431.

155. Milman N, Graudal N, Grode G, Munch E. No effect of high-dose inhaled steroids in pulmonary sarcoidosis: a double-blind, placebo-controlled study. J Intern Med 1994; 236:285–290.

156. Trulock EP, Cooper JD, Kaiser LR, Pasque MK, Ettinger NA, Dresler CM. The Washington University-Barnes Hospital experience with lung transplantation. Washington University Lung Transplantation Group (see comments). JAMA 1991; 266:1943.

157. Cooper JD, Pohl MS, Patterson GA. An update on the current status of lung transplantation: report of the St. Louis international lung transplant registry. In: Terasaki PI, Cecka JM, eds. Clinical Transplants 1993. Los Angeles: UCLA Tissue Type Laboratory, 1994:95–100.

158. Levine SM, Anzueto A, Peters JI, Calhoon JH, Jenkinson SG, Bryan CL. Single lung transplantation in patients with systemic disease. Chest 1994; 105:837.

159. Martinez FJ, Orens JB, Deeb M, Brunsting LA, Flint A, Lynch JP. Recurrence of sarcoidosis following bilateral allogeneic lung transplantation. Chest 1994; 106:1597–1599.

160. Padilla ML, Schilero GJ, Teirstein AS. Sarcoidosis and transplantation. Sarcoidosis 1997; 14:16–22.

161. Scott J, Higgenbottam T. Transplantation of the lungs and heart lung for patients with severe pulmonary complcations from sarcoidosis. Sarcoidosis 1990; 7:9–11.

162. Judson MA. Lung transplantation for pulmonary sarcoidosis. Eur Respir J 1998; 11:738–744.

163. Arcasoy SM, Christie JD, Pochettino A, et al. Characteristics and outcomes of patients with sarcoidosis listed for lung transplantation. Chest 2001; 120:873–880.

164. Barnard J, Newman LS. Sarcoidosis: immunology, rheumatic involvement, and therapeutics. Curr Opin Rheumatol 2001; 13:84–91.

165. Sullivan EJ. Lymphangioleiomyomatosis: a review. Chest 1998; 114:1689–1703.

166. Lie JT. Pulmonary tuberous sclerosis in tuberous sclerosis complex. In: Gomez MR, Sampson JR, Whittemore VH, eds: Tuberous Schlerosis. New York: Oxford University Press, 1999:207–217.

167. Dwyer JM, Hickie JB, Garvan J. Pulmonary tuberous sclerosis. Report of three patients and a review of the literature. QJ Med 1971; 40:115–125.

168. Aubry MC, Myers JL, Ryu JH, et al. Pulmonary lymphangioleiomyomatosis in a man. Am J Respir Crit Care Med 2000; 162:749–752.

169. Foundation L. LAM Foundation Database, 2000.

170. Urban T, Lazor R, Lacronique J, et al. Pulmonary lymphangioleiomyomatosis. A study of 69 patients. Groupe d'Etudes et de Recherche sur les Maladies "Orphelines" Pulmonaires (GERM"O"P). Medicine (Baltimore) 1999; 78:321–337.

171. Johnson S. Rare disease. 1. Lymphangioleiomyomatosis: clinical features, management and basic mechanisms. Thorax 1999; 54:254–264.

172. Moss J, Avila NA, Barnes PM, et al. Prevalence and clinical characteristics of lymphangioleiomyomatosis (LAM) in patients with tuberous sclerosis complex. Am J Respir Crit Care Med 2001; 164:669–671.

173. Franz DN, Brody A, Meyer C, et al. Mutational and radiographic analysis of pulmonary disease consistent with lymphangioleiomyomatosis and micronodular pneumocyte hyperplasia in women with tuberous sclerosis. Am J Respir Crit Care Med 2001; 164:661–668.

174. Costello LC, Hartman TE, Ryu JH. High frequency of pulmonary lymphangioleiomyomatosis in women with tuberous sclerosis complex. Mayo Clin Proc 2000; 75:591–594.

175. Oh YM, Mo EK, Jang SH, et al. Pulmonary lymphangioleiomyomatosis in Korea. Thorax 1999; 54:618–621.

176. Chu SC, Horiba K, Usuki J, et al. Comprehensive evaluation of 35 patients with lymphangioleiomyomatosis. Chest 1999; 115:1041–1052.

177. Kitaichi M, Nishimura K, Itoh H, Izumi T. Pulmonary lymphangioleiomyomatosis: a report of 46 patients including a clinicopathologic study of prognostic factors. Am J Respir Crit Care Med 1995; 151:527–533.

178. Taylor JR, Ryu J, Colby TV, Raffin TA. Lymphangioleiomyomatosis. Clinical course in 32 patients. N Engl J Med 1990; 323:1254–1260.

179. Avila NA, Bechtle J, Dwyer AJ, Ferrans VJ, Moss J. Lymphangioleiomyomatosis: CT of diurnal variation of lymphangioleiomyomas. Radiology 2001; 221:415–421.
180. Taveira-DaSilva AM, Hedin C, Stylianou MP, et al. Reversible airflow obstruction, proliferation of abnormal smooth muscle cells, and impairment of gas exchange as predictors of outcome in lymphangioleiomyomatosis. Am J Respir Crit Care Med 2001; 164:1072–1076.
181. Matsui K, Beasley MB, Nelson WK, et al. Prognostic significance of pulmonary lymphangioleiomyomatosis histologic score. Am J Surg Pathol 2001; 25:479–484.
182. Bonetti F, Chiodera P. Lymphangioleiomyomatosis and tuberous sclerosis: where is the border? Eur Respir J 1996; 9:399–401.
183. Lana R, Sanchez-Alarcos JM, Martinez-Cruz R, Calle M, Alvarez-Sala JL. Lymphangioleiomyomatosis and tuberous sclerosis: a casual association or a causative one? Arch Broncopneumol 1998; 34:463–465.
184. van Slegtenhorst M, de Hoogt R, Hermans C, et al. Identification of the tuberous sclerosis gene TSC1 on chromosome 9q34. Science 1997; 277:805–808.
185. Identification and characterization of the tuberous sclerosis gene on chromosome 16. The European Chromosome 16 Tuberous Sclerosis Consortium. Cell 1993; 75:1305–1315.
186. Povey S, Burley MW, Attwood J, et al. Two loci for tuberous sclerosis: one on 9q34 and one on 16p13. Ann Hum Genet 1994; 58:107–127.
187. Wienecke R, Konig A, DeClue JE. Identification of tuberin, the tuberous sclerosis-2 product. Tuberin possesses specific Rap1 GAP activity. J Biol Chem 1995; 270:16409–16414.
188. Xiao GH, Shoarinejad F, Jin F, Golemis EA, Yeung RS. The tuberous sclerosis 2 gene product, tuberin, functions as a Rab5 GTPase activating protein (GAP) in modulating endocytosis. J Biol Chem 1997; 272:6097–6100.
189. Henry KW, Yuan X, Koszewski NJ, Onda H, Kwiatkowski DJ, Noonan DJ. Tuberous sclerosis gene 2 product modulates transcription mediated by steroid hormone receptor family members. J Biol Chem 1998; 273:20535–20539.
190. Tsuchiya H, Orimoto K, Kobayashi K, Hino O. Presence of potent transcriptional activation domains in the predisposing tuberous sclerosis (Tsc2) gene product of the Eker rat model. Cancer Res 1996; 56:429–433.
191. Lamb RF, Roy C, Diefenbach TJ, et al. The TSC1 tumour suppressor hamartin regulates cell adhesion through ERM proteins and the GTPase Rho. Nat Cell Biol 2000; 2:281–287.
192. Dabora SL, Jozwiak S, Franz DN, et al. Mutational analysis in a cohort of 224 tuberous sclerosis patients indicates increased severity of TSC2, compared with TSC1, disease in multiple organs. Am J Hum Genet 2001; 68:64–80.
193. Cheadle JP, Reeve MP, Sampson JR, Kwiatkowski DJ. Molecular genetic advances in tuberous sclerosis. Hum Genet 2000; 107:97–114.
194. Jones AC, Shyamsundar MM, Thomas MW, et al. Comprehensive mutation analysis of TSC1 and TSC2-and phenotypic correlations in 150 families with tuberous sclerosis. Am J Hum Genet 1999; 64:1305–1315.
195. Smolarek TA, Wessner LL, McCormack FX, Mylet JC, Menon AG, Henske EP. Evidence that lymphangiomyomatosis is caused by TSC2 mutations: chromosome 16p 13 loss of heterozygosity in angiomyolipomas and lymph nodes from women with lymphangiomyomatosis. Am J Hum Genet 1998; 62:810–815.

196. Astrinidis A, Khare L, Carsillo T, et al. Mutational analysis of the tuberous sclerosis gene TSC2 in patients with pulmonary lymphangioleiomyomatosis. J Med Genet 2000; 37:55–57.
197. Carsillo T, Astrinidis A, Henske EP. Mutations in the tuberous sclerosis complex gene TSC2 are a cause of sporadic pulmonary lymphangioleiomyomatosis. Proc Natl Acad Sci USA 2000; 97:6085–6090.
198. Slingerland JM, Grossman RF, Chamberlain D, Tremblay CE. Pulmonary manifestations of tuberous sclerosis in first degree relatives. Thorax 1989; 44:212–214.
199. Carsillo T. Mutations in the TSC2 gene are a cause of sporadic lymphangioleiomyomatosis. Proc Natl Acad Sci USA 2000; 97(11):6085–6090.
200. Bittmann I, Dose TB, Muller C, Dienemann H, Vogelmeier C, Lohrs U. Lymphangioleiomyomatosis: recurrence after single lung transplantation. Hum Pathol 1997; 28:1420–1423.
201. Nine JS, Yousem SA, Paradis IL, Keenan R, Griffith BP. Lymphangioleiomyomatosis: recurrence after lung transplantation. J Heart Lung Trans 1994; 13:714–719.
202. O'Brien JD, Lium JH, Parosa JF, Deyoung BR, Wick MR, Trulock EP. Lymphangioleiomyomatosis recurrence in the allograft after single lung transplantation. Am J Respir Crit Care 1995; 151:2033–2036.
203. Bernstein SM, Newell JD Jr, Adamczyk D, Mortenson RL, King TE Jr, Lynch DA. How common are renal angiomyolipomas in patients with pulmonary lymphangiomyomatosis? Am J Respir Crit Care Med 1995; 152:2138–2143.
204. Avila NA, Chen CC, Chu SC, et al. Pulmonary lymphangioleiomyomatosis: correlation of ventilation-perfusion scintigraphy, chest radiography, and CT with pulmonary function tests. Radiology 2000; 214:441–446.
205. Nguyen-Vu PA, Fackler I, Rust A, et al. Loss of tuberin, the tuberous-sclerosis-complex-2 gene product is associated with angiogenesis. J Cutan Pathol 2001; 28:470–475.
206. Usuki J, Horiba K, Chu SC, Moss J, Ferrans VJ. Immunohistochemical analysis of proteins of the Bcl-2 family in pulmonary lymphangioleiomyomatosis: association of Bcl-2 expression with hormone receptor status. Arch Pathol Lab Med 1998; 122:895–902.
207. Hayashi T, Fleming MV, Stetler-Stevenson WG, et al. Immunohistochemical study of matrix metalloproteinases (MMPs) and their tissue inhibitors (TIMPs) in pulmonary lymphangioleiomyomatosis (LAM). Hum Pathol 1997; 28:1071–1078.
208. Castro M, Shepherd CW, Gomez MR, Lie JT, Ryu JH. Pulmonary tuberous sclerosis. Chest 1995; 107:189–195.
209. O'Callaghan FJ, Shiell AW, Osborne JP, Martyn CN. Prevalence of tuberous sclerosis estimated by capture-recapture analysis. Lancet 1998; 351:1490.
210. Castro M, Shepherd CW, Gomez MR, Lie JT, Ryu JH. Pulmonary tuberous sclerosis. Chest 1995; 107:189–195.
211. Shen A, Iseman MD, Waldron JA, King TE. Exacerbation of pulmonary lymphangioleiomyomatosis by exogenous estrogens. Chest 1987; 91:782–785.
212. Warren SE, Lee D, Martin V, Messink W. Pulmonary lymphangiomyomatosis causing bilateral pneumothorax during pregnancy. Ann Thorac Surg 1993; 55:998–1000.
213. Shuman RL, Engelman R, Kittle CF. Pulmonary lymphangiomyomatosis. Ann Thorac Surg 1979; 27:70–75.

214. Banner AS, Carrington CB, Emory WB, et al. Efficacy of oophorectomy in lymphangioleiomyomatosis and benign metastasizing leiomyoma. N Engl J Med 1981; 305:204–209.

215. Svendsen TL, Viskum K, Hansborg N, Thorpe SM, Nielsen NC. Pulmonary lymphangioleiomyomatosis: a case of progesterone receptor positive lymphangioleiomyomatosis treated with medroxyprogesterone, oophorectomy and tamoxifen. Br J Dis Chest 1984; 78:264–271.

216. Kitzsteiner KA, Mallen RG. Pulmonary lymphangiomyomatosis: treatment with castration. Cancer 1980; 46:2248–2249.

217. Taylor JR, Ryu J, Colby TV, Raffin TA. Lymphangioleiomyomatosis. Clinical course in 32 patients. N Engl J Med 1990; 323:1254–1260.

218. McCarty KS Jr, Mossler JA, McLelland R, Sieker HO. Pulmonary lymphangiomyomatosis responsive to progesterone. N Engl J Med 1980; 303:1461–1465.

219. Eliasson AH, Phillips YY, Tenholder MF. Treatment of lymphangioleiomyomatosis. A meta-analysis. Chest 1989; 96:1352–1355.

220. Johnson SR, Tattersfield AE. Decline in lung function in lymphangioleiomyomatosis. Relation to menopause and progesterone treatment. Am J Respir Crit Care Med 1999; 160:628–633.

221. Moss J, DeCastro R, Patronas NJ, Taveira-DaSilva A. Meningiomas in lymphangioleiomyomatosis. JAMA 2001; 286:1879–1881.

222. Desurmont S, Bauters C, Copin MC, Dewailly D, Tonnel AB, Wallaert B. Treatment of pulmonary lymphangioleiomyomatosis using a GnRH agonist (see comments). Rev Mal Respir 1996; 13:300–304.

223. Johnson SR, Tattersfield AE. Treatment and outcome of lymphangioleiomyomatosis in the UK. Am J Respir Crit Care Med 1997; 155:A327.

224. Bush JK, McLean RL, Sieker HO. Diffuse lung disease due to lymphangiomyoma. Am J Med 1969; 46:645–654.

225. Silverstein EF, Ellis K, Wolff M, Jaretzki AD. Pulmonary lymphangiomyomatosis. Am J Roentgenol Radium Ther Nucl Med 1974; 120:832–850.

226. Wellens F, Estenne M, de Francquen P, Goldstein J, Leclerc JL, Primo G. Combined heart-lung transplantation for terminal pulmonary lymphangioleiomyomatosis. J Thorac Cardiovasc Surg 1985; 89:872–876.

227. Estenne M, de Francquen P, Wellens F, et al. Combined heart-and-lung transplantation for lymphangioleiomyomatosis. Lancet 1984; 1:275.

228. Boehler A, Speich R, Russi EW, Weder W. Lung transplantation for lymphangioleiomyomatosis. N Engl J Med 1996; 335:1275–1280.

229. Flint A, Lynch JP III, Martinez FJ, Whyte RI. Pulmonary smooth muscle proliferation occurring after lung transplantation. Chest 1997; 112:283–284.

229a. Karbowniczek M, Astrindis A, Balsara BR, Testa JR, Lium JH, Colby TV, McCormack FX, Henske EP. Recurrent lymphangiomyomatosis after transplantation: genetic analyses reveal a metastatic mechanism. Am J Respir Crit Care Med 2002 Oct 31 (epub ahead of print) PMID: 12411287 (PubMed, as supplied by publisher).

230. Rimensberger PC, Muller-Schenker B, Kalangos A, Beghetti M. Treatment of a persistent postoperative chylothorax with somatostatin. Ann Thorac Surg 1998; 66:253–254.

231. Kelly RF, Shumway SJ. Conservative management of postoperative chylothorax using somatostatin. Ann Thorac Surg 2000; 69:1944–1945.

232. Demos NJ, Kozel J, Scerbo JE. Somatostatin in the treatment of chylothorax. Chest 2001; 119:964–966.

233. Calabrese PR, Frank HD, Taubin HL. Lymphangiomyomatosis with chylous ascites: treatment with dietary fat restriction and medium chain triglycerides. Cancer 1977; 40:895–897.

234. Yildizeli B, Yuksel M. Chylothorax and lymphangiomyomatosis. Ann Thorac Surg 2000; 69:1640.

235. Shapiro AM, Bain VG, Sigalet DL, Kneteman NM. Rapid resolution of chylous ascites after liver transplantation using somatostatin analog and total parenteral nutrition. Transplantation 1996; 61:1410–1411.

236. Ferrandiere M, Hazouard E, Guicheteau V, et al. Chylous ascites following radical nephrectomy: efficiency of octreotide as treatment of a ruptured thoracic duct. Intens Care Med 2000; 26:484–485.

237. Widjaja A, Gratz KF, Ockenga J, Wagner S, Manns MP. Octreotide for therapy of chylous ascites in yellow nail syndrome. Gastroenterology 1999; 116:1017–1018.

238. Borro JM, Morales P, Baamonde A. Tuberous sclerosis and pregnancy; report of a case with renal and pulmonary involvement. Eur J Obstet Gynecol Reprod Biol 1987; 26:169–173.

239. Brunelli A, Catalini G, Fianchini A. Pregnancy exacerbating unsuspected mediastinal lymphangioleiomyomatosis and chylothorax (letter). Int J Gynaecol Obstet 1996; 52:289–290.

240. Hughes E, Hodder RV. Pulmonary lymphangiomyomatosis complicating pregnancy. A case report. J Reprod Med 1987; 32:553–557.

241. Johnson SR, Tattersfield AE. Pregnancy in lymphangioleiomyomatosis. Am J Respir Crit Care Med 1998; 157:A807.

242. Murata A, Takeda Y, Usuki J, et al. A case of pulmonary lymphangiomyomatosis induced by pregnancy. Nihon Kyobu Shikkan Gakkai Zasshi 1989; 27:1106–1111.

243. Yockey CC, Riepe RE, Ryan K. Pulmonary lymphangioleiomyomatosis complicated by pregnancy. Kans Med 1986; 87:277–288,293.

244. Vassallo R, Ryu JH, Colby TV, Hartman T, Limper AH. Pulmonary Langerhans cell histiocytosis. N Engl J Med 2000; 342:1969–1978.

245. Tazi A, Soler P, Hance AJ. Adult pulmonary Langerhans cell histiocytosis. Thorax 2000; 55:405–416.

246. Favara BE, Feller AC, Pauli M, et al. Contemporary classification of histiocytic disorders. The WHO Committee On Histiocytic/Reticulum Cell Proliferations. Reclassification Working Group of the Histiocyte Society. Med Pediatr Oncol 1997; 29:157–166.

247. Basset F, Soler P, Hance AJ. The Langerhans cell in human pathology. Ann NY Acad Sci 1986; 465:324–339.

248. Mierau GW, Favara BE. S-100 protein immunohistochemistry and electron microscopy in the diagnosis of Langerhans cell proliferative disorders: a comparative assessment. Ultrastruct Pathol 1986; 10:303–309.

249. Emile JF, Wechsler J, Brousse N, et al. Langerhans' cell histiocytosis. Definitive diagnosis with the use of monoclonal antibody O10 on routinely paraffin-embedded samples. Am J Surg Pathol 1995; 19:636–641.

250. Tazi A, Bonay M, Bergeron A, Grandsaigne M, Hance AJ, Soler P. Role of granulocyte-macrophage colony stimulating factor (GM-CSF) in the pathogenesis of adult pulmonary histiocytosis X. Thorax 1996; 51:611–614.

251. Zeid NA, Muller HK. Tobacco smoke induced lung granulomas and tumors: association with pulmonary Langerhans cells. Pathology 1995; 27:247–254.

252. Yu RC, Chu C, Buluwela L, Chu AC. Clonal proliferation of Langerhans cells in Langerhans cell histiocytosis. Lancet 1994; 343:767–768.

253. Yousem SA, Colby TV, Chen YY, Chen WG, Weiss LM. Pulmonary Langerhans cell histiocytosis: molecular analysis of clonality. Am J Surg Pathol 2001; 25:630–636.

254. Bernstrand C, Cederlund K, Sandstedt B, et al. Pulmonary abnormalities at long-term follow-up of patients with Langerhans cell histiocytosis. Med Pediatr Oncol 2001; 36:459–468.

255. Bernstrand C, Cederlund K, Ashtrom L, Henter JI. Smoking preceded pulmonary involvement in adults with Langerhans cell histiocytosis diagnosed in childhood. Acta Paediatr 2000; 89:1389–1392.

256. Delobbe A, Durieu J, Duhamel A, Wallaert B. Determinants of survival in pulmonary Langerhans cell granulomatosis (histiocytosis X). Groupe d'Etude en Pathologie Interstitielle de la Societe de Pathologie Thoracique du Nord. Eur Respir J 1996; 9:2002–2006.

257. Crausman RS, Jennings CA, Tuder RM, Ackerson LM, Irvin CG, King TE Jr. Pulmonary histiocytosis X: pulmonary function and exercise pathophysiology. Am J Respir Crit Care Med 1996; 153:426–435.

258. Friedman PJ, Liebow AA, Sokoloff J. Eosinophilic granuloma of lung. Clinical aspects of primary histiocytosis in the adult. Medicine (Baltimore) 1981; 60:385–396.

259. Hirsch MS, Hong CK. Familial pulmonary histiocytosis X. Am Rev Respir Dis 1973; 107:831–835.

260. Howarth DM, Gilchrist GS, Mullan BP, Wiseman GA, Edmonson JH, Schomberg PJ. Langerhans cell histiocytosis: diagnosis, natural history, management, and outcome. Cancer 1999; 85:2278–2290.

261. Hance AJ, Basset F, Saumon G, et al. Smoking and interstitial lung disease. The effect of cigarette smoking on the incidence of pulmonary histiocytosis X and sarcoidosis. Ann NY Acad Sci 1986; 465:643–656.

262. Schonfeld N, Frank W, Wenig S, et al. Clinical and radiologic features, lung function and therapeutic results in pulmonary histiocytosis X. Respiration 1993; 60:38–44.

263. Collins J. CT signs and patterns of lung disease. Radiol Clin North Am 2001; 39:1115–1135.

264. Keyzer C, Bankier AA, Remmelinck M, Gevenois PA. Pulmonary lymphangiomyomatosis mimicking Langerhans cell histiocytosis. J Thorac Imaging 2001; 16:185–187.

265. Costabel U, Guzman J. Bronchoalveolar lavage in interstitial lung disease. Curr Opin Pulm Med 2001; 7:255–261.

266. Chollet S, Soler P, Dournovo P, Richard MS, Ferrans VJ, Basset F. Diagnosis of pulmonary histiocytosis X by immunodetection of Langerhans cells in bronchoalveolar lavage fluid. Am J Pathol 1984; 115:225–232.

267. Soler P, Chollet S, Jacque C, Fukuda Y, Ferrans VJ, Basset F. Immunocyto-chemical characterization of pulmonary histiocytosis X cells in lung biopsies. Am J Pathol 1985; 118:439–451.

268. Housini I, Tomashefski JF Jr, Cohen A, Crass J, Kleinerman J. Transbronchial biopsy in patients with pulmonary eosinophilic granuloma. Comparison with findings on open lung biopsy. Arch Pathol Lab Med 1994; 118:523–530.

269. Ha SY, Helms P, Fletcher M, Broadbent V, Pritchard J. Lung involvement in Langerhans cell histiocytosis: prevalence, clinical features, and outcome. Pediatrics 1992; 89:466–469.

270. King TE Jr. Restrictive lung disease in pregnancy. Clin Chest Med 1992; 13:607–622.

271. DiMaggio LA, Lippes HA, Lee RV. Histiocytosis X and pregnancy. Obstet Gynecol 1995; 85:806–809.

272. Lombard CM, Medeiros LJ, Colby TV. Pulmonary histiocytosis X and carcinoma. Arch Pathol Lab Med 1987; 111:339–341.

273. Sadoun D, Vaylet F, Valeyre D, et al. Bronchogenic carcinoma in patients with pulmonary histiocytosis X. Chest 1992; 101:1610–1613.

274. Egeler RM, Neglia JP, Puccetti DM, Brennan CA, Nesbit ME. Association of Langerhans cell histiocytosis with malignant neoplasms. Cancer 1993; 71:865–873.

275. Neumann MP, Frizzera G. The coexistance of Langerhans cell granulomatosis and malignant lymphoma may take different forms: report of seven cases with a review of the literature. Hum Pathol 1986; 17:1060–1065.

276. Egeler RM, Neglia JP, Arico M, et al. The relation of Langerhans cell histiocytosis to acute leukemia, lymphomas, and other solid tumors. The LCH-Malignancy Study Group of the Histiocyte Society. Hematol Oncol Clin North Am 1998; 12:369–378.

277. Egeler RM, Neglia JP, Arico M, Favara BE, Heitger A, Nesbit ME. Acute leukemia in association with Langerhans cell histiocytosis. Med Pediatr Oncol 1994; 23:81–85.

278. Etienne B, Bertocchi M, Gamondes JP, et al. Relapsing pulmonary Langerhans cell histiocytosis after lung transplantation. Am J Respir Crit Care Med 1998; 157:288–291.

279. Gabbay E, Dark JH, Ashcroft T, et al. Recurrence of Langerhans cell granulomatosis following lung transplantation. Thorax 1998; 53:326–327.

280. Habib SB, Congleton J, Carr D, et al. Recurrence of recipient Langerhans' cell histiocytosis following bilateral lung transplantation. Thorax 1998; 53:323–325.

281. Igarashi T, Nakagawa A, Nishino M, et al. Improvement of pulmonary eosinophilic granuloma after smoking cessation in two patients. Nihon Kyobu Shikkan Gakkai Zasshi 1995; 33:1125–1129.

282. Morimoto T, Matsumura T, Kitaichi M. Rapid remission of pulmonary eosinophilic granuloma in a young male patient after cessation of smoking. Nihon Kokyuki Gakkai Zasshi 1999; 37:140–145.

283. Yamakami Y, Mieno T, Tashiro T, Moriuchi A, Nasu M. A case of pulmonary lymphangiomyomatosis diagnosed by biopsy of retroperitoneal tumor and treated with hormonal therapy. Nihon Kyobu Shikkan Gakkai Zasshi 1994; 32:261–265.

284. Benyounes B, Crestani B, Couvelard A, Vissuzaine C, Aubier M. Steroid-responsive pulmonary hypertension in a patient with Langerhans' cell granulomatosis (histiocytosis X). Chest 1996; 110:284–286.

285. Yokota S, Tada S, Sugimoto K, et al. A case of pulmonary eosinophilic granuloma with extrapulmonary involvement treated effectively with steroid hormone. Nihon Kyobu Shikkan Gakkai Zasshi 1994; 32:78–83.

286. Giona F, Caruso R, Testi AM, et al. Langerhans' cell histiocytosis in adults: a clinical and therapeutic analysis of 11 patients from a single institution. Cancer 1997; 80:1786–1791.

287. Saven A, Burian C. Cladribine activity in adult Langerhans-cell histiocytosis. Blood 1999; 93:4125–4130.

288. Arzoo K, Sadeghi S, Pullarkat V. Pamidronate for bone pain from osteolytic lesions in Langerhans-cell histiocytosis. N Engl J Med 2001; 345:225.

289. Farran RP, Zaretski E, Egeler RM. Treatment of Langerhans cell histiocytosis with pamidronate. J Pediatr Hematol Oncol 2001; 23:54–56.

290. Brown RE. Bisphosphonates as antialveolar macrophage therapy in pulmonary Langerhans cell histiocytosis? Med Pediatr Oncol 2001; 36:641–643.

11

Medical Management of Pulmonary Vascular Disease

ALLISON C. WIDLITZ and ROBYN J. BARST

Columbia University College of Physicians and Surgeons
New York, New York, U.S.A.

I. Introduction

Pulmonary vascular disease can be classified in many different ways. This variability and diagnostic classification has been problematic. In 1998, at the Primary Pulmonary Hypertension World Symposium, clinical scientists from around the world proposed a new diagnostic classification system (Table 1). It categorizes pulmonary vascular disease by common clinical features reflecting the recent advances in the understanding of pulmonary hypertensive diseases and the similarity between primary pulmonary hypertension and pulmonary arterial hypertension associated with conditions such as collagen vascular diseases, congenital systemic to pulmonary shunts, portal hypertension, HIV infection, and drugs and toxins. The classification separates those cases of pulmonary arterial hypertension from pulmonary venous hypertension and pulmonary hypertension associated with disorders of the respiratory system, pulmonary hypertension due to chronic thrombotic and/or embolic disease, and pulmonary hypertension due to disorders directly affecting the pulmonary vasculature. This diagnostic classification supports the use of many of the therapeutic modalities that have been demonstrated to be efficacious for primary pulmonary hypertension in patients who have pulmonary arterial hypertension associated with these other conditions.

Pulmonary hypertension is defined as a mean pulmonary artery pressure greater than 25 mmHg at rest or greater than 30 mmHg during exercise.

Table 1 Diagnostic Classification of Pulmonary Hypertension

A. *Pulmonary arterial hypertension*
  1. Primary pulmonary hypertension
    a. Sporadic
    b. Familial
  2. Related to
    a. Collagen vascular disease
    b. Congenital systemic to pulmonary shunts
    c. Portal hypertension
    d. HIV infection
    e. Drugs/toxins
      (1) Anorexigens
      (2) Other
    f. Persistent pulmonary hypertension of the newborn
    g. Other

B. *Pulmonary venous hypertension*
  1. Left-sided atrial or ventricular heart disease
  2. Left-sided valvular heart disease
  3. Extrinsic compression of central pulmonary vein
    a. Fibrosing mediastinitis
    b. Adenopathy/tumors
  4. Pulmonary veno-occlusive disease
  5. Other

C. *Pulmonary hypertension associated with disorders of the respiratory system and/or hypoxia*
  1. Chronic obstructive pulmonary disease
  2. Interstitial lung disease
  3. Sleep-disordered breathing
  4. Alveolar hypoventilation disorders
  5. Chronic exposure to high altitudes
  6. Neonatal lung disease
  7. Alveolar-capillary dysplasia
  8. Other

D. *Pulmonary hypertension due to chronic thrombotic and/or embolic disease*
  1. Thromboembolic obstruction of proximal pulmonary arteries
  2. Obstruction of distal pulmonary arteries
    a. Pulmonary embolism (thrombus, ova and/or parasites, foreign material)
    b. In situ thrombosis
    c. Sickle cell disease

E. *Pulmonary hypertension due to disorders affecting the pulmonary vasculature*
  1. Inflammatory
    a. Schistosomiasis
    b. Sarcoidosis
    c. Other
  2. Pulmonary capillary hemangiomatosis

Whether the pulmonary hypertension is due to increased flow or resistance (Table 2) depends on its cause (Table 3). Pulmonary artery wedge pressure will be normal in the absence of left heart obstruction or dysfunction causing pulmonary venous hypertension. To diagnose primary pulmonary hypertension, one must exclude all secondary causes as well as associated disorders (Table 1) and demonstrate a normal pulmonary artery wedge pressure.

Although there is no cure for pulmonary hypertension, recent advances in therapeutic interventions have resulted in significantly improved hemodynamics, quality of life, and survival since the first case of primary pulmonary hypertension was reported over a century ago (1). The therapeutic approach that has evolved over the past two decades for primary pulmonary hypertension is also now being used for the treatment of pulmonary arterial hypertension associated with systemic-to-pulmonary shunts, connective tissue diseases, and other conditions related to pulmonary arterial hypertension, as listed in Table 1. The overall goal of treatment is to increase survival and improve quality of life. The treatment of patients with pulmonary arterial hypertension depends upon an accurate assessment of its cause(s) (Table 1). When an underlying cause is identified, therapy should first be directed at the cause with additional therapy as needed for residual pulmonary hypertension. Underlying diseases associated with pulmonary hypertension complicates the medical management decision making. For example, there is a subset of patients with chronic obstructive pulmonary disease (COPD) and pulmonary hypertension. Although there are no data to support this, we currently believe that if the pulmonary hypertension is out of proportion to the COPD, these patients should be treated with therapy similar to that for primary pulmonary hypertension. Conversely, if there is mild pulmonary hypertension with COPD, the treatment should be directed at the COPD and not the pulmonary hypertension.

II. General Measures

Once a diagnosis of pulmonary arterial hypertension has been confirmed, it is important to counsel the patient regarding physical activity. Patients should

Table 2 Classification of Pulmonary Hypertension

Type	Classification
Hyperkinetic	$P = R \times F$
Pulmonary vascular obstruction or pulmonary venous hypertension	$P = R \times F$

Key: P, pulmonary artery pressure; R, pulmonary vascular resistance; F, pulmonary blood flow.

Table 3 Causes of Pulmonary Hypertension

Type	Causes
Reversible	
Hyperkinetic	VSD or PDA
Pulmonary venous hypertension	Mitral stenosis, pulmonary venous obstruction, or left ventricular failure
Irreversible	
Pulmonary vascular obstruction	Primary pulmonary hypertension
	Eisenmenger's syndrome

Key: VSD, ventricular septal defect; PDA, patent ductus arteriosus.

engage in activities to the extent of their physical capabilities. Physical activity can be associated with marked increases in pulmonary artery pressure (2). Patients should avoid performing isometric exercises and physical activities that produce chest pain, presyncope, or syncope.

Respiratory tract infections cause significant problems for patients with pulmonary hypertension. These infections result in ventilation/perfusion mismatching and subsequent alveolar hypoxia, which can produce a catastrophic event if not aggressively treated. Fever higher than 101°F should be treated with antipyretics to minimize the consequences of increased metabolic demands. Decongestants and other alpha-acting drugs should be avoided due to cardiovascular effects. Annual influenza vaccination and regular pneumococcal vaccination is recommended as a preventive measure unless there are specific contraindications.

Nonsteroidal anti-inflammatory agents during pregnancy should be used with caution, since their maternal use has been implicated in the pathogenesis of pulmonary hypertension of the newborn (3). Appetite suppressants should not be used, since they are known to cause pulmonary arterial hypertension (4). Pregnancy and parturition produce dramatic hemodynamic and hormonal changes that are poorly tolerated by patients with pulmonary hypertension. Abrupt deterioration and death can occur, particularly during the postpartum period (5–7). Due to this experience, pregnancy is contraindicated for patients with pulmonary arterial hypertension. Oral contraceptive agents that contain estrogen should be avoided, if possible, due to the increased risk of thromboembolic events, which could potentially aggravate pulmonary hypertension (8,9). Exposure to high altitude can worsen pulmonary hypertension by producing hypoxic-induced pulmonary vasoconstriction due to alveolar hypoxia. Although airplane travel in a pressurized cabin should be safe, supplemental oxygen therapy may be advisable. Phlebotomy is helpful with cyanotic congenital heart disease, in which severe hypoxemia has produced symptomatic polycythemia. Caution is advised in order to avoid depletion of iron stores and reduction of the circulating blood volume. Diet or medical therapy, if needed, should be used to prevent constipation so as to avoid the effects of the Valsalva maneuver on the venous return to the right side of the heart, which can precipitate syncope.

III. Anticoagulation

Patients with severe pulmonary hypertension are at risk for a thrombotic event due to their sedentary lifestyle, venous insufficiency, dilated right heart chambers, and sluggish pulmonary blood flow. Even a small pulmonary vascular obstruction by thrombus can be life-threatening in patients with compromised pulmonary vascular beds that have little ability to dilate or recruit unused vessels. Patients with pulmonary hypertension frequently die suddenly; not uncommonly, fresh intrapulmonary clots are found on postmortem examination. In primary pulmonary hypertension, chronic anticoagulation has been demonstrated to increase survival rates in adults (10,11). Efficacy of anticoagulation has not been demonstrated in children (12). The usefulness of anticoagulation in patients with Eisenmenger's syndrome has not been studied, but because the pulmonary vascular lesions are the same as in primary pulmonary hypertension, the rationale exists for consideration of low-dose anticoagulation in patients with Eisenmenger's syndrome as well. Warfarin has been the anticoagulant of choice, which was shown in previous studies to improve survival. The optimal dose of warfarin in these studies was not determined although the range of anticoagulation recommended is to achieve an international normalized ratio (INR) of 1.5 to 2.0. However, different clinical circumstances (e.g., documentation of a procoagulant state or chronic thromboembolic disease) may require dose adjustment to maintain a higher INR as clinically indicated. For patients at risk for bleeding (e.g., portal pulmonary hypertension with varices, or calcinosis, Raynaud's phenomenon, esophageal dysmotility, sclerodactyly, teleangectasia (CREST) patients with esophageal dysmotility dose adjustment) may be needed to maintain a lower INR to avoid bleeding. Heparin administered subcutaneously in doses of 5000 to 10,000 U twice daily may be a suitable alternative, although the long-term side effects of heparin, such as osteopenia and thrombocytopenia, can be troublesome. Intravenous heparin use for patients when needed should be used to maintain a PTT of 1.3 to 1.5 times the control. Additionally, low-molecular-weight heparin (Lovenox) in doses of 40 mg subcutaneously once or twice daily is another suitable alternative for adequate anticoagulation. What optimal anticoagulant should be used remains unclear and requires further investigation.

IV. Oxygen

Ventilation/perfusion mismatching occurs in many patients with pulmonary arterial hypertension. This results in hypoxic and hypercapneic pulmonary vasoconstriction, further exacerbating the underlying pulmonary arterial hypertension. Supplemental low-flow oxygen alleviates the arterial hypoxemia and attenuates the pulmonary hypertension in patients with chronic pulmonary parenchymal disease. If patients have significant mixed venous oxygen desaturation with activity caused by increased oxygen extraction in the face of a fixed oxygen delivery, they may benefit from ambulatory supplemental oxygen. Some patients also desaturate with sleep without evidence of obstructive apnea and may benefit from oxygen with sleep. The use of supplemental oxygen with sleep to slow the progression of polycythemia in patients with pulmonary arterial hypertension associated with congenital systemic-to-pulmonary shunts has been suggested (13). Patients with severe right heart failure with hypoxemia at rest resulting from a markedly increased oxygen extraction should be treated with continuous oxygen therapy.

V. Cardiac Glycosides and Diuretics

The efficacy of cardiac glycosides and diuretics in patients with pulmonary arterial hypertension is unknown. Since the cause of death in many patients with pulmonary hypertension is right heart failure, drugs that will improve right ventricular performance are often used, although there are no data to support this practice. The use of digitalis concomitantly with calcium channel blockers may counteract the potentially negative inotropic effects of calcium channel blockers (10). Specific care should be taken to avoid digitalis toxicity, which can be exacerbated with hypoxemia and/or diuretic-induced hypokalemia. Diuretics are useful for reducing the increased intravascular volume and hepatic congestion seen in patients with right heart failure. However, excessive diuresis should be avoided, as patients with a right ventricle that is preload-dependent are at risk for a fall in cardiac output with excessive diuresis. Aggressive monitoring of serum electrolytes is needed to avoid the risks of digitalis toxicity, hypokalemia, and hypomagnesemia.

VI. Vasodilators

The original use of vasodilator agents to treat patients with pulmonary arterial hypertension was initially based on the premise that pulmonary vasoconstriction is present to varying degrees and that even small reductions in right ventricular afterload produce substantial improvement in right ventricular output. This concept is supported by pathological studies demonstrating medial hypertrophy of the muscular pulmonary arteries as an early consistent feature of pulmonary arterial hypertension (14). Wagenvoort and Wagenvoort's early hypothesis that vasoconstriction precedes and contributes to a fixed obstruction (15) initially focused vasodilator therapy on patients with a large vasoconstrictive component, and the failure of acute pulmonary vasodilation was compatible with the concept of a "fixed" irreversible pulmonary vascular bed. The goal of treatment with vasodilators is to reduce pulmonary artery pressure and increase cardiac output without producing symptomatic systemic hypotension. This effect may be achievable with oral calcium channel blockers in approximately 20% of adults (10) and 40% of children (12) with primary pulmonary hypertension.

Acute vasodilator testing is performed during a right-heart catheterization as part of an initial assessment of patients with pulmonary arterial hypertension to determine whether patients fit into the category of "responder" versus "nonresponder" (Fig. 1). A response to acute vasodilator testing is defined as a fall in mean pulmonary artery pressure by $\geq 20\%$ with no change or an acute increase in cardiac output (using nitric oxide, intravenous prostacyclin, or intravenous adenosine). The "responders" represent a group of patients with a more vasoreactive pulmonary arterial bed, perhaps representing a different subset of patients with pulmonary arterial hypertension than "nonresponders" and/or representing patients diagnosed and evaluated earlier in the course of the disease when reversal of muscular hypertrophy occurs. "Nonresponders" may represent those with advanced disease and histopathological changes of intimal proliferation and fibrosis as well as plexiform lesions, which may undergo pulmonary vascular remodeling with long-term prostacyclin treatment.

VII. Calcium Channel Blockers

Calcium channel blockers inhibit calcium influx through the slow channel into cardiac and smooth muscle cells. Their usefulness in primary pulmonary

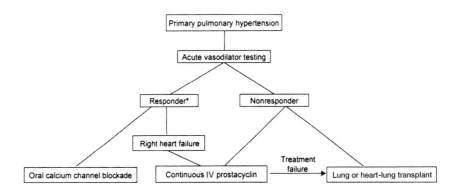

Figure 1 Treatment algorithm of primary pulmonary hypertension prior to the availability of prostacyclin analogs, endothelin receptor antagonists, inhaled nitric oxide as well as other novel therapeutic agents under clinical investigation. (*Responder to testing with inhaled NO or IV. Prostacyclin defined as a fall in the mean pulmonary arterial pressure of $\geq 20\%$ without a fall in the cardiac output.)

hypertension is believed to be based on their ability to cause vasodilation of the pulmonary vascular smooth muscle. Chronic calcium channel blockade is efficacious for patients who demonstrate a response to acute vasodilator testing. In contrast, patients who do not respond acutely fail to respond to long-term calcium channel blockade (10,15) and are unlikely to benefit from chronic therapy. Calcium channel blockers reduce pulmonary artery pressure, increase cardiac output and survival, and improve symptoms and exercise tolerance in responders. Although most studies have used calcium channel blockers at relatively high doses, the optimal dosing for patients with pulmonary arterial hypertension remains unknown. Because of the frequent reporting of significant adverse effects with calcium channel blockade in these patients (e.g., systemic hypotension, right ventricular failure, and death), calcium channel blockers should not be used in patients in whom acute effectiveness has not been demonstrated.

VIII. Prostaglandins

The use of prostacyclin or a prostacyclin analog for the treatment of pulmonary arterial hypertension is supported by a demonstration of an imbalance of thromboxane to prostacyclin metabolites in patients with primary pulmonary hypertension and demonstration of a reduction in prostacyclin synthase in the pulmonary arteries of patients with pulmonary arterial hypertension (16). Nonresponders to acute vasodilator testing are often treated with other vasoactive agents, including chronic intravenous epoprostenol, which surprisingly has resulted in what looks like remodeling of the pulmonary vascular bed (17–22), most likely due to other effects of prostacyclin rather than its vasodilator effects (i.e., antiproliferative effects). This has translated to improved hemodynamics, quality of life, and survival in patients with primary pulmonary hypertension (Fig. 2). Chronic therapy with prostacyclin analogs (e.g., aerosolized iloprost, subcutaneously administered treprostinil, or oral beraprost) will hopefully further our understanding of prostacyclin's mechanisms of action in addition to its vasodilator and antiaggretory properties.

Chronic intravenous epoprostenol has been evaluated in prospective randomized clinical trials of primary pulmonary hypertension and demonstrated improved exercise tolerance, hemodynamics, and survival in patients who were New York Heart Association (NYHA) functional class III or IV (17–19). Chronic intravenous prostacyclin was also studied in patients with pulmonary arterial hypertension associated with the scleroderma spectrum of diseases and demonstrated an improvement in exercise tolerance and hemodynamics in patients who were functional class III or IV (22). The mechanisms of action of the chronic effects of epoprostenol are very likely to be multifactorial, including lowering of the pulmonary artery pressure, increasing cardiac output, and increasing systemic oxygen transport. The

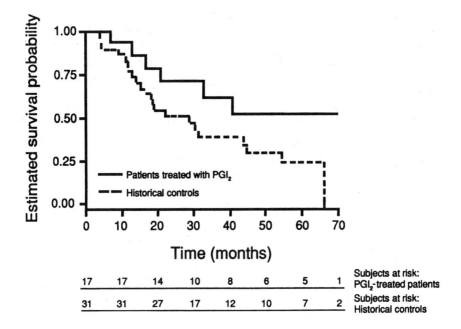

Figure 2 Comparison of survival probabilities between patients treated with prostacyclin and historical controls. Kaplan-Meier observed survival probability curves for New York Heart Association class III and IV patients treated with prostacyclin ($n = 17$) and historical controls from the National Institutes of Health Registry (NYHA class III and IV patients receiving standard therapy including anticoagulant agents, $n = 31$). Survival function was calculated at 6-month intervals for 5 years. Survival was significantly improved in the patients treated with prostacyclin ($p = 0.045$). The 1-, 2-, and 3-year predicted survival rates estimated by the NIH Primary Pulmonary Hypertension Registry equation for the patients treated with prostacyclin were 63.2, 50.4, and 41.1%, respectively; for the historical controls, the predicted survival rates were 65.2, 52.1, an 42.4%, respectively. (From Ref. 18.)

optimal dose of intravenous epoprostenol for pulmonary arterial hypertension remains uncertain. The starting dose is 1 to 2 ng/kg/min with incremental increases, especially during the first several months of initiation. The development of tolerance to the effects of intravenous epoprostenol remains unknown; some patients appear to need periodic dose escalation. A mean dose after 1 year is approximately 20 to 40 ng/kg/min for most patients, although there seems to be significant patient variability of the "optimal" dose (23). Continuous intravenous epoprostenol has also been used to treat patients with pulmonary arterial hypertension associated with congenital systemic-to-pulmonary shunts, portal hypertension, HIV, drugs, toxins and anorexigens, with reported improvement in exercise capacity and hemodynamics, although a survival benefit has not been demonstrated. Because epoprostenol is chemically unstable at neutral pH/room temperature and due to its short half-life (1–2 min), it requires a continuous intravenous system for chronic treatment. Permanent central venous access is required to administer the medication. The delivery system for continuous intravenous epoprostenol is associated with risks, including local infection, sepsis, abrupt drug interruption and line injury, or dislodgment as well as side effects from the drug itself, which include nausea, diarrhea, headache, arthralgias, and facial flushing. The side effects influence the overall risk/benefit of the therapy and have prompted clinical trials using alternative delivery systems that may enhance efficacy, improve safety, and reduce side effects. Clinical trials with the prostacyclin analog treprostinil (administered subcutaneously) have demonstrated improved exercise capacity, hemodynamics, and quality of life. In addition, clinical trials are also evaluating the efficacy of two additional prostacyclin analogs: iloprost (by inhalation) and beraprost (with oral administration). The use of prostacyclin analogs in less severely ill patients will be desirable, as they require less complex delivery systems compared with chronic intravenous epoprostenol.

Treprostinil (Remodulin) is a chemically stable tricyclic benzindene analog of prostacyclin, which also shares the same pharmacological actions as epoprostenol. It is chemically stable at room temperature and has a neutral pH and a half-life of 3 to 4 hr when administered subcutaneously (24). In a randomized trial, subcutaneous treprostinil improved exercise capacity, hemodynamics, and clinical signs and symptoms in patients with primary pulmonary hypertension and pulmonary hypertension associated with connective tissue diseases or congenital heart defects (25,26). Treprostinil (administered subcutaneously) was approved in 2001 by the Food and Drug Administration for the treatment of pulmonary arterial hypertension. Like epoprostenol, subcutaneous treprostinil is started at 1 ng/kg/min and slowly increased to achieve an "optimal dose." Side effects are pain, erythema, and induration at the injection site as well as other prostacyclin-like side effects (e.g., nausea, diarrhea, headache, and flushing).

Iloprost, a more stable synthetic analog of prostacyclin (in open-label uncontrolled trials), has been shown to improve hemodynamics and exercise capacity when administered short- and long-term (27,28). It has a molecular structure similar to that of prostacyclin and works through prostacyclin receptors present in vascular endothelial cells. Iloprost is also more stable than prostacyclin and may be stored at room temperature without any protection from light. It has a half-life of 20 to 30 min (29). Iloprost is used outside of the United States and has not been approved by the Food and Drug Administration (FDA) at the time of this publication. Intravenous iloprost has also been used acutely and chronically in patients with pulmonary arterial hypertension. Although further controlled studies are warranted to compare its efficacy to that of epoprostenol, intravenous iloprost has the benefit of being stable at room temperature and being more affordable than epoprostenol.

Beraprost sodium is an oral prostacyclin analog. It is a chemically stable and orally active prostaglandin I_2 derivative with a substantially longer half-life ($t_{1/2}$: 1.11 $\pm$ 1 hr). The drug has properties similar to those of epoprostenol and increases red blood cell flexibility; it decreases blood viscosity and limits platelet aggregation, produces vasodilatation, and decreases platelet adhesion to the endothelium as well as disaggregating platelets that have already clumped. Its potency is approximately 50% of epoprostenol. Preliminary data from Japan (open-label uncontrolled) suggests that Beraprost, is efficacious, improving hemodynamics and survival in patients with primary pulmonary hypertension (30,31). It has also been suggested to improve hemodynamics and NYHA functional class in patients with primary and secondary pulmonary hypertension (32). Currently, the first multicenter randomized study to evaluate the effects of Beraprost when compared with placebo on disease progression in patients with pulmonary arterial hypertension is under away. Results are anticipated in 2003. Beraprost is used outside of the United States and has not been approved by the Food and Drug Administration at the time of this publication.

IX. Endothelin Receptor Antagonists

Endothelin-1 is the most potent vasoconstrictor identified to date. It has been implicated in the pathogenesis of pulmonary arterial hypertension, providing the rationale for endothelin receptor antagonists as promising drugs for the treatment of pulmonary arterial hypertension (33) (Fig. 3). Plasma ET-1 levels are known to be increased in patients with pulmonary arterial hypertension and inversely correlate with prognosis (34,35). There are at least two different receptor subtypes. ET_A receptors are localized on smooth muscle cells and mediate vasoconstriction and proliferation, while ET_B receptors are found predominantly on endothelial cells and are associated with (1) endothelin-dependent vasorelaxation by the release of vasodilators—i.e., prostacyclin and nitric oxide; (2) clearance of endothelin; and (3) vasoconstriction on smooth muscle cells as well as bronchoconstriction. Both ET_A and ET_B receptors play a fundamental role in pulmonary vasoconstriction, inflammation, proliferation of smooth muscle cells, and fibrosis. In addition, because ET_B receptors may be upregulated on smooth muscle cells in certain pathological conditions as well as "cross talk" occurring between ET_A and ET_B receptors. Whether a dual ET receptor antagonist or a selective ET_A receptor antagonist will prove more efficacious remains to be determined (36,37). The dual oral receptor endothelin antagonist bosentan was approved for the treatment of pulmonary arterial hypertension by the FDA in 2001. The target dose of bosentan is 125 mg bid after being started at 62.5 mg bid for 4 weeks. Randomized clinical trials demonstrated improved exercise capacity measured by the 6-min walk test and improved hemodynamics (35). Adverse events associated with endothelin receptor antagonists include increased levels on liver function enzyme studies,

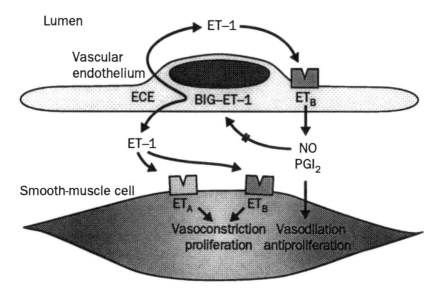

Figure 3 Endothelin system in vascular tissue. ET-1, endothelin-1; BIG-ET-1, proendothelin-1; ECE, endothelin-converting enzyme; NO, nitric oxide; PGl$_2$, prostacyclin.

which may require a decrease in dose or discontinuation of therapy. At the time of publication, bosentan is the only FDA-approved endothelin receptor antagonist. Clinical investigation is also under way to evaluate whether a selective ET$_A$ receptor antagonist such as sitaxsentan will be more efficacious than a dual endothelin receptor antagonist.

X. Nitric Oxide

Nitric oxide activates guanylate cyclase in pulmonary vascular smooth muscle cells, which increases cyclic GMP and decreases intracellular calcium concentration, thereby leading to smooth muscle relaxation (Fig. 4). When inhaled, the rapid combination of nitric oxide with hemoglobin inactivates any nitric oxide diffusing into the blood, preventing systemic vasodilatation. Nitric oxide is therefore a potent and selective pulmonary vasodilator when administered by inhalation. The usefulness of inhaled nitric oxide as well as possible other agents that may increase endogenous levels of nitric oxide (38) may also prove to be beneficial for their antiproliferative effects as well as their vasodilator effects. Although there is considerable experience with the use of inhaled nitric oxide as a short-term treatment for pulmonary hypertension in a variety of clinical situations, the role of inhaled nitric oxide as a chronic therapy for pulmonary hypertension remains under clinical investigation.

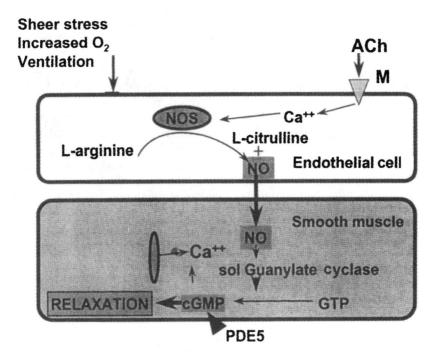

Figure 4 The nitric oxide pathway.

Furthermore, histological studies demonstrating reduced levels of nitric oxide synthase in the pulmonary vasculature of patients with primary pulmonary hypertension provides rationale and justification for the development of gene replacement therapy.

XI. The Future

At present, treatment for pulmonary vascular disease remains challenging, as the exact etiology of the disease is often unknown. If one views pulmonary vascular disease as a multifactorial condition with various mechanisms involved in its pathobiology, the role for distinct agents (i.e., prostacyclin analogues and endothelin receptor antagonists) can be perceived. At the present time, while chronic intravenous epoprostenol remains the "gold standard" of treatment for patients who do not respond to acute vasodilator testing or who are unresponsive to conventional agents, chronic intravenous epoprostenol is invasive and not without risk due to its delivery system. The recent attempt to compound this medication for delivery by oral, subcutaneous, and inhaled routes is a step in the right direction. However, at the present time, it is too early to say if these agents will be as efficacious as chronic intravenous epoprostenol. In addition, the use of endothelin receptor antagonists also appears to be extremely promising. There will likely be many new developments in the next several years as trials with these novel therapeutic agents are completed. Whether these newer agents will, in fact, replace chronic intravenous epoprostenol in selected patients remains unknown. Based on distinct mechanisms of action of these various agents, a role for combination therapy may further improve the efficacy of a patient's pulmonary arterial hypertension regimen—e.g., combining endothelin receptor antagonists with either intravenous epoprostenol or with a prostacyclin analog. Furthermore, future investigations with other agents—such as inhaled nitric oxide, phosphodiesterase inhibitors (e.g., type 5 to increase or maintain cyclic GMP activity or type 3/4 to increase or maintain cyclic AMP activity) substrate loading agents (e.g., arginine to increase nitric oxide production) as well as consideration of elastase inhibitors—should further improve treatment options for patients with pulmonary arterial hypertension. By following a wide variety of approaches, there is considerable promise in the development of novel therapeutic modalities for pulmonary arterial hypertension. In addition to the reversal of vascular remodeling, stimulation or enhancement of normal endothelial cell function may be possible.

XII. Conclusion

As our understanding of the pathogenesis of pulmonary arterial hypertension evolves, newer strategies for its treatment are being developed and implemented. Further clarification of the mechanisms of the development and perpetuation of the pulmonary arterial hypertension process will undoubtedly lead to refinement in treatment strategies for pulmonary arterial hypertension. We hope that by increasing our understanding of the pathogenesis and pathophysiology of pulmonary vascular disease, we will one day be able to prevent or cure pulmonary arterial hypertension as opposed to only providing palliative therapy. Despite this, recent therapeutic advances have significantly improved the outcome for patients with pulmonary vascular disease.

References

1. Romberg E. Über Sklerose der lungen Arterie. Dtsch Arch Klin Med 1891; 48:197–206.
2. Janicki JS, Weber KT, Likoff MJ, Fishman AP. The pressure-flow response of the pulmonary circulation in patients with heart failure and pulmonary vascular disease. Circulation 1985; 72:1270–1275.
3. Levin DL, Fixler DE, Morriss FC, Tyson J. Morphologic analysis of the pulmonary vascular bed in infants exposed in utero to prostaglandin synthase inhibitors. J Pediatr 1978; 92:478–483.

4. Abenhaim L, Moride Y, Brenot F, Rich S, Benichou J, Kurz X, Higenbottam T, Oakley C, Wouters E, Aubier M, Simonneau G, Begaud B. Appetite-suppressant drugs and the risk of primary pulmonary hypertension. N Engl J Med 1996; 335:609–616.

5. McCaffrey RM, Dunn LJ. Primary pulmonary hypertension in pregnancy. Obstet Gynecol Surg 1964; 19:567–592.

6. Demas NW. Maternal death due to primary pulmonary hypertension. Trans Pacif Coast Obstet Gynecol Soc 1972; 40:64–65.

7. Nelson DM, Main E, Crafford W, Ahumada GG. Peripartum heart failure due to primary pulmonary hypertension. Obstet Gynecol 1983; 63:58S–63S.

8. Kleiger RE, Boxer M, Ingham RE, Harrison DE. Pulmonary hypertension in patients using oral contraceptives. Chest 1976; 69:143–147.

9. Oakley C, Somerville J. Oral contraceptives and progressive pulmonary vascular disease. Lancet 1968; 1:890–891.

10. Rich S, Kaufmann E, Levy PS. The effects of high doses of calcium-channel blockers on survival in primary pulmonary hypertension. N Engl J Med 1992; 327:76–81.

11. Fuster V, Steele PM, Edwards WE, Gersh BJ, McGoon MD, Frye RL. Primary pulmonary hypertension: natural history and the importance of thrombosis. Circulation 1984; 70:580–587.

12. Barst RJ, Maislin G, Fishman AP. Vasodilator therapy in primary pulmonary hypertension in children. Circulation 1999; 99:1197–1204.

13. Bowyer JJ, Busst CM, Denison DM, Shinebourne EA. Effect of long-term oxygen treatment at home in children with pulmonary vascular disease. Br Heart J 1986; 55:385–390.

14. Wagenvoort CA, Wagenvoort N. Primary pulmonary hypertension: A pathologic study of the lung vessels in 156 clinically diagnosed cases. Circulation 1970; 42:1163–1184.

15. Wagenvoort CA, Wagenvoort N. Primary Pulmonary Hypertension. New York: Wiley, 1977.

16. Christman BW, McPherson CD, Newman JH, King GA, Bernard GR, Groves BM, Loyd JE. An imbalance between the excretion of thromboxane and prostacyclin metabolites in pulmonary hypertension. N Engl J Med 1992; 327:70–75.

17. Rubin LJ, Mendoza J, Hood M, McGoon M, Barst RJ, Williams WB, Diehl JH, Crow J, Long W. Treatment of primary pulmonary hypertension with continuous intravenous prostacyclin: results of a randomized trial. Ann Intern Med 1990; 112:485–491.

18. Barst RJ, Rubin LJ, McGoon MD, Caldwell EJ, Long WA, Levy, PS. Survival in primary pulmonary hypertension with long-term continuous intravenous prostacyclin. Ann Intern Med 1994; 121:409–415.

19. Barst RJ, Rubin LJ, Long WA, McGoon MD, Rich S, Badesch DB, Groves BM, Tapson VF, Bourge RC, Brundage BH, Koerner SK, Langleben D, Keller CA, Murali S, Uretsky BF, Clayton LM, Jobsis MM, Blackburn SD, Shortino D, Crow JW. For the Primary Pulmonary Hypertension Study Group. A comparison of continous intravenous epoprostenol (prostacyclin) with conventional therapy for primary pulmonary hypertension. N Engl J Med 1996; 334:296–301.

20. McLaughlin VV, Genthner DE, Panella MM, Rich S. Reduction in pulmonary vascular resistance with long-term epoprostenol (prostacyclin) therapy in primary pulmonary hypertension. N Engl J Med 1998; 338:273–277.

21. Berman-Rosenzweig E, Kerstein D, Barst RJ. Chronic prostacyclin therapy for pulmonary hypertension with associated congenital heart defects. Circulation 1999; 99:1858–1865.

22. Badesch DB, Tapson VF, McGoon MD, Brundage BH, Rubin LJ, Wigley FM, Rich S, Barst RJ, Barrett PS, Kral KM, Jobsis MM, Loyd JE, Murali S, Frost A, Girgis R, Bourge RC, Ralph DD, Elliott CG, Hill NS, Langleben D, Schilz RJ, McLaughlin VV, Robbins IM, Groves BM, Shapiro S, Medsger TA Jr. A comparison of continuous intravenous epoprostenol with conventional therapy for pulmonary hypertension secondary to the scleroderma spectrum of disease. Ann Intern Med 2000; 132:425–434.

23. Rich S, McLaughlin VV. The effects of chronic prostacyclin therapy on cardiac output and symptoms in primary pulmonary hypertension. J Am Coll Cardiol 1999; 34(4):1184–1187.

24. Steffen RP, De La Mata M. The effects of 15AU81, a chemically stable prostacyclin analog, on the cardiovascular and renin-angiotensin systems of anesthetized dogs. Prostaglandins Leuko Essent Fatty Acids 1991; 43:277–286.

25. Simonneau G, Barst RJ, Galie N, Naeije R, Rich S, Bourge RC, Keogh A, Oudiz R, Frost A, Blackburn SD, Crow JW, Rubin LJ. Continuous subcutaneous infusion of UT-15, a prostacyclin analogue, in patients with pulmonary arterial hypertension, a double-blind randomized controlled trial. Am J Resp Care 2002; 165:800–804.

26. Barst RJ, Simonneau G, Rich S, Blackburn SD, Naeije R, Galie N, Rubin LJ for the Uniprost PAH Study Group. Efficacy and Safety of chronic subcutaneous infusion of UT-15 (Uniprost) in pulmonary arterial hypertension (PAH). Circulation 2000; 102(18):II-100–II-101.

27. Hoeper MM, Oschewski H, Ghofrani HA, Wilkens H, Winkler J, Borst MM, Niedermeyer J, Fabel H, Seeger W. A comparison of the acute hemodynamic effects of inhaled nitric oxide and aerosolized iloprost in primary pulmonary hypertension. German PPH Study Group. J Am Coll Cardiol 2000; 35:176–182.

28. Olschewski H, Ghofrani HA, Schmehl T, Winkler J, Wilkens H, Hoepper MM, Behr J, Kleber FX, Seeger W. Inhaled Iloprost to treat severe pulmonary hypertension. An uncontrolled trial. German PPH Study Group. Ann Intern Med 2000; 132:435–443.

29. Skuballa W, Raduchel B, Borbruggen H. Chemistry of stable prostacyclin analogues: synthesis of Iloprost. In: Gryglewski RS, Stock G, eds. Prostacyclin and Its Stable Analogue Iloprost. Springer, Berlin: Springer-Verlag, 1987:17–24.

30. Okano Y, Yoshioka T, Shimouchi A, Satoh T, Kunieda T. Orally active prostacyclin analogue in primary pulmonary hypertension. Lancet 1997; 349:1365.

31. Saji T, Ozawa Y, Ishikita T, Matsuura H, Matsuo N. Short-term hemodynamic effect of a new oral prostacyclin analogue, beraprost in primary and secondary pulmonary hypertension. Am J Cardiol 1996; 78(2):244–247.

32. Kuneida T, Nakanishi N, Satoh T, Kyotani S, Okano Y, Nagaya N. Clinical trials of TK-100 in primary and collagen pulmonary hypertension. Jpn J Clin Exp Med 1997; 74:10.

33. Yanagisawa M, Kurihari H, Kimura S, Tomobe Y, Kobayashi M, Mitsui Y, Yazaki Y. A novel potent vasoconstrictor peptide produced by vascular endothelial cells. Nature 1988; 332:411–415.
34. Galie N, Grigoni F, Bacchi-Reggiani L, et al. Relation of Endothelin-1 to survival in patients with primary pulmonary hypertension. Eur J Clin Invest 1996; 26(1):273.
35. Yoshibayashi M, Nishioka K, Nakao K, Saito Y, Matsumura M, Ueda T, Temma S, Shirakami G, Imura H, Mikawa H. Plasma endothelin concentrations in patients with pulmonary hypertension associated with congenital heart defects. Evidence for increased production of endothelin in pulmonary circulation. Circulation 1991; 84(6):2280–2285.
36. Channick RN, Simonneau G, Sitbon O, Robbins IM, Frost A, Tapson VF, Bodesoh DB, Roux S, Rainisio M, Bodin P, Rubin LJ. Effects of the dual endothelin-receptor antagonist bosentan in patients with pulmonary hypertension. Lancet 2001; 358:1119–1123.
37. Barst RJ, Rich S, Horn EM, McLaughlin V, Kerstein D, Widlitz AC, McFarlin J, Dixon R. Efficacy and safety of chronic treatment with selective endothelin-A receptor blockade in pulmonary arterial hypertension (PAH). Circulation 2000; 102(18):II-427.
38. Channick RN, Newhart JW, Johnson FW, Williams PJ, Augur WR, Fedullo PF, Moser KM. Pulsed delivery of inhaled nitric oxide to patients with primary pulmonary hypertension: an ambulatory delivery system and clinical tests. Chest 1996; 109:1545–1549.

12

Lung Volume Reduction Surgery

GERARD J. CRINER and FRANCIS C. CORDOVA

Temple University School of Medicine
and Temple Lung Center
Philadelphia, Pennsylvania, U.S.A.

I. Introduction

Chronic obstructive pulmonary disease (COPD) is a major cause of morbidity and mortality. It currently ranks as the fourth leading cause of death in the world, and further increases in prevalence and mortality are predicted in the coming decades (1). COPD is a heterogeneous disease and includes patients who suffer from emphysema, asthmatic bronchitis, chronic bronchitis, or a mixture of the above. It is estimated that of the 16 million individuals diagnosed as having COPD, approximately 2 million suffer predominately from emphysema. Emphysema is a progressive disorder characterized by destruction of alveolar-capillary exchange units. Emphysema patients have a large economic burden and a markedly impaired quality of life.

Over the past several decades, significant improvements have been made in the care of patients with COPD. These include the development of new bronchodilators, the use of supplemental oxygen, recognition of the benefits of adequate nutrition, and pulmonary rehabilitation—all of which improve patients' quality of life—and the implementation of lung transplantation in selected individuals (1). However, because of the high prevalence of the disease, its progressive nature, and its high morbidity and mortality, the above interventions are still inadequate to treat the large number of patients afflicted with emphysema. Understandably, the promise of lung volume reduction surgery (LVRS) as a novel approach to surgically improve expiratory flow limitation, alleviate dyspnea, improve exercise performance, and, most importantly, improve the quality of life was enthusiastically and broadly embraced by emphysema patients, pulmonologists, and thoracic surgeons.

Since the reintroduction of LVRS 8 years ago, significant amounts of data have accumulated regarding its short- and long-term effects on lung function and exercise performance. Moreover, the introduction of LVRS has also precipitated a new debate on the introduction of surgical therapy in the clinical arena and the need to subject new surgical techniques to clinical investigation via prospective, randomized, and controlled clinical trials.

This chapter summarizes the most recent data regarding the physiological basis for LVRS, the short- and long-term outcomes of LVRS, and the most current guidelines for optimal patient selection.

II. Pathophysiological Basis for Lung Volume Reduction Surgery

The hallmarks of COPD are peripheral airways inflammation and destruction of the lung parenchyma, resulting in the development of emphysema. The abnormal inflammatory response that characterizes COPD is manifest as chronic inflammation in the peripheral airways, lung parenchyma, and pulmonary vasculature. In various regions throughout the lung, inflammatory cells in the forms of macrophages, T lymphocytes (predominately CD8+), and neutrophils are found (2). A variety of cytokines—including leukotriene LTB_4, interleukin 8 (IL-8), tumor necrosis factor alpha (TNF-α), and others—are released, all of which are capable of further damaging lung tissue and perpetuating inflammation (3). Besides inflammation, an imbalance between proteinases and antiproteinases, and oxidatives stresses are additional pathways contributing to the pathogenesis of poorly reversible or nonreversible airflow obstruction and lung tissue destruction (1).

Lung parenchymal destruction in emphysema patients typically manifests itself as centrilobular emphysema, a process that denotes dilatation and destruction of the respiratory bronchioles. In milder forms of the disease, these lesions predominate in the upper lung regions; but in advanced disease states, the lesions appear diffusely throughout the entire lung and also involve destruction of the pulmonary capillary bed.

Expiratory airflow limitation is the hallmark physiological change that occurs in patients with COPD, a key not only to the diagnosis of the disease but to its severity. Expiratory airflow limitation occurs in emphysema due to a reduction in lung elastic recoil (e.g., the driving pressure that promotes expiratory flow) and airways obstruction (caused by hypersecretion of mucus, mucous gland hypertrophy, airways mucosal engorgement, and bronchoconstriction) that inhibits airflow. Emphysema contributes to airflow limitation by reducing lung elastic recoil as a result of lung tissue destruction as well as destruction of alveolar attachments, which limits the patency of the small airways.

As a consequence of expiratory airflow limitation, the volume over which the lung and chest wall operates increases, because the outward recoil of the chest wall is now opposed by significantly less inwardly directed lung recoil, thereby placing the chest wall and inspiratory muscles at mechanical disadvantage. Breathing at elevated lung volumes not only places the inspiratory muscles at a mechanical disadvantage but also increases their elastic load secondary to the development of intrinsic positive end-expiratory pressure ($PEEP_i$). Elevated lung volume and the development of $PEEP_i$ may also adversely affect cardiac function by limiting venous return and increasing right ventricular impedance.

Further compounding the negative consequences of emphysema on respiratory mechanics is the development of abnormal gas exchange. Ventilation perfusion ($\dot{V}/\dot{Q}$) mismatch results in an elevation of physiological dead space, which further increases the patient's ventilatory load in order to maintain normal gas exchange. Figure 1 is a schematic showing the various effects of emphysema on lung and chest wall function.

The physiological derangements described above as a consequence of advanced emphysema are further exacerbated by conditions that provoke greater ventilatory demands—such as exercise, diseases like pneumonia, or

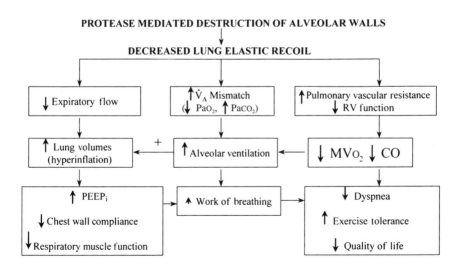

Figure 1 Protease-mediated destruction of alveolar walls. Effects of emphysema on lung and chest wall mechanics. Definitions: $\dot{V}_A$, alveolar ventilation; RV, right ventricular; MV_{O_2}, mixed venous oxygen content; CO, cardiac output; $PEEP_i$, intrinsic positive end-expiratory pressure.

exacerbations of COPD. Since patients with advanced emphysema breathe at rest at the outer limit of the expiratory flow curve, higher ventilatory demands cannot be offset by increased expiratory flow, thereby producing dynamic hyperinflation. This vicious cycle of expiratory airflow limitation, dynamic hyperinflation, $\dot{V}/\dot{Q}$ imbalance, and impaired right ventricular function all contribute to the patient's sense of breathlessness, limited functional performance, and a severely impaired quality of life.

III. History of Lung Volume Reduction Surgery

A. Background

The anatomical consequences of emphysema—producing a hyperinflated thorax, and a depressed and flattened diaphragm—have been the subject of investigation and attempted surgical therapy for the last 50 to 75 years. As a result, early attempts were made to surgically reduce lung volume or make an over-distended and stiffened chest wall more compliant. Several procedures—including costochondrectomy, thoracoplasty, pneumoperitoneum, phrenic nerve interruption, glomectomy, and radical hilar nerve stripping—were all endorsed for short periods of time, based on anecdotal reports of subjective improvement. However, the lack of objective controlled data coupled with a lack of consistent results from other practitioners caused each of the procedures to be abandoned. Only resection of a giant bulla remains a useful intervention when performed in patients without evidence of diffuse emphysema. Resection of an isolated bulla has been shown to decrease dyspnea, improve lung function, increase exercise tolerance, and also improve diaphragmatic function (4–7). It is believed that all of these functional and physiological improvements associated with bullectomy are the results of a surgical reduction in lung volume, which results in improvements in lung, chest wall, and respiratory muscle mechanics (7).

In 1957, Brantigan and colleagues published their experiences with a surgical procedure aimed at downsizing the lung in patients with severe diffuse emphysema (8–10). Brantigan and colleagues (8) hypothesized that in patients with severe emphysema and hyperinflation, downsizing of the lungs would restore toward normal the outward radial traction on the small airways, thereby facilitating expiratory airflow. Brantigan emphasized that the procedure was "an operation directed at restoration of a physiologic principle" and "not concerned with removal of pathological tissue." He performed his procedure through a standard thoracotomy, performing multiple lung resections and plications and also incorporated radical hilar stripping to denervate the lung.

Brantigan and colleagues (10) reported subjective improvement in 75% of patients for periods up to 5 years; however, the procedure was associated with a 16% postoperative mortality. Furthermore, no objective data were provided to supplement the subjective reports of patients improvement. Because of the high mortality and lack of objective data, Brantigan's procedure never gained full acceptance or widespread application.

B. Subsequent Developments

In 1991, Wakabayashi et al. (11) performed thorascopic laser ablation of multiple bullae in 22 patients with diffuse emphysema. CO_2 laser beams were applied to the external surface of the bullae to shrink them, thereby reducing lung volume. These investigators also reported a subjective improvement in patients' symptoms but provided little in the way of objective data. Moreover, his report included not only those with diffuse emphysema but also some patients with isolated bullous disease, thereby potentially overstating the benefits in reporting mean group data for those suffering from nonbullous emphysema.

In 1993, Cooper and colleagues (12) modified the procedure of Brantigan and colleagues and performed bilateral LVRS in 20 consecutive patients by removing 20 to 30% of each lung via stapled resections through a median sternotomy. Postoperatively, they reported a significant increase in FEV_1, an improvement in resting hypoxemia, improved quality of life, and a marked relief of dyspnea. Modifications of Brantigan's technique by Cooper included the use of a median sternotomy; placement of a thoracic epidural for analgesic relief—thereby avoiding the need for systemic narcotics or respiratory depressants; automatic cutting stapling devices, which were buttressed with bovine pericardium to decrease the development of postoperative air leaks at the staple line; and radiographic imaging—including computed tomography (CT) and quantitative lung perfusion scans—which helped target those lung regions with the worst emphysema for resection. Based on the favorable reports presented by Cooper and colleagues, significant interest was rekindled in lung resection for severe emphysema. Soon after his initial report, a number of reports using unilateral or bilateral lung resections via median sternotomy, lateral thoracotomy, or video-assisted thorascopic surgery (VATS) were reported from a number of different centers. Although most of the reports demonstrated positive results with the use of LVRS, a number of problems were encountered in interpreting the data.

C. Controversies Resulting in Developing the National Emphysema Treatment Trial

Problems encountered in reviewing early LVRS reports included inconsistent follow-up of patients, varying surgical techniques used to perform LVRS, variable patient selection criteria, lack of control groups, different endpoints for defining success, and inconsistent and sometimes inadequate characterization of patients receiving LVRS. The effect of incomplete data on biasing the interpretation of data in longitudinal studies was highlighted by Butler et al. (13). These investigators determined the reasons why patients dropped out without further follow-up after LVRS, and assessed the characteristics between those subjects who came back for follow-up compared to those who did not. Patients who did not present for follow-up had a long-term mortality of 27%, considerably greater than those who did comply with follow-up testing (3%, $p < 0.05$). The authors interpreted their data as showing that long-term mortality following LVRS may be biased in the direction of underestimating true mortality if incomplete follow-up is encountered.

Despite limited data, LVRS cases soared in number from 1994 through 1996. An estimated 1212 LVRS operations were performed in Medicare patients between July 1994 and December 1995 (14). At the end of December 1995, LVRS was being performed in 37 states, and the number of claims submitted to Medicare for LVRS peaked in December 1995 to 169 claims per month. The average Medicare reimbursement per procedure was $31,398. Based on the projected number of patients suffering from emphysema who conceivably could be candidates for LVRS, it was estimated that expenditures by Medicare for LVRS could be as high as $1 billion.

Following implementation of a specific ICD-9 code for LVRS, Medicare identified 722 claims for LVRS that used the code between October 1995 and January 1996 (15). Of these patients, approximately 30% ($n = 215$) died within 18 months of LVRS, a mortality rate considerably higher than that reported or projected by the available published medical data at that time (15). Analysis by Medicare also demonstrated that Medicare beneficiaries receiving LVRS used hospital rehabilitation or long-term care facilities considerably more following LVRS compared to the calendar year preceding LVRS. These factors were used by Medicare officials to underscore in an outcomes report that published studies may be biased toward being more favorable than truly reflected in patients who actually received LVRS. Furthermore, Medicare officials hypothesized that since LVRS patients appeared to be a high risk for postoperative mortality, a control group was necessary in order to distinguish between the impact of LVRS in comparison to the impact of the disease itself.

In December of 1995, the Health Care Financing Administration (HCFA) issued a noncoverage policy for all LVRS procedures (based on the lack of medical evidence and potential for excessive morbidity and mortality among Medicare beneficiaries) (15). The HCFA asked the Center for Health Care Technology (CHCT), a part of the Agency for Health Care Policy and Research, to undertake a complete review of the available evidence, both published and unpublished, on the effects of LVRS. In April 1996, the CHCT report was released, based on the analysis of approximately 2800 patients reported to them from 27 institutions. The report concluded that "the available data did not permit a scientific conclusion regarding the risks and benefits of LVRS." The report further commented that "some patients appeared to benefit from LVRS, at least in the initial postoperative period," but that a "significant amount of data was incomplete, with limited follow-up." They recommended a controlled clinical trial be undertaken to further assess the efficacy of this procedure, both its long- and short-term effect, in a comprehensive manner. Moreover, they recommended a prospective trial comparing LVRS to optimized medical treatment while simultaneously providing Medicare financial coverage.

Later on in that same month of April 1996, HCFA and the National Heart, Lung, and Blood Institute (NHLBI) both signed an agreement to participate in such a study, with Medicare providing reimbursement for the clinical costs of the trials. This unique partnership between Medicare and the NHLBI broke new ground, and the study became known as the National Emphysema Treatment Trial (NETT).

The NETT has been promoted as precedent-setting in establishing a cooperative effort between the nation's largest insurance payer and its premiere scientific agency for research in pulmonary disease with the hope of providing a model for future assessment of new medical or surgical interventions. It was also the intention that Medicare beneficiaries be provided controlled access to a promising but in some respects unproven surgical procedure while scientifically valid data were collected to further guide clinical use and reimbursement decisions.

Circumstances surrounding the suspension of reimbursement for LVRS payment by Medicare; the requirement for participation in a prospective, randomized, controlled trial evaluating the effectiveness of a new surgical procedure in order to receive LVRS financial coverage; coupled with the pressures placed upon physicians by a severely impaired and desperate patient population were factors contributing to making the issue of LVRS and the NETT one of controversy and heightened interest.

IV. Outcome of Lung Volume Reduction Surgery

In general, numerous published studies to date have shown that LVRS in carefully selected patients with diffuse emphysema led to an improvement in lung function, exercise capacity, and quality of life. In addition, LVRS has also been shown to decrease the need for supplemental oxygen and steroid therapy and to improve dyspnea. However, the impact of LVRS on these different outcome measures are variable across different institutions, and the magnitudes of physiological and subjective improvement are modest compared to the initial report by Cooper and colleagues (12). The beneficial effects appear to peak at 3 to 6 months following LVRS and are maintained for an additional 3 to 4 years, followed by a gradual decline in lung function similar to the progressive decline encountered with the natural history of emphysema. The variability in clinical outcome reported following LVRS is due to multiple factors, including different selection criteria (homogeneous versus hetero-genous emphysema, preoperative pulmonary rehabilitation versus no rehabi-litation, etc.), different surgical techniques used between investigators (laser versus stapled resection, unilateral versus bilateral); and differences in outcome measures reported (pre- versus postbronchodilator expiratory flow rate, 6-min walk test versus cardiopulmonary exercise study). Outside of a prospective, multicenter, randomized trial on LVRS, the currently reported outcome on LVRS should be interpreted with these limitations in mind. In this review, both the short- and long-term effects of LVRS on lung function, gas exchange, cardiopulmonary exercise, and quality of life are reviewed in detail.

A. Short-Term Results (<12 Months)

Spirometry

Early reports detailing the benefits of LVRS focused on the improvement in forced expiratory airflow, specifically, forced vital capacity (FVC) and forced expiratory volume in 1 sec (FEV_1). When Cooper and colleagues (12) reported their experience in their first 20 patients who underwent bilateral LVRS via sternotomy, the mean improvements in FEV_1 and FVC were 82 and, 27%, respectively. In their follow-up study on 150 patients, the postoperative increases in FEV_1 and FVC 6 months after LVRS were reported as 51 and 20%, respectively (16). However, the magnitude of the increases in FEV_1 after surgery reported by other investigators have been variable, ranging between 13 and as high as 96% compared to baseline (17–25). It is important to remember that not all patients show an improvement in spirometry after LVRS, which may not be apparent in studies reporting only group mean data. In one study, 34% of the patients who underwent bilateral LVRS via median sternotomy had less than 20% improvement in FEV_1 3 to 6 months after surgery (22). Table 1 summarizes postoperative changes in spirometry reported by published studies to date. The variability in postoperative changes in FEV_1 after LVRS are highlighted in Figure 2.

Several factors may contribute to the variability in improvement in spirometry after LVRS. From the mechanistic viewpoint, taking into account the coupling of the lung and chest wall properties, the extent of air trapping as measured by residual volume/total lung capacity has been proposed as one of the best predictors of the magnitude of improvement in FVC and FEV_1 after LVRS (26). From clinical studies published to date, several preoperative factors have been suggested as important in predicting the magnitude of improvement in spirometry after LVRS. These include the pattern of distribution of emphysema (27–29), the type of surgical techniques utilized (30–33) and whether unilateral or bilateral LVRS was performed (30,34). Each of these factors is discussed separately in the subsequent sections.

Lung Volumes

As the name implies, the aim of LVRS is to remove 20 to 30% of each lung to reduce lung volume and thereby decrease hyperinflation and air trapping due to emphysema. On average, both TLC and RV are reduced by 10 to 20% and 15 to 30%, respectively, at 3 to 6 months after bilateral LVRS. Likewise, the reported decreased in lung volume is variable, with the decrease in TLC ranging from 1 to 23% and RV between 3 and 46%, as shown in Table 1. In

Table 1 Short-Term Changes in Spirometry, Lung Volumes, Diffusion Capacity, and Gas Exchange After Bilateral LVRS

Author	Procedure	Number of patients/ follow-up	FEV$_1$ (% change)	FVC (% change)	RV (% change)	TLC (% change)	D$_{LCO}$ (% change)	Pa$_{O_2}$ ($\triangle$mmHg)	Pa$_{CO_2}$ ($\triangle$mmHg)
Cooper, 1995	MS	20/20	82	27	−39	−22	NA	6	−1
Argenziano, 1997	MS and thoracoster-notomy	85/51	58	41	NA	NA	NA	NA	NA
Bingisser, 1996	VATS	20/20	42	29	−23	−16	NA	4	−2
Daniel, 1996	MS	26/17	49	23	−14	−14	NA	4	−2
Gaissert, 1996	MS	33/33	85	NA	NA	NA	NA	−6	−5
Gelb, 1996	VATS	12/12	68	18	−30	−18	196	NA	NA
Kotloff, 1996	MS	80/56	41	20	−28	NA	NA	NA	NA
	VATS	40/34	41	25	−23				
Benditt, 1997	MS	21/21	30	17	−22	−7	NA	5	−4
Brenner, 1997	VATS	145/130	62	40	−28	−19	63	−1	−1
Bousamra, 1997	MS(42)	45/37	59	37	NA	NA	NA	NA	NA
Cordova, 1997	MS	69/25	37	22	−27	−11	14	NA	−2
Martinez, 1997	MS	17/17	38	17	−25	−13	10	NA	NA
Stammberger, 1997	VATS	42/36	43	18	−13	−2	NA	7	−2
Weder, 1997	VATS	50/50	34−81	34−60	−20 to −30	−9	NA	4 to 7	−2 to −4
Wisser, 1998	MS	15	60	33	−22	−11	NA	3	−6
	VATS	15	62	35	−29	−8	NA	3	−1

Table 1 *Continued*

Author	Procedure	Number of patients/ follow-up	FEV₁ (% change)	FVC (% change)	RV (% change)	TLC (% change)	DLco (% change)	Pao₂ (ΔmmHg)	Paco₂ (ΔmmHg)
Albert, 1998	MS	46/46	33	52	−22	−10	24	3	−3
Ferguson, 1998	MS	27/18	32	14	−28	−15	−4	1	−3
Hazelrigg, 1998	MS	29	40	NA	−28	NA	15	9	−1
	VATS	50	41	NA	−37	NA	10	2	−5
Ingenito, 1998	VATS	29/29	33	18	NA	NA	NA	NA	NA
Ko, 1998	MS	19	28	NA	−7	NA	NA	11	−1
	VATS	23	62	NA	−11	NA	NA	−2	−9
Norman, 1998	MS	14/14	26	11	−27	−16	NA	1	0
Scharf, 1998	MS	9/9	61	30	−35	−13	18	NA	NA
Stammberger, 1998	VATS	40/40	55	42	−25	−17	0	6	−3
Tschernko, 1998	VATS	8/8	38	24	−28	−9	NA	NA	NA
Anderson, 1999	MS	80/20	21	NA	NA	NA	NA	NA	NA
Thurnheer, 1999	VATS	70/70	23–57	17–47	−15 to −28	−6–18	−2 to 5	5	−2 to −3

Key: FEV₁, forced expiratory volume in 1 sec; FVC, forced vital capacity; TLC, total lung capacity; RV, residual volume; DL_{CO}, lung diffusion capacity for carbon monoxide; Pao₂, arterial partial pressure of oxygen; Paco₂, partial pressure of carbon dioxide; MS, median sternotomy; VATS, video-assisted thoracic surgery; NA, not available.
Source: Ref. 125.

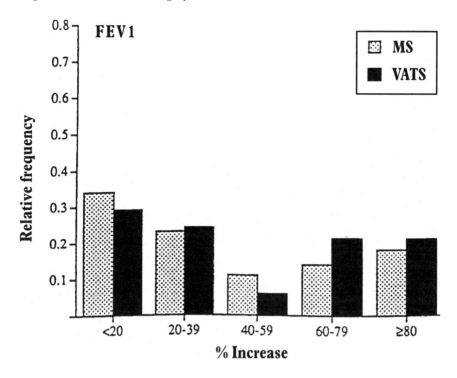

Figure 2 The magnitude of postoperative changes in FEV₁ after LVRS either by median sternotomy or video-assisted thoracoscopic surgery can be variable among individual patients. (From Ref. 22.)

general, decreases in TLC and RV following bilateral LVRS are greater following bilateral stapled LVRS than unilateral (34) or laser surgical resection (33). Thus the amount of lung tissue removed and the surgical techniques utilized account for some of the variability of the reported decreases in lung volumes after surgery.

The reduction in lung volume following LVRS also results in decreases in the dimensions of the thoracic cage. Using radiography and CT of the chest, Lando and colleagues showed that the conformational changes in the rib cage dimension was mainly due to decreases in the middle to lower anteroposterior rib cage diameters (35). These changes in the dimensions of the thoracic cage are seen 3 months post-LVRS and are maintained for at least 1 year post-LVRS.

Diffusion Capacity

The effect of LVRS on diffusion capacity (DL_{CO}) has not been consistently reported in the majority of studies. Some studies reported a slight increase in DL_{CO} while others showed no significant change after surgery. In an animal model of emphysema, the DL_{CO} decreases in proportion to the amount of lung tissue removed (36). In a recent report from the National Emphysema Treatment Trial (NETT), patients who underwent bilateral LVRS who had a preoperative $DL_{CO} < 20\%$ of predicted and an $FEV_1 < 20\%$ had a 30-day mortality rate of 16% compared to no deaths over the same time period in patients who were treated medically (Fig. 3) (37). Based on this initial analysis of the NETT data, the entry criteria have been modified to exclude patients who have an FEV_1 of <20% of predicted and either homogenous emphysema, or very low diffusion capacity (<20% of predicted). In essence, patients with very severe emphysema and homogenous emphysema involvement should be referred for lung transplantation.

Arterial Blood Gas

The initial report on the effect of LVRS on gas exchange showed a modest increase in the partial pressure of oxygen in the arterial blood (Pa_{O_2}) and a decrease in the partial pressure of carbon dioxide in arterial blood (Pa_{CO_2}). Cooper and colleagues showed a increase in Pa_{CO_2} from the baseline value of 64 mmHg to 70 mmHg with no significant change in Pa_{CO_2} at 6 months postsurgery in their first 20 patients (12). In their subsequent report of 101 patients, the Pa_{O_2} increased by a mean of 8 mmHg after surgery, while the mean Pa_{CO_2} decreased by 4 mmHg (16). Other investigators have since reported similar improvements in arterial blood gases after surgery (38–41) while still others reported contradictory responses in arterial blood gases post-LVRS, characterized by a significant increase in Pa_{O_2} without changes in Pa_{CO_2} (42,43) or vice versa—that is, no significant postoperative changes in Pa_{O_2} but a modest decrease in Pa_{CO_2} (44–47). The response of an individual patient is even more variable, with a wide range of changes in Pa_{O_2} (-17 to 29 mmHg) and Pa_{CO_2} (-11 to $+5$) reported after LVRS (48).

The conflicting reports by different centers on the effect of LVRS on gas exchange are unclear but are likely to be multifactorial and related to differences in patient selection, surgical techniques, and inaccuracies in measuring Pa_{O_2} in patients receiving supplemental oxygen via nasal cannula. In 46 patients who underwent bilateral LVRS via median sternotomy, Albert and colleagues (48) showed no correlation between changes in Pa_{O_2} and Pa_{CO_2}, with preoperative arterial blood gas values, severity of airflow obstruction, the degree of hyperinflation or air trapping and the severity of diffusion impairment. In addition, there was also no correlation between the changes in Pa_{O_2} and Pa_{CO_2} and postoperative changes in FEV_1, RV, TLC, and DL_{CO}. In contrast, Shade and colleagues (49) showed that changes in Pa_{CO_2} significantly correlated with changes in FEV_1 ($r = -0.56, p = 0.0007$), maximal inspiratory pressure PL_{max} ($r = -0.46, p = 0.009$), DL_{CO} ($r = -0.47, p = 0.009$), and RV/TLC ($r = -0.40, p = 0.02$). In addition, decreases in Pa_{CO_2} after surgery also correlated with increases in minute ventilation and tidal volume during maximum exercise. Moreover, this study also showed that patients with the

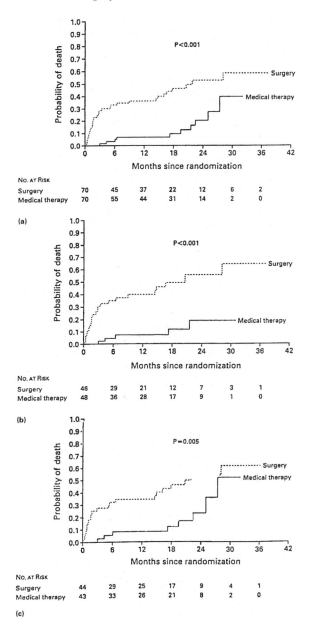

Figure 3 Kaplan-Meier estimates of the probability of death in patients who underwent bilateral LVRS versus medical therapy alone in the NETT study. (a) Intention-to-treat analysis of patients with FEV_1 <20% of predicted with either homogeneous emphysema pattern or diffusion capacity <20% of predicted. (b) Subgroup with FEV_1 <20% of predicted with homogeneous emphysema pattern. (c) Subgroup with FEV_1 <20% of predicted with diffusion capacity <20%. The difference between two treatment groups were significant by log-rank test. (From Ref. 37.)

highest baseline Pa_{CO_2} had the greatest declines in Pa_{CO_2} and the greatest increases in DL_{CO} and PI_{max} post-LVRS.

The exact mechanism(s) responsible for the improvements in gas exchange post-LVRS are unclear but are thought to be due to either improvements in $\dot{V}/\dot{Q}$ matching after resection of the most diseased portions of the lung or to an increase in alveolar ventilation (50).

Oxygen Requirement

Some studies have reported a reduction in the requirement for supplemental oxygen use after LVRS. Some 3 to 6 months after LVRS, several studies have reported a reduction in the number of patients requiring supplemental oxygen, anywhere from 16 to 42% (12,16,38,51). Since other studies do not show a significant increase in Pa_{O_2} postsurgery, as previously discussed although not directly reported, the percentage of patients who are actually able to be weaned off of supplemental oxygen successfully is probably less than that reported. In 101 patients who underwent bilateral LVRS who were followed for at least 1 year, the number of patients who required long-term supplemental oxygen at rest decreased from 52 to 16% at 6 months after surgery (16). To a lesser degree, LVRS also lowered the number of patients who required supplemental oxygen during exercise from 92% before surgery to 44% at 6 months postsurgery. Of 56 patients from the same report who were followed up to 1 year postsurgery, most of those who were successfully weaned from supplemental oxygen were able to maintain an oxygen-free status (16).

In a study looking at oxygen requirements during exercise before and after LVRS using the American Thoracic Society recommendation for long-term use of oxygen, Bousama and colleagues (52) showed in their series of 45 patients (bilateral 43), that oxygen requirement during exercise was essentially unchanged after LVRS. Interestingly, 10 of their patients stopped using oxygen because of decreased dyspnea despite documented oxygen desaturation during exercise. More data are needed to determine the actual percentage of patients who have a reduced need for supplemental oxygen after LVRS, both at rest with and exercise, and to assess the durability of this response over time.

Six-Min Walk Test

The improvement in exercise capacity is one of the most important outcome measures reported in LVRS studies. The 6-min walk test, a timed measure of distance walked, is commonly used as a simple, reproducible measure of functional capacity. In general, the distance walked in 6 min is significantly increased at 3 to 6 months after LVRS. The average reported percent increase in 6-min walk distance ranges from 15 to 103% (16,23,39,47,51,53), as shown in Table 2. This wide variability in reported increases in 6-min walk distance may be due in part to the inherent limitations of the test itself (learning effect) and the uncontrolled effect of preoperative pulmonary rehabilitation in some of the reported studies.

Table 2 Changes in Cardiopulmonary Exercise Capacity After Lung Volume Reduction Surgery

Author	Number of patients	6-min walk test (% change)	Maximal work (% change)	$\dot{V}_{O_2 max}$ (% change)	$\dot{V}_{E max}$ (% change)	$V_{T max}$ (% change)	F_b (% change)
Bingisser, 1996	20	59[a]	52	30	31	NA	NA
Benditt, 1997	21	NA	46	25	27	43	0
Cordova, 1997	25	35	48	25	29	34	−12
Keller, 1997	25	15	41	22	17	20	−4
Martinez, 1997	17	103	NA	NA	NA	2	−22
Wisser, 1997	30	NA	28	NA	NA	NA	NA
Criner, 1998	20	20	33	37	38	19	−13
Ferguson, 1998	27	18	20	3	30	25	4
Stammberger, 1998	40	52	43	28	31	39	−4
Tschernko, 1998	8	NA	100	27	NA	25	−15

Key: $\dot{V}_{O_2 max}$, maximum oxygen consumption; $\dot{V}_{E max}$, maximum minute ventilation; $V_{T max}$, maximum tidal volume; F_b, respiratory rate.
[a] 12-minute walk distance
Source: Ref. 125.

Cardiopulmonary Exercise Test

An increase in exercise capacity after LVRS as reflected by the 6-min walk test is supported by similar improvements reported during cardiopulmonary testing. Several authors have shown that maximum oxygen consumption ($\dot{V}_{O_2 max}$), total exercise time, maximum workload, and maximum minute ventilation ($\dot{V}E$) are significantly increased 3 to 6 months after unilateral (43) or bilateral LVRS (23,47,54,55) Table 2. In addition, the increase in $\dot{V}E$ at a given workload is mainly achieved by an incremental increase in tidal volume with only a minimal increase in respiratory rate. The increase in exercise capacity is due mainly to increases in maximum ventilation and resting ventilatory reserve, which is thought to be due in part to increases in inspiratory and expiratory flow both at rest and during exercise (23,47,56–58). This favorable ventilatory pattern during exercise also leads to a decrease in dead space ventilation during exercise (54). Stammberger and associates (58) showed that the increase in $\dot{V}_{O_2 max}$ and $\dot{V}E_{max}$ after LVRS correlates with increases in FEV_1 and the decreases in hyperinflation as measured by RV/TLC.

LVRS may also improve exercise performance by favorably affecting cardiac function. Benditt and colleagues (54) showed that the heart rate is lower at a given workload and the oxygen pulse is higher after LVRS compared to baseline. Cordova et al. (23) also showed significant increases in oxygen pulse during exercise in 25 patients for up to 1 year after LVRS. The mechanism of the improvement in oxygen pulse is unclear, but it is thought to be caused by improvements in both right and left ventricular function due to a lower end-expiratory lung volume and possibly a decrease in pulmonary vascular resistance.

Overall, the improvement in exercise capacity after LVRS is likely due to a combination of an improvement in expiratory airflow, reduction in the degree of hyperinflation and improvement in respiratory muscle function and possibly in cardiac function as well.

Medications

Several investigators have reported that a significant number of patients are able to discontinue oral corticosteroids after LVRS (16,38,51). In Cooper's study, 53% of the patients were on steroids preoperatively, but only 17% required oral steroids after 6 months and 19% at 1 year after bilateral LVRS (16). Of their initial 20 patients, only 11% needed oral corticosteroids 2 years post-LVRS, as compared to 42% preoperatively (16). Miller and others (38) also reported a significant decrease in the number of patients who required oral corticosteroids after LVRS (66 versus 28%). Unfortunately, studies reported to date on steroid withdrawal lack a control group, and specific details on steroid use and withdrawal were not provided. Furthermore, some studies required prednisone withdrawal or weaning to <20 mg/day during the preoperative period, which may also have contributed to successful steroid weaning after

LVRS. Further studies are needed to clarify this finding before firm conclusions can be drawn.

Dyspnea

Several investigators have reported a significant decrease in dyspnea after both unilateral and bilateral LVRS (16,38,51,56). Using the indexes of the Medical Research Council (MRC) for both dyspnea and transitional dyspnea, Cooper and others were able to show a significant decrease in dyspnea after LVRS independent of the effect of pulmonary rehabilitation (59). Using the MRC dyspnea index alone, Argenziano and colleagues showed comparable decreases in patients who underwent unilateral versus bilateral LVRS (25). In contrast, using the same MRC dyspnea scale, McKenna and associates (34) showed that the percentage of patients undergoing unilateral LVRS who complained of dyspnea with mild exertion (an MRC score of 3-stops for breath every few minutes; a score of 4-housebound) decreased from 73 to 44% postoperatively, whereas only 12% of patients who underwent bilateral LVRS experienced the same degree of dyspnea after surgery. In this study, patients who had bilateral LVRS had higher increases in FEV_1 than those who had unilateral LVRS, suggesting perhaps that a higher gain in lung function could account for superior symptomatic relief from disabling dyspnea after bilateral LVRS compared to the unilateral procedure. However, in the study by Brenner et al. (32), a weak correlation was found between the changes in FEV_1 and dyspnea index after LVRS. Indeed, 10 of 37 patients who had minimal or no improvement in FEV_1 exhibited significant decreases in the MRC scale of dyspnea (less dyspneic) post-LVRS. Martinez and colleagues reported similar observations (56). In 17 patients who showed a significant improvement in dyspnea, 6 had a less than 20% improvement in FEV_1 after bilateral LVRS. Bingisser and colleagues (41) showed moderate correlations between changes in the dyspnea score with FEV_1 ($r = -0.44$, $p < 0.01$), residual volume ($r = -0.44$, $p < 0.01$), and an improvement in exercise capacity ($r = -0.73$, $p < 0.01$). Overall, the improvement in dyspnea after LVRS is probably multifactorial and due to physiological changes such as an increase in expiratory airflow, decrease in hyperinflation, increase in respiratory muscle strength (53,59), and decrease in respiratory drive (60).

Quality of Life

The short-term effect of LVRS on quality of life (QOL), using either disease-specific health questionnaires or general health-related quality-of-life measures have been reported by several investigators (16,21,23,61,62). Among the general health-related quality-of-life measures commonly used are the Medical Outcomes Survey—Short Form 36 (SF-36), the Nottingham Health Profile, and the Sickness Impact Profile (SIP). The Chronic Respiratory Disease Questionnaire and the St. George's Respiratory Questionnaire are commonly used disease-specific questionnaires in COPD patients. In Cooper's initial reports of 20 patients and subsequent report of 150 patients who underwent bilateral LVRS, both the SF-36 and Nottingham Heath Profile showed a significant improvement 6 months post-LVRS. Specifically, improvements in measures of vitality, social and physical functioning, general health, and ability to perform various roles were reported in these studies. Using only the SF-36, Hazelrigg et al. showed a similar improvement in quality of life following both staged thoracoscopy and median sternotomy (21). The improvement in social functioning has been correlated with spirometric improvement, and the improvement in exercise capacity has shown correlation with an improvement in physical functioning (47). Using the SIP questionnaire, a tool that measures 136 items of the patient's perception of his or her daily activities, we found that the total scores and the patient's physical and psychological categories of SIP scores—relating to mobility, ambulation, social interaction, alertness and emotional well-being—were improved 3 to 6 months after surgery (23). Moreover, the improvement in SIP scores was associated with reduced hyperinflation, possibly resulting in a more efficient pattern of breathing and dyspnea (62).

B. Long-Term Results (>12 Months)

Spirometry

It is clear from the preceding discussion that LVRS results in short-term improvement in lung function, exercise capacity, and quality of life. In some patients, it also improves gas exchange and may decrease the need for supplemental oxygen. However, because emphysema is a slowly progressive disease, data on the stability of these short-term gains in lung function after LVRS are limited. In addition, serious concerns regarding the effect of LVRS on the rate of decline of FEV_1 have been raised by Brenner and colleagues (63). In the study by Brenner et al., the highest rate of decline in FEV_1 was seen in patients who experienced the greatest improvement in FEV_1 during the initial 6 months after surgery. Those patients who had the least improvement in FEV_1 after surgery had the lowest rate of decline.

To date only few published studies have addressed the long-term stability of lung function after LVRS. In our report, 13 initial patients who underwent bilateral LVRS via median sternotomy had increases in FEV_1 3 months after LVRS that were sustained at 12 months of follow-up. In 6 of 13 patients with data at 18 months postsurgery, the FEV_1 remained higher compared to baseline $(0.91 \pm 0.37$ versus 0.69 ± 0.02 L, $p<0.12)$ (23). Gelb and colleagues showed similar sustained improvements in FEV_1 and FVC at 12 months postsurgery when compared to baseline data (64). However, both FEV_1 and FVC 12 months post-LVRS were significantly lower when compared to 6 months post-LVRS, suggesting that the improvement in lung function post-LVRS peaks at 6 months. The same trend in FEV_1 was reported in 12 patients by the same authors with up to 24 months of follow-up (65). The initial maximum increase in FEV_1 at 6 months post-LVRS was followed by a gradual decline in FEV_1, but it still remained higher at 24 months post-LVRS compared to the preoperative value (0.88 ± 0.08 versus 1.19 ± 0.13 L, $p < 0.02$). More recently, the same group of investigators reported lung function in 26 patients 5 years after bilateral LVRS via VATS (66). Increases in $FEV_1 > 200$ mL or $FVC > 400$ mL at 1, 2, 3, 4, and 5 years after LVRS were seen in 73, 46, 35, 27, and 8% of these patients. The annual rate of decline in FEV_1 was 141 ± 60 mL/year, with the fastest rate of decline in the initial 1 to 2 years post-LVRS. In 5 patients with serial spirometries (3.8 ± 0.4 performed in the year prior to LVRS), the rate of decline in FEV_1 was similar to their post-LVRS values. In 11 patients who survived beyond 5 years, the FEV_1 decreased by 149 ± 157 mL the first year post-LVRS and 78 ± 59 mL/year over 4 to 4.5 additional years. Based on this study, only 9 of 26, 7 of 26, and 2 of 26 patients had sustained clinical and physiological improvement at 3, 4, and 5 years respectively. In the author's analysis, only the preoperative FVC separated those patients who achieved significant long-term improvement beyond 3 years. Thus it appears that the improvement in lung function is maintained 3 to 4 years post-LVRS in some patients, but unfortunately the annual of rate of decline in FEV_1 is not increased following LVRS.

The long-term effects of LVRS on patients with cigarette-induced emphysema do not seem to apply to patients with emphysema due to alpha$_1$-antitrypsin deficiency. In a study by Cassina et al. (24), the physiological outcome of 12 patients with alpha$_1$-antitrypsin deficiency and 18 patients with smoking-related emphysema were compared following bilateral targeted LVRS. There were no significant differences in these groups in 6-min walk test or performing dyspnea score, although the FEV_1 was lower in the alpha$_1$-antitrypsin group (24 versus 31% of predicted, $p < 0.05$). After LVRS, both groups of patients showed significant short-term improvements in dyspnea score, 6-min walk test performance, and pulmonary function tests. However, the improvements in lung function in the group with alpha$_1$-antitrypsin deficiency returned to baseline at 6 to 12 months after LVRS. Moreover, the FEV_1 decreased further at 24 months, despite optimal medical therapy (Fig. 4). In contrast, patients with centrilobular emphysema (smoker's emphysema) had a slower decline in FEV_1 following the initial improvement at 6 months. At the end of 2 years, the FEV_1 remained significantly higher in the smoker's emphysema group than preoperative baseline.

The reason for accelerated rate of decline in FEV_1 in patients with alpha$_1$-antitypsin deficiency compared to those with smoker's emphysema is unclear. It has been suggested that perhaps basal adhesions in the group with alpha$_1$-antitrysin deficiency after LVRS may lead to impaired diaphragmatic function. Alternatively, differences in lung fiber composition and in the architecture of the connective tissue stroma may predispose patients with panacinar emphysema to lose lung function more rapidly after LVRS.

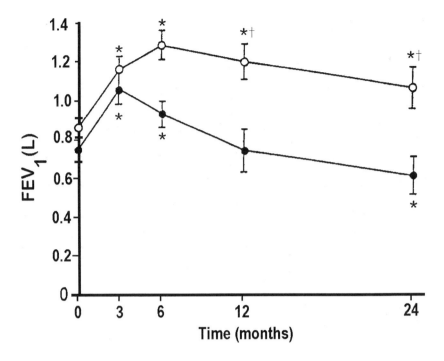

Figure 4 Changes in FEV$_1$ before and after bilateral LVRS in patients with smoking-induced emphysema (open circle) ($n = 18$) compared to patients with alpha$_1$-antitrypsin deficiency (close circle $n = 12$). In patients with alpha$_1$-antitrypsin deficiency. The initial improvement in FEV$_1$ at 3 months is lost at 12 months after surgery. In constrast, patients with smoking-induced emphysema had sustained improvement in FEV$_1$ up to 24 months postsurgery. (From Ref. 24.)

Lung Volumes

The decreases in residual volume and total lung capacity post-LVRS appear to be maintained for at least 2 years (8,23,66). Cooper et al. showed that the initial decreases in RV and TLC reported in their first cohort of 20 patients were maintained at 2 years after LVRS (16). Similarly, we showed a sustained decrease in lung volumes in 6 patients with 18 months of follow-up (23). Gelb and associates (65) showed similar sustained decrease in RV and TLC at 2 years in 12 patients who underwent bilateral LVRS via VATS. However at 3 years after LVRS, the same authors showed that not all patients exhibited sustained decreases in lung volumes; only 9 of 26 patients had significantly lower RV and TLC at the 3 years post-LVRS (67). In 10 short-term responders (<2 years) who died, RV and TLC reverted to preoperative values. Thus, similar to spirometric data, sustained decreases in lung volumes occur in only some but not all patients at 3 to 4 years post-LVRS.

Diffusion Capacity

Limited data are available regarding the effects of LVRS on diffusion capacity during long-term follow-up. In 12 patients followed up to 24 months post-LVRS, the diffusion capacity at 2 years remained significantly higher compared to the preoperative value (43 versus 18% of predicted, $p < 0.001$) (65). In 9 patients who were considered long-term responders, the diffusion capacity/ alveolar volume ratio remained significantly higher compared to baseline (67).

Gas Exchange and Oxygen Requirements After Lung Volume Reduction Surgery

In studies that showed initial significant increases in Pa_{O_2} and decreases in Pa_{CO_2} after LVRS, very few data have been published regarding its long-term stability. In 18 patients who underwent bilateral LVRS via thoracoscopy, the measured Pa_{O_2} at baseline, 3 months, and 24 months were 63.3 ± 2.6, 70.1 ± 2.7, and 64.7 ± 3.1 mmHg respectively. The short-term increase in Pa_{O_2} at 3 months was no longer seen at 2 years after LVRS (20). Similar decreases in Pa_{O_2} to near the baseline values was reported by Gelb and associates in 12 patients at 24 months following bilateral LVRS via thoracoscopy (65).

Similar long-term changes in Pa_{CO_2} after LVRS have been reported. The initial decreases in Pa_{CO_2} at 3 months post-LVRS were lost at 24 months in follow-up, although patients with markedly heterogeneous emphysema were likely to maintain decreases in Pa_{CO_2} at 24 months compared to patients with homogeneous emphysema (20).

As one would expect, the need for supplemental oxygen depends on the magnitude of increase in Pa_{O_2} after LVRS. In Cooper's initial cohort of 20 highly selected patients, 26% required long-term oxygen therapy at baseline compared to zero patients at 12 and 24 months after bilateral LVRS (16). However, the number of patients who required supplemental oxygen during exercise increased from 5% at 12 months to 32% at 24 months. Beyond 2 years, increasing number of patients required supplemental oxygen. In 18 of 26 patients who were oxygen-dependent preoperatively, 78, 50, 33, and 22% of patients were weaned from oxygen therapy at 1, 2, 3, and 4 years after LVRS respectively (67).

Six-Min Walk Test

There are few data available regarding the long-term stability in exercise performance after LVRS. The initial increase in 6-min walk distance seen at 3 to 6 months appears to be maintained at 2 years post-LVRS despite a slight downward trend in FEV_1 (16). We similarly showed sustained increases in 6-min walk distance in 12 patients at 12 months, and in 6 patients at 18 months after bilateral LVRS via sternotomy (23). Hamacher and colleagues showed similar sustained improvements in 6-min walk distance at 24 months post-

LVRS in patients with heterogenous emphysema who underwent bilateral LVRS via thoracoscopy (20). Interestingly, in patients with alpha$_1$-antitrypsin deficiency, the 6-min walk distance at 24 months follow-up remained significantly higher compared to the preoperative value despite an FEV$_1$ that was lower than baseline (24) (Fig. 5).

It is unclear to what extent continued pulmonary rehabilitation plays in the maintenance of the initial gain in exercise capacity, since the majority of authors do not prescribe maintenance exercise routinely after surgery. We previously had shown that the initial gain in functional capacity was sustained by using a maintenance exercise program (55).

Cardiopulmonary Exercise Test

Symptom-limited cardiopulmonary exercise is a better measure of exercise capacity since it does not have the inherent limitations of the 6-min walk test. For one thing, the protocol of performing the 6-min walk test is not well standardized across various studies. In addition, the 6-min walk test is subject

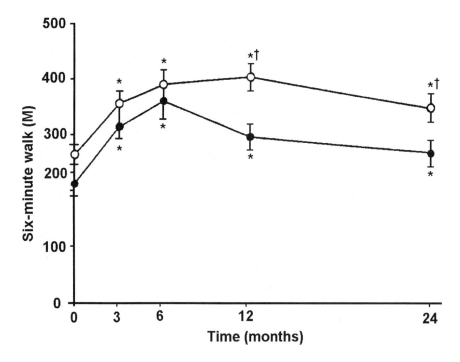

Figure 5 Changes in six-min walk distance before and after bilateral LVRS in patients with smoking-induced emphysema (open circle) ($n = 18$) compared to patients with alpha$_1$-antitrypsin deficiency (close circle $n = 12$). Sustained improvement in exercise capacity in both groups of patients up to 24 months postsurgery. (From Ref. 24.)

to a learning effect—that is, patients are able to walk more efficiently with repeated testing even without a specific intervention. Unfortunately, long-term data on the stability of cardiopulmonary exercise are limited. In 10 patients followed up to 12 months after bilateral LVRS via median sternotomy, total exercise time, $\dot{V}_{O_2 \, max}$, $\dot{V}_{E_{max}}$, and tidal volume at peak exercise remained higher compared to baseline values, although there was a downward trend in $\dot{V}_{E_{max}}$ at 12 months and $\dot{V}_{O_2 max}$ starting at 6 to 12 months (Fig. 6) (23). Gelb and associates (65) showed a similar downward trend in exercise capacity in 7 patients at 24 months after bilateral LVRS via thoracoscopy. At 24 months follow-up only, $\dot{V}_{O_2 max}$ remained significantly higher compared to baseline, while $\dot{V}_{E_{max}}$ and VT_{max} drifted down to preoperative values. At 36 months follow-up, only 9 of 26 (35%) patients showed a persistent improvement in exercise capacity. At 5 years post-LVRS, only 2 of 26 patients showed sustained a clinical benefit, from LVRS (66).

Medications

Of Cooper's original cohort of 20 patients, 42% were steroid dependent preoperatively, whereas only 6 and 11% required systemic steroids at 1 and 2

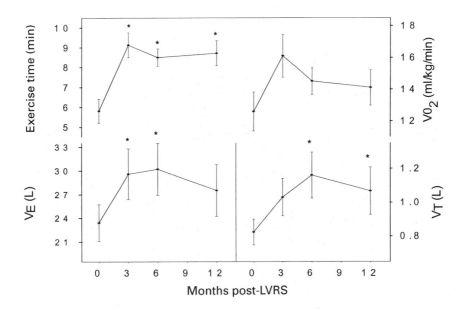

Figure 6 Changes in exercise parameters in 10 patients who underwent bilateral LVRS. Total exercise time and tidal volume were significantly increased at 3 to 6 months post-LVRS and maintained up to 12 months follow-up. The $\dot{V}_{O_2 max}$ were higher at all time points after surgery compared to baseline but did not reach statistical significance maximum minute ventilation ($\dot{V}_{E_{max}}$) was significantly higher at 3 to 6 months post-LVRS. (From Ref. 23.)

years following LVRS (16). In the absence of data from prospective randomized trials, specific guidelines for corticosteroids use, withdrawal, and the use of objective criteria to assess response to therapy, the current data on systemic steroid requirement after LVRS remains anecdotal.

Dyspnea and Quality of Life

Like the declines reported in lung function and exercise capacity over time, the decrease in dyspnea after LVRS also wanes over time, but not necessarily in tandem with the decrement in lung function. Using the Fletcher scale, 12 of 13 patients had an improvement in dyspnea following LVRS (11 unilateral, 2 bilateral). At 2-year follow-up, only 4 of 12 patients continued to enjoy symptomatic relief from dyspnea. No patients maintained an improvement in dyspnea at 48 months follow up (40). In 26 patients with severe emphysema who underwent bilateral LVRS via VATS, Gelb et al. reported a greater than 1 grade decrease in dyspnea scale at 6 months post-LVRS. At 2, 3, 4, and 5 years in follow-up, only 69, 46, 27, and 15% of patients were able to maintain an improvement in dyspnea, respectively (66).

In previously cited studies reporting the long-term outcome following LVRS, too much emphasis has been placed on the stability of physiological changes to the exclusion of the long-term impact of LVRS on the quality of life. Since no correlation has been reported between the improvement in quality of life and the physiological changes after LVRS, the decrement in lung function and quality of life may not necessarily occur at the same time point. We have previously reported that the improvement in the quality of life as measured using the SIP score is maintained for up to 18 months after bilateral LVRS (23).

C. Prospective, Randomized, Clinical Trials

The majority of studies that have reported the results of LVRS are limited by not being prospective, randomized, or controlled trials. Several trials have been reported that have used a control group; a few recent trials are not only prospective and randomized but also include appropriate controls.

Meyers and colleagues (68) reported a retrospective study comparing 22 patients who were candidates for LVRS but were denied the operation secondary to the cessation of Medicare funding, with 65 contemporaneous and comparable LVRS recipients. Patients denied surgery were similar in all baseline measurements to those who received LVRS. A comparison was made between the two groups at 12 and 24 months after baseline data were obtained. Patients who underwent LVRS in comparison to those who were denied LVRS, realized improvements in the need for supplemental oxygen at rest and during exercises decreased steroid requirements were also noted. Furthermore, the authors found that survival for the patients receiving LVRS was 100% at 12 months and 64% at 36 months, in contrast to patients receiving LVRS, in whom the survival was 89% at 12 months and 83% at 36 months.

Although this study's strength was that it had a comparable control group, it was limited because of its small number of subjects, its failure to randomize subjects or to provide follow-up in all subjects in both groups, and the incompleteness of the data collected (i.e., lack of figures regarding quality of life, frequency of hospital admissions, lung volumes, and exercise testing).

Wilkens et al. (69) similarly reported the outcomes of LVRS in comparison to a patient group receiving optimized medical therapy. In this report, 57 patients with emphysema who met standard criteria for LVRS were divided into two groups, according to their own decision, to immediately undergo LVRS or to postpone LVRS for a period $\geqslant 12$ months. There was no significant differences in baseline lung function between the two groups; however, there was a tendency for better functional status in the patient group who postponed LVRS. Significant improvements were observed in the LVRS group compared to the group who decided to postpone LVRS (e.g., control group) in measurements of FEV_1, total lung capacity, residual volume, dyspnea score, and 6-min walk distance on follow-up visits. Failure to randomize, variability in LVRS technique (22 had bilateral LVRS, 6 patients had unilateral LVRS), and short duration of follow-up (i.e., $\leqslant 18$ months) limited the author's conclusion that LVRS is more effective than medical treatment for improvement in dyspnea, lung function, and exercise capacity in patients with severe emphysema.

Recently, however, the results of three prospective, randomized, controlled trials of bilateral LVRS to optimized medical therapy including pulmonary rehabilitation have been reported. Criner and colleagues (55) recruited 200 patients with severe emphysema for a prospective, randomized trial of pulmonary rehabilitation versus bilateral LVRS with stapling resection of 20 to 40% of each lung. Spirometry, lung volumes and diffusing capacity, arterial blood gases, 6-min walk tests, symptom-limited exercise testing, and quality of life were measured in all patients at baseline and after 8 weeks of rehabilitation. The patients were then randomized to either 3 additional months of rehabilitation, or to undergo LVRS. Of 37 patients who met study criteria and were enrolled into the trial, 18 were assigned to the medical arm; 15 of these 18 completed 3 months of additional pulmonary rehabilitation. A total of 32 patients underwent LVRS (19 in the surgical arm and 13 who crossed over from the medical arm). After 8 weeks of pulmonary rehabilitation, pulmonary function tests remained unchanged compared to baseline data. However, there was a trend toward a higher 6-min walk distance (285 ± 96 versus 269 ± 91 m, $p = 0.14$), and total exercise time on maximum exercise testing was significantly longer compared with baseline (7.4 ± 2.1 versus 5.8 ± 1.7 min, $p < 0.001$). Among 15 patients who were randomized to the medical arm and completed 3 months of additional rehabilitation, there was a trend toward a higher maximum oxygen consumption ($\dot{V}_{O_2 max}$, 13.3 ± 3 versus 12.6 ± 3.3 mm/min, $p < 0.08$). In contrast, 3 months post-LVRS, FVC

$(2.79 \pm 0.59$ versus 2.36 ± 0.55 L, $p < 0.001$) and FEV_1 $(0.85 \pm 0.3$ versus 0.65 ± 0.16 L, $p < 0.05$) increased, while TLC $(6.53 \pm 1.3$ versus 7.65 ± 2.1 L, $p < 0.01$) and residual volume (RV, 3.7 ± 1.2 versus 4.9 ± 1.1 L, $p < 0.01$) decreased when compared with 8-week postrehabilitation data. Moreover, Pa_{CO_2} decreased significantly 3 months post-LVRS compared with 8-week postrehabilitation data. The 6-min walk distance, total exercise time, and $\dot{V}_{O_2max}$ were higher after LVRS but did not reach statistical significance. However, when 13 patients who had crossed over from the medical to the surgical arm were included in the analysis, the increases in 6-min walk distance $(337 \pm 99$ versus 282 ± 100 m, $p < 0.01$) and $\dot{V}_{O_2max}$ $(13.8 \pm 4$ versus 12.0 ± 3 mL/kg/min, $p < 0.01$) 3 months post-LVRS were highly significant when compared to postrehabilitation data. The sickness impact profile, which was used as a general measure of life, significantly improved 8 weeks after rehabilitation, with the improvements maintained during 3 months of additional maintenance rehabilitation. Further improvement was noted in the quality of life observed 3 months after LVRS compared with the initial improvement observed 8 weeks after rehabilitation. Following LVRS, there were three postoperative deaths (9.4%); one patient died before surgery (2.7%). After LVRS, the number of hospitalizations, the need for mechanical ventilation and for systemic steroid requirements were reduced. The authors concluded that bilateral LVRS and the addition of pulmonary rehabilitation improved static lung function, gas exchange, and quality of life compared with pulmonary rehabilitation alone but also further suggested larger and longer-term studies to evaluate the risks, benefits, and durability of LVRS over time.

An additional prospective, randomized, and controlled trial involving a small number of patients followed for a shorter period of time has also been reported by Geddes et al. (18). A total of 174 subjects were initially evaluated; of these, 24 were subsequently randomized to receive medical therapy and 24 patients to undergo LVRS. After 15 patients had been randomized, the criteria were modified to exclude patients with a $DL_{CO_2} < 30\%$ of predicted, or a 6-min walk test below 150 m, because deaths were reported in 5 such patients (3 treated with LVRS and 2 treated medically). All potentially eligible patients were given intensive medical therapy and completed a smoking cessation program and a 6-week outpatient rehabilitation program before randomization to LVRS or medical treatment. Six months after randomization, the mean FEV_1 had increased by 70 mL in the surgical group and decreased by 80 mL in the medical group ($p = 0.02$). Median shuttle walk distance increased by 50 m in the surgical group and decreased by 20 m in the medical group ($p = 0.02$). The quality of life did not differ between the two groups at 12-month follow up.

The authors reported that 5 out of 24 patients in the surgical group died (mortality 21%), as did 3 in the medical group (12%, $p = 0.43$). In addition, 5 of the 19 surviving patients in the surgical group had no benefit from the treatment.

Overall, both of the above studies have contributed to the literature in that they were prospective, randomized, controlled trials, demonstrating that LVRS has a short-term beneficial effect on static lung function, exercise capacity, gas exchange, and quality of life, in contrast to optimized medical therapy, including pulmonary rehabilitation. However, the studies were limited by their small numbers, their short periods of observation (3 to 6 months), and the failure to characterize those patients who benefited from LVRS compared to those who did not.

Most recently, preliminary data has been reported from the National Emphysema Treatment Trial (NETT)—a randomized, multicentered clinical trial comparing LVRS with optimized medical treatment, including rehabilitation (37). As previously stated, this study is supported by the National Heart, Lung, Blood Institute, and the center for Medicare and Medicaid services (formally HCFA). The main goal of the trial is to compare survival rates and exercise capacity 2 years after LVRS with results obtained with medical treatment only. Another important goal of the trial is to identify selection criteria for LVRS. Inclusion criteria in this trial were broad enough to include evaluations of subgroups of patients who had traditionally been considered candidates for LVRS but were present in only small numbers in previously reported trials.

In this initial report, a total of 1033 patients had been randomized to receive LVRS or medical therapy by June 2001. In 69 patients who had an FEV_1 less than 20% of predicted, with either a homogeneous distribution of emphysema on high resolution computed tomography (HRCT) of the chest (chest CT), or carbon monoxide diffusing capacity $\leqslant 20\%$ of the predicted value, the 30-day mortality after surgery was 16%, as compared with a mortality of 0% in the medically treated patients ($p < 0.01$). As compared to medically treated patients, survivors of LVRS had only small improvements at 6 months in the maximum symptom-limited exercise testing workload ($p = 0.06$), the 6-min walk distance ($p = 0.03$), and FEV_1, ($p < 0.001$) but a similar health-related quality of life. The results of an analysis of functional outcomes in all patients, which accounted for deaths and missing data, did not favor one form of treatment over the other. In an additional analysis, patients who had all three high-risk characteristics (e.g., $DL_{CO} < 20\%$ of predicted; severe, diffuse homogeneous pattern of emphysema on chest CT; and $FEV_1 \leqslant 20\%$ of predicted), had a 30-day mortality rate following LVRS of 25%.

These data suggest that patients who fit the above profile are not suitable candidates for LVRS because they are at high risk of death; even if they do survive, they are unlikely to receive significant physiological or functional benefit. Since this report, the NETT has been modified to exclude patients exhibiting these characteristics from enrolling into the trial. However, patients who did not meet the above exclusion criteria continued to be enrolled into the trial. The results of LVRS compared to medical treatment in the larger cohort of patients (e.g., approximately 86% of patients randomized into NETT) who did not meet the above criteria are unknown at the present time.

V. Techniques of Lung Volume Reduction Surgery

A variety of surgical techniques have been used in LVRS. These techniques include median sternotomy with bilateral stapling resection (12), VATS performed unilaterally (42,44) or bilaterally with stapling lung resection (21,31), and unilateral VATS with laser ablation of emphysematous tissue (11,70). As previously mentioned, the goal of LVRS is targeted resection of 20 to 30% of the severely emphysematous lung as identified on the preoperative HRCT scan, quantitative ventilation/perfusion $\dot{V}/\dot{Q}$ scan, and intraoperative assessment by the thoracic surgeon.

The type of surgery, whether median sternotomy or VATS, depends largely on the preference of the individual surgeon and the availability of surgical expertise within institutions (30). Bilateral LVRS—whether performed via median sternotomy, or VATS—leads to similar improvements in lung function and exercise capacity (21,22,31), although VATS may be associated with a lower postoperative morbidity and mortality (71). Laser surgery is currently no longer recommended for LVRS because of less than satisfactory results compared to stapled resection (30). In a study by McKenna and coworkers (33) comparing the efficacy of neodymium-yttrium aluminum garnet (Nd-YAG) contact laser surgery to stapled lung resection in 72 patients who underwent unilateral LVRS, there was no difference in postoperative morbidity and mortality between the two groups. However, patients who underwent stapled lung surgery had significantly higher improvements in lung function than did the laser ablation group (FEV$_1$ 33 versus 13%).

A. Bilateral Versus Unilateral Lung Volume Reduction Surgery

In appropriately selected patients, bilateral LVRS is preferred over the unilateral procedure because of greater short-term improvements in lung function after surgery, with comparable perioperative mortality (21,25,34). More importantly, bilateral LVRS via VATS results in better 2-year survival than unilateral LVRS. In a study of 260 COPD patients who underwent LVRS via VATS (bilateral VATS, 159; unilateral VATS, 110), the overall survival at 2 years was 86.4% after bilateral LVRS compared to 72.6% in patients who underwent unilateral LVRS ($p = 0.001$) (72). On the other hand, a recent report involving 673 patients who underwent LVRS showed no survival advantage in patients who underwent bilateral LVRS compared to unilateral LVRS (73). At the present time, because of the better functional outcome reported in patients who have undergone bilateral compared to unilateral LVRS, bilateral LVRS is the preferred surgical approach. Unilateral LVRS should be considered only in patients with an asymmetrical distribution of emphysema and pleural adhesions from prior thoracic surgery (25,30).

VI. Physiological Mechanisms of Improvement with Lung Volume Reduction Surgery

Over the last several years, preliminary data have accumulated regarding proposed mechanisms for the improvement in lung function and exercise performance in some patients following LVRS. These mechanisms have included an increase in airflow secondary to an increase in lung elastic recoil and an increase in airway conductance, an increase in respiratory muscle strength, a decrease in central neural drive, and improved right ventricular systolic function following LVRS.

Approximately 70 years ago, Christie (74) hypothesized that the essential physiological disturbance in emphysema was a loss in lung elasticity, which precipitated an increase in functional residual capacity (FRC) and resulted in hyperinflation and thereby adverse effects on the primary and accessory muscles of inspiration. Butler et al. (75) further demonstrated that, in emphysema patients, when the FRC increased, measurements of airway conductance were reduced. In the 1960s, Rogers et al. (76) demonstrated the effect of removing bullae on airway conductance and the conductance/volume ratio in patients who had isolated large bullae occupying more than one-third of a hemithorax, and in three patients with severe diffuse emphysema without discernible bullae on chest radiographic imaging. In all patients who underwent lung resection, there was a decrease in FRC and an increase in airway conductance and the ratio of airway conductance to volume. This change was sustained for years in patients who had isolated large bullae removed, but the beneficial effects abated over a period of approximately 10 to 15 months in patients who had more diffuse emphysema. The authors speculated that the removal of the bullae precipitated an increase in lung elastic recoil, which triggered an increase in peripheral airway diameter and length, thereby increasing the lung elastic pressure measured at any given lung volume.

A. Effect of Lung Volume Reduction Surgery on Lung Recoil

Recent theoretical models have also implicated an increase in lung elastic recoil as the crucial element responsible for the improvements observed post-LVRS. Fessler and Permut (26) provided a theoretical model supporting the notion that LVRS improves airflow limitation primarily by restoring the balance between the lung and the chest wall as a result of decreasing residual volume more than total lung capacity in patients with severe emphysema and hyperinflation. They surmised that since total lung capacity is reached when the force generated by maximum inspiratory contraction balances the elastic recoil of the lungs and the chest wall, this balance of forces occurs at a lower total lung capacity (TLC) following LVRS. At the lower lung volumes encountered post-LVRS, the inspiratory muscles would be optimized to generate a greater force and lung elastic recoil pressure would also be greater. The authors concluded that these two features of LVRS—increased lung elastic recoil at TLC and the increased ability of the inspiratory muscles to generate force—are the two most likely physiological factors to explain the beneficial effects of LVRS. However, these two factors do not necessarily explain the increase in vital capacity observed post-LVRS. The authors further hypothesized that the ratio of residual volume/total lung capacity (RV/TLC) reflects the mismatch in size of the lungs to the chest walls observed in patients with severe emphysema, and that the magnitude and direction of the change in vital capacity is dominated by the reduction in RV/TLC that occurs following LVRS. Although the above analysis provides keen insight into the determinants of airflow limitation, the potential mechanistic benefits of LVRS outlined by these authors have not been subjected to retrospective or prospective validation.

Substantial data, however, do exist that demonstrate an improvement in lung elastic recoil post-LVRS. Sciurba et al. (45) studied 20 patients with diffuse emphysema following unilateral ($n = 17$) or bilateral ($n = 3$) LVRS. In all patients, static lung elastic recoil pressure curves were generated using transpulmonary pressure (e.g., the difference between esophageal pressure mouth pressure) over a range of lung volumes from TLC to FRC. The authors found that the mean coefficient of retraction, an indicator of lung elastic recoil, increased from $1.3 \pm 0.6\,cmH_2O$ before surgery to $1.8 \pm 0.8\,cmH_2O$ after surgery, ($p < 0.001$). Moreover, the 16 patients who had the greatest postoperative increases in lung recoil also achieved a greater distance in performance of the 6-min walk test than did the 4 patients in whom lung recoil did not increase ($p = 0.02$). The authors found that the increases in lung elastic recoil post-LVRS were associated with significant reductions in TLC, RV, and FRC ($p < 0.001$). Gelb and colleagues (19) corroborated the findings of Sciurba and colleagues in showing that LVRS produces at least a short-term increase in lung elastic recoil, but they extended these results in also showing an increase in airways conductance. Gelb et al. prospectively investigated 12 consecutive patients who underwent bilateral LVRS and measured lung function, static lung elastic recoil, and airway conductance 2 weeks before and 5 to 6 months after LVRS. After LVRS, they found significant reductions in TLC, FRC, and RV. Lung elastic recoil pressure increased markedly at TLC, 10.3 ± 0.5 to $14.6 \pm 1.0\,cmH_2O$, ($p < 0.001$), as did maximal expiratory airflow in every patient. Further analysis of the maximum expiratory flow–static elastic recoil pressure curves indicated that conductance of the S segment (Gs) increased from 0.2 ± 0.03 to 0.27 ± 0.03 L/sec/cmH$_2$O ($p < 0.01$) and critical transmural pressure ($P_{TM}{}^1$), decreased from 3.1 ± 0.2 to $2.4 \pm 0.2\,cmH_2O$ ($p < 0.02$). Furthermore, mean airway conductance increased from 0.14 to 0.22 L/sec/cmH$_2$O ($p < 0.001$). The authors concluded that the improvement in maximum airflow was attributable to both an increased lung elastic recoil, causing an increase in driving pressure, as well as to its secondary effects on tethering open the peripheral airways, thereby causing an increased airways conductance, an increased conductance of the S segment, and a decrease in transluminal pressure. More recently, Gelb et al. (66) showed, in two long-term responders to LVRS (survived $\geqslant 5$ years after surgery), that lung elastic recoil pressures remained increased, as did maximum expiratory flow and conductance of the S segment, compared to preoperative values.

Not all investigators, however, agree that LVRS produces an improvement in airflow by tethering open the small airways or decreasing dynamic compression causing small airway collapse. Ingenito et al. (46) used a mathematical model based on a Taylor expansion of the Pride-Permit equation of flow limitation to examine changes in tests of spirometry and pulmonary mechanics pre- and postoperative bilateral LVRS in 37 patients. They used this mathematical model to examine the relative contributions of changes in lung compliance, lung recoil pressure, small airway conductance, and small airway closing pressure to changes in expiratory flow. The investigators found that the improvement in expiratory flows after LVRS was largely due an increase in lung recoil pressures, and that large improvements in FEV_1 occurred without significant changes in small airway conductance or small airway closing pressure. Moreover, they found that large changes in recoil pressure occurred without changes in lung compliance, supporting the previous arguments of Fessler and Permut that resizing of the lung to the chest wall—that is, a disproportionate reduction in RV to TLC—is the primary mechanism by which LVRS improves lung, chest wall, and respiratory muscle function.

Regardless of the mechanism of the improvement in small airway function, it appears that large and small airway ventilation is improved following LVRS. Travaline et al. (50) used xenon-133 washout curves during lung scintigraphy in patients with severe emphysema. (FEV_1 $0.69 \pm 0.04 \, L$, RV/TLC $65 \pm 2\%$), both before and 3 months post-LVRS. Xenon-133 washout curves during lung scintigraphy exhibit a biphasic pattern; the first component of the washout curve corresponds to an initial rapid washout phase, which reflects larger airways emptying. A second component reflects a slower washout phase, which represents gas elimination from smaller peripheral airways. The authors found that the mean improvement in washout of the large and small airways after LVRS was significantly greater compared to baseline values and that there was no relationship with respect to post-LVRS washout and the lung regions that had or had not been operated on. The increase in small airways ventilation correlated strongly with the increase in FEV_1 ($r = 0.66$, $p < 0.0001$), and decrease in RV/TLC ($r = -0.67$; $p < 0.0001$). Moreover, the increase in small airways ventilation correlated with a decrease in Pa_{CO_2} ($r = -0.39$; $p = 0.003$). The authors concluded that small airways ventilation is improved following bilateral LVRS regardless of the region of lung resection.

B. Effect of Lung Volume Reduction Surgery on Diaphragm Strength

Respiratory muscle strength is reduced in patients with severe emphysema. Most of the reduction in respiratory muscle strength is believed related to the degree of underlying hyperinflation. COPD patients may also have generalized muscle weakness that may be attributable to the inflammatory process occurring in these patients coupled with immobility, which causes disuse atrophy, and also the compounding effect of high-dose systemic steroids. Regardless of the above mechanisms, however, the effect of LVRS on respiratory muscle strength and breathing pattern has been a significant focus of attention.

The adverse effects of hyperinflation on diaphragmatic and inspiratory mechanics have been extensively reported. These include: foreshortening of diaphragm precontraction length, a reduced radius of curvature of the diaphragm, impaired diaphragmatic blood flow, decreased diaphragmatic insertional rib cage action, and a decrease in the area of apposition of the costal diaphragmatic fibers with the lateral chest wall (77–80). A treatment modality, such as LVRS, which simultaneously decreases ventilatory workload and improves respiratory pump function, could have the combined advantage of diminishing ventilatory workload while simultaneously improving maximum ventilatory capacity. Several studies have reported on the effects of LVRS on respiratory muscle recruitment during exercise and on inspiratory muscle strength. Bloch et al. (81) reported in 19 patients with severe emphysema that abdominal paradoxical motion monitored by respiratory inductive plethsmography decreased significantly during restful breathing after bilateral or unilateral LVRS. Benditt et al. (57) examined breathing patterns and respiratory muscle recruitment both before and after LVRS by examining changes in pleural and gastric pressures. Post-LVRS, reductions in expiratory esophageal and gastric pressures at rest and at exercise were observed, suggesting an increased diaphragmatic contribution to breathing. Although both studies suggest an improvement in diaphragmatic strength is responsible for the changes in breathing pattern post-LVRS, no measurements of diaphragmatic strength were provided.

Other studies that examined the effects of LVRS on respiratory muscle strength, however, produced conflicting results. Teschler et al. (82) examined the effects of LVRS on inspiratory muscle strength in 17 severely obstructed, hyperinflated, COPD patients. Twelve of the patients had unilateral LVRS. Investigators found that mean PI_{max} increased by 52%, and $Pdi_{max\ sniff}$ (transdiaphragmatic pressure during maximum sniff maneuver) increased by 28% 1 month postoperatively. On the other hand, Martinez et al. (56) measured maximum mouth and transdiaphragmatic pressures in 17 patients before and after bilateral LVRS. They found a 21% increase in PI_{max} after LVRS but no significant change in $Pdi_{max\ sniff}$. Finally, Keller and colleagues (43) found no effect unilateral LVRS on PI_{max} in 25 subjects despite finding significant changes in spirometry, lung volumes, 6-min walk tests, and ventilatory function during maximum exercise testing.

Why LVRS produced conflicting results on respiratory muscle strength in the preceding reports is unclear, but several reasons can be offered. All of the above studies reported on only a small number of subjects; further, there was significant variability in not only the techniques used to measure respiratory muscle strength but also in the time point post-LVRS at which the tests were performed. Furthermore, the effects of a reduction in systemic steroid use or dose or whether pulmonary rehabilitation or correction of metabolic abnormalities may have contributed to the patient's sense of well being and or respiratory muscle strength were not commented on.

Criner and colleagues (53) reported on the effects of LVRS in 20 patients who had measurements of maximum static inspiratory and expiratory mouth pressures and transdiaphragmatic pressures during maximum static inspiratory efforts and during supermaximal bilateral electrophrenic twitch stimulation. Nineteen of the subjects had bilateral LVRS and one had unilateral LVRS. Measurements of respiratory muscle strength, PI_{max}, 74 ± 28 versus 50 ± 18 cmH_2O, $p < 0.002$; $Pdi_{max\ combined}$, 80 ± 25 versus 56 ± 29 cmH_2O, $p < 0.01$; $Pdi_{max\ sniff}$ 71 ± 7 versus 46 ± 27 cmH_2O, $p < 0.01$; and Pdi_{twitch}, 15 ± 5 versus 7 ± 5 cmH_2O, $p < 0.01$) were all greater, post-LVRS. Inspiratory muscle workload as measured by the tension time index for the diaphragm was lower following LVRS $(0.07 \pm 0.09 \pm 0.03, p < 0.03)$. On multiple regression analysis, Criner et al. found that increases in PI_{max} post-LVRS correlated significantly with decreases in RV and FRC trapped gas after LVRS $(r = 0.67, p < 0.03)$. Despite a significant correlation between a reduction in end-expiratory lung volume and an increase in PI_{max} post-LVRS, he failed to demonstrate a correlation between changes in transdiaphragmatic pressures with a reduction in lung volume. He hypothesized that a small number of subjects with a lesser degree of variability in PI_{max} measurement than measurements of transdiaphragmatic pressures between subjects may have accounted for his inability to determine such a relationship.

In a subsequent study by the same group (83), however, it was determined that the effect of bilateral LVRS on diaphragmatic length, hypothesizing that LVRS, by reducing lung volume, increases diaphragmatic precontraction length, which would precipitate an increase in diaphragmatic force generation. To determine the effects of LVRS on diaphragmatic length, Criner et al. measured diaphragmatic length at TLC using plain chest radiographs in 25 patients before LVRS and 3 to 6 months post-LVRS. A subgroup of 7 patients had diaphragmatic length measurements made on chest x-rays using films made within a year before LVRS evaluation. The measurements of diaphragmatic length included right hemidiaphragm silhouette length, diaphragm length on PA chest x-ray (PADL) and the length of the most vertically oriented position of the right hemidiaphragm muscle, vertical dimension of diaphragm length (VDML). Diaphragmatic dome height was determined from (1) the distance between the dome and transverse diameter at the level of the manubrium and (2) the highest point of the dome referenced horizontally to the vertebral column. Post-LVRS, they found that PADL increased by $4\%(13.9 \pm 1.9$ cmH_2O to 14.5 ± 1.7 cmH_2O; $p = 0.02)$, and VDML increased by 44% (from 2.08 ± 1.5 cmH_2O to 3.0 ± 1.6 $cmH_2O, p = 0.01)$ and diaphragmatic dome height increased by more than 10%. In contrast, diaphragmatic lengths were similar in subjects with chest x-rays made before LVRS and 1 year prior to evaluation. An increase in diaphragmatic length also correlated directly with postoperative reductions in TLC and RV and also with increases in transdiaphragmatic pressure made during maximum sniff assessment ($Pdi_{max\ sniff}$). The investigators concluded that diaphragmatic lengthening is one of the most likely mechanisms resulting in the improvements in diaphragmatic strength observed following LVRS.

Schrager et al. (84) confirmed the effects of LVRS on restoring the normal diaphragmatic length relationship in emphysematous rats. Five months after LVRS was performed in the elastase-induced emphysema rodent model, in situ diaphragmatic length and the length at which maximum diaphragmatic twitch force was generated were longer in animals undergoing bilateral LVRS than in those undergoing sham surgery. Moreover, Cassart et al. (85) performed three-dimensional (3D) reconstructions of the diaphragm using spiral CT of the chest in 11 patients with severe emphysema before and 3 months after LVRS and compared the results to those from 11 normal subjects matched for age, sex, height, and weight. They found that post-LVRS, reduction in lung volume correlated with a more cephalad displacement of the diaphragm and an increase in the area of apposition of the more vertical portion of the diaphragm costal fibers with the chest wall.

This improvement in diaphragmatic and inspiratory muscle function post-LVRS has also been hypothesized to account for a decrease in central neural drive, which may account for a reduction in dyspnea. Lahrmann (86) found a decrease in central diaphragmatic drive assessed by root mean square analysis of the esophageal electromyogram, which correlated with a reduction in dyspnea. Laghi et al. (87) also found that net diaphragmatic neuromechanical coupling, quantified as the quotient of tidal volume (normalized to total lung capacity) to the tidal volume change in Pdi (normalized to Pdi_{max}) improved post-LVRS and also correlated with a reduction in dyspnea ($r = 0.76$, $p = 0.08$). These studies indicate that an improvement in diaphragmatic function may signal an improvement in the electromechanical action of the diaphragm, thus resulting in a reduction in dyspnea.

C. Effect of Lung Volume Reduction Surgery on Pulmonary Hemodynamics

Information regarding the effects of LVRS on pulmonary hemodynamics and cardiac function is limited. Conceptually, LVRS may have varying and even conflicting effects on pulmonary hemodynamics. On the one hand, LVRS may cause a reduction in pulmonary vascular resistance by enabling pulmonary capillary recruitment, secondary to reducing peripheral vascular compression by hyperinflated lung zones or increasing extra-alveolar vascular tethering secondary to increased lung elastic recoil. Moreover, a reduction in end-expiratory lung volume and especially dynamic hyperinflation during exercise may improve right ventricular preload and decrease the development of large swings in intrathoracic pressure, which may embarrass both right and left ventricular performance. On the other hand, resection of lung tissue could decrease the vascular bed, thereby leading to an increase in pulmonary vascular resistance in patients who already have moderate to severe underlying emphysema.

Sciurba and colleagues (45) reported an improvement in right ventricular systolic function when estimated by echocardiographic assessment in 20 patients following unilateral or bilateral LVRS. However, two small studies utilizing right heart catheterization both before and after bilateral LVRS found no significant changes in pulmonary hemodynamic measurements either at rest or during exercise compared to baseline assessment (88,89). In contrast, however, Weg et al. (90) found a rise in group mean pulmonary artery systolic pressure in 9 patients post LVRS compared to baseline data. However, this trend was not exhibited in all 9 patients; 3 of the 9 individuals did not have a significant increase in PA systolic pressure and 2 of the 9 patients had a reduction in pulmonary vascular resistance, not an increase, post-LVRS. In fact, mean pulmonary vasculature resistance was not different for the group post-LVRS in comparison to preoperative data.

Reasons for the discrepancy is findings between the above studies is not clear but may have much to do with the patients selected in regard to the magnitude and extent of underlying emphysema and the amount of lung tissue resected. Powell et al. (91) have shown in a rabbit model of emphysema that LVRS induced sustained increases in PVR in animals with more severe emphysema who had larger resections of lung tissue in contrast to animals with milder forms of emphysema and less extensive resection. Overall, the effects of LVRS on pulmonary hemodynamics and cardiac function are not clear-cut at the present time and more extensive study is required.

VII. Complications of Lung Volume Reduction Surgery

The mortality rates post-LVRS range from as low as 0% to as high as 23% (12,16,18,22,34,55). In carefully selected patients and with an experienced surgeon, postoperative mortality rate is approximately 5% (16,73). The causes of postoperative complications and mortality are shown in Table 3. The most common postoperative complications after LVRS are air leaks, postoperative respiratory failure, and the development of nosocomial pneumonia.

Techniques to decrease the incidence and duration of air leaks have been described (92,93). Recently, postoperative gastrointestinal complications have been reported as a potential serious complication following LVRS (71,94). Diabetes mellitus, steroid use, low preoperative hematocrit value, and the use of parenteral meperidine analgesia have been shown to be predictive of serious gastrointestinal complications after LVRS (94). Rare complications reported to date include the formation of giant bullae (95), metalloptysis (coughing of staples) (96), and acute myocardial infarction (97).

Table 3 Common Causes of Postoperative Morbidity and Mortality Following Bilateral Thoracoscopic Lung Volume Reduction Surgery

Complications	Bilateral LVRS ($N = 343$)
Air leak (%)	68
Pneumonia (day)	14
GI complications (%)	8.3
Tracheostomy (%)	6.2
Arrhythmia (%)	8.9
Heimlich valve at discharge (%)	6.0
Reoperation for bleeding (%)	3.1
Operative mortality	
Respiratory failure (%)	2
Cardiac related (%)	1.5
Sepsis (%)	0.9
Multiorgan failure (%)	1.2
Pneumonia (%)	0.9

Source: Ref. 73.

The impact of a particular surgical technique on the incidence of postoperative complications is now coming to light with widespread use of LVRS. Roberts and colleagues (71) reported the incidence of postoperative complications in 136 patients who underwent bilateral LVRS either via median sternotomy (MS) ($n = 86$) or via the thoracoscopic approach (VATS, $n = 50$). In the VATS group, 38 patients had a bilateral procedure in the same sitting while 12 patients underwent staged procedure. The MS patients were older compared to those in the VATS group (63.9 ± 6.8 versus 59.3 ± 9.4, $p < 0.005$) but were otherwise equally matched for severity of emphysema and functional impairment. Life-threatening events in this study included perforated bowel, pneumonia, aspiration, cardiac arrest, mediastinitis, empyema, tension pneumothorax, seizure, and postoperative bleeding. Patients who had bilateral LVRS via median sternotomy suffered more life-threatening complications (22.1 versus 6%, $p = 0.01$) after surgery than did VATS patients. Moreover, MS patients were likely to be reintubated after the surgery, had a longer stay in the intensive care unit (ICU), and were more likely to require tracheostomy.

VIII. Patient Selection

A. General Criteria

In most reported case series, only about 20 to 25% of patients with severe emphysema who were referred for surgery were deemed to be good LVRS candidates after preoperative evaluation (16,55). Despite numerous published reports, there are no established inclusion and exclusion criteria. More recently, interim analysis from the National Emphysema Treatment Trial (NETT) showed higher postoperative mortality in patients who have an $FEV_1 <20\%$ of predicted with either a homogeneous emphysema pattern on CT scan of the chest or a diffusion capacity $<20\%$ of predicted (37). The reported 30-day mortality in this subgroup of emphysema patients was 16%, compared with no deaths in the 70 medically treated patients. Overall, patients who are considered for LVRS should have spirometric and radiographic evidence of advanced emphysema and remain symptomatic despite optimal medical therapy, including pulmonary rehabilitation. This means that the pulmonary function testing should show evidence of severe, nonreversible airflow obstruction with a FEV_1 in the range of 25 to 45% of predicted evidence of hyperinflation and air trapping, total lung capacity $\geqslant 100\%$ of predicted, and residual volume $\geqslant 150\%$ of predicted. The chest radiograph and HRCT scan should demonstrate emphysematous changes and hyperinflation. A quantitative $\dot{V}/\dot{Q}$ scan is used to quantify variable regions of perfusion within each lung field. The HRCT scan in conjunction with the quantitative $\dot{V}/\dot{Q}$ scan serve to identify lung regions with severe emphysema that can become targets for resection. The role of LVRS in the overall management of patients with advanced COPD is shown in Figure 7.

Exclusion criteria include age above 75 years, tobacco usage within 6 months prior to evaluation, evidence of hypercapnia ($Pa_{CO_2} >55$ mmHg), and moderate to severe pulmonary hypertension (mean PA systolic pressure

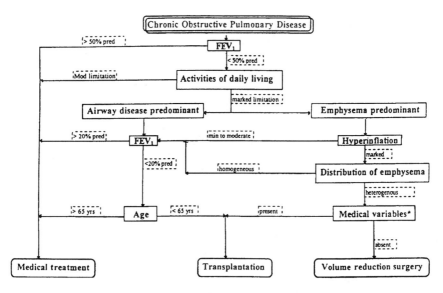

Figure 7 Proposed evaluation of patients with advanced COPD. Medical variables include (1) $Pa_{CO_2} > 55$ mmHg, (2) pulmonary artery mean >35 mmHg, (3) pleural space adhesions, (4) comorbid medical conditions. (From Ref. 126.)

$\geqslant 50$ mmHg). Patients who are obese (body weight $>125\%$ of predicted ideal body weight), undernourished (body weight $<75\%$ of predicted ideal body weight), and who are ventilator-dependent are also similarly excluded. Published inclusion and exclusion criteria used in NETT are listed in Tables 4 and 5, respectively (98). Preoperative testing commonly used to evaluate potential LVRS candidates is shown in Table 6.

Table 4 Inclusion Criteria from the National Emphysema Treatment Trial

Assessment	Criteria
History and physical examination	Consistent with emphysema BMI, $\leqslant 31.1$ kg/m^2 (men) or $\leqslant 32.3$ kg/m^2 (women) at randomization Stable with $\leqslant 20$ mg prednisone (or equivalent)
Radiographic	HRCT scan evidence of bilateral emphysema
Pulmonary function (prerehabilitation)	FEV$_1$, $\leqslant 45\%$ predicted ($\geqslant 15\%$ predicted if age $\geqslant 70$ years) TLC, $\geqslant 100\%$ predicted RV, $\geqslant 150\%$ predicted
Arterial blood gas level (prerehabilitation)	P$_{CO_2}$, $\leqslant 60$ mmHg (Denver criterion: P$_{CO_2}$, $\leqslant 55$ mmHg) P$_{O_2} \geqslant 45$ mmHg (Denver criterion P$_{O_2} \geqslant 30$ mmHg) on room air
Cardiac assessment	Approval for surgery prior to randomization by cardiologists if any of the following are present: unstable angina; LVEF cannot be estimated from the echocardiogram; LVEF $<45\%$; dobutamine-radionuclide cardiac scan indicates coronary artery disease or ventricular dysfunction; arrhythmia (>5 PVCs per minute; cardiac rhythm other than sinus; PACs at rest)
Exercise	Postrehabilitation 6-min walk of $\geqslant 140$ m; able to complete 3 min unloaded pedaling in exercise tolerance test (pre- and postrehabilitation)
Smoking	Plasma cotinine level $\leqslant 13.7$ ng/mL (or arterial carboxyhemoglobin $\leqslant 2.5\%$ if using nicotine products) Nonsmoking for 4 months prior to initial interview and throughout screening

Key: BMI, body mass index; FEV$_1$, forced expiratory volume in 1 sec; HRCT, high-resolution computed tomography; LVEF, left ventricular ejection fraction; PAC, premature atrial contraction; P$_{CO_2}$, partial arterial carbon dioxide pressure; P$_{O_2}$, partial arterial oxygen pressure; PVC, premature ventricular contractions; RV, residual volume; TLC, total lung capacity.
Source: Ref. 98.

In general, emphysema patients who appear to achieve good results from LVRS have the following characteristics: heterogeneous bullous changes in the lung on CT scan (27,99), presence of severe hyperinflation and air trapping (32), absence of severe hypercapnia and pulmonary hypertension (100), and ability to participate in outpatient pulmonary rehabilitation (38). Conversely,

Table 5 Exclusion Criteria from the National Emphysema Treatment Trial—Patients with an FEV_1 <20% and with Either Homogeneous Emphysema Pattern on High-Resolution CT Scan of the Chest or a Diffusion Capacity of <20% Are Now Excluded from the Study

History	Criteria
Previous surgery	Lung transplant
	LVRS
	MS or lobectomy
Cardiovascular	Dysrhythmia that might pose a risk during exercise or training
	Resting bradycardia (<50 beats per minute): frequent multifocal PVCs; complex ventricular arrhythmia; sustained SVT
	History of exercise-related syncope MI within 6 months and LVEF <45%
	Congestive heart failure within 6 months and LVEF <45%
	Uncontrolled hypertension (systolic, >200 mm; diastolic, >110 mm)
Pulmonary	History of recurrent infections with clinically significant sputum production
	Pleural or interstitial disease that precludes surgery
	Clinically significant bronchiectasis
	Pulmonary nodule requiring surgery
	Giant bulla (>1/3 volume of lung)
	Pulmonary hypertension: peak systolic PPA, ≥45 mmHg (Denver criterion; ≥50 mmHg) or mean PPA, ≥35 mmHg (Denver criterion: ≥38 mmHg). (Right heart catheter is required to rule out pulmonary hypertension if peak systolic PPA on echocardiogram is ≥45 mmHg)
	Requirement for >6 L_{O_2} to keep saturation ≥90% with exercise
Radiographic	CT evidence of diffuse emphysema judged unsuitable for LVRS
General	Unplanned weight loss of >10% usual weight in 90 days prior to enrollment
	Evidence of systemic disease or neoplasia expected to compromise survival during 5-year period
	6-min walk distance ≤s140 m after rehabilitation

Key: CT, computed tomography; LVEF, left ventricular ejection fraction; LVRS, lung volume reduction surgery; MI, myocardial infarction; MS, median sternotomy; PPA, pulmonary artery pressure; PVC, premature ventricular contractions; SVT, supraventricular tachycardia.
Source: Ref. 98.

Table 6 Preoperative Diagnostic Test for LVRS

Severity and distribution of emphysema
   Chest radiograph
   High-resolution CT of the chest
   Quantitative lung ventilation/perfusion scan

Pulmonary function tests
   Spirometry
   Lung volume measurements
   Diffusion capacity
   Arterial blood gas

Exercise test
   6-min walk test
   Cardiopulmonary exercise test

Cardiac assessment
   ECG
   Cardiac echocardiogram
   Dobutamine-radionuclide cardiac scan if indicated
   Right- and left-heart catheterization (selected patients)

preoperative hypercapnia of $\geqslant 45\,mmHg$, 6-min walk test of $\leqslant 200\,m$ either pre- or postrehabilitation (100), and very low FEV_1 with either homogeneous or diffusion capacity of $<20\%$ have been shown to be strong predictors of increased mortality after LVRS (37). However, we believe that patients should not be excluded for LVRS in the presence of mild to moderate hypercapnia alone. We recently showed that patients with moderate to severe hypercapnia exhibit a significant improvement in spirometry, gas exchange, and quality of life after bilateral LVRS (101). Although hypercapnic patients showed a lower preoperative FEV_1, lower DL_{CO}, lower Pa_{O_2}/FI_{O_2} ratio, and a lower 6-min walk distance compared to normocapnic patients, the percentage of improvements in FVC, FEV_1, TLC, RV, and RV/TLC were comparable to those in eucapnic patients. Moreover, there was no difference in morbidity and mortality between hypercapnic and eucapnic COPD patients.

One of the reasons for the wide range of improvement in pulmonary function studies that have been published to date is the variability in pattern and distribution of emphysema across patients. In general, emphysema can be divided into three histopathological types, although an overlap of histopathological subtypes is commonly seen in patients with end-stage emphysema. The most common histopathological type of emphysema due to smoking is centrolobular emphysema, which predominantly involves the upper lung zones. In contrast, the predominant histopathological subtype of emphysema seen in hereditary protease deficiency is the panlobular type, which predominantly involves both lower lobes. The third type of emphysema, known as paraseptal emphysema, tends to occur adjacent to fibrous septa or pleura. These different anatomical type of emphysema, especially the centriolobular and the panlobular types, may be seen on HRCT scan of the chest as a heterogeneous distribution of emphysema, with primary involvement of either the upper or lower lung zones, respectively. The same qualitative information on the distribution of emphysema can also be obtained by the quantitative $\dot{V}/\dot{Q}$ scan. Lung areas with severe emphysematous changes will show decreased regional perfusion when compared to other lung zones. Intuitively, it makes sense that emphysematous patients with heterogeneous involvement would benefit most from LVRS, since the most diseased portion of lung is resected, thereby improving ventilation to the relatively better preserved lung zones, akin to the physiological changes following bullectomy. Several reports have shown that morphological grading of the distribution of emphysema may help predict the extent of improvement in expiratory airflow following LVRS (27,99,102).

In general, patients who have a heterogeneous pattern of emphysema appear to have a greater improvement in lung function post-LVRS than patients with a homogeneous pattern. Since, to a certain extent, the idea of LVRS can be thought of as a conceptual extension of the rationale behind bullectomy, it is easy to imagine that patients with a heterogenous emphysema pattern will have areas of the lung that are more severely destroyed relative to the rest of the lung parenchyma. The most diseased portions of the lung identified by HRCT of the chest or quantitative $\dot{V}/\dot{Q}$ lung scanning are identified as target areas for resection. Indeed, 30% of the patients evaluated for LVRS by Cooper's group were excluded from surgery because of a diffuse pattern of emphysema, without focal areas that could be targeted for resection (16). In a study specifically evaluating the impact of the distribution of emphysema on lung function after LVRS, Wisser and coworkers (27) reported lung function in 47 patients who underwent bilateral LVRS according to the distribution of their emphysema on their preoperative chest CT scan. The degree of emphysema heterogeneity (DHG) was divided into grades 1 through 4 (DHG 1 to 4), with the higher grade representing marked heterogeneity of emphysema. The degree of heterogeneity was found to correlate with the extent of improvement in spirometry after LVRS ($r^2 = 0.11, p = 0.04$). The changes in FEV_1 after LVRS according to the assigned to the heterogeneity grade, DHG 1, 2, 3, and 4, were $60 \pm 20\%$, $42 \pm 10\%$, $82 \pm 20\%$, and $160 \pm 29\%$, respectively. In a similar study but using a simplified classification of emphysema, as shown in Figure 8, functional improvement after LVRS was greatest in patients with markedly heterogeneous emphysema, with an increase in FEV_1 of $81 \pm 17\%$, compared to $44 \pm 10\%$ for intermediate heterogenous emphysema and $34 \pm 6\%$ for homogenous emphysema (Fig. 9) (28). It is also important to remember that patients with homogenous emphysema on CT scan also had a significant improvement in lung function after LVRS.

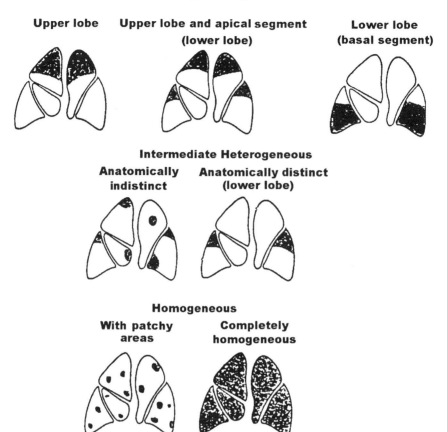

Figure 8 Different patterns of emphysema according to the distribution of alveolar destruction. (From Ref. 109.)

B. Extended Indications for Lung Volume Reduction Surgery

Ventilator-Dependent Emphysema Patients

The prognosis of ventilator-dependent COPD patient is poor, with several studies reporting 30 to 49%, 2- to 3-year survival rates (103). Unfortunately, ventilator-dependent COPD patients are often excluded from LVRS evaluation because of pre-existing respiratory failure, significant pulmonary hypertension, and deconditioning. We recently reported on three ventilator-dependent COPD patients who were successfully weaned from mechanical ventilation after LVRS (104). All three had severe COPD ($FEV_1 - 0.41$ L in two patients), chronic hypercapnia ($Pa_{CO_2} - 55$ mmHg in two patients and

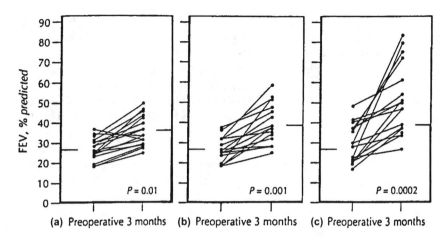

Figure 9 Changes in FEV_1 before and 3 months after bilateral thoracoscopic LVRS in patients with (a) homogeneous emphysema, ($n = 17$, $p = 0.01$), (b) intermediately heterogeneous emphysema, ($n = 16$, $p = 0.001$), (c) markedly heterogenous emphysema ($n = 18$, $p = 0.0002$). (From Ref. 109.)

70 mmHg in one patient), and significant respiratory muscle weakness (mean maximum inspiratory mouth pressure of $29 \, cmH_2O$). In addition, all three patients had evidence of cor pulmonale by echocardiogram.

All three patients had had multiple episodes of intubation and mechanical ventilation due to acute exacerbations of their underlying COPD; at the time of LVRS evaluation, they have been on mechanical ventilation anywhere from 11 to 16 weeks. All three patients had been on oral steroids, which were weaned to lowest possible dose prior to LVRS. All patients were admitted to our Ventilator Rehabilitation Unit, which is a noninvasive respiratory care unit emphasizing respiratory and whole-body reconditioning so as to maximize the condition of patients weaning from prolonged mechanical ventilation. However, despite aggressive medical care, all three patients failed multiple attempts at weaning.

After LVRS, there was a significant improvement in gas exchange parameters, as evidenced by an increase in Pa_{O_2}/FI_{O_2} and reduction in Pa_{CO_2}. In addition, there was a significant improvement in FVC and maximum inspiratory mouth pressure. Postoperative complications included persistent air leaks and one tension pneumothorax. All patients were successfully weaned from mechanical ventilation after 10 to 21 days and were discharged home.

Since this initial report, we have performed LVRS in three additional ventilator-dependent COPD patients and have reported their clinical outcome on prolonged follow-up (mean 12 months) (105). Of the 6 patients we have reported to date, one died 3 months post-LVRS from sepsis and multiple system organ failure. Schmid and others (106) reported a patient with severe emphysema and mitral stenosis who was originally scheduled to undergo combined LVRS and mitral valve replacement. However, due to intraoperative complications, LVRS was postponed. The postoperative course was complicated, including cardiac tamponade, bilateral pneumothoraces, and a large left bronchopleural fistula. Based on this stormy postoperative course, the authors concluded that extubation was impossible. The patient subsequently underwent LVRS on the third and tracheostomy on the fifth postoperative days. The patient was decannulated 18 days after LVRS. Hansson et al. (107) described a dramatic case of a 51-year-old male who developed bilateral pneumothoraces, respiratory failure requiring mechanical ventilation, and massive bilateral air leaks who underwent LVRS as an "emergency and lifesaving procedure." Not only did the patient survive but his FEV_1 at 3 months increased by almost 100%. Like those in our case series, the patient in this report showed a substantial improvement in respiratory function 3 months after LVRS. Unlike those in our case series, the patient in this report was on the ventilator for only a short period of time and therefore may not have been deconditioned or undernourished, as typically seen in patients on prolonged mechanical ventilation. Nevertheless, the authors concluded that LVRS facilitated successful weaning of their patient.

More recently Murtuza et al. (108) reported a patient with severe emphysema who was admitted with acute respiratory failure. The patient had had two previous episodes of airway intubation and mechanical ventilation and had been on nocturnal nasal intermittent positive-pressure ventilation for 12 months. During her hospital stay, she was increasingly difficult to ventilate despite permissive hypercapnia. CT of the chest showed regional heterogenous emphysema predominantly affecting both upper lobes. She underwent bilateral LVRS via a "clamshell" incision on the 18th hospital day. On the 12th postoperative day, she was able to sustain spontaneous ventilation for an extended period of time, and was successfully extubated on the 19th postoperative day. She was discharged on the 30th postoperative day with oxygen therapy and nocturnal noninvasive positive-pressure ventilation.

Based on our experience and that of other investigators, LVRS in a select group of ventilator-dependent COPD patients may improve gas exchange, spirometry, and respiratory muscle function so as to improve functional status and the ability to be weaned from ventilator support. We believe that only patients a with heterogenous distribution of emphysema should be considered for LVRS. Patients with mild to moderate hypercapnia may undergo LVRS without an increase in morbidity or mortality (101). We would like to emphasize, however, that our series of patients, described above, were treated in a special unit geared toward reconditioning the ventilated patients. Therefore we recommend that surgery in ventilator-dependent COPD should be done only in centers with a multidisciplinary team that includes pulmonologists; respiratory, physical, occupational, and speech therapists; a psychologist, and nutritionists skilled in the care of ventilator-dependent patients in order to optimize the patient's overall condition prior to LVRS.

Lung Cancer/Nodules

Both benign and malignant nodules have been detected in patients referred for LVRS either during routine preoperative workup [chest radiograph and conventional CT or HRCT (109–112) at the time of surgery] or after histopathological review (113,114). The overall incidence of pulmonary nodules in patients who are referred for LVRS evaluation is between 11 to 40% (109–112). The incidence of lung cancer in patients who undergo simultaneous LVRS and lung resection is reported to be between 5 and 6% (109–112,115). In one of the largest case series reported to date, McKenna and Fischel et al. (110) reported 53 lung masses in 51 of 325 patients who underwent LVRS. On histological diagnosis, 43 lesions (in 42 patients) were found to be benign and 11 lesions were non-small-cell lung cancer. The benign lesions included 20 calcified nodules, 17 granulomas, 4 fibrotic nodules, and 1 hematoma. Two patients had both a granuloma and lung cancer. Of the 11 patients with clinical stage 1 lung cancer, 3 patients were referred for lung cancer and LVRS, 7 patients were diagnosed by CT during evaluation, and 1 patient was diagnosed after histopathological analysis. Thus the incidence of lung cancer by routine chest CT in the course of LVRS evaluation was 2%.

CT is the single best ancillary test to diagnose unsuspected pulmonary nodules in patients who are undergoing LVRS evaluation. In one study involving 148 LVRS candidates, preoperative CT scans detected 18 pulmonary nodules that were suspicious for primary lung cancer (112); 16 of these lesions were resected during LVRS. Nine non-small-cell carcinomas were detected in 8 patients, yielding a 5% incidence of lung cancer. The median size of the malignant lesions was 1.6 cm (range 1.0 to 3.8 cm), whereas the benign lesions were 1.0 cm (range 0.7 to 2.0 cm).

In another study involving 281 patients who underwent LVRS, 147 nodules were identified in 111 (40%) patients (109). The majority of lung nodules were identified preoperatively by chest CT. However, 14 were identified intraoperatively and another 14 were only identified after careful histological analysis. Of these nodules, 57 were calcified and were thought to be benign. Twelve nodules were resected and pathological analysis confirmed the benign nature of the lesions. The other remaining nodules were followed clinically and were reported to be stable in size with a mean follow-up of 23 months. On the other hand, there were 20 noncalcified lesions on CT scan, which were also followed clinically. Nineteen of these nodules remained radiographically stable after 18.5 months of follow-up, and one nodule was eventually diagnosed as squamous cell carcinoma, resulting in the patient's demise 18 months after the nodule was initially identified. Overall, a total of 78 nodules were resected in this study, of which 61 (78.2%) were benign and 17 (21.8%) were neoplastic. The most common benign diagnosis was granuloma (29), fibrosis (17), and hematoma (5). Among the neoplastic lesions, adenocarcinoma (7), squamous cell carcinoma (3), and large cell carcinoma (2) topped the list. One case each of bronchoalveolar carcinoma, beta-cell lymphoma, carcinoid, mesothelioma, and renal cell metastasis was found. The overall incidence of malignancy in the 281 patients was 6.4% (18 patients). The size of the primary lung cancer ranged from 0.5 to 3.2 cm with a mean size of 1.6 cm. The size of the primary lung cancer not detected radiographically was 0.76 cm. This study emphasizes that chest CT is not capable of diagnosing all lung lesions, especially less than 0.75 cm in size.

Based on the above studies involving 754 patients, the incidence of pulmonary nodules in the course of LVRS workup was 24%. Of these, 4.7% were unsuspected primary lung cancer. The majority of the diagnosed lung cancers are in their early stages and can be resected with curative intent. Thus preoperative CT may serve a dual role, not only to characterize the pattern of parenchymal destruction due to emphysema but also to detect early, potentially curable lung cancers. The wide range in the reported incidence of pulmonary nodules may reflect different study populations, varying definitions of pulmonary nodules among authors, different methods of detection, and the variable incidence of benign pulmonary nodules based on geographic location. Further investigation is required.

Preoperative Evaluation of Lung Nodules for Resection and LVRS

Before LVRS was made possible by advances in thoracic surgical techniques and modern cardiothoracic anesthesia, the majority of patients with severe COPD and pulmonary nodules would have been deemed inoperable using standard preoperative criteria for lung resection owing to their limited pulmonary reserve. For example, one recent study showed successful postoperative recovery and short-term improvement in lung function in 11 patients who underwent combined LVRS and resection of pulmonary nodules (111). If two of the standard preoperative criteria for lung resection were applied to these patients (postoperative FEV_1 of <40% and oxygen desaturation with exercise to <89%), all 11 would have been classified as at very high risk for lung resection, and surgical resection would not have been considered. If an FEV_1 of <0.6 L and a predicted postoperative DL_{CO} of <40%, were applied to the same patient group, 4 of 11 and 4 of 9 patients, respectively, would have been deemed inoperable surgical candidates. Thus current experience suggests that standard preoperative criteria for pulmonary nodule resection may not predict postoperative respiratory insufficiency in highly select severe COPD patients if resection of the lung nodule is combined with LVRS. Moreover, several studies have shown no increase in mortality and morbidity in patients who undergo combined pulmonary nodule surgery and LVRS compared to LVRS alone (109–112,115).

During preoperative evaluation, patients who are considered for pulmonary nodule resection and LVRS should have the following questions answered: (1) Is the patient a good candidate for LVRS? (2) Is the tumor accessible via bronchoscopy or transthoracic needle biopsy for preoperative histologic diagnosis? (3) Is the nodule located in an area of the lung with the worst emphysema? (4) Are there any hilar or mediastinal nodes that are suspicious for metastasis on CT scan? These questions should be answered during the preoperative evaluation period to optimize lung cancer surgery and to preserve residual lung function.

It is important to remember that all of the patients with severe COPD who were reported to have pulmonary nodule resection and LVRS were initially referred for LVRS evaluation. Once the patient fulfills the preoperative clinical criteria for LVRS, as previously discussed, careful interpretation of the HRCT scan for regional heterogeneity of emphysema is conducted, since the expected improvement in lung function after LVRS should counterbalance the lung tissue removal during lung nodule resection.

The majority of reported patients who have undergone lung nodule resection and LVRS have not undergone preoperative bronchoscopy or had transthoracic needle biopsy performed. This is because most of the nodules are small and located at the periphery of the lung parenchyma, making the yield of bronchoscopy very low. Additionally, the presence of significant bullous lung disease increases the risk of pneumothorax, a severe consequence, rendering transthoracic needle biopsy an infrequently used technique in these patients. The usefulness of these two procedures needs to be evaluated on a case-by-case basis. In certain clinical situations, a preoperative histological diagnosis may be required. Moreover, a preoperative diagnosis of lung cancer should include a complete staging evaluation to look for unsuspected metastases or other significant medical problems (e.g., cardiac dysfunction).

The location of the pulmonary nodule is very important in planning the type of thoracic surgery. Ideally lobectomy with hilar node sampling is the preferred surgical technique, rather than simple wedge resection, for stage I lung cancer. Previous studies have shown that lobectomy for stage I non-small-cell lung carcinoma improves survival and decreases the incidence of local recurrence (116). However, if the lung cancer is located in an area of relatively normal lung parenchyma, lobectomy may lead to postoperative respiratory insufficiency. In this circumstance, wedge resection may be the procedure of choice to avoid loss of remaining functioning lung tissue (117). If the lung cancer is located in an area of the lung that is extensively destroyed by emphysema, then a lobectomy, the surgical choice for optimal lung cancer surgery, is the preferred surgical procedure (116,118).

An accurate assessment of hilar and mediastinal lymph nodes for metastatic disease is important for both the treatment and prognosis of primary lung cancer. This is even more important in this group of patients who are undergoing LVRS and clinical stage I lung cancer surgical resection, since mediastinal and subcarinal lymph nodes are inadequately exposed when median sternotomy is used. Although chest CT has good negative predictive accuracy in the evaluation of mediastinal lymph node metatasis, it does not completely rule out mediastinal metastases in patients with stage I disease. In a recent study involving 575 patients with clinical stage I non-small-cell lung carcinoma who underwent lobectomy and systematic mediastinal lymphadenectomy, 79 patients (14%) had positive mediastinal lymph metastases on pathological examination (119). In addition, 54 of the 79 patients had intraoperatively normal-appearing mediastinal lymph nodes. The authors concluded that systematic staging of the mediastinal lymph nodes is necessary in all patients with resectable clinical stage 1 lung cancer. To avoid this dilemma, preoperative mediastinoscopy should be considered, especially if median sternotomy is the planned surgical approach.

Outcome of Combined Pulmonary Nodule Resection in Patients Undergoing Lung Volume Reduction Surgery

Based on the basic guidelines of lung cancer surgery and LVRS previously discussed, several investigators have reported encouraging early results of combined solitary pulmonary nodule resection and LVRS in patients with severe emphysema.

McKenna and associates reported 51 patients who underwent combined LVRS and pulmonary nodule resection within a larger series of 325 patients who underwent LVRS (110). The clinical outcomes of 11 patients with clinical stage I non-small-cell lung cancer who underwent either wedge resection (8) or lobectomy with lymph node dissection combined with LVRS were reported in detail. There were no reported perioperative deaths or major complications. The average length of hospital stay was 8.7 days. Despite substantial lung resection in addition to the standard LVRS procedure (20–30% of each lung was resected), the group mean FEV_1 significantly increased to 1079 mL after surgery, compared to a baseline value of 654 mL. No patients showed any decline in FEV_1 postoperatively. In 4 cancer patients who underwent lobectomy (3 patients with right upper lobe (RUL) and 1 patient with right lower lobe (RML)), substantial increases in FEV_1 were also observed. Using the Medical Outcome Study SF-36, the authors reported that 7 of 11 patients experienced a significant decline in perceived dyspnea postoperatively. The range of follow-up was between 2 and 22 months, with a mean of 9.7 months. In 5 patients who had >12 months of follow-up, no tumor recurrences were documented.

In another large series of 281 severe COPD patients who underwent LVRS, Hazelrigg and others (109) identified 148 nodules, 78 of which were resected. Seventeen of the resected nodules were found to be neoplastic on histopathological examination. Interestingly, 9 of the 17 resected neoplastic lesions were not diagnosed preoperatively; 2 turned out to be primary lung cancer. Of the 17 nodules, 13 were primary lung cancer. Among the 13 patients with lung cancer, 10 had pathological stage I disease, 2 had stage II, and 1 had stage IV disease. All patients underwent wedge resection and nodal dissection if malignancy was recognized intraoperatively. The reported overall in-hospital mortality for the 281 patients was 5%. There were 5 deaths in the neoplastic group during follow-up: 1 with metastatic renal cell carcinoma, 1 unresectable mesothelioma, 2 with progression of primary lung carcinoma, and 1 with a stroke 10 months after surgery. Twelve patients were disease-free with a mean follow-up of 14.3 months. No lung function data were provided in this study.

Do patients who undergo combined LVRS and lung nodule resection have higher perioperative morbidity and mortality? This question was answered in part by a retrospective study reported by Ojo and Martinez (111), who compared the clinical outcome of 11 patients who had combined lung nodule resection and LVRS (LVRS group), with a cohort of age and sex-matched lung cancer patients who had undergone standard lobectomy during the same period (control group). The rate of postoperative complications and the length of hospital stay between the two study groups were comparable. The LVRS group had very limited lung reserve prior to surgical resection, while the control group had normal baseline lung function. In the LVRS group, mean FEV_1 was $26 \pm 2\%$ of predicted and all patients had oxygen desaturation on 6-min walk test. In addition, 2 patients had a $Pa_{CO_2} > 45\,mmHg$. At 3 months follow-up, the LVRS and nodule resection groups had 47 and 25% increases in FEV_1 and FVC, respectively. Moreover, all study patients reported less dyspnea after surgery as measured by the Transitional Dyspnea Index. The study was limited by the small number of patients and by its retrospective design. In addition, the study groups may not have been comparable, since only 3 patients from the LVRS group who had stage I non-small-cell lung carcinoma underwent tumor wedge resection.

The issue of whether hypoxemia, hypercapnia (defined as $Pa_{CO_2} > 45\,mmHg$). and preoperative steroid dependence would preclude combined lung nodule resection surgery and LVRS was recently addressed by in a study of 21 patients with severe emphysema and concomitant pulmonary nodules (115). Seven patients were deemed inappropriate candidates for combined LVRS and pulmonary nodule resection based on inclusion and exclusion criteria previously discussed. Mediastinoscopy was performed only if suspicious lymph nodes ($>1\,cm$) were detected on CT scan. The surgical approach was tailored to the anatomical distribution of the lesion in relation to the preoperative targeted emphysematous areas of the lung. Seven patients underwent unilateral resection through a posterolateral thoracotomy, one through a VATS. Three had bilateral LVRS via median sternotomy and 3 through bilateral anterior thoracosternotomy. Due to concern for the development of persistent air leaks and bronchopleural fistula, routine intraoperative hilar nodal sampling was not routinely performed. Twelve of the pulmonary nodules were within the target areas of emphysema resection, while the remaining 4 nodules required separate wedge resection.

In 14 patients, with severe emphysema (mean FEV_1 $24 \pm 5\%$) who underwent combined LVRS and pulmonary nodule resection, 10 patients were oxygen dependent, 5 had hypercapnia, and 5 were steroid dependent. The mean age of the study group was 69 ± 2 years old, with 7 patients older than 70 years old and the oldest being age 80. Sixteen lesions were resected and 9 lesions were non-small-cell carcinoma. All patients were extubated in the operating room. Three patients had prolonged air leaks (>14 days); one of these required surgical repair. One patient had postoperative ileus and another experienced a transient neurological event. There was one postoperative death in a patient who had prior ipsilateral lung operation; it was attributed to a large bronchopleural fistula. At 6 months follow-up, significant improvements in FEV_1, dyspnea score, and 6-min walk test were documented. Moreover, there was a significant decrease in Pa_{CO_2} after surgery, from a baseline of 46.8 ± 2.9 to 39.6 ± 1.7 mmHg postoperatively. One patient had a mediastinal recurrence 12 months after surgery from two separate lesions found to be bronchoalveolar carcinoma. The rest of the patients were alive and well at a mean follow-up of 22.6 months (range 12 to 35 months).

In almost of the patients described above, limited resection or segmentectomy was utilized for fear of further loss of lung function. However, in a randomized trial comparing surgical outcome of lobectomy versus segmentectomy in stage I non-small-cell lung cancer, segmentectomy or limited resection was associated with an increased risk of local recurrence and a reduction in both overall and disease-free survival (116). Whether patients with advanced emphysema can tolerate optimal surgery for stage I non-small-lung cancer is not clear. This problem is compounded by the fact that the degree of improvement in lung function after LVRS is poorly predicted by preoperative static lung function and cardiopulmonary exercise testing.

In an attempt to determine outcome following combined lobectomy for lung cancer treatment and LVRS, Demeester et al (118) recently reported their experience with 5 patients who underwent combined lobectomy and LVRS. The mean age of the 5 patients was 62 years (range 53–70), 3 were male, 2 were oxygen-dependent, and 1 was on prednisone 30 mg/day. Of these patients, 4 had preoperative diagnoses of lung cancer and 2 were found to have concomitant cardiac disease on noninvasive cardiac evaluation. One patient required angioplasty before LVRS and lobectomy, the other patient had low cardiac ejection fraction but no active ischemia was identified. All patients, except one underwent 6 to 8 weeks of pulmonary rehabilitation prior to surgery. All patients underwent intraoperative bronchoscopy and 4 patients with preoperative diagnosis of lung cancer also underwent mediastinoscopy. A median sternotomy was used in 4 patients and 1 patient underwent bilateral staged thoracotomy because of prior pleurectomy on the left for treatment of recurrent spontaneous pneumothorax. Two patients had lobectomy of the right middle lobe in addition to LVRS. After surgery, all patients were reported to have significant improvement in lung function. There were no deaths; however, 3 of 5 patients had postoperative complications. One patient developed pneumothorax and retained airway secretions, requiring reintubation and mechanical ventilation for 24 hr. Two patients had postoperative bleeding into the extrapleural space created by pleural tents. Both patients improved with conservative management and did not require further surgical intervention. Four patients had pathological stage 1 lung cancer; 1 patient had stage II lung cancer and received adjuvant radiation therapy. No recurrence was detected in any patients with mean follow-up of 19 months.

Overall, all prior studies showed that combined pulmonary nodule resection and LVRS can be done in a highly select group of COPD patients who are deemed good candidates for LVRS. Although most of the studies are small and limited by retrospective design, it appears that perioperative morbidity and mortality are acceptable and not different than in patients who undergo LVRS alone. Since untreated lung cancer confers a 100% mortality and there is no other treatment that can potentially cure stage 1 non-small-cell lung cancer, surgery seems to be a rationale approach to consider in selected patients with severe COPD who are deemed to be good LVRS candidates. However, it is premature to conclude that wedge resection with limited nodal dissection offers a survival advantage comparable to standard lobectomy with hilar and mediastinal dissection in the surgical treatment of lung cancer. Additional studies are needed to compare the various surgical types of treatment with/or without the use of neoadjuvant chemo- or radiotherapy.

Cardiovascular Procedures

Since COPD patients are typically males in their sixth decade of life with greater than 50 pack-years of smoking history, it is not uncommon to uncover significant concomitant cardiac disease in the course of LVRS evaluation. However, the diagnosis of coronary artery disease (CAD) may not be readily apparent, since most patients with severe COPD are forced to live sedentary lives due to incapacitating breathlessness brought on by a limited ventilatory reserve. Thus these patients may either have asymptomatic cardiac disease that is masked by severe lung disease or they may present with atypical symptoms such as frequent COPD exacerbations not readily amenable to standard medical therapy. Indeed, the incidence of asymptomatic but significant CAD in patients who undergo LVRS evaluation has been estimated to be as high as 15% in one study (120). Our data confirm the high prevalence of silent ischemic heart disease in COPD patients as reported by others. Since the inception of our LVRS and lung-transplant program, we screened 336 patients with severe COPD between June 1993 and August 1998. A total of 115 patients underwent left-heart catheterization as part of their routine evaluation. Of 115 patients, 105 were asymptomatic for CAD, 6 had a previous history of CAD, 2 had symptoms of CAD, and 2 had abnormal exercise stress tests. A total of 33 patients (30%) had angiographic evidence of significant CAD. Twenty of the 33 patients had severe CAD (17%); 10 of these were completely asymptomatic and underwent only routine cardiac catheterization. The true incidence of COPD and CAD is probably higher, since patients who have a history of myocardial infarction or congestive heart failure are often excluded from LVRS evaluation.

Combined Lung Volume Reduction Surgery and Coronary Artery Bypass Grafting

The technical feat of combined pulmonary resection and cardiac surgery has been successfully performed in only a small number of patients. In the pre-

LVRS era, the majority of combined cardiothoracic surgeries involving coronary artery bypass with resection of lung tissue have been reported only in cases requiring resection of suspected malignant pulmonary nodules. Since the reintroduction of LVRS, several investigators, including our group, have reported the feasibility of combined LVRS and coronary artery bypass grafting (120). The concept of combined major thoracic and cardiac surgery is appealing because a single combined procedure avoids the risk of a second major operation and may result in reduced overall hospitalization and medical costs and improved patient survival. In addition, LVRS may make coronary artery bypass possible in patients with severe emphysema by significantly improving lung function postoperatively, thus decreasing postoperative morbidity and mortality due to respiratory failure.

Furukawa et al. (121) reported a 60-year-old male with peripheral vascular disease and triple-vessel coronary artery disease with greater than 90% blockage who also had severe COPD (FEV_1 29%) who underwent bilateral LVRS and four vessel coronary artery bypass grafting. Ten months after surgery, he was off supplemental oxygen, his FEV_1 increased to 1.3 L, he had no further angina, and all bypass grafts were patent. Successful coronary artery bypass grafting $3\frac{1}{2}$ months after bilateral LVRS has also been reported (122). However, cardiopulmonary bypass can potentially contribute to postoperative morbidity. There is a danger of pulmonary hemorrhage due to anticoagulation during cardiopulmonary bypass. Some authors recommend resection after reversal of anticoagulation with protamine sulfate (123). In a recent review from the University of Toronto, among 19 patients who underwent resection during cardiopulmonary bypass, only 1 patient suffered from a bleeding requiring reexploration (124). The greater application of off-bypass coronary artery grafting may avoid the risk of perioperative hemorrhage and extend the application of combined coronary artery revasculization with LVRS in selected candidates. Currently, there are no comprehensive data making it possible to evaluate the true risks and benefits of combined LVRS and coronary artery revascularization in patients with severe lung and heart disease.

IX. Summary

LVRS promises to be an important palliative surgical tool in improving lung mechanics, alleviating dyspnea, and improving exercise tolerance in patients suffering from severe, progressive emphysema whose condition was previously maximized on medical therapy, including rehabilitation. A number of recent studies have shown that LVRS has important physiological and functional improvements enabling an improved quality of life in patients suffering from severe emphysema. However, many questions still remain regarding LVRS—specifically, characterization of the appropriate candidate, variability in LVRS response, durability of the beneficial effects of LVRS, the best surgical approach to performing LVRS, and the best tests that not only allow the characterization of patients likely to benefit from the procedure but also make it possible to gauge the extent of optimal resection.

The National Emphysema Treatment Trial (NETT) is currently under way and has the potential to define the optimum patient for LVRS, the durability of LVRS response, the mechanisms important in improving lung and exercise tolerance after LVRS, and ultimately the effect of LVRS in contrast to medical therapy on survival. Hopefully, information from NETT in combination with other investigations will help define the place of LVRS in the treatment of patients with severe emphysema.

References

1. Pauwels RA, Buist AS, Calverly PMA, Jenkins CR, Hurd SS, on behalf of the Gold Scientific Commitee. Global strategy for the diagnosis, management, and prevention of chronic obstructive pulmonary disease: NHLBI Global Initiative for Chronic Obstructive Lung Disease (GOLD) workshop Summary. Am J Respir Crit Care Med 2001; 163:1256–1276.
2. Saetta M, DiStefano A, Tuato G, Facchini FM, Corbino L, Mapp CE, et al. CD 8 + T-lymphocytes in the peripheral airways of smokers with chronic obstructive pulmonary disease. Am J Respir Crit Care Med 1998; 157:822–826.
3. Saetta M, Turato G, Maestrelli P, Mapp CE, Fabbri LM. Cellular and structural basis of chronic obstructive pulmonary disease. Am J Respir Crit Care Med 2001; 163:1304–1309.
4. Pride N, Hugh-Jones P, O'Brien EN, Smith LA. Changes in lung function following the surgical treatment of bullous emphysema. Am J Med 1970; 153:49–69.
5. Fitzgerald MX, Keelan PJ, Cugell DW, Gaensler EA. Long-term results of surgery for bullous emphysema. J Thorac Cardiovasc Surg 1974; 68:566–587.
6. Connolly JE, Wilson A. The current status of surgery of bullous emphysema. J Thorac Cardiovasc Surg 1989; 97:351–361.
7. Travaline J, Addonizio VP, Criner GJ. Effect of bullectomy on diaphragm strength. Am J Respir Crit Care Med 1995; 152:1697–1701.
8. Brantigan OC, Mueller E. Surgical treatment of pulmonary emphysema. Ann Surg 1957; 23:789–804.
9. Pompeo E, Marino M, Nofroni I, Matteucci G, Cladio M. Reduction pneumoplasty versus respiratory rehabilitation in severe emphysema. Ann Thorac Surg 2000; 70:948–954.
10. Brantigan OC, Mueller E, Kress MB. A surgical approach to pulmonary emphysema. Am Rev Respir Dis 1959; 80:194–202.
11. Wakabayashi A. Thorocoscopic laser pneumoplasty in the treatment of diffuse bullous emphysema. Ann Thorac Surg 1995; 60:936–942.
12. Cooper J, Trulock EP, Triantafillou AN, et al. Bilateral pneumonectomy (volume reduction) for chronic obstructive pulmmonary disease. J Thorac Cardiovasc Surg 1995; 109:106–119.
13. Butler CW, Sundyer M, Wood DE, Curtis JR, Albert RK, Benditt JO. Underestimation of mortality following lung volume reduction surgery resulting from incomplete follow-up. Chest 2001; 119:1056–1060.

14. Huizenga HG, Ramsey SD, Albert RK. Estimated growth of lung volume reduction surgery among medicare enrollees. Chest 1998; 114:1583–1587.

15. Shalala DE. Report to Congress: lung volume reduction surgery and medicare coverage policy implication of recently published evidence, 1998. Federal Pub 1998; Vol. 1.

16. Cooper JD, Patterson GA, Sundaresan RS, Trulock EP, Yusen RD, Pohl M, Lefrak S. Results of 150 consecutive bilateral lung volume reduction procedures in patients with severe emphysema. J Thorac Cardiovasc Surg 1996; 112:1319–1330.

17. Eugene J, Ott RA, Gogia HS, Santos CD, Zeit R, Kayaleh RA. Video-thoracic surgery for treatment of end-stage bullous emphysema and chronic obstructive pulmonary disease. Am Surg 1995; 61:934–936.

18. Geddes D, Davies M, Koyama H, Hansell D, Pastorino V, Pepper J, et al. Effect of lung volume reduction surgery in patients with severe emphysema. N Engl J Med 2000; 343:239–245.

19. Gelb AF, Zamel N, McKenna RJ, Brenner M. Mechanism of short-term improvement in lung function after emphysema resection. Am J Respir Crit Care Med 1996; 154:945–951.

20. Hamacher J, Bloch KE, Stammberger U, Schmid RA, Laube I, Russi EW, et al. Two years' outcome of lung volume reduction surgery in different morphologic emphysema types. Ann Thorac Surg 1999; 68:1792–1798.

21. Hazelrigg SR, Boley TM, Magee MJ, Lawyer CH, Henkle JQ. Comparison of staged thoracoscopy and median sternotomy for lung volume reduction. Ann Thorac Surg 1998; 66:1134–1139.

22. Kotloff RM, Tino G, Bavaria JE, Palevskey HI, Hansen-Flaschen J, Wahl PM, Kaiser LR. Bilateral lung volume reduction surgery for advanced emphysema: a comparison of median sternotomy and thoracoscopic approaches. Chest 1996; 110:1399–1406.

23. Cordova FC, O'Brien GM, Furukawa S, Kuzma AM, Travaline J, Criner GJ. Stability of improvements in exercise performance and quality of life following bilateral lung volume reduction surgery in severe COPD. Chest 1997; 112:907–915.

24. Cassina PC, Teschler H, Konietzko N, Theegarten D, Stamatis G. Two year results after lung volume reduction surgery in antitrypsin deficiency vs smoker's emphysema. Eur Respir J 1998; 12:1028–1032.

25. Argenziano M, Thomashow B, Jellen PA, Rose EA, Steinglass KM, Ginsburg ME. Functional comparison of unilateral versus bilateral lung volume reduction surgery. Ann Thorac Surg 1997; 64:321–327.

26. Fessler HE, Permutt S. Lung volume reduction surgery and airflow limitation. Am J Respir Crit Care Med 1998; 157:715–722.

27. Wisser W, Klepetko W, Kontrus M, Bankier A, Senbaklavaci O, Kaider A, Wanke T, Tschernko E, Wolner E. Morphological grading of the emphysematous lung and its relation to improvement after lung volume reduction surgery. Ann Thorac Surg 1998; 65:793–799.

28. Russi EW, Bloch KE, Weder W. Functional and morphological heterogeneity of emphysema and its implication for selection of patients for lung volume reduction surgery. Eur Respir J 1999; 14:230–236.

29. Baldwin JC, Miller CC, Prince RA, Espada R. Chest radiograph heterogeneity predicts functional improvement with volume reduction surgery. Ann Thorac Surg 2000; 70:1208–1211.

30. Klepetko W. Surgical aspects and techniques of lung volume reduction surgery for severe emphysema. Eur Respir J 1999; 13:919–925.
31. Wisser W, Tschernko E, Senbaklavaci O, Kontrus M, Wanke T, Wolner E, Klepetko W. Functional improvement after lung volume reduction sternotomy versus videoendoscopic approach. Ann Thorac Surg 1997; 63:822–828.
32. Brenner M, McKenna RJ, Gelb A, Osann KE, Schein MJ, Panzera J, Wong H, Berns MW, Wilson A. Objective predictors of response for stapled versus laser emphysematous lung reduction. Am J Respir Crit Care Med 1997; 155:1295–1301.
33. McKenna RJ, Brenner M, Gelb A, Mullin M, Singh N, Peters H, Panzera J, Calmese J, Schein MJ. A randomized, prospective trial of stapled lung reduction versus laser bullectomy for diffuse emphysema. J Thorac Cardiovasc Surg 1996; 111:317–322.
34. McKenna RJ, Brenner M, Fischel RJ, Gelb A. Should lung reduction for emphysema be unilateral or bilateral? J Thorac Cardiovasc Surg 1996; 112:1331–1339.
35. Lando Y, Boiselle PM, Shade D, Travaline J, Furukawa S, Criner GJ. Effect of lung volume reduction surgery on bony thorax configuration in severe COPD. Chest 1999; 116:30–39.
36. Chen JC, Serna DL, Brenner M, Powell LL, Huh J, McKenna RJ, Fischel RJ, Gelb A, Monti J, Burney T, Gaon MD, Aryan H, Wilson A. Diffusion capacity limitations of the extent of lung volume reduction surgery an animal model of emphysema. J Thorac Cardiovasc Surg 1999; 117:728–735.
37. National Emphysema Treatment Trial Research Group. Patients at high risk of deaths after lung volume reduction surgery. N Engl J Med 2001; 345:1075–1081.
38. Miller JL, Lee RB, Mansour KA. Lung volume reduction surgery: lessons learned. Ann Thorac Surg 1996; 61:1464–1469.
39. Teschler H, Thompson AB, Stamatis G. Short and long-term functional results after lung volume reduction surgery for severe emphysema. Eur Respir J 1999; 13:1170–1176.
40. Roue C, Mal H, Sleiman C, Fournier M, Duchatelle JP, Baldeyrou P, et al. Lung volume reduction in patients with severe diffuse emphysema. Chest 1996; 110:28–34.
41. Bingisser R, Zollinger A, Hauser M, Bloch KE, Russi EW, Weder W. Bilateral volume reduction surgery for diffuse pulmonary emphysema by video-assisted thoracoscopy. J Thorac Cardiovasc Surg 1996; 1996:875–882.
42. Naunheim KS, Keller CA, Krucylak PE, et al. Unilateral video-assisted thoracic surgical lung reduction. Ann Thorac Surg 1996; 61:1092–1098.
43. Keller CA, Ruppel G, Hibbett A, Osterloh J, Naunheim K. Thoracoscopic lung volume reduction surgery reduces dyspnea and improves exercise capacity in patients with emphysema. Am J Respir Crit Care Med 1997; 156:60–67.
44. Keenan RJ, Landreneau RJ, Sciurba FC, Ferson PF, Holbert JM, Brown ML, et al. Unilateral thoracoscopic surgical approach for diffuse emphysema. J Thorac Cardiovasc Surg 1996; 111:308–316.
45. Sciurba FC, Rogers RM, Keenan R, Slivka WA, Gorgsan J, Ferson PF, et al. Improvement in pulmonary function and elastic recoil after lung reduction surgery for diffuse emphysema. N Engl J Med 1996; 334:1095–1129.
46. Ingenito EP, Loeing SH, Moy ML, Mentzer SJ, Swanson SJ, Reilly JJ. Interpreting improvement in expiratory flows after lung volume reduction surgery

in terms of flow limitation theory. Am J Respir Crit Care Med 2001; 163:1074–1080.

47. Ferguson GT, Fernandez E, Zamora MR, Pomerantz M, Buchholz J, Make B. Improved exercise performance following lung volume reduction surgery for emphysema. Am J Respir Crit Care Med 1998; 157:1195–1203.

48. Albert RK, Benditt JO, Hildebrandt J, Wood DE, Hlastala MP. Lung volume reduction surgery has variable effects on blood gases in patients with emphysema. Am J Respir Crit Care Med 1998; 158:71–76.

49. Shade D, Cordova FC, Lando Y, Travaline J, Furukawa S, Kuzma AM, Criner GJ. Relationship between resting hypercapnia and physiologic parameters before and after lung volume reduction surgery in severe chronic obstructive pulmonary disease. Am J Respir Crit Care Med 1999; 159:1405–1411.

50. Travaline JM, Maurer AH, Charkes ND, Urbain JL, Furukawa S, Criner GJ. Quantitation of regional ventilation during the washout phase of lung scintigraphy: measurement in patients with severe COPD before and after bilateral lung volume reduction surgery. Chest 2000; 118:721–727.

51. Daniel TM, Chan BBK, Bhaskar V, Parekh JS, Walters PE, Reeder J, Truwit JD. Lung volume reduction surgery: case selection, operative techniques, and clinical results. Ann Surg 1996; 223:526–533.

52. Bousamra M, Haasler G, Lipchik RJ, Henry D, Chammas JH, Rokkas CK, et al. Functional and oximetric assessment of patients after lung reduction surgery. J Thorac Cardiovasc Surg 1997; 113:675–682.

53. Criner GJ, Cordova FC, Leyenson V, Roy B, Travaline J, Sundarshan S, et al. Effect of lung volume reduction surgery on diaphragm strength. Am J Respir Crit Care Med 1998; 157:1578–1585.

54. Benditt JO, Lewis S, Wood DE, Klima L, Albert RK. Lung volume reduction surgery improves maximal O_2 consumption, maximal minute ventilation, O_2 pulse, and dead space-to-tidal volume ratio during leg cycle ergometry. Am J Respir Crit Care Med 1997; 156:561–566.

55. Criner GJ, Cordova FC, Furukawa S, Kuzma AM, Travaline JM, Leyenson V, O'Brien GM. Prospective randomized trial comparing bilateral lung volume reduction surgery to pulmonary rehabilitation in severe chronic obstructive pulmonary disease. Am J Respir Crit Care Med 1999; 160:2018–2027.

56. Martinez FJ, Montes de Oca M, Whyte RI, Stetz J, Gay SE, Cerfolio RJ. Lung volume reduction improves dyspnea, dynamic hyperinflation, and respiratory muscle function. Am J Respir Crit Care Med 1997; 155:1984–1990.

57. Benditt JO, Wood DE, McCool FD, Lewis S, Albert RK. Changes in breathing and ventilatory muscle recruitment patterns induced by lung volume reduction surgery. Am J Respir Crit Care Med 1997; 155:279–284.

58. Stammberger U, Bloch KE, Thurnheer R, Bingisser R, Weder W, Russi EW. Exercise performance and gas exchange after bilateral video-assisted thoracoscopic lung volume reduction for severe emphysema. Eur Respir J 1998; 12:785–792.

59. Tschernko E, Wisser W, Wanke T, Rajek MA, Kritzinger M, Lahrmann H, Kontrus M, Benditte H. Changes in ventilatory mechanics and diaphragm function after lung volume reduction surgery in patients with COPD. Thorax 1997; 52:545–550.

60. Celli BR, Montes de Oca M, Mendez R, Stetz J. Lung reduction surgery in severe COPD decreases central drive and ventilatory response to C_{O_2}. Chest 1997; 112:902–906.

61. Moy ML, Ingenito EP, Mentzer SJ, Evans RB, Reilly JJ. Health-related quality of life improves following pulmonary rehabilitation and lung reduction surgery. Chest 1999; 115(2):383–389.

62. Leyenson V, Furukawa S, Kuzma AM, Cordova F, Travaline J, Criner GJ. Correlation of changes in quality of life after lung volume reduction surgery with changes in lung function, exercise, and gas exchange. Chest 2000; 118:728–735.

63. Brenner M, McKenna RJ, Gelb A, Fischel RJ, Wilson A. Rate of FEV_1 change following lung volume reduction surgery. Chest 1998; 113:652–659.

64. Gelb A, Brenner M, McKenna RJ, Zamel N, Fischel RJ, Epstein JD. Lung function 12 months following emphysema resection. Chest 1996; 110:1407–1415.

65. Gelb A, Brenner M, McKenna RJ, Fischel RJ, Zamel N, Schein MJ. Serial lung function and elastic recoil 2 years after lung volume reduction surgery for emphysema. Chest 1998; 113:1497–1506.

66. Gelb A, McKenna RJ, Brenner M, Epstein JD, Zamel N. Lung function 5 years after Lung volume reduction surgery for emphysema. Am J Respir Crit Care Med 2001; 163:1562–1566.

67. Gelb A, McKenna RJ, Brenner M, Schein MJ, Zamel N, Fischel RJ. Lung function 4 years after lung volume reduction surgery for emphysema. Chest 1999; 116:1608–1615.

68. Meyers BF, Yusen RD, Lefrak S, Patterson G, Pohl M, Richardson V, Cooper J. Outcomes of Medicare patients with emphysema selected for, but denied, a lung volume reduction operation. Ann Thorac Surg 1998; 66:331–336.

69. Wilkens H, Demertzis S, Konig J, Leitnaker CK, Shafer HJ, Sybrecht GW. Effect of lung volume reduction surgery in patients with severe emphysema. Eur Respir J 2000; 16:1043–1049.

70. Lewis RJ, Caccavale RJ, Sisler GE. VATS-Argon beam coagulator treatment of diffuse end-stage bilateral disease of the lung. Ann Thorac Surg 1993; 55:1394–1399.

71. Roberts JR, Bavaria JE, Wahl P, Wurster A, Friedberg JS, Kaiser L. Comparison of open and thoracoscopic bilateral volume reduction surgery: complication analysis. Ann Thorac Surg 1998; 66:1759–1765.

72. Serna DL, Brenner M, Osann KE, McKenna RJ, Chen JC, Fischel RJ, Jones BU, Gelb AF, Wilson AF. Survival after unilateral versus bilateral lung volume reduction surgery for emphysema. J Thorac Cardiovasc Surg 1999; 118:1101–1109.

73. Naunheim K, Kaiser L, Bavaria JE, Hezelrigg SR, Magee MJ, Landreneau RJ, Keenan RJ, Osterloh JF, Boley TM, Keller CA. Long-term survival after thoracoscopic lung volume reduction: a multi-institutional review. Ann Thorac Surg 1999; 68:2026–2032.

74. Christie RB. The elastic properties of the emphysematous lung and their significance. J Clin Invest 1934; 13:295–321.

75. Butler J, Caro G, Alcala R, DuBois A. Physiological factors affecting airway resistance in normal subjects and in patients with obstructive lung disease. J Clin Invest 1960; 39:584–590.

76. Rogers RM, DuBois AR, Blakemore WS. Effect of removal of bullae on airway conductance and conductance volume ratios. J Clin Invest 1968; 157:715–722.

77. Smith J, Bellemare F. Effect of lung volume on in vivo contraction characteristics of human diaphragm. J Appl Physiol 1987; 62:1893–1900.

78. Minh V, Dolan GF, Konopka RF, Moser KM. Effect of hyperinflation on inspiratory function of the diaphragm. J Appl Physiol 1976; 40:67–73.

79. Evanich MJ, Franceo MJ, Lourenco RV. Force output of the diaphragm as a function of the phrenic nerve firing rate and lung volume. J Appl Physiol 1973; 35:208–212.
80. Kim MJ, Druz WS, Danon J, Machnach W, Sharp JT. Mechanics of the canine diaphragm. J Appl Physiol 1976; 41:369–382.
81. Bloch KE, Li Y, Zhang J, Bingisser R, Kaplan V, Weder W, Russi EW. Effect of surgical lung volume reduction on breathing patterns in severe pulmonary emphysema. Am J Respir Crit Care Med 1997; 156:553–560.
82. Teschler H, Stamatis G, El-Raouf Farhat AA, Meyer FJ, Costabel U, Konietzko N. Effect of surgical lung volume reduction surgery on respiratory muscle function in pulmonary emphysema. Eur Respir J 1996; 9:1779–1784.
83. Lando Y, Boiselle PM, Shade D, Furukawa S, Kuzma AM, Travaline J, Criner GJ. Effect of lung volume reduction surgery on diaphragm strength length in severe chronic obstructive pulmonary disease. Am J Respir Crit Care Med 1999; 159:796–805.
84. Schrager JB, Kim D, Hashami Y, Lankford E, Wahl P, Stedman H, Levine S, Kaiser L. Lung volume reduction surgery restores the normal diaphragmatic length-tension relationship in emphysematous rats. J Thorac Cardiovasc Surg 2001; 121:217–224.
85. Cassart M, Hamacher J, Verbandt Y, Wildermuth S, Rischer D, Russi EW, de Francquen P, Cappello M, Weder W, Estenne M. Effects of lung volume reduction surgery for emphysema on diaphragm dimensions and configuration. Am J Respir Crit Care Med 2001; 163:1171–1175.
86. Lahrmann H, Wild M, Wanke T, Tschernko E, Wisser W, Klepetko W, Zwick H. Neural drive to the diaphragm after lung volume reduction surgery. Chest 1999; 116:1593–1600.
87. Laghi F, Jubran A, Topeli A, Fahey PJ, Garrity ER, Arcidi JM, de Pinto DJ, Edwards LC. Effect of lung volume reduction surgery on neuromechanical coupling of the diaphragm. Am J Respir Crit Care Med 1998; 157:475–483.
88. Kubo K, Koizumi T, Fujimoto K, Matsuzawa Y, Yamanda T, Haniuda M, Takahashi S. Effects of lung volume reduction surgery on exercise pulmonary hemodynamics in severe emphysema. Chest 1998; 114:1575–1582.
89. Oswald-Mammosser M, Kessler R, Massard G, Wilhm JM, Weitzenblum E, Lonsdorfer J. Effects of lung volume reduction surgery on gas exchange and pulmonary hemodynamics at rest and during exercise. Am J Respir Crit Care Med 1998; 1998:1020–1025.
90. Weg IL, Rossoff L, McKeon K, Grayer LM, Scharf SM. Development of Pulmonary hypertension after lung volume reduction surgery. Am J Respir Crit Care Med 1999; 159:552–556.
91. Powell LL, Serna DL, Brenner M, Gaon M, Jalal R, Stemmer E, Chen JC. Pulmonary vascular pressures increases after lung volume reduction surgery in rabbits with more severe emphysema. J Surg Res 2000; 92:157–164.
92. Cooper JD. Technique to reduce air leaks after resection of emphysematous lung. Ann Thorac Surg 1994; 57:1038–1039.
93. McKenna RJ, Fischel RJ, Brenner M, Gelb A. Use of the Heimlich valve to shorten hospital stay after lung volume reduction surgery for emphysema. Ann Thorac Surg 1996; 51:1115–1117.

94. Centindag I, Boley TM, Magee MJ, Hazelrigg SR. Postoperative gastrointestinal complications after lung volume reduction operations. Ann Thorac Surg 1999; 68:1029–1033.

95. Igbal M, Rossoff L, McKeon K, Graver M, Scharf SM. Development of giant bulla after lung volume reduction surgery. Chest 1999; 116:1809–1811.

96. Oey I, Waller DA. Metalloptysis: a late complication of lung volume reduction surgery. Ann Thorac Surg 2001; 21:819–848.

97. Hogue CW, Stamos T, Winters K, Moulton M, Krucylak PE, Cooper JD. Acute myocardial infarction during lung volume reduction surgery. Anesth Analg 1999; 88:332–334.

98. The National Emphysema Treatment Trial Research Group. Rationale and design of the National Emphysema Treatment Trial. Chest 1999; 116:1750–1761.

99. Slone RM, Pligram TK, Gierarda DS, Sagel SS, Glazer HS, Yusen RD, Cooper JD. Lung volume reduction surgery: comparison of preoperative radiologic features and clinical outcome. Radiology 1997; 204:685–693.

100. Szekely LA, Oelberg DA, Wright C, Johnson DC, Wain J, Trotman-Dickenson B, Shepard JA, Kanarek DJ, Systrom D, Ginns LC. Preoperative predictors of operative morbidity and mortality in COPD patients undergoing bilateral lung volume reduction surgery. Chest 1997; 111:550–558.

101. O'Brien GM, Furukawa S, Kuzma AM, Cordova FC, Criner GJ. Improvements in lung function, exercise, and quality of life in hypercapneic COPD patients. Chest 1999; 115:75–84.

102. Maki DD, Miller WT, Aronchick JM, Gefter WB, Kotloff RM. Advanced emphysema: preoperative chest radiograph findings as predictors of outcome following lung volume reduction surgery. Radiology 1999; 212:49–55.

103. Criner GJ, Kreimer DT, Pidlaoan L. Patient outcome following prolonged mechanical ventilation via tracheostomy. Am J Respir Crit Care Med 1993; 147:A874.

104. Criner, G. J., O'Brien, G., Furukawa, S, Cordova, F., Swartz, M., Fallahnejad, M, D'Alonzo, G. Lung volume reduction surgery in ventilator-dependent COPD patients. Chest 1996; 110:877–884.

105. Criner GJ, Cordova F, Furukawa S, Kuzma AM, Kreimer DT, Travaline J, O'Brien G. Prolonged follow-up of lung volume reduction surgery (LVRS) in ventilator-dependent COPD patients. Am J Respir Crit Care Med 1997; A602.

106. Schmid R A, Vogt P, Stocker R, Zalunardo M, Russi EW, Weder W. Lung volume reduction surgery for a patient receiving mechanical ventilation after a complex cardiac operation. J Thorac Cardiovasc Surg 1998; 115:236–237.

107. Hansson B, Jorens PG, van Schil P, van Kerckhoven W, van den Brande F, Eyskens E. Lung volume reduction surgery as an emergency and life-saving procedure. Eur Respir J 1997; 10:2650–2652.

108. Murtuza B, Keogh BF, Simonds AK, Pepper JR. Lung volume reduction surgery in a ventilated patient with severe pulmonary emphysema. Ann Thorac Surg 2001; 71:1037–1038.

109. Hazelrigg, SR, Boley TM, Weber D, Magee MJ, Naunheim KS. Incidence of lung nodules found in patients undergoing lung volume reduction. Ann Thorac Surg 1997; 64:303-306.

110. McKenna RJ, Fischel RJ, Brenner M, Gelb A. Combined operations for lung volume reduction surgery and lung cancer. Chest 1996; 110:885–888.

111. Ojo TC, Martinez F, Paine R III, Christensen PJ Curtis J, Weg JG, Kazerooni EA, Whyte R. Lung volume reduction surgery alters management of pulmonary nodules in patients with severe COPD. Chest 1997; 112:1494–1500.

112. Rozenshtein A, White CS, Austin JHM, Romney BM, Protopapas Z, Krasna MJ. Incidental lung carcinoma detected at CT in patients selected for lung volume reduction surgery to treat severe pulmonary emphysema. Radiology 1998; 207:487–490.

113. Duarte IG, Gal AA, Mansour KA, Lee RB, Miller JI. Pathologic findings in lung volume reduction surgery. Chest 1998; 113:660–664.

114. Keller CA, Naunheim KS, Osterloh J, Espiritu J, McDonald JW, Ramos RR. Histopathologic diagnosis made in lung tissue resected from patients with severe emphysema undergoing lung volume reduction surgery. Chest 1997; 111:941–947.

115. DeRose JJ, Argenziano M, El-Amir N, Jellen PA, Gorenstein LA, Steinglass KM, Thomashow B, Ginsburg ME. Lung reduction operationand resection of pulmonary nodules in patients with severe emphysema. Ann Thorac Surg 1998; 65:314–318.

116. Ginsburg, R. J., Rubinstein, L. V., and Lung cancer study group. Randomized trial of lobectomy versus limited resection for T1 N0 non-small cell lung cancer. Ann Thorac Surg 1995; 60:615–623.

117. Landreneau RJ, Sugarbaker DJ, Mack MJ, Hazelrigg SR, Luketich JD, Fetterman L, Liptay MJ, Bartley S, Boley TM, Keenan RJ, Ferson PF, Weyant RJ, Naunheim KS. Wedge resection versus lobectomy for stage 1 (T1 N0 M0) non-small cell lung cancer. J Thorac Cardiovasc Surg 1997; 113:691–698.

118. DeMeester SR, Patterson GA, Sundaresan RS, Cooper JD. Lobectomy combined with volume reduction for patients with lung cancer and advanced emphysema. J Thorac Cardiovasc Surg 1998; 115:681–688.

119. Takizawa T, Terashima M, Koike T, Akamatsu H, Kurita Y, Yokoyama A. Mediastinal lymph node metastasis in patients with clinical stage 1 peripheral non-small-cell lung cancer. J Thorac Cardiovasc Surg 1998; 113:248–252.

120. Thurnheer R, Muntwyler J, Stammberger U, Bloch KE, Zollinger A, Weder W, Russi EW. Coronary artery disease in patients undergoing lung volume reduction surgery for emphysema. Chest 1997; 112:122–128.

121. Furukawa S, Criner GJ, O'Brien G, Kuzma AM, Jeevanandam JB, McClurken JB, Addonizio VP. Ischemic heart disease does not preclude surgery for chronic obstructive lung disease. Am J Respir Crit Care Med 1997; A608.

122. Liopyris P, Triantafillou AN, Sundt TM III, Block MI, Cooper J. Coronary artery bypass grafting after bilateral lung volume reduction operation. Ann Thorac Surg 1997; 63:1790–1792.

123. Ulicny KS Jr, Schmelzer V, Flege JB. Concomitant cardiac and pulmonary operation: the role of cardiopulmonary bypass. Ann Thorac Surg 1992; 54:289–295.

124. Rao V, Todd TRJ, Weisel RD, Komeda M, Cohen G, Ikonomidis JS, Christakis GT. Results of combined pulmonary resection and cardiac operation. Ann Thorac Surg 1996; 62:342–347.

125. Flaherty KR, Martinez FJ. Lung volume reduction surgery for emphysema. Clin Chest Med 2000; (21)4:819–848.

126. Yusen RD, Lefrak SS, Trulock ER. Evaluation and preoperative management of lung volume reduction surgery candidates. Clinics in Chest Medicine 1997; 18(2):199–224.

13

Pulmonary Thromboendarterectomy

WILLIAM R. AUGER, PETER F. FEDULLO, KIM M. KERR, DAVID P. KAPELANSKI, and STUART W. JAMIESON

University of California, San Diego
San Diego Medical Center
San Diego, California, U.S.A.

I. Introduction

Chronic thromboembolic (CTE) obstruction of the main, lobar, and segmental pulmonary arteries represents a rare and atypical sequela of acute pulmonary embolism. Depending on the extent of pulmonary vascular involvement, the duration of obstruction, and what is likely the development of small vessel hypertensive changes in the unobstructed pulmonary vascular bed over time, pulmonary hypertension and cor pulmonale may ensue. If this clinical entity is overlooked or left untreated, right ventricular decompensation and death becomes inevitable. However, increased physician awareness and diagnostic advances over the past few decades have resulted in greater recognition of chronic thromboembolic pulmonary hypertension (CTEPH). And it is with the demonstration that surgical removal of the thrombus residua can substantially reduce pulmonary pressures and improve right ventricular function—a procedure referred to as a pulmonary thromboendarterectomy (PTE)—that CTEPH is now appreciated to be a form of pulmonary hypertension that is potentially correctable by surgical means.

II. Historical Perspective

The concept of "pulmonary heart disease" due to chronic thrombotic occlusion of the small pulmonary arteries can be traced back to the early decades of the twentieth century (1,2). Owen and colleagues have further suggested that this "rare condition" may result from "unrecognized emboli" and should be considered in cases of severe congestive heart failure of undetermined cause (3). In a 1956 review of the topic, Ball et al. (4) identified in the literature over 200 reported cases of massive thrombosis of the large pulmonary arteries, the first report being attributed to Helie in 1837 (5). However, these were autopsy reports and, for the most part, the finding of organized thrombus in the pulmonary vessels was in association with other diseases—such as pulmonary tuberculosis, congenital heart disease, and lung carcinoma; only occasionally was it appreciated in the absence of another disorder. Attention to the syndrome of chronic thrombotic occlusion of the major pulmonary arteries, and the antemortem diagnosis of this disease, were advanced by the case reports of Carroll (6), Owen et al. (3), Ball et al. (4), and later Hollister and Cull (7). It was also suggested that the "syndrome occurs more often than indicated by the number of cases reported" (7). In the series of five patients described by Carroll, two patients underwent cardiac catheterization, confirming the presence of pulmonary hypertension, and angiography was performed in one patient, documenting the enlarged right heart chambers and complete occlusion of the left pulmonary artery. In this same patient, a biopsy of the left pulmonary artery was performed, providing the first antemortem tissue diagnosis of organized thromboembolic involvement of a major pulmonary artery.

Though Hollister and Cull maintained that surgical removal of the organized thrombus may be feasible by embolectomy or endarterectomy, the first planned surgical treatment for chronic pulmonary embolic disease was reported in 1958 by Hurwitt and colleagues (8). Utilizing the technique of caval inflow occlusion, access to the thromboembolic material was through an incision in the main pulmonary artery. During the brief period of blood flow interruption, organized thrombus adherent to the vessel wall was "scooped out." However, cardiac arrest ensued and the patient was not successfully resuscitated. An autopsy disclosed extensive organized thromboembolic disease involving virtually all the lobar vessels. This first surgical experience provided an important lesson. It illustrated the distinction between acute and organized thromboembolic disease, the latter incorporated into the vessel wall and necessitating an endarterectomy rather that an embolectomy to achieve a successful surgical outcome.

The first successful pulmonary thromboendarterectomy (PTE) using endarterectomy instruments was reported by Synder in 1961 (9). This was a unilateral endarterectomy with a thoracotomy approach. The first PTE in which cardiopulmonary bypass was used was reported in 1964 by Castleman et al. (10), while Houk and colleagues (11) are credited with the first bilateral PTE via a transverse sternotomy.

Once it became apparent that chronic thromboembolic occlusion of the major pulmonary vessels was a potentially treatable form of pulmonary hypertension and cor pulmonale, several small series describing surgical successes appeared in the literature in the 1960s and early 1970s (12–14). Following this, Cabrol and colleagues in Paris (15), Sabiston's group at Duke University (16), and Moser, Utley, and later, Daily at the University of California, San Diego (17,18), took the lead in defining the diagnostic approach to patients with chronic thromboembolic disease, in refining the surgical techniques in treating these patients, and in describing some of the unique postoperative challenges encountered as a result of this surgery. Beginning in 1987, Daily et al. published several reports that laid the foundation for the current state of the art of pulmonary thromboendarterectomy. An early report describes a novel approach to myocardial protection during PTE surgery (19), which substantially reduced the incidence of postoperative phrenic nerve paresis and overall mortality rates. In 1989, Daily and colleagues outlined a standard approach for the surgical procedure (20). The essential aspects of the surgery involved a median sternotomy, myocardial protection consisting of single-dose cold-blood cardioplegia and a cooling jacket placed around the ventricles, periods of intermittent circulatory arrest at a maximum duration of 20 min, and dissection of both the right and left pulmonary arteries within the pericardial space to optimize exposure of the major pulmonary vessels without entering the pleural space. And finally, further modifications in surgical techniques came about with alterations in the surgical instruments used (21). The development of specific dissectors with suctioning capabilities allowed continuous removal of blood from the operative field during an endarterectomy. Consequently, periods of circulatory arrest could be substantially shortened, with a resultant decline in the incidence of several postoperative difficulties.

Throughout the 1990s, there were few changes in the essential surgical aspects of performing a pulmonary thromboendarterctomy. Jamieson et al. proposed an alternative method of placing incisions in the pulmonary arteries, thereby improving exposure within the left pulmonary artery and minimizing the risk of vascular tears (22). Zund and colleagues suggested that PTE surgery could be performed using normothermic cardiopulmonary bypass (23). This group also advocated transection of the superior vena cava to improve exposure of the right pulmonary artery. Experience with this approach, however, has been limited.

The last two decades have witnessed an expanded worldwide experience in the diagnosis and treatment of patients with chronic thromboembolic pulmonary hypertension (24–32). This experience underscores the increased recognition of this disease and the growing understanding that surgery can be a lifesaving remedy in appropriately selected patients.

III. Natural History

The evolution from an acute pulmonary embolus, or emboli, to the involvement of major pulmonary arteries (segmental, lobar, or larger vessels) with organized thrombotic residua is poorly understood. It is generally appreciated that this sequence of events is an uncommon sequela following acute thromboembolic occurrences. Though estimates vary, it appears that less than 0.1% of acute pulmonary embolic survivors in the United States will develop hemodynamically significant residua that will ultimately warrant surgical intervention (32).

Defining an underlying predisposition to develop chronic thromboembolic disease has been elusive in most patients. In those individuals with established disease, identification of an impairment in fibrinolysis (33,34) or defining a prothrombotic tendency occurs rarely. The presence of a lupus anticoagulant and/or high-titer anticardiolipin antibodies can be detected in 10 to 24% of patients with chronic thromboembolic pulmonary hypertension (35,36). Cumulatively, hereditary thrombophilias such as protein C, protein S, and antithrombin III deficiencies are established in less than 5% of patients. The presence of factor V Leiden has been reported in 4 to 6.5% of CTEPH patients (36,37), while the incidence of other thrombophilic states such as factor II mutation, the prothrombin 20210 G/A gene mutation, elevated factor VIII levels, and hyperhomocystinemia has yet to be completely defined.

An explanation for the development of pulmonary hypertension in the presence of chronic thromboemboli has changed over the past decade. It was previously suggested that the progressive rise in pulmonary vascular resistance was a result of occlusion or narrowing of the proximal pulmonary vascular bed with recurrent, unresolved thromboemboli. Though this may the pathophysiological pathway in some, the observation that lung perfusion studies in most patients change little over time, while at the same time pulmonary hypertension develops, has prompted an alternate explanation. Though speculative, it is believed the gradual rise in pulmonary vascular resistance is at least partially attributed to the development of small vessel hypertensive changes in the vascular bed uninvolved with proximal CTE disease. Supporting evidence includes the poor correlation between the degree of pulmonary hypertension and the extent of central pulmonary artery obstruction or partial vascular occlusion as assessed by angiography. In addition, examining biopsied lung tissue of CTE patients, Moser and Bloor demonstrated that small vessel hypertensive arteriopathy, similar to that seen in primary pulmonary hypertension patients, was found in the vascular bed uninvolved with proximal CTE disease (38). Furthermore, following PTE surgery, lung perfusion studies typically document a low perfusion state in nonendarterectomized (i.e., uninvolved with chronic thrombus) lung regions with "hyperperfusion" observed in areas from which organized thromboembolic material has been surgically removed. Presumptively, this represents a shifting of blood flow from regions of high vascular resistance to lung regions of lower resistance, a phenomenon referred to as "pulmonary vascular steal" (39). Although this may represent a loss of normal vasoreactivity in the endaterectomized vascular bed, the findings in Moser's lung biopsy study makes it equally plausible that the small vessel disease in the unobstructed lung has established a region of relatively higher vascular resistance. Consequently, it is currently believed that most patients with CTEPH have suffered an acute, anatomically significant pulmonary embolic event or events that incompletely resolved. With the loss of pulmonary vascular reserve, modest pulmonary hypertension would be present at rest and would worsen with exercise because of the loss of adaptive mechanisms. Over a period of time, as a result of the direct effect of these elevated pressures and flows on the unobstructed pulmonary vascular bed or as a result of yet undiscovered mediator-related effects, a secondary arteriopathy develops in the distal vessels. These pathophysiological changes result in a progressive cycle of worsening pulmonary hypertension, declining cardiac function, and diminished exercise capabilities.

Survivorship of untreated patients suffering with chronic thromboembolic pulmonary hypertension is particularly poor and correlates with the level of pulmonary hypertension at the time of presentation. Riedel and colleagues showed that thromboembolic patients presenting with a mean pulmonary artery pressure between 31 to 40 mmHg, a 50% survival rate over a 10-year period was demonstrated. If the initial mean pulmonary artery pressure was 41 to 50 mmHg, the survival rate declined to 20% over 10 years; it declined to 5% for a mean pulmonary artery pressure greater than 50 mmHg. In this latter group, 2-year survival was only 20% (40). A recent report has substantiated these early observations. Lewczuk et al. showed that in a group of 49 CTE patients deemed unsuitable for surgery who received continuous anticoagulation therapy, prognosis was adversely affected by the presence of pulmonary hypertension (mean PA pressure greater than 30 mmHg), the coexistence of chronic obstructive pulmonary disease, and poor exercise tolerance (41).

IV. Clinical Presentation

The frequent absence of an apparent acute thromboembolic event in the past and the unpredictable time course of developing pulmonary hypertension accounts for the variable and often subtle manner in which patients present clinically. The patient's age, the presence of other comorbid diseases, and an individual's state of conditioning (i.e., athletic versus sedentary) will further influence the timing and degree of clinical difficulties experienced by the CTE patient at the time of initial presentation. The most common presenting complaints are exertional dyspnea and a progressive decline in exercise tolerance. The basis for this seems to be a limitation in cardiac output related to the elevation in pulmonary vascular resistance, along with an increase in dead-space ventilation. A nonproductive cough, atypical chest pains (usually pleuritic in character), and palpitations are variably reported by patients with chronic thromboembolic pulmonary hypertension. Hemoptysis is an infrequent occurrence. A change in voice quality or hoarseness may result from left vocal cord dysfunction, a consequence of the recurrent laryngeal nerve compressed between the aorta and an enlarged left main pulmonary artery. Late in the course of the disease, as right ventricular function is unable to accommodate normal metabolic demands, exertion-related dizziness, syncope provoked by a sudden fall in venous return (e.g., coughing or bending over), resting dyspnea, and exertional chest pain can be observed.

For otherwise healthy individuals accustomed to higher levels of activity, a change in exercise tolerance is generally recognized at an earlier stage of pulmonary hypertension than those who lead more sedentary lives. These same individuals will usually blame their symptoms on deconditioning or advancing age. The presence of another medical condition, such as mild parenchymal lung disease or intrinsic heart disease, can further complicate the initial presentation. In such a situation, a decline in exercise tolerance is often attributed to an exacerbation of the known disease state. And finally, exertional dypnea is nonspecific to chronic thromboembolic disease. Such a complex interplay of circumstances contributes to the usual diagnostic delay in this disorder. For these reasons, patients with CTEPH typically have been labeled with an alternative diagnosis during the course of their initial evaluation, such as new-onset "asthma," valvular heart disease, or psychogenic dyspnea. It has also been demonstrated that the delay in achieving the correct diagnosis from the onset of cardiopulmonary symptoms ranges between 2 and 3 years (24,32).

Physical examination findings reflect the stage at which CTE patients present in the course of their disease. In the absence of right heart dysfunction, exam findings attributable to CTEPH can be subtle. The classic findings of pulmonary hypertension—a right ventricular lift, an accentuated pulmonic component of the second heart sound, a right ventricular S_4 gallop, and tricuspid regurgitation—can be difficult to discern. This is particularly the case if the clinician is not considering the possibility of CTEPH. An obese patient or one who presents with coexisting cardiopulmonary disease can also make these exam findings difficult to detect. Jugular venous distension, severe tricuspid regurgitation, a right ventricular S_3 gallop, hepatomegaly, ascites, peripheral edema, and cyanosis are physical signs suggestive of more significant right heart dysfunction. For patients with a history of lower extremity venous thrombosis, edema, and venous stasis skin discoloration may be evident. The presence of pulmonary flow mumurs (42) can also be demonstrated in approximately 30% of patients with chronic thromboembolic pulmonary hypertension. These bruits result from turbulent flow across narrowed, partially obstructed large pulmonary arteries, are high-pitched and blowing in quality, are auscultated over the lung folds rather than the precordium, and are most apparent during an end-inspiratory, breath-holding maneuver. These bruits, however, are not unique to chronic thromboembolic disease. They have been described in other disease states associated with focal narrowing of large pulmonary arteries, such as congenital branch stenoses and pulmonary arteritis. They are not a finding in primary pulmonary hypertension (PPH), which is a common competing diagnosis.

V. Diagnostic Evaluation

The initial evaluative studies in the assessment of a patient complaining of exertional dyspnea or a change in exercise tolerance may provide few clues to the presence of pulmonary hypertension due to chronic thromboembolic disease. Routine hematological and blood chemistry tests are generally unremarkable early in the course of CTEPH. Long-standing hypoxemia may result in a secondary polycythemia. A modest thrombocytopenia and a prolonged activated partial thromboplastin time (in the absence of heparin anticoagulation) can be observed in those patients with a lupus anticoagulant. Liver function studies may be abnormal from hepatic congestion in the setting of significant right ventricular dysfunction and elevation of right atrial pressure. A poor cardiac output and consequent reduction in renal blood flow may manifest itself in an elevation of blood urea nitrogen, serum creatinine, and uric acid levels (43).

Pulmonary function testing is frequently obtained in the evaluation of patients complaining of exertional dyspnea. Lung volume and airflow abnormalities attributable to CTEPH are relatively minor; therefore these studies are most useful in excluding coexisting parenchymal or obstructive airways disease. Approximately 20% of patients demonstrate mild to moderate lung restriction due to the presence of parenchymal scarring from prior lung infarction (44). A modest reduction in single-breath diffusing capacity for carbon monoxide (DL_{CO}) can be present in CTEPH (45), though a normal value does not exclude the diagnosis. Severe reduction in DL_{CO} (i.e., <50% predicted) is rarely a feature of major vessel CTE disease and should suggest an alternative diagnosis that significantly involves the small pulmonary vascular bed (46). Resting blood gas analysis frequently shows an arterial oxygen level (Pa_{O_2}) to be within normal limits, though dead-space ventilation is often elevated. With exercise, many CTEPH patients will experience a decline in Pa_{O_2} and an abnormal increase in dead-space ventilation. The hypoxemia seems to be related to ventilation perfusion inequalities and an insufficient cardiac output, reflected in a low mixed venous oxygen saturation (47). Hypoxemia at rest in this patient population implies severe compromise of right heart function or the presence of a right-to-left shunt through a patent foramen ovale.

Depending on the stage of the disease, chest radiographic findings in CTEPH can range from relative few and subtle irregularities to several distinct abnormalities suggestive of the diagnosis (48). In the absence of coexisting parenchymal lung disease, the lung fields are typically free of infiltrates, though regions of hypoperfusion or hyperperfusion—the latter sometimes appearing as a prominent interstitial pattern—may be present. Peripheral lung field opacities consistent with scarring from previous infarctions can be seen in hypoperfused lung regions, frequently accompanied by pleural thickening. Pleural effusions are uncommon unless right ventricular dysfunction, a high right atrial pressure, volume overload and ascites are prominent clinical features. Enlargement of the right ventricle and pulmonary outflow tract are evident on lateral films with obliteration of the retrosternal space. Dilatation of the central pulmonary vessels is reflective of long-standing pulmonary hypertension. Unlike the symmetrical enlargement of the proximal vessels in small vessel pulmonary hypertension, CTEPH patients often demonstrate irregularly shaped, asymmetrically enlarged pulmonary arteries (49). The discrepancy in the size of the central pulmonary vessels may be so dramatic that agenesis of one of the main pulmonary arteries is suggested (50). Also, the unusual contour of the pulmonary vessels is frequently interpreted as adenopathy, which is an important distinction to be made.

In the absence of an apparent pulmonary cause for a patient's exertional dyspnea, a cardiac etiology and, more specifically, a pulmonary vascular source should be explored. Echocardiography is an effective noninvasive study to screen for the presence of pulmonary hypertension. As an initial diagnostic tool, it is also helpful in excluding significant left ventricular dysfunction or mitral valve disease, which may be the basis for the elevated pulmonary pressures. Available technology allows for the estimate of pulmonary artery systolic pressure with Doppler assessment of the degree of tricuspid regurgitation in addition to an estimate of the cardiac output. Right heart chamber enlargement, paradoxical interventricular septal motion, and encroachment of an enlarged right ventricle on left ventricular filling are consequences of pulmonary hypertension, which can be further demonstrated by echocardiography (51). The venous injection of "contrast" or agitated saline during an echocardiogram will sometimes detect the presence of intracardiac shunting, as with a patent foramen ovale or septal defect. In those patients with only mild pulmonary hypertension and right ventricular enlargement at rest, echocardiography during exercise may document a substantial rise in pulmonary artery pressures, along with an abnormal increase in right heart size.

Once the diagnosis of pulmonary hypertension has been established or is strongly suspected, the focus of the evaluation turns to distinguishing between major vessel occlusive disease and small vessel pulmonary vascular disease. In most cases, a lung ventilation perfusion ($\dot{V}/\dot{Q}$) scan is a noninvasive means of achieving this end. Patients with major-vessel CTE disease will exhibit multiple segment–sized or larger perfusion defects in lung regions with normal ventilation (Fig. 1). This is in contrast to the normal or subsegmental "mottled" perfusion pattern seen in small vessel disease such as primary pulmonary hypertension (52). However, during the process of organization, proximal vessel thromboemboli may recanalize or narrow the vessel in such a way that radiolabeled macroaggregated albumin may pass beyond the point of partial occlusion. Two additional observations can be made about perfusion

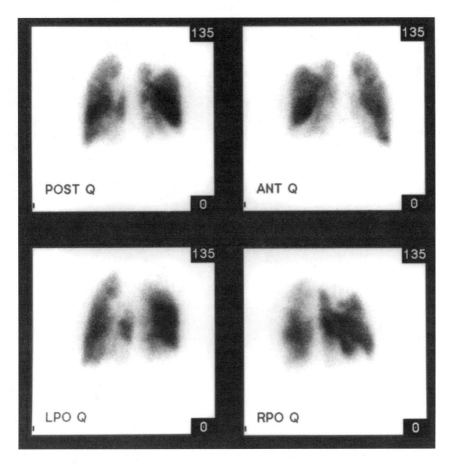

Figure 1 Lung perfusion scan in a patient with chronic thromboembolic pulmonary hypertension. Ventilation study was normal.

scans in CTEPH patients. "Gray zones," or regions of relative hypoperfusion, are frequently observed; as a result, lung perfusion studies often underestimate the degree of vascular obstruction caused by proximal vessel chronic thromboembolic disease (53). Furthermore, the finding of mismatched segmental perfusion defects is not specific for chronic thromboembolic disease. Other disease entities that lead to occlusion of the central pulmonary arteries can present such a pattern on $\dot{V}/\dot{Q}$ scan. Extrinsic compression of the central pulmonary arteries (as seen with mediastinal adenopathy or fibrosis), primary pulmonary vascular tumors, and large vessel arteritis are examples of such competing considerations. Consequently, additional imaging studies are necessary to define the pulmonary vascular anatomy and to establish diagnosis.

Over the past decade, with available high-speed technology, computed tomography (CT) of the chest has been increasing utilized in the evaluation of the pulmonary vascular bed. CT findings in chronic thromboembolic disease include a mosaic perfusion of the lung parenchyma; pulmonary vessel enlargement with variation in the size of segmental vessels, appearing relatively small in affected lung regions; peripheral, scar-like densities in hypoattenuated lung regions; and the presence of mediastinal collateral vessels (54–57). Related to the presence of pulmonary hypertension are enlarged central pulmonary arteries, right atrial and right ventricular enlargement, pleural and pericardial effusions, and ascites with accompanying liver engorgement. With contrast enhancement and distinct from the intraluminal defects seen with acute thrombemboli, chronic thrombus will typically appear to line the larger pulmonary vessels in either a concentric or eccentric fashion (Fig. 2).

    The role of CT in the evaluation of patients with suspected chronic thromboembolic disease is yet to be fully defined. CT imaging has considerable value in those cases where there is a possible alternative explanation for encroachment on the major pulmonary vessels. Examples include hilar or mediastinal adenopathy, such as that seen in fibrosing mediastinitis (58,59); adenopathy with parenchymal lung lesions suggestive of sarcoidosis or carcinoma (60); and intraluminal occlusive or partially occlusive lesions involving the pulmonary outflow tract or main pulmonary arteries character-istic of primary pulmonary vascular tumors (59,61). In addition, CT imaging of the chest provides useful anatomical information on the status of the lung parenchyma in patients with coexisting emphysematous or restrictive lung disease. Problematic, however, is the observation that chronic thromboemboli usually organize and become endothelialized in such a manner that their presence on CT angiography may not be apparent. Consequently, the absence of "lining thrombus" involving the central pulmonary arteries does not exclude the diagnosis of chronic thromboembolic disease or the possibility of surgical intervention. Conversely, the demonstration of centrally located thrombus does not uniformly confirm the diagnosis of surgically accessible chronic

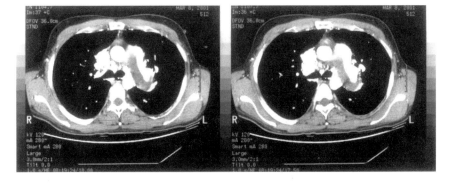

Figure 2 Contrast CT scan in a CTEPH patient. Thrombus lines the enlarged left main pulmonary artery.

thromboembolic disease. Central thrombus demonstrated by CT has been described in PPH and other types of end-stage lung disease (62,63). Surgical endarterectomy in these cases not only presents a substantial mortal risk but is unlikely to mitigate the existing pulmonary hypertension. Historical information is typically helpful in establishing the correct diagnosis and, for most of these patients, the perfusion lung scan shows either a normal perfusion pattern or one with minimal defects (Fig. 3).

Given the diagnostic shortcomings with other imaging modalities, pulmonary angiography, in the vast majority of cases, is the most reliable means of defining the extent and proximal location of suspected chronic thromboembolic lesions. Though performance of angiography in the setting of pulmonary hypertension often is viewed with trepidation, the risks can be minimized in skilled hands and with appropriate precautions (64,65). For CTEPH patients, the benefit of pulmonary arteriography is in establishing the diagnosis and providing critical information for determining surgical candidacy. The angiographic appearance of CTE disease reflects the complex pattern of organization and recanalization that occurs following an acute thromboembolic event. Consequently, chronic thromboemboli are angiographically distinct from the well-defined intraluminal filling defects seen with acute pulmonary emboli. Several angiographic patterns have correlated with the presence of chronic thrombus. These include vascular webs or band-like narrowings, intimal irregularities, "pouching defects," abrupt and often angular narrowing of major pulmonary arteries, and obstruction of pulmonary vessels, frequently at their point of origin and in the absence of an apparent intraluminal filling defect (66). In most CTE patients, two or more of these angiographic findings are present and are distributed in both lung fields (Fig. 4).

Competing diagnoses can present angiographic findings similar to those seen in major vessel chronic thromboembolic disease. Band-like vessel narrowing is a feature of medium or large vessel pulmonary arteritis (Takayasu's arteritis) (67,68); when primarily involving numerous segmental vessels, it is a hallmark finding in congenital stenosis of the pulmonary arteries (69). Total or partial obstruction of the central pulmonary vessels— particularly in the case of unilateral disease—may be the consequence of extravascular pathology (lymphadenopathy, carcinoma, fibrosis) or intravascular occlusive disease (primary pulmonary vascular tumor).

Despite the values of pulmonary angiography in this patient population, there remains a subgroup of patients where the diagnosis of CTE disease and surgical accessibility of the CTE lesions are not completely addressed with angiography alone. In approximately 20 to 25% of CTEPH patients, visualization of the vascular intima with pulmonary angioscopy has proven to be a useful evaluative tool (70). This fiberoptic device can be introduced into the pulmonary vascular bed through a central venous access; with inflation of a balloon tied to the tip of the angioscope, blood flow is briefly interrupted allowing the walls of the pulmonary arteries to be visualized. The angioscopic appearance of organized thromboemboli consists of roughening or pitting of

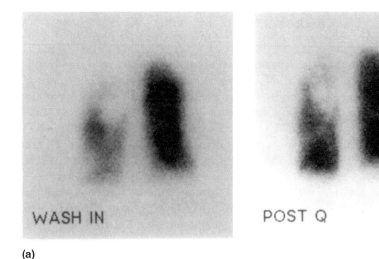

(a)

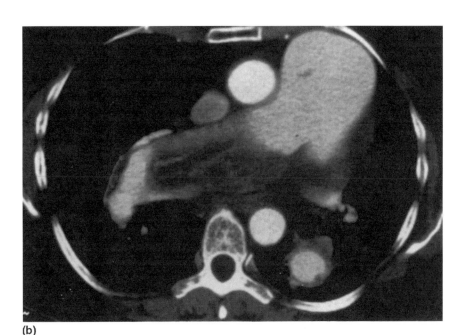

(b)

Figure 3 (a) Lung ventilation/perfusion scan in a patient with severe pulmonary hypertension (PVR) (1659 dynes/sec/cm^5). Poor ventilation of the left lung (upper panel) with left upper lobe perfusion defects. Right-lung perfusion is essentially normal. (b) Contrast CT scan in the same patient shown in Figure 3a showing extensive thrombus involving the right main pulmonary artery (PA) and lining the left descending PA. (c) Large amount of thrombus removed with endarterectomy, though without "tails" from lobar or segmental vessels. No hemodynamic improvement (postoperative PVR 1506 dynes/sec/cm^5) or change in lung scan resulted from the operation.

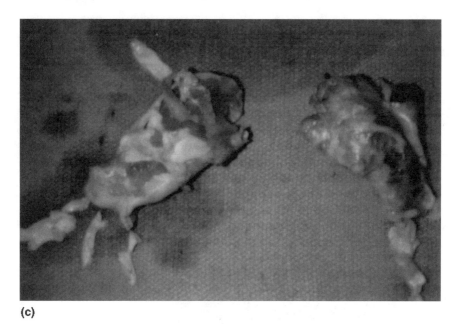

(c)

Figure 3 Continued.

the intimal surface, "bands" traversing the vascular lumen, irregularly shaped vessel ostia, and "recanalization" or the presence of multiple channels where a single lumen should occur (Fig. 5). This procedure has proved most useful in confirming operability in patients with severe pulmonary hypertension who would not have been deemed surgical candidates based on angiographic findings alone and in predicting a beneficial hemodynamic outcome in patients with modest pulmonary hypertension in whom pulmonary angiography did not precisely define the proximal extent of CTE disease (71).

Important in the selection of suitable candidates for pulmonary thromboendarterectomy is defining the presence of coexisting cardiac disease. In those patients at risk for coronary artery disease or in whom echocardiography has revealed previously undetected left ventricular dysfunction or valvular heart disease, coronary arteriography and left heart catheterization provide essential supplemental information in the assessment of the CTEPH patient.

VI. Pulmonary Thromboendarterectomy

Patients with suspected chronic thromboembolic pulmonary hypertension undergo evaluation with the goals of (1) establishing the need for surgical intervention, (2) determining the surgical accessibility of the chronic

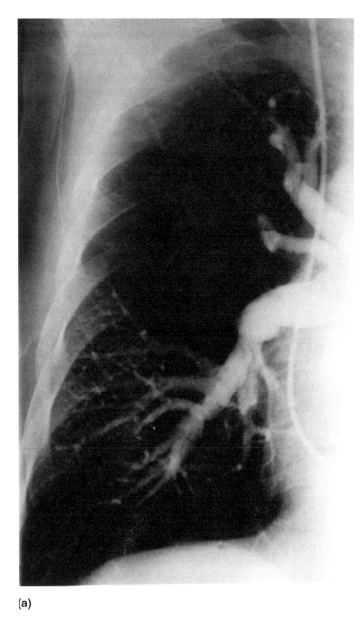

(a)

Figure 4 (a and b) PA and lateral views, right pulmonary arteriogram in a CTEPH patient. Features of chronic thromboembolic disease include the narrowed and irregularly shaped interlobar vessel; the occluded middle lobe, anterior and posterior upper lobe arteries; and a "pouch defect" (arrows) at the origin of the lower lobe arteries.

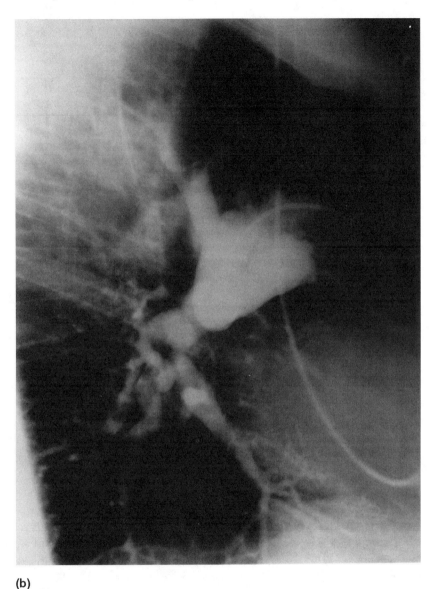

(b)

thromboemboli, and (3) assessing the risk of surgery in the individual patient. The majority of patients who ultimately go on to surgery exhibit a pulmonary vascular resistance greater than 300 dynes/sec/cm^{-5}. At centers reporting their experience with PTE surgery, preoperative pulmonary vascular resistance is typically in the range of 700 to 1100 dynes/sec/cm^5 (24–32). At this level of pulmonary hypertension, a patient's impairment at rest and with exercise can

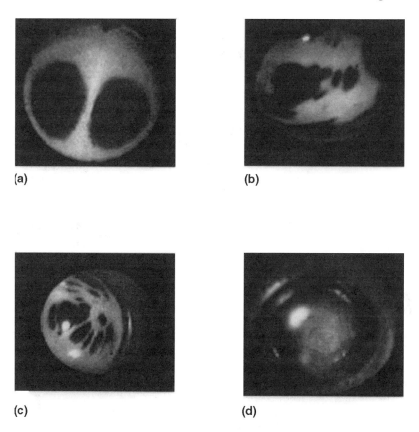

(a)   (b)

(c)   (d)

Figure 5 Pulmonary angioscopic views of the vascular intima. (a) Smooth white intima at the bifurcation of a normal pulmonary artery. (b and c) Appearance of recanalization in an organized thrombus. (d) Semiorganized thrombus lining a pulmonary artery.

be considerable; in the absence of surgical intervention, prognosis is poor (40,41). For those patients with less severe pulmonary hypertension, surgery is considered based on individual circumstances. For some with CTE disease, mild to moderate pulmonary pressures at rest can become significantly elevated with exertion. Though not as yet fully substantiated, it is suspected that these high pressures and/or flow states over a prolonged period of time contribute to the development of a small vessel arteriopathy in the unobstructed vascular bed. With time, pulmonary hypertension worsens and the need to proceed with surgery becomes more pressing. Patients with this hemodynamic profile often find their functional status unacceptable, and with the knowledge that their pulmonary pressures and right heart function will deteriorate, will elect to have surgery. However, in the absence of surgical intervention at this stage of CTE disease, diligent follow-up of an individual's symptoms and hemodynamic status is imperative. And for those with minimal or mild pulmonary hemodynamic difficulties, the decision to undergo a pulmonary thromboendarterectomy is one based on an assessment of risks and possible long-term benefits of surgery. In this category are patients with involvement of one main pulmonary artery, those with vigorous lifestyle expectations (e.g., athletes), and those who live at altitude. Symptomatic limitation in this group is usually a function of elevated dead-space and minute ventilatory demands and a restriction on maximal cardiac output with exercise.

An absolute criterion for surgery is the presence of accessible chronic thrombi as assessed by pulmonary angiography or angioscopy. The experience of the surgical team will dictate what can be considered "accessible." Current surgical techniques allow removal of organized thrombi in the main and lobar levels, extending to the proximal segmental vessels. However, dissection of segmental-level thrombus requires greater surgical skill and experience. In either situation, an accurate determination of accessible disease, and a prediction that the removal of these lesions will reduce right ventricular afterload and pulmonary pressures, are essential to a successful surgical outcome. Especially in those patients with severe pulmonary hypertension and right ventricular dysfunction preoperatively, failure to endarterectomize sufficient thromboembolic material to reduce the pulmonary vascular resistance is associated with a greater perioperative mortality rate and poorer long-term outcome (72,73).

The third consideration in assessing surgical candidacy is the presence of comorbid conditions that may adversely affect perioperative mortality or morbidity. Coexisting coronary artery disease, parenchymal lung disease, renal insufficiency, hepatic dysfunction, or the presence of a hypercoaguable state may complicate patient management during the postoperative period. However, the reversal of pulmonary hypertension and right ventricular dysfunction with PTE surgery will often improve hepatic and renal function postoperatively; for those patients with coronary artery or valvular heart disease, coronary artery bypass grafting or valve replacement can be performed at the time of the thromboendarterectomy without an increase in surgical risk (74). Consequently, advanced age or the presence of collateral disease is not an absolute contraindication to pulmonary thromboendarterectomy, although both age and disease do impact risk assessment and affect postoperative management strategies. One exception seems to be the presence of severe parenchymal or obstructive lung disease. The postoperative course in these patients is frequently complicated by prolonged ventilatory support, and the cardiopulmonary benefits of thromboendarterectomy often result in minimal symptomatic improvement. The limitations of surgery in this patient population require careful disclosure to the individual and his or her family prior to proceeding with the thromboendarterectomy.

Though details of the surgical procedure have been described elsewhere (75,76), there are several features of the operation that should be highlighted.

Surgical success is founded on the concept that a true endarterectomy to remove the organized thrombi is to be accomplished, not an embolectomy. Removal of nonadherent, partially organized thrombus within the lumen of the central pulmonary arteries is ineffective in reducing right ventricular afterload. An endarterectomy involves identification of the endothelialized thrombus, and creation of a dissection plane—often down to the media of the vessel—to adequately free the thrombotic residua from the central vascular bed.

The operation is performed through a median sternotomy. This allows access to the central pulmonary vessels of both lungs. As patients with significant CTEPH will have bilateral disease, the advantages to this approach are evident. A sternotomy also avoids the pleural space and potential disruption of pleural adhesions and the hypertrophic bronchial blood vessels that develop as a result of chronically obstructed pulmonary arteries. Furthermore, if other cardiac procedures are required, such as coronary artery or valve surgery, adequate exposure with this approach is already achieved. Between January 2000 and August 2001, a total of 200 CTEPH patients underwent PTE surgery at the University of California, San Diego (UCSD). In this group, 57 patients (30.3%) underwent right atrial exploration and closure of a patent foramen ovale; 20 patients (10%) required coronary bypass graft surgery; and 2 patients (1%) required valve surgery (pulmonary valvuloplasty, tricuspid valve repair with annuloplasty ring) in addition to their pulmonary thromboendarterectomy.

Cardiopulmonary bypass (CPB) with periods of circulatory arrest is essential to ensure optimal exposure of the pulmonary vascular intima in a bloodless field. The significant back-bleeding created by bronchial arterial blood flow is mitigated by interruption of CPB. These circulatory arrest periods are limited to 20 min, with resumption of blood flow and restoration of mixed venous O_2 saturation between each interruption. With experience, endarterectomy of either the right or left pulmonary vessel can usually be completed within the time constraint of one arrest period. This exposure allows the circumferential dissection of thromboembolic residua from the involved lobar, segmental, and subsegmental vessels (Fig. 6).

Safeguards to ensure tissue integrity are an integral component of this surgical procedure, allowing circulatory arrests to be accomplished without adverse consequences. Though standard flow for cardiopulmonary bypass is used, the patient is systemically cooled to 20 °C. Hemodilution to a hematocrit in the range of 18 to 25% is performed to decrease blood viscosity during hypothermia and to optimize capillary blood flow. Additional cerebral protection is provided by surrounding the head with ice and a cooling blanket; phenytoin is administered intravenously during the cooling period to reduce the risk of perioperative seizure activity. When the patient's temperature reaches 20 °C, the aorta is cross-clamped and a single dose of cold cardioplegic solution is administered. Further myocardial protection is achieved with the use of a cooling jacket wrapped around the heart. Following cross-clamping of the aorta, thiopental is then administered until the electroencephalogram

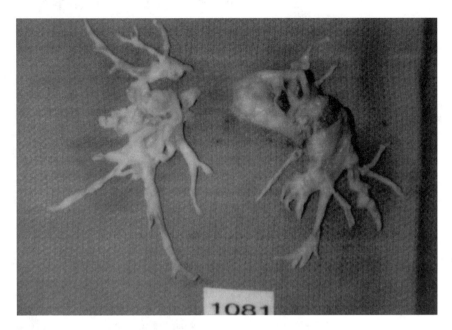

Figure 6 Chronic thromboembolic material removed at the time of thromboendarterectomy.

(EEG) becomes isoelectric. When the patient is cooled to the optimal level of hypothermia, periods of circulatory arrest can be initiated. During these periods, all monitoring lines to the patient are turned off to prevent air aspiration, and the patient is exsanguinated. The endaterectomy can proceed at this point, usually first on the right side, then on the left. After completion of the endarterectomy, cardiopulmonary bypass is resumed and rewarming commenced. A gradient of 10 °C is maintained between the perfusate and body temperature during rewarming; doses of methylprednisolone and mannitol are administered at this point in the operation. Given the high incidence of sinus arrest within the first 24 hr postendarterectomy, atrial and ventricular epicardial wires are placed; mediastinal chest tubes also are left in place to evacuate any accumulated blood during the first 2 to 3 postoperative days. Following rewarming and successful defibrillation of the heart, cardiopulmonary bypass is discontinued and mechanical ventilation resumed.

Over the past few years, modifications of the surgical approach have been suggested in an effort to decrease risk and improve hemodynamic outcome. Dartevelle and colleagues have suggested the use of intraoperative video-assisted angioscopy to increase visibility in the distal pulmonary arteries, potentially allowing surgical intervention in patients with previously inaccessible disease (77). Division rather than retraction of the superior vena cava to improve exposure of the right pulmonary artery has been advocated by

Zund et al. (23). Selective antegrade cerebral perfusion during circulatory arrest has been proposed to decrease the risk of neurological sequelae (78).

VII. Postoperative Care

Several problems encountered following PTE surgery are similar to those experienced by patients undergoing other forms of cardiac surgery. Coagulation disorders, arrhythmias, wound infections, delirium, pleural and pericardial effusions, atelectasis, and nosocomial infections are among the difficulties faced by this patient population (79). Table 1 depicts the incidence of the more common complications in 200 operated patients at UCSD between January 2000 and August 2001. One of the most difficult problems following PTE surgery, and one which substantially contributes to postoperative mortality, is the development of reperfusion lung injury (80). The exact pathophysiological basis for this lung injury remains uncertain, though both clinically and biochemically it seems to demonstrate features of a localized form of high-permeability, neutrophil-mediated lung damage. The onset of this acute lung injury typically occurs within the first 24 hr postoperatively, though it may appear up to 72 hr after surgery. It is highly variable in severity, ranging from mild to moderate hypoxemia in most affected patients to profound alveolar hemorrhage, which is most often fatal. Seemingly unique to this form of lung injury is that it is usually limited to endarterectomized lung regions. It is in these same lung regions that pulmonary arterial blood flow is preferentially redistributed, causing a greater degree of transpulmonary shunting and hypoxemia. This phenomenon, referred to as pulmonary vascular "steal" (39), further complicates the postoperative management of patients suffering from reperfusion lung injury.

The management of reperfusion lung edema is, to a large extent, supportive until resolution occurs. High-dose corticosteroids have been used to

Table 1 Postoperative Complications in 200 PTE Patients Who Underwent Surgery at UCSD Between January 2000 and August 2001

Complication	Number of patients	%
Reperfusion lung Injury	65	32.5
Persistent pulmonary hypertension[a]	28	14.4
Atrial fibrillation-flutter	26	13.0
Delirium	21	10.5
Nosocomial lung infection	21	10.5
Wound infection	6	3.0

[a] Postoperative pulmonary vascular resistance > 500 dyne/sec/cm^{-5}; complete perioperative hemodynamic values available in 195 patients.

modulate the inflammatory component of the process, though their effectiveness is unpredictable and frequently minimal. Positional changes occasionally improve $\dot{V}/\dot{Q}$ mismatch, though again this is not a uniformly useful intervention. The use of inverse-ratio ventilation, a low-volume ventilatory strategy to minimize the risk of ongoing alveolar damage or incremental levels of positive end-expiratory pressure have variably proved useful in improving $\dot{V}/\dot{Q}$ relationships and gas exchange when conventional ventilator therapy has failed. In extreme situations, extracorporeal support (ECCO2R) has been used successfully in patients where aggressive conventional measures have been inadequate to maintain oxygenation. In a recent study of 47 patients undergoing PTE surgery, the postoperative avoidance of positive inotropic catecholamines and vasodilators, along with a strategy of low-volume (<8 mL/ kg) ventilation, resulted in a lower incidence of reperfusion pulmonary edema (81).

Persistent pulmonary hypertension following PTE surgery is a particularly difficult management problem and, like reperfusion lung injury, remains a major cause of postoperative mortality. In the immediate postoperative period, those patients left with residual pulmonary hypertension can exhibit significant hemodynamic instability. This situation results not only from persistently elevated right ventricular afterload but also from the adverse physiological consequences of prolonged cardiopulmonary bypass, deep hypothermia, a residual metabolic acidosis, and hypoxemia. Management goals focus on minimizing systemic oxygen consumption, optimizing right ventricular preload, and providing inotropic support. Pharmacological attempts at right ventricular afterload in this patient population often is ineffectual, as pulmonary vascular resistance is fixed and risks provoking a decrease in systemic vascular resistance, systemic blood pressure, and coronary artery perfusion pressure. Inhaled nitric oxide has a theoretical advantage in this setting, with its pulmonary vasodilatory properties and negligible systemic effects. However, anecdotal experience with this intervention in the setting of persistent postoperative pulmonary hypertension has been disappointing. If the patient survives the immediate postoperative period, long-term pulmonary vasodilator therapy, such as the continuous intravenous administration of epoprostenol, should be considered (82).

VIII. Outcome Following Pulmonary Thromboendarterectomy

Though early reports describing the surgical treatment of CTEPH acknowledged the postoperative improvement in pulmonary hemodynamics, it was frequently cited that the mortal risk of the procedure was high. In a 1984 review of the world's experience with PTE surgery, Chitwood and colleagues described 85 patients having undergone this operation between 1960 and 1983. The combined mortality rate of this group was 22%, with one center in their review with a postoperative mortality rate of 40% (83). Despite these early figures, progress in the surgical approach to these patients was sustained primarily because medical therapies were ineffective, surgery had the potential of substantially improving pulmonary hemodynamics, and survival in untreated patients was poor. To date, it is estimated that approximately 2000 thromboendarterectomy procedures have been performed worldwide, with over 1400 of these at the University of California, San Diego (84). In reported series of PTE patients since 1996, in-hospital mortality rates range between 5 and 24% (24–31,76). In the 31-year history of thromboendarter-ectomy operations at UCSD, a trend of declining mortality rates has been noted (73). Between 1970 and 1983, the group of 17 patients undergoing PTE surgery at UCSD exhibited a 17.6% in-hospital mortality rate. From January 1984 to November 1989, the mortality rate in 171 operated patients was 15.2%. With the current medical-surgical team providing care for the PTE patients, the mortality rate between the end of 1989 and 1992 was 7.2% of 207 operated patients; since 1993, an additional 1022 patients have undergone surgery with an in-hospital mortality rate of 6.7%.

The factors affecting perioperative mortality have not been completely defined. In global terms, it has been suggested that experience in patient selection as well as in the surgical and postoperative management of the patients can positively influence mortality figures. Moser and colleagues reported several factors that appeared to impact survivorship postoperatively: New York Heart Association (NYHA) functional class IV status preopera-tively, age older than 70 years, morbid obesity, the presence of significant comorbid diseases, the severity of preoperative pulmonary vascular resistance, the presence of right ventricular failure as manifest by high right atrial pressures, and "perhaps" the duration of pulmonary hypertension (85). Recently, Hartz et al. found that a preoperative pulmonary vascular resistance greater than 1100 dynes/sec/cm^5 and a mean pulmonary artery pressure greater than 50 mmHg predicted a higher operative mortality (26). However, this observation was not substantiated in the report of D'Armini and colleagues (31). They were unable to demonstrate that the preoperative severity of pulmonary hypertension or the degree of cardiac failure correlated with early postoperative death. Tscholl et al., in a study of 69 PTE patients, showed that older age, increased right atrial pressure, decreased cardiac output, a higher NYHA functional class, a greater number of involved pulmonary segments, and higher pulmonary vascular resistance (>1136 dynes/sec/cm^5) influenced hospital mortality (86). Mares and colleagues also demonstrated that postoperative management strategies could affect outcome (81). Combining a low tidal volume (<8 mL/kg) ventilator strategy with the avoidance of positive inotropic catecholamines and vasodilators in the postoperative period, this group was able to achieve lower in-hospital mortality rates (9.1 versus 21.4%).

Attributable causes of death following PTE surgery vary considerably and relate to the complexities of the surgical procedure and to the postoperative difficulties experienced by this patient population. Cardiac arrest, uncontrollable mediastinal bleeding, cerebrovascular accidents, myocardial injury, massive pulmonary hemorrhage, sepsis syndrome, and multiorgan failure are among the causes of death cited (18,22,26,28–31,86). However, most deaths postendarterectomy have resulted from unremitting reperfusion lung injury or persistent pulmonary hypertension and right ventricular failure. At UCSD, between January 1984 and November 1995, one or both of these postoperative complications accounted for 54.2% of the deaths in 651 patients (73).

In the majority of CTEPH patients undergoing thromboendarterectomy surgery, the hemodynamic and functional outcomes have been outstanding. With restoration of blood flow to previously occluded lung regions, an immediate reduction in right ventricular afterload occurs, resulting in a decline in pulmonary arterial pressures and an augmentation in cardiac output. This postoperative improvement in pulmonary hemodynamics has been reported by several groups (22,26–30,77,81,87); data available from UCSD between January 2000 and August 2001 are presented in Table 2. Postoperative echocardiographic findings further document the improvement in cardiac function and pulmonary hemodynamics following surgery. Dittrich and colleagues performed two-dimensional echocardiography 8 ± 8 days before and 6 ± 4 days after PTE surgery in 30 patients. They demonstrated a significant decrease in end-diastolic right ventricular size postoperatively, accompanied by a more normal position of the interventricular septum, a moderate increase in left ventricular end-diastolic size, a reduction in right atrial size, and a reduction in the caliber of the inferior vena cava (88). Menzel et al. reported similar findings in 14 patients within 18 ± 12 days post thromboendarterectomy (89).

The long-term results following PTE surgery have been similarly impressive. Sustained hemodynamic improvement (>3 months postoperatively) has been reported by numerous groups, accompanied by substantial gains in functional status when compared to their preoperative state

Table 2 Perioperative Hemodynamics in 200 PTE Patients[a] Who Underwent Surgery at UCSD Between January 2000 and August 2001

	Preoperative	Postoperative	p value[b]
Mean PA pressure (mmHg)	$46.4 +/- 9.8$	$29.3 +/- 10.5$	$p < 0.001$
PA systolic pressure (mmHg)	$76.2 +/- 16.1$	$49.2 +/- 17.4$	$p < 0.001$
Cardiac output (L/min)	$3.58 +/- 1.18$	$5.50 +/- 1.56$	$p < 0.001$
PVR (dyne/sec/cm^{-5})	$960 +/- 423$	$331 +/- 249$	$p < 0.001$

[a] Complete pre- and postoperative hemodynamic numbers available in 195 patients; postoperative values within 72 hr following surgery. [b] Two-tailed student's t-test.
Key: PA, pulmonary artery; PVR, pulmonary vascular resistance.

(25,31,77,90,91). A corresponding improvement in gas exchange over time also has been noted (92,93).

In a large cross-sectional study, Archibald and coworkers examined functional status and quality-of-life issues in a cohort of 308 patients having undergone PTE surgery between 1970 and 1994 (94). At an average of 3.3 years following surgery (range 1–16 years), 93% of 306 respondents identified their functional status as NYHA class I or II. Most patients (63% of 303 respondents) reported no dyspnea walking on a level surface; 73.2% of patients noted their dyspnea to be "much improved" when asked to rate their shortness of breath since surgery; and 89.6% of 275 respondents were no longer using supplemental oxygen, with the mean duration of oxygen use post PTE of 7.1 weeks (range 1–64 weeks). In the evaluation of employment status, 133 patients, or 43.3% of the surveyed group, returned to work following their PTE surgery. Though 51 of these individuals were employed prior to the operation, 82 patients were able to resume gainful employment. Sixty three patients, or 20.5% of the respondents, were disabled prior to surgery and remained disabled. This study also examined long-term survivorship in this patient population. With data obtained in 532 patients, there was a 75% probability of survival beyond 6 years. The majority of posthospital deaths in this cohort were unrelated to pulmonary vascular difficulties; however, persistent pulmonary hypertension or recurrent pulmonary emboli contributed to 22 of the 51 deaths.

IX. Future Directions

Pulmonary thromboendarterectomy has proven to be an effective means of treating selected patients with chronic thromboembolic pulmonary hypertension. And despite the tremendous advances in the diagnostic approach, surgical management, and postoperative care of these patients, there remain numerous questions to be answered to further reduce the morbidity and mortality of this disease process. The predisposition to chronic thromboembolic disease in some patients suffering an acute pulmonary embolus and the subsequent hemodynamic progression over time remains a mystery in most individuals. The ability to identify those CTE patients with extensive, coexisting small vessel pulmonary vascular disease who would not benefit from PTE surgery continues to be a challenge even for the most experienced diagnostician. If surgery fails to improve pulmonary hemodynamics and a patient is left with significant pulmonary hypertension, the ideal approach to long-term therapy has yet to be defined. Finally, this patient population offers a unique opportunity to enhance our understanding of the mechanisms underlying acute lung injury. With these insights, novel therapeutic interventions and management strategies can be evaluated with the hope of positively impacting patient outcome.

References

1. Ljungdahl M. Gibt es eine chronische embolistierung der lungenarterie? Dtsch Arch Klin Med 1928; 102:1–23.
2. McMichael J. Heart failure of pulmonary origin. Edinburgh Med J 1948; 55:65.
3. Owen WR, Thomas WA, Castleman B, Bland EF. Unrecognized emboli to the lungs with subsequent cor pulmonale. N Engl J Med 1953; 249:919–926.
4. Ball KP, Goodwin JF, Harrison CV. Massive thrombotic occlusion of the large pulmonary arteries. Circulation 1956; 14:766–783.
5. Helie M. Inflammation de l'artere pulmonaire. Mort subite. Bull Soc Anat Paris. 1837; 12:254.
6. Carroll D. Chronic obstruction of major pulmonary arteries. Am J Med 1950; 9:175–185.
7. Hollister LE, Cull VL. The syndrome of chronic thrombosis of the major pulmonary arteries. Am J Med 1956; 21:312–320.
8. Hurwitt ES, Schein CJ, Rifkin H, Lebendiger A. A surgical approach to the problem of chronic pulmonary artery obstruction due to thrombosis or stenosis. Ann Surg 1958; 147:157–165.
9. Synder WA, Kent DC, Baisch BF. Successful endarterectomy of chronically occluded pulmonary artery: clinical report and physiologic studies. J Thorac Cardiovasc Surg 1963; 45:482–489.
10. Castleman B, McNeeley BU, Scannell G. Case records of the Massachusetts General Hospital, Case 32-1964. N Engl J Med 1964; 271:40–50.
11. Houk VN, Hufnagel CH, McClenathan JE, Moser KM. Chronic thrombotic obstruction of major pulmonary arteries: report of a case successfully treated by thromboendarterectomy and a review of the literature. Am J Med 1963; 35:269–282.
12. Moser KM, Houk VN, Jones RC, Hufnagel CH. Chronic, massive thrombotic obstruction of pulmonary arteries: analysis of four operated cases. Circulation 1965; 32:377–385.
13. Nash ES, Shapiro S, Landau A, Barnard CN. Successful thromboembolectomy in long-standing thromboembolic pulmonary hypertension. Thorax 1966; 23:121–130.
14. Moor GF, Sabiston DC Jr. Embolectomy for chronic pulmonary embolism and pulmonary hypertension: case report and review of the problem. Circulation 1970; 41:701–708.
15. Cabrol C, Cabrol A, Acar J, Gandjbakhch I, Guiraudon G, Laughlin L, Mattei M-F, Godeau P. Surgical correction of chronic postembolic obstructions of the pulmonary arteries. J Thorac Cardiovasc Surg 1978; 76:620–628.
16. Sabiston DC, Jr, Wolfe WG, Oldham HN Jr, Wechsler AS, Crawford FA Jr, Jones KW, Jones RH. Surgical management of chronic pulmonary embolism. Ann Surg 1977; 185:699–712.
17. Utley JR, Spragg RG, Long WB, Moser KM. Pulmonary endarterectomy for chronic thromboembolic obstruction: recent surgical experience. Surgery 1982; 92:1096–1102.
18. Moser KM, Daily PO, Peterson K, Dembitsky W, Vapnek JM, Shure D, Utley J, Archibald C. Thromboendarterectomy for chronic, major-vessel thromboembolic

pulmonary hypertension: immediate and long-term results in 42 patients. Ann Intern Med 1987; 107:560–565.

19. Daily PO, Dembitsky WP, Peterson KL, Moser KM. Modifications of techniques and early results of pulmonary thromboendarterectomy for chronic pulmonary embolism. J Thorac Cardiovasc Surg 1987; 93:221–233.

20. Daily PO, Dembitsky WP, Iversen S. Technique of pulmonary thromboendarterectomy for chronic pulmonary embolism. J Card Surg 1989; 4:10–24.

21. Daily PO, Dembitsky WP, Daily RP. Dissectors for pulmonary thromboendarterectomy. Ann Thorac Surg 1991; 51:842–843.

22. Jamieson SW, Auger WR, Fedullo PF, Channick RN, Kriett JM, Tarazi RY, Moser KM. Experience and results with 150 pulmonary thromboendarterectomy operations over a 29-month period. J Thorac Cardiovasc Surg 1993; 106:116–127.

23. Zund G, Pretre R, Niederhauser U, Vogt PR, Turina MI. Improved exposure of the pulmonary arteries for thromboendarterectomy. Ann Thorac Surg 1998; 66:1821–1823.

24. Simonneau G, Azarian R, Brenot F, Dartevelle PG, Musset D, Duroux P. Surgical management of unresolved pulmonary embolism: a personal series of 72 patients. Chest 1995; 107:52S–55S.

25. Mayer E, Dahm M, Hake U, Schmid FX, Pitton M, Kupferwasser I, Iversen S, Oelert H. Mid-term results of pulmonary thromboendarterectomy for chronic thromboembolic pulmonary hypertension. Ann Thorac Surg 1996; 61:1788–1792.

26. Hartz RS, Byme JG, Levitsky S, Park J, Rich S. Predictors of mortality in pulmonary thromboendarterectomy. Ann Thorac Surg 1996; 62:1255–1259.

27. Nakajima N, Masuda M, Mogi K. The surgical treatment for chronic pulmonary thromboembolism: our surgical experience and current review of the literature. Ann Thorac Cardiovasc Surg 1997; 3:15–21.

28. Gilbert TB, Gaine SP, Rubin LJ, Sequeira AJ. Short-term outcome and predictors of adverse events following pulmonary thromboendarterectomy. World J Surg 1998; 22:1029–1032.

29. Ando M, Okita Y, Tagusari O, Kitamura S, Nakanishi N, Kyotani S. Surgical treatment for chronic thromboembolic pulmonary hypertension under profound hypothermia and circulatory arrest in 24 patients. J Card Surg 1999; 14:377–385.

30. Rubens F, Wells P, Bencze S, Bourke M. Surgical treatment of chronic thromboembolic pulmonary hypertension. Can Respir J 2000; 7:49–57.

31. D'Armini AM, Cattadori B, Monterosso C, Klersy C, Emmi V, Piovella F, Minzioni G, Vigano M. Pulmonary thromboendarterectomy in patients with chronic pulmonary hypertension: Hemodynamic characteristics and changes. Eur J Cardiothorac Surg 2000; 18:696–702.

32. Fedullo PF, Auger WR, Channick RN, Kerr KM, Rubin LJ. Chronic thromboembolic pulmonary hypertension. Clin Chest Med 2001; 22:561–581.

33. Rich S, Levitsky S, Brundage BH. Pulmonary hypertension from chronic pulmonary thromboembolism. Ann Intern Med 1988; 108:425–434.

34. Olman MA, Marsh JJ, Lang IM, Moser KM, Binder BR, Schleef RR. The endogenous fibrinolytic system in chronic large-vessel thromboembolic pulmonary hypertension. Circulation 1992; 86:1241–1248.

35. Auger WR, Permpikul P, Moser KM. Lupus anticoagulant, heparin use, and thrombocytopenia in patients with chronic thromboembolic pulmonary hypertension: a preliminary report. Am J Med 1995; 99:392–396.

36. Wolf M, Soyer-Neumann C, Parent F, Eschwege V, Jaillet H, Meyer D, Simonneau G. Thrombotic risk factors in pulmonary hypertension. Eur Respir J 2000; 15:395–399.
37. Sompradeekul S, Fedullo PF, Le DT. Congenital and acquired thrombophilias in patients with chronic thromboembolic pulmonary hypertension (abstr). Am J Respir Crit Care Med 1999; 159:A358.
38. Moser KM, Bloor CM. Pulmonary vascular lesions occurring in patients with chronic major vessel thromboembolic pulmonary hypertension. Chest 1993; 103:685–692.
39. Olman MA, Auger WR, Fedullo PF, Moser KM. Pulmonary vascular steal in chronic thromboembolic pulmonary hypertension. Chest 1990; 98:1430–1434.
40. Riedel M, Stanek V, Widimsky J, Prerovsky I. Long-term follow-up of patients with pulmonary thromboembolism: late prognosis and evolution of hemodynamic and respiratory data. Chest 1982; 81:151–158.
41. Lewczuk J, Piszko P, Jagas J, Porada A, Wojciak S, Sobkowicz B, Wrabec K. Prognostic factors in medically treated patients with chronic pulmonary embolism. Chest 2001; 119:818–823.
42. Auger WR, Moser KM. Pulmonary flow murmurs: a distinctive physical sign found in chronic pulmonary thromboembolic disease (abstr). Clin Res 1989; 37:145A.
43. Voelkel MA, Wynne KM, Badesch DB, Groves BM, Voelkel NF. Hyperuricemia in severe pulmonary hypertension. Chest 2000; 117:19–24.
44. Morris TA, Auger WR, Ysrael MZ, Olson LK, Channick RN, Fedullo PF, Moser KM. Parenchymal scarring is associated with restrictive spirometric defects in patients with chronic thromboembolic pulmonary hypertension. Chest 1996; 110:399–403.
45. Steenhuis LH, Groen HJM, Koeter GH, van der Mark Th W. Diffusion capacity and haemodynamics in primary and chronic thromboembolic pulmonary hypertension. Eur Respir J 2000; 16:276–281.
46. Elliott CG, Colby TV, Hill T, Crapo RO. Pulmonary veno-occlusive disease associated with severe reduction of single-breath carbon monoxide diffusing capacity. Respiration 1988; 53:262–266.
47. Kapitan KS, Buchbinder M, Wagner PD, Moser KM. Mechanisms of hypoxemia in chronic thromboembolic pulmonary hypertension. Am Rev Respir Dis 1989; 139:1149–1154.
48. Woodruff WW III, Hoeck BE, Chitwood WR Jr, Lyerly HK, Sabiston DC Jr, Chen JT. Radiographic findings in pulmonary hypertension from unresolved embolism. AJR 1985; 144:681–686.
49. D'Alonzo GE, Bower JS, Dantzker DR. Differentiation of patients with primary and thromboembolic pulmonary hypertension. Chest 1984; 85:457–461.
50. Moser KM, Olson LK, Schlusselberg M, Daily PO, Dembitsky WP. Chronic thromboembolic occlusion in the adult can mimic pulmonary artery agenesis. Chest 1989; 95:503–508.
51. Dittrich HC, McCann HA, Blanchard DG. Cardiac structure and function in chronic thromboembolic pulmonary hypertension. Am J Cardiac Imaging 1994; 8:18–27.
52. Lisbona R, Kreisman H, Novales-Diaz J, Derbekyan V. Perfusion lung scanning: Differentiation of primary from thromboembolic pulmonary hypertension. AJR 1985; 144:27–30.

53. Ryan KL, Fedullo PF, Davis GB, Vasquez TE, Moser KM. Perfusion scan findings understate the severity of angiographic and hemodynamic compromise in chronic thromboembolic pulmonary hypertension. Chest 1988; 93:1180–1185.

54. King MA, Bergin CJ, Yeung D, Belezzouli E, Olson L, Ashburn W, Auger WR, Moser KM. Chronic pulmonary thromboembolism: detection of regional hypoperfusion with CT. Radiology 1994; 191:359–363.

55. Schwickert HC, Schweden F, Schild HH, Piepenburg R, Duber C, Kauczor H-U, Renner C, Iversen S, Thelen M. Pulmonary arteries and lung parenchyma in chronic pulmonary embolism: Preoperative and postoperative CT findings. Radiology 1994; 191:351–357.

56. Tardivon AA, Musset D, Maitre S, Brenot F, Dartevelle P, Simonneau G, Labrune M. Role of CT in chronic pulmonary embolism: comparison with pulmonary angiography. J Comput Assist Tomogr 1993; 17:345–352.

57. Bergin CJ. Chronic thromboembolic pulmonary hypertension: The disease, the diagnosis, and the treatment. Semin Ultrasound CT MR 1997; 18:383–391.

58. Berry PF, Buccigrossi D, Peabody J, Peterson KL, Moser KM. Pulmonary vascular occlusion and fibrosing mediastinitis. Chest 1986; 89:296–301.

59. Bergin CJ, Hauschildt JP, Brown MA, Channick RN, Fedullo PF. Identifying the cause of unilateral hypoperfusion in patients suspected to have chronic pulmonary thrombo-embolism: diagnostic accuracy of helical CT and conventional angio-graphy. Radiology 1999; 213:743–749.

60. Cho SR, Tisnado J, Cockrell CH, Beachley MC, Fratkin MJ, Henry DA. Angiographic evaluation of patients with unilateral massive perfusion defects on the lung scan. Radiographics 1987; 7:729–745.

61. Anderson MB, Kriett JM, Kapelanski DP, Tarazi R, Jamieson SW. Primary pulmonary artery sarcoma: a report of six cases. Ann Thorac Surg 1995; 59:1487–1490.

62. Moser KM, Fedullo PF, Finkbeiner WE, Golden J. Do patients with primary pulmonary hypertension develop extensive central thrombi Circulation 1995; 91:741–745.

63. Russo A, De Luca M, Vigna C, De Rito V, Pacilli M, Lombardo A, Armillotta M, Fanelli R, Loperfido F. Central pulmonary artery lesions in chronic obstructive pulmonary disease. A transesophageal echocardiographic study. Circulation 1999; 100:1808–1815.

64. Nicod P, Peterson K, Levine M, Dittrich H, Buchbinder M, Chappuis F, Moser K. Pulmonary angiography in severe chronic pulmonary hypertension. Ann Intern Med 1987; 107:565–568.

65. Pitton MB, Duber C, Mayer E, Thelen M. Hemodynamic effects of nonionic contrast bolus injection and oxygen inhalation during pulmonary angiography in patients with chronic major-vessel thromboembolic pulmonary hypertension. Circulation 1996; 94:2485–2491.

66. Auger WR, Fedullo PF, Moser KM, Buchbinder M, Peterson KL. Chronic major-vessel thromboembolic pulmonary artery obstruction: appearance at angiography. Radiology 1992; 182:393–398.

67. Yamato M, Lecky JW, Hiramatsu K, Kohda E. Takayasu's arteritis: radiographic and angiographic findings in 59 patients. Radiology 1986; 161:329–334.

68. Kerr KM, Auger WR, Fedullo PF, Channick RN, Moser KM. Large vessel pulmonary arteritis mimicking chronic thromboembolic disease. Am J Respir Crit Care Med 1995; 152:367–373.

69. D'Cruz IA, Agustsson MH, Bicoff JP, Weinberg M, Arcilla RA. Stenotic lesions of the pulmonary arteries: clinical and hemodynamic findings in 84 cases. Am J Cardiol 1964; 13:441–450.

70. Shure D, Gregoratos G, Moser KM. Fiberoptic angioscopy: Role in the diagnosis of chronic pulmonary arterial obstruction. Ann Intern Med 1985; 103:844–850.

71. Sompradeekul S, Fedullo PF, Kerr KM, Channick RN, Auger WR. The role of pulmonary angioscopy in the preoperative assessment of patients with thromboembolic pulmonary hypertension (CTEPH) (abstr). Am J Respir Crit Care Med 1999; 159:A456.

72. Daily PO, Dembitsky WP, Iversen S, Moser KM, Auger W. Risk factors for pulmonary thromboendaterectomy. J Thorac Cardiovasc Surg 1990; 99:670–678.

73. Auger WR, Fedullo PF, Moser KM, Channick RN, Kapelanski DP, Jamieson SW. In-hospital mortality has decreased for patients undergoing pulmonary thrombo-endarterectomy (abstr). Am J Respir Crit Care Med 1996; 153:A92.

74. Thistlethwaite PA, Auger WR, Madani MM, Pradhan S, Kapelanski DP, Jamieson SW. Pulmonary thromboendarterectomy combined with other cardiac operations: Indications, surgical approach, and outcome. Ann Thorac Surg 2001; 72:13–19.

75. Daily PO, Dembitsky WP, Jamieson SW. The evolution and the current state of the art of pulmonary thromboendarterectomy. Semin Thorac Cardiovasc Surg 1999; 11:152–163.

76. Jamieson SW, Kapelanski DP. Pulmonary thromboendarterectomy. Curr Probl Surg 2000; 37:165–252.

77. Dartevelle P, Fadel E, Chapelier A, Macchiarini P, Cerrina J, Parquin F, Simonneau, Simonneau G. Angioscopic video-assisted pulmonary endarterectomy for post-embolic pulmonary hypertension. Eur J Cardiothorac Surg 1999; 16:38–43.

78. Zeebregts CJ, Dossche KM, Morshuis WJ, Knaepen PJ, Schepens MA. Surgical thromboendarterectomy for chronic thromboembolic pulmonary hypertension using circulatory arrest with selective antegrade cerebral perfusion. Acta Chir Belg 1998; 98:95–97.

79. Fedullo PF, Auger WR, Dembitsky WP. Postoperative management of the patient undergoing pulmonary thromboendaterectomy. Semin Thorac Cardiovasc Surg 1999; 11:172–178.

80. Levinson RM, Shure D, Moser KM. Reperfusion pulmonary edema after pulmonary thromboendarterectomy. Am Rev Respir Dis 1986; 134:1241–1245.

81. Mares P, Gilbert TB, Tschernko EM, Hiesmayr M, Muhm M, Herneth A, Taghavi S, Klepetko W, Lang I, Haider W. Pulmonary artery thromboendarterectomy: a comparison of two different postoperative treatment strategies. Anesth Analg 2000; 90:267–273.

82. McLaughlin VV, Genthner DE, Panella MM, Hess DM, Rich S. Compassionate use of continuous prostacyclin in the management of secondary pulmonary hypertension: a case series. Ann Intern Med 1999; 130:740–743.

83. Chitwood WR, Sabiston DC Jr, Wechsler AS. Surgical treatment of chronic unresolved pulmonary embolism. Clin Chest Med 1984; 5:507–536.

84. Fedullo PF, Auger WR, Kerr KM, Rubin LJ. Chronic thromboembolic pulmonary hypertension. N Engl J Med 2001; 345:1465–1472.

85. Moser KM, Auger WR, Fedullo PF. Chronic major vessel thromboembolic pulmonary hypertension. Circulation 1990; 81:1735–1743.

86. Tscholl D, Langer F, Wendler O, Wilkens H, Georg T, Schafers H-J. Pulmonary thromboendarterectomy—risk factors for early survival and hemodynamic improvement. Eur J Cardiothorac Surg 2001; 19:771–776.
87. Mayer E, Kramm T, Dahm M, Moersig W, Eberle B, Duber C, Menzel T, Oelert H. Early results of pulmonary thrombo-endarterectomy in chronic thromboembolic pulmonary hypertension. Z Kardiol 1997; 86:920–927.
88. Dittrich HC, Nicod PH, Chow LC, Chappuis FP, Moser KM, Peterson KL. Early changes of right heart geometry after pulmonary thromboendarterectomy. J Am Coll Cardiol 1988; 11:937–943.
89. Menzel T, Wagner S, Mohr-Kahaly S, Mayer E, Kramm T, Fischer TA, Brauninger S, Meinert R, Oelert H, Meyer J. Reversibility of changes in left and right ventricular geometry and hemodynamics in pulmonary hypertension. Echocardiographic characteristics before and after thromboendarterectomy. Z Kardiol 1997; 86:928–935.
90. Moser KM, Auger WR, Fedullo PF, Jamieson SW. Chronic thromboembolic pulmonary hypertension: clinical picture and surgical treatment. Eur Respir J 1992; 5:334–342.
91. Kramm T, Mayer E, Dahm M, Guth S, Menzel T, Pitton M, Oelert H. Long-term results after thromboendarterectomy for chronic pulmonary embolism. Eur J Cardiothorac Surg 1999; 15:579–584.
92. Kapitan KS, Clausen JL, Moser KM. Gas exchange in chronic thromboembolism after pulmonary thromboendarterectomy. Chest 1990; 98:14–19.
93. Tanabe N, Okada O, Nakagawa Y, Masuda M, Kato K, Nakajima N, Kuriyama T. The efficacy of pulmonary thromboendarterectomy on long-term gas exchange. Eur Respir J 1997; 10:2066–2072.
94. Archibald CJ, Auger WR, Fedullo PF, Channick RN, Kerr KM, Jamieson SW, Kapelanski DP, Watt CN, Moser KM. Long-term outcome after pulmonary thromboendarterectomy. Am J Respir Crit Care Med 1999; 160:523–528.

14

Lung Transplantation

ADAANI E. FROST

Baylor College of Medicine
Houston, Texas, U.S.A.

I. History

Chronic lung diseases affect 29 million Americans (1). The limitations of medical management for end-stage crippling lung disease have been a physical burden to millions of patients and an intellectual and emotional burden to their treating physicians. The prevalence of non-neoplastic lung disease, with its associated mortality and morbidity, coupled with surgical innovation, fostered the early canine experiments in lung transplantation in the 1950s. This was followed by the first human lung transplant, undertaken by Hardy in 1963 (2). Although the patient died 18 days postoperatively, this landmark operation provided proof of the surgical feasibility of lung transplantation. Subsequent transplants during the 1960s and 1970s refined surgical techniques but ultimately failed to confer prolonged survival (the longest survival being about 10 months). Deaths were due to rejection, infection, and bronchial dehiscence.

The former two problems, rejection and infection, are different sides of the same coin and reflect the limitations of steroids and azathioprine in controlling rejection while predisposing to bacterial, viral and fungal infection. The availability of the first calcineurin inhibitor (cyclosporine) in 1980 and the more recent (1990–2001) availability of many novel immunosuppressants have substantially improved complications related to acute and chronic rejection.

The complication of bronchial dehiscence was a major stumbling block in the evolution of lung transplantion. It is a function of interruption/impairment of the microvascular supply of the bronchus and is affected by surgical technique, organ preservation methods, and control of vasculitis of the donor bronchial microvasculature—in other words, rejection. To address this complication, extensive experimentation was undertaken. Animal models demonstrated that optimum preservation was achieved with the lung inflated (3,4) and prostacyclin (5) included in the flush. Surgical refinements suggested that the integrity of the bronchus could be improved by careful preservation of peribronchial tissue and the use of an omental pedicle at the anastomotic site or sites. This pedicle provided structural support and an additional source of perfusion until graft healing was established. In addition, it was recognized that high-dose steroids impaired bronchial healing (6). The development and clinical availability of cyclosporine in 1981 possibly permitted steroid dose reduction perioperatively and also clearly contributed to the control of transplant rejection/vasculitis. These innovations improved survival and resulted in the first successful long-term single- (7) and then double-lung transplant (8) survivors, operated on by the Toronto Lung Transplant Group in 1983 and 1986 respectively.

Since that time approximately 13,000 single-, double-, or heart-lung transplants have been performed worldwide for patients with end-stage lung diseases (9). This chapter reviews the indications, surgical options, complications, and results of this novel therapy for non-neoplastic lung disease.

II. Indications

In very general terms, lung transplantation is an option for patients with severe lung disease who have received or are receiving optimum therapy with limited expectation of improvement and substantial risk of death within 1 to 2 years. This cautious wording reflects the fact that many lung diseases worsen inexorably in spite of therapy and consideration for transplantation should not be left to the eleventh hour. A joint effort sponsored by the National Institutes of Health (NIH), including transplant physicians and surgeons, to delineate general guidelines for selection of patients for lung transplantation was developed, adopted, and published simultaneously in 1998 in three major pulmonary and transplant journals (10–12). The consideration of a patient for transplantation involves determining first if he or she is sick enough to warrant consideration for transplantation. In other words, does the expected mortality of the disease within 12 to 18 months exceed the mortality associated with transplantation? Second, is the patient well enough to be considered for transplant? This requires evaluation for potential comorbidities and risk factors predictive of poor outcome. Third and finally, the patient has to have been optimally managed both for the underlying pulmonary disease process and for any comorbidities. While this third area is not really the purview of the transplant center, most major lung transplant centers have also become expert in state-of-the-art treatment and novel experimental therapies for end-stage pulmonary parenchymal and pulmonary vascular disease.

General and disease-specific guidelines were developed by the NIH, American Society of Transplantation (AST), International Society for Heart and Lung Transplantation (ISHLT), and American Thoracic Society (ATS) consensus group and are summarized below with the addition of recent further information.

A. General Recommendations for Lung Transplantation

1. Age limits, There is a trend toward increasing mortality with advancing age demonstrated by the United Network for Organ Sharing/International Society for Heart and Lung Transplantation database (UNOS/ISHLT) (13). This fact, coupled with the paucity of organs, led to the recommendation to restrict heart-lung transplants to those $\leqslant 55$ years, bilateral lung transplants to those $\leqslant 60$ years, and single-lung transplant to those $\leqslant 65$ years.

2. Symptomatic osteoporosis results in substantial morbidity (14,15). This should be treated aggressively pre- and posttransplantation, and patients should be evaluated individually for their acceptability for transplant. Symptomatic osteoporosis is considered a relative contraindication to transplantation.

3. Severe musculoskeletal disease with thoracic deformity can substantially affect respiratory mechanics and successful surgical implantation; it is therefore considered a relative contraindication to transplantation.

4. Similarly, progressive neuromscular disease is considered an absolute contraindication to lung transplantation.

5. Obesity and cachexia. Recipient weight can be calculated as body-mass index (BMI) or as percent ideal body weight. By both parameters, obesity and cachexia have been associated with worse outcome. Weight $<70\%$ or $>130\%$ ideal is considered a contraindication to transplantation and an indication for structured weight loss or weight gain (9,16).

6. Patients must be free of substance addiction for at least 6 months, with appropriate monitoring.

7. Psychosocial issues that may result in noncompliance with treatment regimens are considered relative contraindications to transplantation.

8. Invasive mechanical ventilation has been clearly established as highly predictive of poor outcome; this is considered a relative contraindication to transplantation.

9. Treated tuberculosis is not a contraindication to transplantation. Atypical mycobacteria and fungi, however, need to be considered on an individual basis and probably preclude unilateral transplantation.

10. Significant nonpulmonary organ disease is considered a contra-indication to transplantation. This is defined as a creatinine clearance of $<50 \, mg/mL/min$; significant coronary artery disease or left ventricular dysfunction that is not treatable (this does not preclude heart-lung transplant); liver cirrhosis or hepatitis B antigen positivity; and systemic diseases refractory to therapy (particularly if associated with end-organ damage)—for example, refractory collagen vascular disease or uncontrolled diabetes.

B. Disease-Specific Recommendations for Transplantation

Noninfected Obstructive Lung Disease

FEV_1 has been demonstrated to correlate with survival in obstructive lung disease in a linear fashion (17). In this group, particularly the pure emphysema patients, survival is difficult to predict on an individual basis. The literature indicates that patients with alpha$_1$-antitrypsin deficiency–associated emphysema with a FEV_1 of less than 15% predicted have a 2-year survival of 43% (18). Current guidelines recommend earlier referral (e.g., at an FEV_1 of 30%). Data on earlier listing and transplantation, however, indicate that the emphysema patients, because of their prolonged (albeit disabled) survival, have the least survival benefit from transplantation within the current guidelines (19). It therefore behooves the referring or transplanting physician to assess for other risk factors prior to proceeding to transplantation or to defer the transplanta-tion. Hospitalizations for exacerbations of chronic obstructive pulmonary disease associated with hypercapnia in the preceding year should precipitate immediate referral. These patients have an 11% in-hospital mortality and a 12-month survival of 51% (20). These data also suggest that hypercapnia, (defined as Pa_{CO_2} of 50 mmHg) with hospitalizations and/or the following associated factors should precipitate referral for consideration of lung transplant evaluation: (1) reduced serum albumin; (2) declining BMI; (3) increasing oxygen requirements; (4) presence of cor pulmonale (defined as clinical diagnosis by a physician or any two of the following: right ventriclular hypertrophy or right atrial enlargement on electrocardiography (ECG), enlarged pulmonary arteries on chest x-ray, pedal edema, jugular venous distention, or mean pulmonary artery pressure > 20 mmHg by right heart catheterization). These recommendations dovetail fairly nicely with the recent interim report from the National Emphysema Treatment Trial Research Group (21). This study identified patients with an $FEV_1 \leqslant 20\%$ as those individuals with an unacceptably high 30-day mortality rate after lung volume reduction surgery (16%). This contrasts sharply with a mortality of 0% in similarly defined high-risk patients managed medically. The presence of the additional risk factors of homogeneous emphysema pattern on computed tomography (CT) and a low diffusing capacity for carbon monoxide

(DL_{CO}) $\leqslant 20\%$ of predicted was associated with a 30-day mortality of 25%. This study and the role of lung volume reduction surgery in the management of non-neoplastic lung disease are discussed in Chapter 12. It is reasonable, however, to say that the conclusions of that study further help to define a high-risk population and one for whom lung transplantation is the only surgical option.

Cystic Fibrosis

These patients represent between 18 and 20% of all patients undergoing transplantation (9). They also have a very high pretransplant mortality on the waiting list (19). This reflects delayed referral and the precipitous deterioration that occurs with infection. Risk factors predictive of higher mortality within 2 years have been developed. Data from 673 patients suggest that female sex, younger age, an FEV_1 of less than 30% predicted, a Pa_{O_2} below 55 mmHg, or a P_{CO_2} greater than 50 mmHg are associated with a 2-year mortality rate of greater than 50% (22). Subsequent studies have indicated greater variability in survival in those with an FEV_1 of $<30\%$ predicted, possibly reflecting improved patient care protocols (23). The cystic fibrosis (CF) database, which includes information on more than 30,000 patients, emphasizes the importance of other factors such as race, ethnicity, and the presence of symptoms at time of diagnosis (24). This database corroborates the adverse impact of female sex on survival and the adverse impact of Hispanic or black/other ethnicity/race on survival. Nonwhite status conferred a 1.48 to 1.85 increased risk of death in this multivariate analysis. The presence of diabetes mellitus (25) may also be an independent risk factor for both poor outcome and declining spirometry. While the published guidelines for transplantation in the CF population have not yet been modified to reflect this more recent information, these factors should be included in the assessment of patients for referral and transplant.

The existing guidelines for consideration of CF patients for lung transplantation include the following:

1. $FEV_1 \leqslant 30\%$ predicted or rapid progressive deterioration with $FEV_1 > 30\%$ predicted. Progressive deterioration is defined by an increasing frequency of hospitalizations, rapid fall in FEV_1, massive hemoptysis, and increasing cachexia in spite of optimum nutritional supplementation and diabetic management.
2. Resting hypoxemia ($Pa_{O_2} < 55$ mmHg) on room air; resting hypercapnia ($Pa_{CO_2} \geqslant 50$ mmHg).
3. Rapid deterioration in a young female patient even in the absence of some of the above physiological parameters.

In the original guidelines for selection of lung transplant candidates, the issue of the impact of infection/colonization with multiply resistant organisms and *Burkholderia cepacia* was reviewed at length. This organism is by definition multiply resistant. The term *multiply resistant* has been specifically defined as applying to an organism that is resistant to all agents in two of the following classes of antibiotics: the betalactams, aminoglycosides, and quinolones. *Panresistant* organism are resistant in vitro to all groups of antibiotics (26). Both panresistant and multiply resistant organisms occur in patients with CF referred for transplant, and although they should be carefully considered, these organisms do not represent absolute contraindications to transplantation. In spite of in vitro resistance, broad-spectrum antibiotic coverage usually leads to an acceptable outcome.

The preceding statements, however, do not apply in the case of *B. cepacia*. The adverse impact on pretransplant survival in CF patients colonized with *B. cepacia* has been well reported (27) and is recognized as the "*cepacia* syndrome*.*" The increased mortality posttransplant demonstrated in patients infected with multiply or panresistant organisms is attributable entirely to *B. cepacia* (28). Extensive epidemiological and microbiological, evaluations have recently demonstrated that deaths due to the *B. cepacia* complex appear to be related to a specific genomovar type (29). The ability of most general labs to reliably identify *B. cepacia* is limited, and the subcategorizing by genomovar is largely confined to one major reference lab. Therefore it would be wise to have organisms identified as *B. cepacia* reevaluated by the reference lab and if possible a determination made as to whether or not the patient has the genomovar III. This is the strain of *B. cepacia* associated with a strikingly increased transplant perioperative (30 versus 0%) and 1-year mortality (50 versus 17%). While *B. cepacia* is not listed as an absolute contraindication to lung transplantation, each center must consider this recent information in the context of their lab, the patient, and their center-specific survival data.

Idiopathic Pulmonary Fibrosis and the Idiopathic Interstitial Pneumonias

This category includes those patients with fibrosing lung disorders of various categories, most importantly idiopathic pulmonary fibrosis (IPF). The histological correlate of the clinical diagnosis of IPF is usual interstitial pneumonia (UIP). There are many forms of idiopathic interstitial lung disease, which have recently been subcategorized (30). The diagnostic groups for the IPFs include nonspecific interstitial pneumonia (NSIP), acute interstitial pneumonia (AIP), desquamative interstitial pneumonia (DIP), and its more commonly seen variant respiratory bronchiolitis-associated interstitial lung disease (RSBILD). While these manifestations of interstitial pneumonia generally have a much better likelihood of response to therapy (steroids, smoking cessation) as well as different radiological and histological features, a substantial number of patients progress to end-stage lung disease. The unique histological and clinical features of the various ILDs are detailed in preceding chapters. Because of the potential for response to therapy with non-UIP forms of ILD, this is an important differentiation. However the refractory nature of UIP/IPF to therapy dictates that patients with known or suspected IPF should be referred relatively early for consideration of transplantation. Historically, these patients have had the highest mortality on the waiting list for transplant.

Based on this mortality, patients with a diagnosis of IPF receive a 90-day "head start" bonus at time of transplant listing. Median survival from diagnosis to death in patients with IPF is 5 years. Using the same model as for other lung-transplant candidates, one would like to identify those patients at substantial risk of death within 2 years, as these are the individuals who should be immediately referred and evaluated for lung transplantation.

Attempts to develop reliable algorithms for predicting survival have resulted in rather ponderous models that include clinical, radiological, and physiological parameters (31) (a "CRP" score). These parameters include increasing age, smoking status, nail-bed clubbing, profusion score on chest x-ray, presence of pulmonary hypertension, total lung capacity (as percent predicted), and Pa_{O_2} at maximal exercise. These different factors are given different weight for a total maximum potential score of 100. Based on this model the calculated two-year survival of patients with CRP scores of 20, 40, 50, 60, and 80 are 95, 75, 55, 25, and <1% respectively. This scoring system interestingly indicates improved survival in individuals who are current or former (as opposed to "never") smokers. A score of 50 (with an associated 2-year survival of 55%) is achieved easily; an example of such a CRP score would be a patient over the age of 50, who had never smoked, has clubbing and moderate interstitial changes on chest x-ray, a total lung capacity of <70% predicted, and modest hypoxemia ($Pa_{O_2} < 65$ with maximal exercise). Older age and worse radiological or clinical disease increase the CRP score markedly. The original consensus guidelines made the point that most patients with IPF do not even present with symptoms until they have a reduction in TLC to <70%. Therefore patients presenting with symptoms (cough and shortness of breath) will usually meet criteria for a CRP score of 50 or more and have a 2-year survival based on this model of only 55%. The infrequent response to therapy (which almost defines true UIP/IPF) requires, therefore, that patients be referred for consideration of transplantation even while they are embarking on a trial of therapy. A favorable response to therapy will allow transplant to be delayed or deferred. Protracted high-dose steroids, while not a contra-indication to transplantation in these patients, can sometimes increase the risk of unrecognized opportunistic infections (32) and certainly do contribute to muscle wasting and debility. Therefore extended therapy in the absence of benefit should be avoided. Therefore the consensus recommendation for transplantation in these patients is the presence of symptomatic progressive disease in spite of therapy. This generally occurs once the patients has a reduction in VC to <70% predicted or a reduction in diffusion capacity below 60% of predicted. Consideration of the other risk factors delineated above should be factored in when considering a patient for transplantation.

Systemic Disease with Pulmonary Fibrosis

Pulmonary fibrosis occurs in numerous other systemic conditions, including collagen vascular disease, postchemotherapy, sarcoid, etc. These patients do not fit so neatly into an algorithmic approach to determine when they should be transplanted; they should be considered on the basis of their history and pattern of disease progression. Sarcoid particularly can have a relapsing and remitting pattern. When the patient is considered for transplantation, however, there should be no evidence of significant impact of the systemic disease process on other organs. The previously mentioned guidelines for disease severity (hypoxemia, hypercapnia, declining FVC, and TLC, etc.) should be applied to this group of patients.

Pulmonary Hypertension Without Congenital Heart Disease

Pulmonary hypertension can be primary or related to other diseases such as thromboemboli or it may be medication-related, AIDS-related, or secondary to collagen vascular disease. Severe pulmonary hypertension irrespective of its cause is a marker of severe disease and is associated with a poor prognosis. The pathology, physiology, and medical management of pulmonary vascular disease is covered in earlier chapters. Therapies developed in the last 10 years have resulted in a major impact on the natural history of pulmonary hypertension and hence on the role and timing of lung transplantation. Vasodilator therapy with epoprostenol has been shown to increase median survival from 2.9 years in New York Heart Association (NYHA) class III patients to almost 6 years (33). Additional therapies including a recent FDA-approved oral endothelin antagonist may prove to have similar long-term survival benefits. Current recommendations are to initiate optimum therapy and careful follow-up of these high-risk patients. Failure to improve or progression of symptoms in NYHA class III or IV patients is an indication for transplantation. In general terms, the higher the PA pressure, the lower the cardiac output; and the higher the right atrial pressure, the sicker the patient and the greater the mortality. However, these factors are not predictive of response to therapy. Extremely ill patients with florid right heart failure have responded well to vasodilator therapy. In fact, the greatest survival benefit occurring in the initial study of chronic epoprostenol therapy in primary pulmonary hypertension (PPH) was seen in those individuals who were NYHA class IV (34). The data from PPH has been extrapolated to those individuals with secondary pulmonary hypertension. Improvement in cardiac output and exercise tolerance has been demonstrated in patients with secondary pulmonary hypertension due to the scleroderma spectrum of disease. However, it is not clear that vasodilator therapy will demonstrate a similar survival benefit in this patient population.

Pulmonary Hypertension Secondary to Congenital Heart Disease (Eisenmenger's Syndrome)

Patients with pulmonary hypertension secondary to congenital heart disease behave differently than those with primary pulmonary hypertension or those with other causes of their PH. Even within the diagnostic category of

Eisenmenger's, patients with different forms of congenital heart disease have different rates of disease progression. Each patient must be assessed individually. Hemodynamic parameters are not as predictive in this patient population of survival as in the PPH patient population. In general terms, however, deterioration in patients on optimum therapy who are NYHA class III or IV should be an indicator of the need for transplant. The definition of optimum therapy is reviewed in the chapter on management of pulmonary vascular disease. However, vasodilator therapies (prostacyclins and oral endothelin antagonists) currently under review in this diagnostic group may prove useful in delaying transplantation. Novel data suggest that markers of endothelial cell disturbance such as von Willebrand factor activity may be useful in following the severity of disease and the likelihood of survival on an individual patient basis (35). In addition, elevated uric acid levels and serial measurements showing increasing levels have been found by univariate and multivariate analysis to be independent predictors of mortality in patients with Eisenmenger's syndrome. While not a factor to consider in isolation, this is a relatively simple and inexpensive test that can be done serially to help identify those Eisenmenger's patients at increased risk of mortality (36). The elevation in uric acid is apparently due to a disturbance in uric acid clearance as opposed to increased production (37).

III. Surgical Options

The surgical options for lung transplantation include single, bilateral sequential, heart-lung, or bilateral living lobar lung transplantation. These surgical approaches reflect issues of donor availability and the nature of the underlying lung disease necessitating transplantation. There are mounting data that bilateral sequential lung transplantation has advantages over single-lung transplantation for both exercise tolerance and late graft survival. However, the lack of ready availability of double-lung blocks and the prolonged wait required to get such a block as opposed to a single lung (a two- to fourfold increase in waiting time) dictates that patients who do not require double-lung transplantation receive single-lung transplants. Patients who must receive double-lung blocks are those with septic lung disease, such as CF or bronchiectasis. Due to the perioperative hemodynamic instability seen with single-lung transplantation for primary pulmonary hypertension, patients with this diagnosis usually receive bilateral sequential single-lung transplants rather than single-lung transplants. There is a general sense that younger patients with severe emphysema, most notably those with alpha$_1$-antitrypsin deficiency–associated emphysema, have difficulty with massive enlargement of the native lung and compromise of the transplant when they receive single-lung transplants. Many centers now transplant these patients with double-lung blocks. The donor organ in all the above instances is procured as a double-lung block but the operation is performed as a bilateral sequential single-lung transplant from a single donor.

Heart-lung transplantation is still done at some centers for cystic fibrosis. Overwhelmingly, however, heart-lung transplantation is reserved for patients with severe lung disease (usually pulmonary vascular disease) associated with cardiac disease that is not surgically correctable. This is often due to complex congenital heart disease with Eisenmenger's physiology. The waiting time for a heart-lung block is even greater than for a double-lung block.

Living-lobar transplantation was pioneered initially to provide a surgical alternative to younger patients at high risk of mortality (CF patients) while awaiting cadaveric organ transplant (38). After careful medical, physiological, ethical, and psychological evaluation, a lower lobe is removed from each of two donors (one right and one left lower lobe donor). Historically the donors have most often been parents or siblings. The two lobes are then implanted in a single recipient who undergoes bilateral native lung pneumonectomies at the time of organ procurement. The results of this surgical approach have been approximately equivalent to those of a cadaveric organ transplant with no mortality reported to date in the donors.

All donors, cadaveric and living, are assessed for the intrinsic normalcy of the lung to be explanted. This is undertaken by chest x-ray, evaluation of blood gases in the context of ventilatory parameters, ventilatory mechanics, and bronchoscopy. Cadaveric donors must be free of active sepsis, HIV, viral hepatitis, malignancy (though isolated skin cancers are acceptable), and history of lung disease. A smoking history and the age of the donor are evaluated in the context of the recipient and other indices of possible donor lung disease.

IV. Complications

The complications of lung transplantation are those related to the surgery itself, to the preservation of the organ, to rejection, and to the complications of immunosuppression.

A. Surgical Complications

These are fairly obvious and are a function of complicated cardiothoracic surgery in high-risk patients. Complications include bleeding, pneumothorax, protracted chest tube drainage, phrenic nerve injury, and anastomotic obstructions which can occur at the bronchus, the pulmonary artery, and at the attachment of the donor venous pedicle to the left atrium. Bronchial anastomotic obstructions are fairly common and can occur as a complication of ischemia, surgical technique, or discrepancy between donor and recipient bronchial size. These are readily recognized bronchoscopically and usually managed simply with balloon dilation and placement of endobronchial stents. Pulmonary arterial anastomotic problems are relatively infrequent and more commonly manifest as immediate perioperative bleeding from the posterior aspect of the pulmonary artery anastomosis. Pulmonary venous anastomotic complications present with immediate perioperative worsening of gas exchange, and a picture of progressive pulmonary edema in the transplanted lung. The diagnosis is made by transesophageal echocardiogram (TEE) (39). This complication can be fatal and, if severe, requires surgical revision. Milder degrees of obstruction require no intervention. To avoid this complication many centers undertake intraoperative TEE assessment of the venous anastomosis.

B. Organ Preservation

Preservation solutions and methods continue to evolve. Increasingly there is evidence supporting the use of low potassium or "extracellular" preservation solutions for optimum preservation of the lung (40). Maintenance of surfactant and alveolar integrity by preserving the lung in inflation has been shown to minimize preservation injury. There is conflicting evidence about the utility or vasodilator and free-radical scavengers (prostacyclin) prior to flush though most centers feel that this is useful in minimizing graft injury and facilitating perfusion of small vessels with the preservation fluid. Preservation injury when it occurs is really ischemia-reperfusion injury characterized by a radiological and clinical picture of low wedge pulmonary edema/pulmonary infiltrates, or acute respiratory distress syndrome (ARDS). Histologically there is disturbance of the alveolar membrane, polymorphonuclear leukocyte infiltrates, and varying degrees of hyaline membrane and intralaveolar fibrin deposition that resolves to varying degrees with time. This is aggravated by prolonged ischemic time (41). Once reperfusion injury occurs, management is limited to minimization of barotrauma using low tidal volumes, high-PEEP mechanical ventilation (42), and supportive measures. In the case of patients with alpha$_1$-antitrypsin deficiency, since the injury is perpetuated by unopposed neutrophil activation, there is a theoretical role for use of alpha$_1$-antitrypsin replacement therapy.

C. Rejection

While acute rejection is a relatively rare cause of death, the augmented immunosuppression that it necessitates produces the many adverse effects listed below. In addition, there is a clear correlation between the frequency and severity of acute rejection, the onset of late acute rejection (43), and the development of bronchiolitis obliterans. Bronchiolitis obliterans is a fibrosing process in the small airways that leads to progressive respiratory compromise due to airway obstruction and is the single greatest cause of death beyond the first year of transplant. It increases in frequency and severity with time and accounts for more than 50% of deaths occurring after 3 years posttransplant.

D. Complications of Immunosuppression

These complications are direct (a consequence of the impact of impaired immunity) and indirect, (due to drug side-effects unrelated to immunosuppressive efficacy).

The two most obvious complications of impaired immunity are infection and malignancy. Infectious complications account for about 50% of deaths occurring within the first year posttransplant. Malignancy occurs in from 5 to 10% of transplant recipients. Most commonly, sun exposure–related skin cancers occur. However other malignancies have been reported, most importantly posttransplant lymphoproliferative disease (PTLD). This is related largely to clonal expansion of infected and immortalized B cells associated with Epstein-Barr virus. It occurs most commonly in EBV-naive recipients of EBV-positive organs. However, it also occurs with endogenous EBV-reactivation thought to be a consequence of aggressive immunosuppression with calcineurin inhibitors and antilymphocyte products. The frequency of PTLD in recipients of lung transplant is between 4 and 8%.

Indirect complications of immunosuppressive therapy are listed in Table 1.

V. Outcomes

Outcomes following lung and heart-lung transplantation are clearly affected by the various factors listed above. The most recent graft and patient survival

Table 1 Side-Effects of Immunosuppressive Drugs

Osteoporosis, osteonecrosis	Steroids, cyclosporine
Systemic hypertension	Calcineurin inhibitors
Renal insufficiency	Calcineurin inhibitors
Glaucoma, cataracts	Steroids
Serum sickness	Antilymphocyte products
Gingival hypertrophy	Cyclosporine (with calcium channel blockers)
Hepatotoxicity	Azathioprine, calcineurin inhbitors
Nausea and diarrhea	Mycophenolate
Hyperglycemia	Tacrolimus
Hirsutism	Cyclosporine
Bone marrow suppression: anemia, leukopenia, thrombocytopenia	Sirolimus, mycophenolate mofetil, antilymphocyte products
Hyperlipidemia	Sirolimus
Hemolytic uremic syndrome	Calcineurin inhibitors, [sirolimus ?]
Multifocal leukoencephalopathy, neuropathy	Calcineurin inhibitors

rates published by the United Network for Organ Sharing (UNOS) include 1-, 3-, and 5-year survivals following lung transplant at 77, 58, and 44%, respectively (44). Survivals for recipients of heart-lung transplantation for the same periods were 60, 51, and 42%, respectively. This underscores the importance of careful recipient selection to ensure that one disabling disease is not replaced with another disabling and frequently mortal condition. These survival statistics, it should be emphasized, have dramatically improved within the last 10 years. Further improvement in surgical techniques and in our understanding and management of acute and chronic rejection should result in survival statistics that will rival those of renal transplantation. Until that time, lung transplantation remains a realistic and appropriate therapy for carefully selected patients with end-stage pulmonary and pulmonary vascular disease.

References

1. Lenfant C. US Department of Health and Human Services, NHLBI report of the Task Force on Behavioral Research in Cardiovascular, Lung and Blood Health and Disease. U.S. Public Health Service. Bethesda, MD: National Institutes of Health, 1998:17.
2. Hardy JD, Webb WR, Dalton ML, et al. Lung homotransplantation in man. JAMA 1963; 186(12):1065.
3. Haniuda M, Hasegawa S, Shiraishi T, et al. Effectsof inflation volume during lung preservation on pulmonary capillary permeability. J Thorac Cardiovasc Surg 1996; 112(1):85–93.
4. Hausen B, Ramsamooj R, Hewitt CW, et al. The importance of static lung inflation during organ storage: the impact of varying ischemic intervals in a double lung rat transplantation model. Transplantation 1996; 62(12):1720–1725.
5. Jurmann MJ, Dammehnayn L, Schafer HJ, et al. Prostacyclin as an additive to single crystalloid flush: improved pulmonary preservation in heart-lung transplantation. Transplant Proc 1987; 19(5):4103–4104.
6. Lima O, Cooper JD, Peters WJ, et al. Effects of methylprednisolone and azathioprine on bronchial healing following lung autotransplantation. J Thorac Cardiovasc Surg 1981; 82(2):211–215.
7. Anonymous. Unilateral lung transplantation for pulmonary fibrosis. Toronto Lung Transplantation Group. N Engl J Med 1986; 314(18):1140–1145.
8. Patterson GA, Cooper JD, Goldman BE, et al. Technique of successful clinical double-lung transplantation. Ann Thorac Surg 1988; 45(6):626–633.
9. Hosenpud JD, Bennett LE, Keck BM, Boucek MM, Novick RJ. The Registry of the International Society for Heart and Lung Transplantation: Eighteenth official report—2001. J Heart Lung Transplant 2001; 20:805–815.
10. Maurer JR, Frost AE, Estenne M, Higenbottam T, Glanville AR. International guidelines for the selection of lung transplant candidates. Transplantation 1998; 66(7):951–956.
11. Maurer JR, Frost AE, Estenne M, Higenbottam T, Glanville AR. International guidelines for the selection of lung transplant candidates. J Heart Lung Transplant 1998; 17(7):703–709.

12. Maurer JR, Frost AE, Estenne M, Higenbottam T, Glanville AR. International guidelines for the selection of lung transplant candidates. The American Society of Transplant Physicians (ASTP)/ The American Thoracic Society (ATS)/ The European Respiratory Society (ERS)/The International Society for Heart and Lung Transplantation (ISHLT). Am J Respir Crit Care Med 1998; 158(1):335–339.

13. Hosenpud JD, Bennett LE, Keck BM, Boucek MM, Novick RJ. The Registry of the International Society for Heart and Lung Transplantation: eighteenth official report—2001. J Heart Lung Transplant 2001; 20:805–815.

14. Spira A, Gutierrez C, Chaparro C, Hutcheon MA, Chan CKN. Osteoporsis and lung transplantation—a prospective study. Chest 2000; 117:476–481.

15. Shane E, Papadopoulos A, Staron RB, Addesso V, Donovan D, McGregor C, Schulman LL. Bone loss and fracture after lung transplantation. Transplantation 1999 27;68(2):220–227.

16. Madill J, Gutierrez C, Grossman J, Allard J, Chan C, Hutcheon M, Keshavjee SH. Nutritional assessment of the lung transplant patient: body mass index as a predictor of 90-day mortality following transplantation. J Heart Lung Transplant 2001; 20(3):288–296.

17. Hansen EF, Vestbo J, Phanareth K, Kok-Jensen A, Dirksen A. Peak flow as predictor of overall mortality in asthma and chronic obstructive pulmonary disease. Am J Respir Crit Care Med 2001; 163(3):690–693.

18. Seersholm N, Dirksen A, Kok-Jensen A. Airway obstruction and two year survival in patients with severe alpha₁-antitrypsin deficiency. Eur Respir J 1994; 7:1985–1987.

19. Hosenpud JD, Bennett LE, Keck BM, Edwards EB, Novick RJ. Effect of diagnosis on survival benefit of lung transplantation for end-stage lung disease. Lancet 1998; 351:24–27.

20. Connors AF Jr, Dawson NV, Thomas C, Harrell FE Jr, Desbiens N, Fulkerson WJ, Kussin P, Bellamy P, Goldman L, Knaus WA for the SUPPORT investigators. Outcomes following acute exacerbation of severe chronic obstructive lung disease: the SUPPORT investigators. Am J Respir Crit Care Med 1996; 154:959–967.

21. National Emphysema Treatment Trial Research Group. Patients at high risk of death after lung-volume-reduction surgery. N Engl J Med 2001 345(15):1075–1083.

22. Kerem E, Reisman J, Corey M, Canny GJ, Levison H. Prediction of mortality in patients with cystic fibrosis. N Engl J Med 1992 30; 326(18):1187–1191.

23. Milla CE, Warwick WJ. Risk of death in cystic fibrosis patients with severely compromised lung function. Chest 1998; 113:1230–1234.

24. O'Connor GT, Quinton HB, Kahn R, Robichaud P, Maddock J, Lefver T, Detzer M, Brooks JG for the Northern New England Cystic Fibrosis Consortium. Case-mix adjustment for evaluation of mortality in cystic fibrosis. Pediatr Pulmonol 2002; 33(2):99–105.

25. Rosenecker J, Hoflger R, Steinkamp G, Eichler I, Smaczny C, Ballmann M, Posselt HG, Bargon J, Von der Hardt H. Diabetes mellitus in patients with cystic fibrosis: the impact of diabetes mellitus on pulmonary function and clinical outcome. Eur J Med Res 2001; 27:6(8):345–350.

26. North American Cystic Fibrosis Foundation Concepts in Care Consensus Conference. Microbiology and infectious diseases in cystic fibrosis. 1994; 5(1):1–25.

27. Tablan OC, Chorba TL, Schidlow DV, et al. *Pseudomonas cepacia* colonization in patients with cystic fibrosis: risk factors and clinical outcome. J Pediatr 1985: 107:382–387.

28. Chapparo C, Maurer J, Gutierrez CA, Krajden M, Chanc C, Winton T, Keshavjee S, Scavuzzo M, Tullis E, Hutcheon M, Keston S. Infection with *Burkholderia cepacia* in cystic fibrosis: outcome following lung transplantation. Am J Respir Crit Care Med 2001; 163(1):43–48.

29. Aris RM, Routh JC, LiPUma JJ, Heath DG, Gilligan PH. Lung transplantation for cystic fibrosis patients with *Burkholderia cepacia* complex. Survival linked to genomovar type. Am J Respir Crit Care Med 2001 164(11):2102–2106.

30. Anonymous. Idiopathic pulmonary fibrosis: diagnosis and treatment. International Consensus Statement. Am J Respir Crit Care Med 2000; 161:646–664.

31. King TE, Tooze JA, Schwarz MI, Brown KR and Cherniack RM. Predicting survival in idiopathic pulmonary fibrosis. Scoring system and survival model. Am J Respir Crit Care Med 2001; 164(7):1171–1181.

32. Milstone AP, Brumble LM, Loyd JE, Ely EW, Roberts JR, Pierson RN III, Dummer JS. Active CMV infection before lung transplantation: risk factors and clinical implications. J Heart Lung Transplant 2000; 19(8):744–750.

33. Shapiro SM, Oudiz RJ, Cao T, Romano MA, Beckmann XJ, Georgiou D, Mandayam S, Ginzton LE, Brundage BH. Primary pulmonary hypertension: improved long-term effects and survival with continuous intravenous epoprostenol infusion. J Am Coll Cardiol 1997; 30(2):343–349.

34. Barst RJ, Rubin LJ, Long WA, Walker A, McGoon MD, Rich S, Badesch DB, Groves BM, Tapson VF, Bourge RC, Brundage BH, Koerner SK, Langleben D, Keller CA, Murali S, Uretsky BF, Clayton LM, Jobsis MM, Blackburn SD, Shortino D, Crow JW. A comparison of continuous intravenous epoprostenol (prostacyclin) with conventional therapy for primary pulmonary hypertension. N Engl J Med 1996; 334(5):296–301.

35. Lopes AA, Maeda NY. Circulating von Willebrand factor antigen as a predictor of short-term prognosis in pulmonary hypertension. Chest 1998; 114(5):1276–1282.

36. Oya H, Nagaya N, Satoh T, Sakamaki F, Kyotani S, Fujita M, Nakanishi N, Miyatake K. Haemodynamic correlates and prognostic significance of serum uric acid in adult patients with Eisenmenger syndrome. Heart 2000; 84:53–58.

37. Ross EA, Perloff JK, Danovitch BM, Child JS, Canobbio MM. Renal function and urate metabolism in late survivors with cyanotic congenital heart disease. Circulation 1986; 73:396–400.

38. Woo MS, MacLaughlin EF, Horn MV, Wong PC, Rowland JM, Barr ML, Starnes VA. Living donor lobar lung transplantation: the pediatric experience. Pediatr Transplant 1998; 2(3):185–190.

39. Schulman LL, Anandarangam T, Leibowitz DW, Ditullio MR, McGregor CC, Galantowicz ME, Homma S. Four-year prospective study of pulmonary venous thrombosis after lung transplantation. J Am Soc Echocardiogr 2001; 14(8): 806–812.

40. Thabut G, Vinatier I, Brugiere O, Leseche Gy, Loirat Ph, Bisson A, Marty J, Fournier M, Mal H. Influence of preservation solution on early graft failure in clinical lung transplantation. Am J Respir Crit Care Med. 2001; 164(7):1204–1208.

41. Snell GI, Rabinov M, Griffiths A, Williams T, Ugoni A, Salamonsson R, Esmore D. Pulmonary allograft ischemic time: an important predictor of survival after lung transplantation. J Heart Lung Transplant 1996 Feb; 15(2):160–168.
42. The Acute Respiratory Distress Syndrome Network. Ventilation with lower tidal volumes as compared with traditional tidal volumes for acute lung injury and the acute respiratory distress syndrome. N Engl J Med 2000; 342(18):1301–1308.
43. Husain AN, Siddiqui MT, Holmes EW, Chandrasekhar AJ, McCabe M, Radvany R, Garrity ER. Analysis of risk factors for the development of bronchiolitis obliterans syndrome. Am J Respir Crit Care Med 1999; 159(3):829–833.
44. 2000 Annual Report of the U.S. Scientific Registry for Transplant Recipients and the Organ Procurement and Transplantation Network: Transplant Data: 1990–1999. Rockville, MD: U.S. Department of Health and Human Services, Health Resources and Services Administration, Office of Special Programs, Division of Transplantation; Richmond, VA: United Network for Organ Sharing.

15

Comorbidities in Advanced Lung Disease

JANET R. MAURER

CIGNA HealthCare
Hartford, Connecticut, U.S.A.

I. Introduction

Coexisting chronic illnesses are present in many patients with advanced lung disease. In some diseases the comorbidities are a manifestation of a systemic illness; in others comorbidities may be secondary to the pulmonary process. For example, cystic fibrosis patients can develop focal biliary cirrhosis resulting in symptomatic hepatic failure as part of their illness; alternatively, pulmonary hypertension patients can develop hepatic cirrhosis from chronic hepatic congestion, which, in turn, is secondary to right heart failure. A third category of comorbidity comprises conditions that are not directly related to the pulmonary disease process but occur at a significant rate in the pulmonary disease population. These comorbidities often occur because of similar risk factors, such as smoking or age. This chapter concentrates on this last category of comorbidity.

II. Impact of Comorbidities

It is difficult to find information about the prevalence of comorbid diseases that occur in patients with COPD or other chronic lung processes. Van Manen et al.

asked this question of a population of patients at least 40 years old who were followed by general practitioners and had a diagnosis of asthma or COPD. In the study, 290 patients with irreversible airway obstruction and 421 controls answered a questionnaire. A total of 73% of the COPD group and 63% of the controls reported at least one other illness. Predominant illnesses in both groups were locomotive diseases, hypertension, sleeping disorders, and cardiac disease (1). However, in the COPD group, locomotive diseases, insomnia, sinusitis, migraine headaches, depression, peptic ulcers, and cancer were significantly more common. The large population-based studies necessary to better understand the prevalence of comorbidity in COPD patients are unfortunately lacking. Information regarding the incidence of comorbidities in other chronic lung processes is also sparse. Despite the often relentlessly progressive course of idiopathic pulmonary fibrosis, for example, Panos et al. found that less than 50% of victims were recorded as dying from the disease itself. Other common causes of death included heart failure (possibly related to the pulmonary fibrosis), bronchogenic carcinoma, ischemic heart disease, infection, and pulmonary embolism (2). Coultas and Hughes also found that patients with interstitial disease often did not have their disease listed as the immediate cause of death. In the New Mexico population studied by Coultas and Hughes, cardiovascular disease (30.2%) and neoplasms (13.2%) were commonly listed as the cause of death (3). This suggests a high rate of comorbid illness in this population, which is not surprising, since the population with pulmonary fibrosis are primarily in their sixth, seventh, and eighth decades.

Much more information has been published regarding the impact of comorbidities in COPD patients. A Spanish study sought to create a model to predict the likelihood of recurrent admissions in COPD patients by identifying risk factors for exacerbations. In the model, which was later validated in a separate population, FEV_1 explained a part of the risk for recurrent admission; however, the other two major risks were age and presence of comorbid illness (4). In a more recent publication, Miravitlles et al. specifically identified ischemic heart disease as a major comorbid factor in exacerbations with relapse that ultimately resulted in admissions (5). Dewan et al. found, in contrast, that comorbidities did not affect outcomes in a Veterans Administration Hospital population they studied. They retrospectively reviewed records from 107 patients hospitalized over a 24-month period. A treatment failure was defined as a return visit that required a change in antibiotic if the patient returned within 4 weeks. By logistic regression analysis, treatment failures were associated with several COPD-related parameters but not with age or presence of comorbidities (6).

The role of comorbidities in mortality is well supported. Various studies have suggested that around half the deaths in patients with advanced COPD are due to causes other than the lung disease (7). Two studies from the same Italian investigators have addressed this issue. In the first study, Fuso et al. reviewed records of 590 COPD admissions from the 1980s and analyzed 23 clinical and laboratory variables to determine risk factors for death. Logistic regression analysis was used to assess the contribution of factors found initially to have a univariate relationship. The four significant predictors were alveolar-arterial oxygen gradient, age, atrial fibrillation, and ventricular arrhythmias (8). In their second study, this group followed COPD patients with severe disease (FEV_1 $34 \pm 16\%$ predicted) after hospital discharge to assess the impact of comorbidities over a longer term. The most frequent comorbidities observed were hypertension (28%), diabetes (14%), and ischemic heart disease (10%) (9). The median survival of this group of 270 patients was 3.1 years and the deaths were predicted by age, electrocardiographic (ECG) signs of right ventricular hypertrophy, chronic renal failure, and ECG signs of myocardial ischemia/infarction. Two other prospective studies in which patients with severe COPD were followed to approximately 50% mortality identified comorbid medical illnesses as significant predictors of death (10,11). The only recent study that has not associated COPD mortality with comorbidities was published by Yohannes et al. This group followed 137 elderly patients with "symptomatic, disabling" COPD for 30 months, at which time 32% had died. Predictors of death in this group were not comorbid diseases but rather level of disability as measured by activities of daily living, prebronchodilator lung function, presence of long-term oxygen therapy, and body mass index (12). The next sections explore specific comorbidities that have been identified as important in patients with chronic lung disease.

III. Cardiac and Vascular Comorbidities

Atrial and ventricular arrhythmias, coronary artery disease, peripheral vascular disease, hypertension, and congestive heart failure have all been identified as significant comorbidities in the patients with obstructive lung disease. Fewer data have been published about the population with interstitial lung disease; however, both Panos et al. and Coultas and Hughes noted in separate reports that cardiac disease accounted for 20 to 30% of deaths in these patients (2,3). Because of the paucity of published information regarding pulmonary fibrosis, the remainder of this section refers to cardiovascular complications in COPD.

A. Atrial and Ventricular Arrhythmias

Supraventricular arrhythmias, commonly associated with obstructive lung disease, vary from multifocal atrial tachycardia to atrial fibrillation to supraventricular tachycardias. Predisposing factors include arrhythmogenic medications, hypoxemia, and underlying intrinsic cardiac disease. In the case of multifocal atrial tachycardia (MAT), the prevailing theory to explain the mechanism is that the underlying disease and metabolic disturbances result in delayed afterdepolarizations, which lead to "triggered" activity (13).

MAT is uncommon but occurs primarily in elderly and very ill patients with decompensated pulmonary or cardiac disease. Diagnosis requires at least three different nonsinus P waves in the same lead, an atrial rate greater than 100 beats per minute and an isoelectric baseline between P waves (14). The incidence has been reported at between 0.13 and 0.4% in hospitalized patients (15). MAT itself is not lethal; however, it is associated with a poor prognosis because of the severity of underlying disease. In one study reporting mortality of COPD patients admitted to an intensive care unit (ICU), 87% of those with multifocal atrial tachycardia compared to only 23.5% of those without died during their ICU stay (16). Other studies suggest similar high mortality rates, ranging from 38 to 62% in hospitalized patients with MAT (17). Treatment of MAT is notoriously difficult. Correction of precipitating causes, while theoretically sound, is often hard to accomplish. The proposed mechanism of "triggered" activity or abnormal automaticity has led to the use of pharmacological interventions, including calcium channel blockers, beta blockers, and magnesium. Several small studies have been reported using verapamil, metoprolol, and magnesium and each has been shown to reduce the heart rate in the majority of patients reported (14,17–19). More recently, small series of medically refractory patients have undergone radiofrequency catheter ablation with a good response in the short term reported in the majority of cases. Ueng et al. reported 6-month follow-up with improved quality of life, improved left ventricular function, and decreased cost of care (20).

Pharmacological therapy used in COPD may be implicated in both atrial and ventricular arrhythmias. Theophylline, now a second-line drug, has a strong association with both atrial and ventricular arrhythmias, especially at toxic levels. Sessler and Cohen studied 16 inpatients with toxic levels of theophylline by continuous cardiac monitoring to record arrhythmias. Sinus tachycardia, which resolved as the drug blood levels fell, was the most common effect, but runs of supraventricular tachycardia occurred in 4 patients, atrial fibrillation in 1, and MAT in 1. Ventricular ectopy occurred in 13 patients, and 1 patient had sustained ventricular tachycardia requiring conversion (21). Infusion of aminophylline to therapeutic levels has been shown to increase plasma catecholamine levels, reduce atrioventricular (AV) and His-Purkinje conduction intervals, reduce sinoatrial conduction time, reduce corrected sinus node recovery time, and reduce atrial effective refractory period (22).

Selective $beta_2$ agonists alone or in combination with theophylline are also potentially arrhythmogenic. Seider et al. used Holter monitoring to compare arrhythmias of patients using either inhaled terbutaline or ipratropium bromide, which is not considered arrhythmogenic. Fourteen patients participated in this double-blind crossover trial. Interestingly, no difference in arrhythmias was observed between the different medications (23). Hall et al. randomly assigned 22 patients with $FEV_1 > 1\,L$ to receive either nebulized salbutamol or saline four times a day on 2 consecutive days while undergoing cardiac monitoring. While both groups had high rates of arrhythmias, there was no difference between beta agonist and placebo treatments (24). In another study, COPD and asthma patients with known ischemic heart disease underwent Holter monitoring while receiving inhaled salbutamol at increasing doses over a 25-hr period. No significant changes in arrhythmias or myocardial ischemia were observed (25). By contrast, a combination of drugs may not be so benign. Eidelman et al. tested the arrhythmogenic potential of salbutamol combined with theophylline in a group of patients with severe COPD. Patients had significantly more arrhythmias when theophylline was added to salbutamol; 76% had runs of supraventricular tachycardia and 24% had runs of ventricular tachycardia. The change in ventricular arrhythmias from baseline was not statistically significant, however (26). Similarly, drugs with longer half-lives pose potential risks. Cazzola et al. studied inhaled salmeterol (50 µg) and formoterol (12 and 24 µg) in 12 COPD patients with pre-existing arrhythmias and hypoxemia. Formoterol at 24 µg resulted in an increase of premature atrial and ventricular premature beats (27).

Arrhythmias often complicate chest surgery in COPD patients. Surgeries for bronchogenic carcinoma and other pathology are commonly performed in these patients. Sekine et al. studied supraventricular arrhythmias and mortality in COPD patients undergoing resections for non-small-cell carcinoma. In a retrospective chart review of 244 patients undergoing resections, 78 had pulmonary function criteria consistent with COPD. In the COPD group, nearly 60% developed supraventricular arrhythmias, compared to 27% in the control group. More than three-quarters of the arrhythmias were atrial fibrillation, and COPD patients tended to be resistant to first-line antiarrhythmic therapy. Arrhythmias were not an independent risk factor for death, but they did predict a significant increase in length of stay (28). In this group, major resection, either pneumonectomy or lobectomy, was also a risk factor. Elderly patients are at particular risk with large resections. Dyszkiewicz et al. found that patients above 70 years of age who underwent pneumonectomy had a 78.5% risk of arrhythmia (29).

Cardiac surgery is complicated by an approximate 50% risk of atrial arrhythmias whether or not underlying pulmonary disease is present. However, the presence of obstructive airway disease is an independent risk factor for the development of atrial fibrillation (30).

Increasingly, exercise programs are included as part of the usual management of patients with advanced disease. Does exercise precipitate arrhythmias in these patients, particularly if they have severe disease and hypoxemia? Stewart and colleagues studied the effect of maximal exercise in 122 patients with severe COPD. At rest, 10 had supraventricular arrhythmias and 13 had ventricular premature beats. With exercise, 6 patients had supraventricular arrhythmias and 24 had premature ventricular beats. Arrhythmias at rest were correlated with arrhythmias on exercise but were not correlated with severity of disease or desaturation. Potentially serious arrhythmias were uncommon (31).

Finally, it should be noted that some patients with hypoxemic COPD have been reported to have a subclinical autonomic neuropathy. Theoretically this could be associated with a prolonged QTc interval and a risk of ventricular arrhythmia and sudden death. Stewart et al. found that half of a group of 34 patients with hypoxemia had subclinical autonomic neuropathy. At 2 years, there were seven deaths in that group compared with two in the nonneuropathy group (32).

B. Systemic Hypertension

Systemic hypertension occurs commonly in the North American population, so it is not surprising that it would occur commonly in patients with COPD. The choice of antihypertensive medication is, of course, important. Beta blockers, if used at all, should be selective for cardiac and vascular receptors; angiotensin-converting enzyme inhibitors may also be problematic because of the frequent cough complication. Meier et al. reviewed a population of predominantly male hypertensives from a Veterans Affairs clinic population. Of the 7526 patients reviewed, 1553 (around 20%) had COPD or asthma as a comorbidity (33).

C. Coronary Artery Disease/Congestive Heart Failure

Despite the high prevalence of ischemic heart disease and COPD individually, it is difficult to get an estimate of the rates at which the two occur as comorbidities, even though smoking is a major risk factor for both. Havranek et al. reviewed charts of a Medicare population as a subgroup of the National Heart Failure project. Of 34,587 cases, one-third were found to have COPD as a comorbid condition (34). Behar et al. from the SPRINT study group reported a 7% prevalence of COPD in that cohort of 5839 patients with acute myocardial infraction (35).

Probably of more importance are issues in diagnosis and treatment when the two disease processes occur together, particularly when congestive failure occurs in conjunction with COPD. Because of the similarity of symptoms and the often unusual x-ray appearance of heart failure in the presence of abnormal lung structure, differentiating between a heart failure decompensation and COPD acute exacerbation remains difficult in many cases. Maisel et al. addressed this issue in a large multicenter study by measuring B-type natriuretic peptide—secreted by the left ventricle when it is volume-over-loaded—in 1586 patients presenting to the emergency room with acute dyspnea. Approximately half the group were ultimately diagnosed with heart failure as opposed to pulmonary and other noncardiac processes. B-type natriuretic peptide levels alone were more accurate than any historical physical finding or other laboratory values in making the diagnosis of congestive heart failure. Using a cutoff level of 100 pg/mL, the positive predictive value was 83.4%, and levels less than 50 pg/mL had a negative predictive value of 96% (36). Further studies will be necessary to determine if this or similar tests will be a valuable adjunct in differential diagnosis.

Beta agonists are a mainstay of the management of obstructive lung disease and beta blockers are a mainstay of coronary artery disease management, particularly in the environment of post–acute myocardial infarction. However, in each case, the side effects potentially worsen the disease in the other organ. Au et al. reported a nested, case-controlled study from a larger Veterans Administration study in which 630 patients with either unstable angina or acute myocardial infarction were identified. Using pharmacy records, the authors compared this group with a control group in terms of those that had filled a beta-agonist prescription within 90 days of their acute event. Filling a beta-agonist prescription was associated with increased risk of experiencing a coronary event, even when adjusting for age and other cardiac risk factors. In addition, the risk increased with the number of canisters dispensed (37).

Beta blockers, on the other hand, are now the standard of care in post–myocardial infarction management and often used in congestive heart failure. A recent Cochrane report evaluated the use of cardioselective beta blockers in patients with COPD; 11 studies of single-dose treatment and 8 studies of longer-duration treatment were reviewed. In neither the single-dose studies nor the longer-term studies was there a significant impact on airway function. Further, there was no evidence that selective beta blockers impacted the effect of beta agonists on airway response (38). The opposite question is whether cardioselective beta blockers are effective in preventing cardiac events in the presence of the use of beta agonists for pulmonary disease. Chen et al. addressed this question in a study of elderly patients using data from the Cooperative Cardiovascular Project. This study evaluated the relationship between beta-blocker use at discharge on 1-year post–myocardial infarction mortality in (1) patients with COPD or asthma on beta agonists; (2) patients with COPD or asthma not using beta agonists; (3) patients with severe COPD; and (4) patients without COPD. The total number of study patients was 54,962. Beta-blocker use conferred a reduced mortality on groups 2 and 4 but not on groups 1 and 3 (39). This question is clearly important and deserves to be explored in a prospective study, with particular attention paid to the causes of death.

COPD patients requiring coronary artery bypass grafting are often thought to face an increased risk of mortality. Michalopoulos et al. conducted a prospective case-controlled study to assess the impact of mild or moderate COPD—patients with severe disease were not included in this study—on the outcome of elective bypass surgery. The morbidity and mortality rates in this study were similar between the study and control groups (40). However, two other studies show increased risk related to COPD. Clough et al. looked at prospective cohort data using a regional cardiac surgery database. A total of 27,239 consecutive patients undergoing cardiac surgery were reviewed and comorbid conditions were documented. The outcome measure was in-hospital mortality rate. COPD was present in 10.9% of patients and was a significant predictor of in-hospital death, with an odds ratio of 1.57 (95% CI 1.29–1.91) even when adjustments were made for disease and other patient characteristics (41). A Dutch study published around the same time showed a significant risk for impaired 5-year survival in patients with COPD undergoing bypass surgery (42).

D. Abdominal Aortic Aneurysms

Abdominal aortic aneurysms (AAA) occur at an increased incidence in COPD patients. COPD also appears to be an independent predictor of their growth and rupture. While the mechanism of this association is not entirely clear, one author theorized it may be due to increased release of elastase activity related to nicotine (43). In another study of the natural history of AAA, Lindholt et al. prospectively followed 141 men with AAA who were identified from a population of 4404 men. The mean annual expansion in the COPD patients in the study group was 2.74 mm/year compared to 2.72 mm/year in non-COPD patients. However, expansion was significantly greater in those patients who used oral steroids compared to those who did not: 4.7 compared to 2.6 mm/year. A correlation with elastase levels was not found (44). These authors suggest that expansion is related more to medication use than to serum elastase levels. Van Laarhoven et al. attempted to determine the prevalence of AAA in COPD patients by prospectively performing abdominal ultrasounds on 362 consecutive patients above age 65 presenting at an emergency room with COPD exacerbation. The study group had a prevalence of 9.9% AAA > 30 mm in diameter (45). Patients with more severe COPD were more likely to have significant aortic dilatation.

Several studies have addressed the risks of open surgical repair in COPD patients; fewer data have been published about the success and long-term durability of endovascular repair. In 1986, Crawford et al. identified COPD as a variable predictive of both early and late death in a series of 605 repairs of thoracoabdominal aneurysms. This series comprised a total of 54 early and 151 late deaths (46). Satta et al. also found COPD to be predictive of early deaths (47). A large study from the Cleveland Clinic also reported that COPD—and several other comorbidities along with advanced age—was associated both with early complications and long-term mortality (48). But a more recent report by Axelrod et al. suggests no increased risk. The authors reviewed national records from Veterans Administration Hospitals and identified 1053 patients who had undergone open AAA repair. Mortality in elective repairs was similar between COPD and non-COPD patients (3.7%), but the length of stay of COPD patients was 2 days longer. Ruptured aneurysms were associated with COPD, but this did not result in a significantly higher risk of death (49). Eskandari et al. argue that even oxygen dependency is not a contraindication to open repair. They report 14 such patients who underwent elective repair. The mean FEV_1 was 34% predicted. No perioperative deaths were recorded, and the mean length of stay was 5.9 days (50). Studies evaluating endovascular repair techniques are ongoing (51,52). Endovascular approaches are very promising, particularly for patients with significant comorbidities.

E. Cerebrovascular Disease

A relationship between COPD and cerebrovascular disease is not well established. Arbix et al. studied a population of 1473 consecutive patients with ischemic stroke. Risk factors were analyzed. Hypertension was the most frequent risk factor in strokes overall, occurring in 52% of patients, followed by atrial fibrillation and diabetes, occurring in 27 and 20% of patients, respectively. COPD was identified as the most common risk factor in atherothrombotic strokes, with an odds ration of 2.63. It was not a separate risk factor in lacunar strokes or those of cardioembolic etiology (53). In a review of ischemic strokes after general surgery at the Mayo Clinic, COPD also emerged as one of the two greatest risks, with an adjusted odds ratio of 10.04 (95% Cl 1.9–53.14) (54).

IV. Pulmonary Embolism

Many patients with chronic lung disease have major risk factors for pulmonary embolism in that they are older and often live very sedentary lives (55). The prevalence of pulmonary embolism in this group is difficult to measure; however, the impact of pulmonary embolism has been documented in several studies.

Like decompensated congestive heart failure, acute pulmonary embolism presents with many of the same symptoms as an exacerbation of the underlying lung disease. Making a correct diagnosis can be a challenge. Traditional diagnostic approaches, particularly ventilation/perfusion ($\dot{V}/\dot{Q}$) scanning, are particularly unreliable in the presence of underlying lung disease. In a study of 108 COPD patients suspected of having pulmonary emboli, Lesser et al. found that clinical assessment, x-ray, $D(a - A)_{O_2}$, and Pa_{CO_2} were unable to distinguish the 21 patients subsequently found to have emboli. $\dot{V}/\dot{Q}$ scans were usually intermediate in probability and thus nondiagnostic. However, in cases of either high-probability scans or normal/near normal scans, the $\dot{V}/\dot{Q}$ studies had high positive predictive value and high negative predictive value, respectively (56). Another study evaluated the clinical probability estimate and a series of diagnostic tests in the COPD population with suspected pulmonary emboli: $\dot{V}/\dot{Q}$ scans, spiral computed tomography, D-dimer testing, and angiography. The usefulness of the clinical probability estimate and each of these studies with the exception of the $\dot{V}/\dot{Q}$ scan were similar between populations with and without COPD (57). The diagnostic role of magnetic resonance imaging is unclear (58).

Pulmonary embolism has a negative impact on outcomes in patients with parenchymal lung disease. Carson et al. prospectively followed 1487 patients who had lung scans because of suspected pulmonary embolism for 1 year and determined death rates in those with and without confirmed embolism. By 1 year, 23.8% of patients with confirmed pulmonary embolism had died, compared to 18.9% of patients without. Of particular interest, those patients with both COPD and pulmonary embolism had a death rate of 53.3% at 1 year (59). Poulsen et al. in a similar but retrospective study assessed outcome of 588 persons clinically suspected of having pulmonary embolism. Follow-up was between 1 and 2 years. In this group, one-third had confirmed pulmonary emboli. A comorbidity (including COPD) was an independent predictor for a confirmed diagnosis; however, death rates were similar in groups with and without pulmonary embolism (60).

Fatal pulmonary embolism is a missed diagnosis premortem in more than half the cases. In a recent autopsy series, pulmonary embolism went undiagnosed more often in patients with comorbidities. Only 13% of COPD patients with fatal pulmonary embolism and 33% of patients with congestive heart failure and pulmonary embolism were diagnosed premortem (61). Similarly, critically ill COPD patients are at high risk of pulmonary embolism. In a Polish study, 10.9% of COPD patients in an ICU had pulmonary emboli, and pulmonary emboli were the cause of death in 40.6% of the COPD patients who died in the ICU. A high index of suspicion is necessary to achieve better detection of this often overlooked and lethal complication in patients with underlying lung disease or other comorbidity (62).

V. Gastroesophageal Reflux Disease

The potential role of gastroesophageal reflux disease (GERD) has been investigated in several pulmonary processes, most notably asthma, COPD, and pulmonary fibrosis. GERD and asthma have the largest literature and have generally been noted to occur frequently in the same patients (63). The prevalence of GERD symptoms in asthma patients has been documented to be more than 75% in some studies (64,65). Some evidence suggests that reflux material and specifically acid reflux can produce bronchoconstriction (66,67). However, the mechanisms of the airway hyperresponsiveness are not fully defined. Boeree et al. reported a double-blind, placebo-controlled trial in which patients with both asthma and GERD were randomized to receive either omeprazole or placebo. The authors were unable to detect an improvement in pulmonary symptoms in those patients who had had relief of acid reflux (68).

The role of GERD and particularly its impact on pulmonary function is less clear in COPD patients. While a retrospective population survey study in a group of veterans showed an increased prevalence of pulmonary disease in those with reflux esophagitis (69), a small study in which airway resistance was measured during acid perfusion of the esophagus did not cause bronchoconstriction in a group of COPD patients (70). These patients, however, had relatively normal esophageal function and are not necessarily the same as the population of COPD patients who report symptomatic reflux. Mokhlesi et al. undertook a prospective questionnaire-based, cross-sectional analytical survey to assess the association between reflux symptoms and COPD. The survey was undertaken in a population of veterans; a control group from the general internal medicine clinic was used. Significant symptoms (occurring more than once a week) of heartburn, dysphagia, and chronic cough were reported more frequently by COPD patients. In addition, 26% of COPD patients associated their pulmonary symptoms with reflux symptoms. There was a nonsignificant trend toward a higher rate of symptoms in COPD patients with $FEV_1 < 50\%$ (70). In a follow-up to the previous study, Mokhlesi and colleagues assessed the swallowing function of patients with COPD and hyperinflation compared to a control population. They used videofluoroscopic techniques and were able to demonstrate than COPD patients used protective techniques against aspiration more frequently than controls. These included longer duration of airway closure and earlier laryngeal closure relative to the cricopharyngeal opening as compared to controls (72). In another evaluation of cricopharyngeal function in COPD patients, however, severe dysfunction was seen in 17 of 22 patients, primarily among the elderly (73). The discrepancy between these two studies speaks to the fact that the COPD population is a heterogenous population, may not be able to addressed simplistically in terms of comorbidities like GERD, and may require individualized approaches to management.

Another study addressed the impact of GERD on pulmonary function in elderly patients. In this study, 27 patients with reflux and 29 without reflux (documented by pH monitoring) had spirometry. Patients with reflux symptoms had slightly lower vital capacities than those without reflux, particularly if the reflux was moderate or severe (74). The association of restrictive disease and GERD has been made not only in elderly patients but also by several authors studying other patient groups since at least the early 1970s (75,76). In 1976, Mays et al. prospectively evaluated 131 patients with pulmonary fibrosis and 270 controls with upper gastrointestinal series. Of 131 pulmonary fibrosis patients, 48 had reflux, a statistically significantly higher rate than found in controls (77). More recently, Tobin et al. investigated 17 patients with idiopathic pulmonary fibrosis using esophageal pH monitoring and documented abnormal acid levels in 16 of the patients, a significantly higher rate than the 50% found in controls (78). These investigators also noted that pulmonary fibrosis patients with GERD often do not have typical symptoms and that the episodes often occur at night. Ing points out, however, that despite the increasing information linking pulmonary fibrosis and reflux disease, no data have shown a causal effect (79). To establish this presumably would require prospective, long-range studies of patients with known significant reflux disease. Nevertheless, it is reasonable to treat symptomatic or asymptomatic reflux aggressively when it is documented in patients with pulmonary fibrosis.

VI. Cancer

Recently published data estimate more than 12 million Americans have at least moderate obstructive lung disease (80). It is the fourth leading cause of death, and cancer is the second leading cause of death. Cancer deaths per year number almost 550,000, and COPD deaths more than 124,000 (81). Thus it is likely that COPD is a significant comorbidity in many cancer victims. Again, however, few data document such a relationship. Coebergh et al. published data from the Netherlands in which the prevalence of serious comorbidity was ascertained at diagnosis in patients with unselected cancers. Over a 3-year period, from 1993 to 1996, data from 34,000 patients were registered. Clinical data regarding comorbidities were collected from clinical records. Comorbid conditions as a percent of new cancer diagnoses ranged from 12% in those less than 45 years old to 63% in those more than 75 years old. The highest incidence was in patients with lung cancers (58%). COPD was among the most frequent comorbidity complicating (across the range of tumors) cancers and ranged from 3 to 25% of newly diagnosed cancer cases (82). A study from the National Institute on Aging and the National Cancer Institute assessed the prevalence of comorbidities in the elderly. Cancers of the breast, cervix, ovary, prostate, colon, stomach, and urinary bladder were included in the study of 7600 patients. As in the previous study, data were collected from medical records. Hypertension, heart disease, and arthritis were the most commonly reported comorbidities; COPD and diabetes less common (83). In hematological malignancies, where pulmonary function is often of concern because of treatment toxicity, again few data have been published. Van Spronsen et al. studied 194 patients with Hodgkin's lymphoma and 904 with non-Hodgkin's lymphoma using the same registry used in the Coebergh study. Comorbidity was low (less than 20%) in the population below age 60 but present in 56% of those above age 60. It was present in 43% of non-Hodgkins patients between 60 and 70 years old and 61% of patients above age 70. COPD was present in approximately 10% of these patients (84). Interestingly, patients with comorbidity received less chemotherapy and had lower survival in the first months after diagnosis, though in this study no correlations to specific comorbidities were made.

One would expect COPD to have its greatest impact as a comorbidity in patients with lung cancer. Sekine et al. retrospectively reviewed data from 244 patients with non-small-cell lung cancer who underwent pulmonary resection. COPD was identified by spirometry preoperatively in 78 of the patients; others were considered to not have COPD. Postoperative complications occurred more frequently in COPD patients; 5-year survival in the COPD patients was 36.2%, compared to 41.2% in the non-COPD patients (27). A Spanish study assessed the frequency of comorbidity in operable lung cancer in relation to the presence of symptoms and age. Between 1993 and 1997, 2992 consecutive patients were studied. Of those, 2189 had one or more comorbidities. Some 50% of lung cancers were associated with the most frequently found comorbidity, COPD; in 32% of patients with COPD, the FEV_1 was less than 70% predicted. Age and presence of symptoms was associated with the presence of COPD (85). The Dutch study cited earlier has also yielded information about lung cancer and comorbidities. Janssen-Heijnen et al. reviewed 3864 lung cancer cases registered from 1993 to 1995 from their population-based registry. COPD was the second most common comorbidity, reported in 22% of patients, and was barely superseded by cardiovascular disease, which occurred in 23% of patients. The rate of resection of localized non-small-cell tumor in patients above age 70 in those with COPD was only 67%, compared to 94% in those without identified comorbidities (86). This suggests an association of less aggressive treatment in the presence of comorbidity and deserves further exploration.

Since the 1950s, a link between pulmonary fibrosis and lung cancer has been suggested (87,88). Several more recent studies have also reported such a correlation.

In Japan, this association has been reported by Nagai and others (89,90). Hubbard et al. used the United Kingdom General Practice Research Database to compare patients with cryptogenic fibrosing alveolitis (idiopathic pulmonary fibrosis) with controls in terms of their rates of lung cancer. Patients with diagnoses of connective tissue diseases were eliminated, leaving 880 patients with fibrosing alveolitis and 5884 controls. A diagnosis of fibrosing alveolitis was accepted only if physical exam and chest x-ray were compatible. The authors found that the relative risk for cancer in fibrosing alveolitis was 7.36 (95% Cl 1.54–35.19) even when smoking was taken into account (91). However, this association has not been supported in U.S.-based studies (92,93). A recent review points out the difficulty of assessing available studies because of the different criteria used to identify a diagnosis of pulmonary fibrosis (94). This is another area where further study will be required before a definitive answer becomes available.

VII. Cognitive Functioning

In two studies in the 1990s, Incalzi et al. reported that significant impairment in verbal and verbal memory tasks could be found in almost half of a group of 36 patients with COPD who had hypoxia and hypercapnia but who were using supplemental oxygen. The impairments were significantly correlated with age and with duration of chronic respiratory failure. The first report was particularly disturbing because of the apparent development of cognitive defects despite appropriate oxygen use (95,96). Stuss et al. also found a correlation between hypoxia and particularly hypercapnia and problems with delayed memory, complex attention, and speed of information processing. No evidence of general dementia was found, but the more subtle impairments led the authors to emphasize the importance of early diagnosis and treatment of hypoxia (97). Finally, Kozora et al. compared the neuropsychological function in three groups: mild Alzheimer's patients, COPD patients with mild hypoxemia, and normal controls. Patients with Alzheimer's disease performed worse than the other groups in most cases. COPD patients had lower letter fluency and lower verbal fluency than controls, though not in the clinically impaired range. In most cases the changes were subtle and not severe enough to impair normal functioning (98). Physicians and family caregivers need to be aware of the possibility of mildly impaired functioning in COPD patients, particularly in the performance of certain mental tasks. These findings underscore the importance of maintaining adequate arterial oxygen levels.

VIII. Summary

The cost of care of COPD represents a significant portion of our health care dollars. Medicare expenditures for COPD patients are 2.4 times as great as the per capita expenditures for all Medicare beneficiaries (99). Strassels et al. reported that only 25% of the expense for COPD patients was direct COPD-related expense (100). The rest presumably is due to comorbid conditions. A third case-controlled study assessing health care utilization and costs in COPD patients demonstrated that health utilization was approximately double that of age- and sex-matched controls, with much of the excess attributable to other smoking-related illness (101). The role of comorbid illness in patients with COPD and other chronic, advanced lung disease is an important consideration in all phases of the patient's management. Alternatively, COPD appears as a significant comorbidity and negative prognostic factor in many common chronic illnesses. Constant awareness of the likelihood of coexistence of two or more chronic illnesses is necessary to assure that all comorbidities are addressed and optimal medical management is achieved.

References

1. van Manen JG, Bindels PJ, Ijzermans CJ, van der Zee JS, Bottema BJ, Schade E. Prevalence of comorbidity with a chronic airway obstruction and controls over the age of 40. J Clin Epidemiol 2001; 54:287–293.
2. Panos RJ, Mortenson RL, Niccoli SA, King TE Jr. Clinical Deterioration in patients with idiopathic pulmonary fibrosis: causes and assessment. Am J Med 1990; 88:396–404.
3. Coultas DB, Hughes MP. Accuracy of mortality data for interstitial lung diseases in New Mexico, USA. Thorax 1996; 51:717–720.
4. Miravitlles M, Guerrero T, Mayordomo C, Sanchez-Agudo L, Nicolau F, Segu JL. Factors associated with increased risk of exacerbation and hospital admission in a cohort of ambulatory COPD patients: a multiple logistic regression analysis. The EOLO Study Group. Respiration 2000; 67:495–501.
5. Miravitlles M, Murio C, Guerrero T. Factors associated with relapse after ambulatory treatment of acute exacerbations of chronic bronchitis. DAFNE Study Group. Eur Respir J 2001; 17:928–933.
6. Dewan NA, Rafique S, Kanwar B, Satpathy H, Ryschon K, Tillotson GS, Niederman MS. Acute exacerbation of COPD: factors associated with poor treatment outcome. Chest 2000; 11762–11771.
7. Gerardi D, ZuWallack R. Non-pulmonary factors affecting survival in patients completing pulmonary rehabilitation. Monaldi Arch Ches Dis 2001; 56:331–335.

8. Fuso L, Incalzi RA, Pistelli R, Muzzolon R, Valente S, Pagliari G, Gliozzi F, Ciappi G. Predicting mortality of patients hospitalized for acutely exacerbated chronic obstructive pulmonary disease. Am J Med 1995; 98:272–277.

9. Antonelli IR, Fuso L, DeRosa M, Forastiere F, Rapiti E, Nardecchia B, Pistelli R. Co-morbidity contributes to predict mortality of patients with chronic obstructive pulmonary disease. Eur Respir J 1997; 10:2794–2800.

10. Connors AF Jr, Dawson NV, Thomas C, Harrell FE Jr, Desbiens N, Fulkerson WJ, Kussin P, Bellamy P, Goldman L, Knaus WA. Outcomes following acute axacerbation of severe chronic obstructive lung disease. The SUPPORT investigators (Study to Understand Prognoses and Preferences for Outcomes and Risks of Treatments). Am J Respir Crit Care Med 1996; 154:959–967.

11. Almagro P, Calbo E, Ochoa de Exhaguen A, Barreiro B, Quintana S, Heredia JL, Garau J. Mortality after hospitalization for COPD. Chest 2002; 121:1441–1448.

12. Yohannes AM, Baldwin RC, Connolly M. Mortality predictors in disabling chronic obstructive lung disease in old age. Age Aging 2002; 31:137–140.

13. McCord J, Borzak S. Multifocal atrial tachycardia. Chest 1998; 113:203–209.

14. Schwartz M, Rodman D, Lowenstein SR. Recognition and treatment of multifocal atrial tachycardia: a critical review. J Emerg Med 1994; 12:353–360.

15. Scher DL, Arsura EL. Multifocal atrial tachycardia: mechanisms, clinical correlates, and treatment. Am Heart J 1989; 118:574–580.

16. Tsai YH, Lee CJ, Lan RS, Lee CH. Multifocal atrial tachycardia as a prognostic indicator in patients with severe chronic obstructive pulmonary disease requiring mechanical ventilation. Changgeng Yi Xue Za Zhi 1991; 14:163–167.

17. Levine JH, Michael JR, Guarnieri T. Treatment of multifocal tachycardia with verapamil. N Engl J Med 1985; 312:21–25.

18. Arsura E, Lefkin AS, Scher DL, Solar M, Tessler S. A randomized, double-blind, placebo-controlled study of verapamil and metoprolol in treatment of multifocal atrial tachycardia. Am J Med 1988; 85:519–524.

19. McCord JK, Borzak S, Davis T, Gheorghiade M. Usefulness of intravenous magnesium for multifocal atrial tachycardia in patients with chronic obstructive pulmonary disease. Am J Cardiol 1998; 81:91–93.

20. Ueng KC, Lee SH, Wu DJ, Lin CS, Chang MS, Chen SA. Radiofrequency catheter modification of atrioventricular junction in patients with COPD and medically refractory multifocal atrial tachycardia. Chest 2000; 117:52–59.

21. Sessler CN, Cohen MD. Cardiac arrhythmias during theophylline toxicity. A prospective, continuous electrocardiographic study. Chest 1990; 98:672–678.

22. Eiriksson CE Jr, Writer SL, Vestal RE. Theophylline-induced alterations in cardiac electrophysiology in patients with chronic obstructive pulmonary disease. Am Rev Respir Dis 1987; 135:322–326.

23. Seider N, Abinader EG, Oliven A. Cardiac arrhythmias after inhaled bronchodilators in patients with COPD and ischemic heart disease. Chest 1993; 104:1070–1074.

24. Hall IP, Woodhead MA, Johnston ID. Effect of high-dose salbutamol on cardiac rhythm in severe chronic airflow obstruction: a controlled study. Respiration 1994; 61214–61218.

25. Rossinen J, Partanen J, Stenius-Aarniala B, Nieminen MS. Salbutamol inhalation has no effect on myocardial ischaemia, arrhythmias and heart-rate variability in patients with coronary artery disease plus asthma or chronic obstructive pulmonary disease. J Intern Med 1998; 243:361–366.

26. Eidelman DH, Sami MH, McGregor M, Cosio MG. Combination of theophylline and salbutamol for arrhythmias in severe COPD Chest 1987; 91:808–812.

27. Cazzola M, Imperatore F, Salzillo A, Di Perna F, Calderaro F, Imperatore A, Matera MG. Cardiac effects of formoterol and salmeterol in patients suffering from COPD with preexisting cardiac arrhythmias and hypoxemia. Chest 1998; 114:411–415.

28. Sekine Y, Kesler KA, Behnia M, Brooks-Brunn J, Sekine E, Brown JW. COPD may increase the incidence of refractory supraventricular arrhythmias following pulmonary resection for non-small cell lung cancer. Chest 2001; 120:1783–1790.

29. Dyszkiewicz W, Pawlak K, Gasiorowski L. Early post-pneumonectomy complications in the elderly. Eur J Cardiothorac Surg 2000; 17:246–250.

30. Ad N, Snir E, Vidne BA, Golomb E. Potential preoperative markers for the risk of developing atrial fibrillation after cardiac surgery. Semin Thorac Cardiovasc Surg 1999; 11:308–313.

31. Cheong TH, Magder S, Shapiro S, Martin JG, Levy RD. Cardiac arrhythmias during exercise in severe chronic obstructive pulmonary disease. Chest 1990; 97:793–797.

32. Stewart AG, Waterhouse JC, Howard P. The QTc interval, autonomic neuropathy and mortality in hypoxaemic COPD. Respir Med 1995; 89:79–84.

33. Meier JL, Lopez J, Siegel D. Prevalence and treatment of hypertension complicated by comorbid conditions. J Clin Hypertens 1999; 1:209–211.

34. Havranek EP, Masoudi FA, Westfall KA, Wolfe P, Ordin DL, Krumholz HM. Spectrum of heart failure in older patients: results from the National Heart Failure project. Am Heart J 2002; 143:412–417.

35. Behar S, Panosh A, Reicher-Reiss H, Zion M, Schlesinger Z, Goldbourt U. Prevalence and prognosis of chronic obstructive pulmonary disease among 5,839 consecutive patients with acute myocardial infarction. SPRINT Study Group. Am J Med 1992; 93:637–641.

36. Maisel AS, Krishnaswamy P, Nowak RM, McCord J, Hollander JE, Duc P, Omland T, Storrow AB, Abraham WT, Wu AHB, Clopton P, Steg PG, Westheim A, Knudsen CW, Perez A, Kazanegra R, Hermann HC, McCullough PA. Rapid measurement of B-type natriuretic peptide in the emergency diagnosis of heart failure. N Engl J Med 2002; 347:161–167.

37. Au DH, Curtis JR, Every NR, McDonell MB, Fihn SD. Association between inhaled beta-agonists and the risk of unstable angina and myocardial infarction. Chest 2002; 121:846–851.

38. Salpeter SS, Ormiston T, Salpeter E, Poole P, Cates C. Cardioselective beta blockers for chronic obstructive pulmonary disease (Cochrane Review). Cochrane Database Syst Rev 2002; 2:CD003566.

39. Chen J, Radford MJ, Wang Y, Marciniak TA, Krumholz HM. Effectiveness of beta-blocker therapy after acute myocardial infarction in elderly patients with chronic obstructive pulmonary disease or asthma. J Am Coll Cardiol 2001; 37:1950–1956.

40. Michalopoulos A, Geroulanos S, Papadimitriou L, Papadakis E, Triantafillou K, Papadopoulos K, Palatianos G. Mild or moderate chronic obstructive pulmonary disease risk in elective coronary artery bypass grafting surgery. World J Surg 2001; 25:1507–1511.

41. Clough RA, Leavitt BJ, Morton JR, Plume SK, Hernandez F, Nugent W, Lahey SJ, Ross CS, O'Connor GT. The effect of comorbid illness on mortality outcomes in cardiac surgery. Arch Surg 2002; 137:428–432.

42. van Domburg RT, Takkenberg JJ, van Herwerden LA, Venema AC, Bogers AJ. Short-term and 5-hear outcome after primary isolated coronary artery bypass graft surgery: results of risk stratification in a bilocation center. Eur J Cardiothorac Surg 2002; 21:733–740.

43. Murphy EA, Danna-Lopes D, Sarfati I, Rao SK, Cohen JR. Nicotine-stimulated elastase activity release by neutrophils in patients with abdominal aortic aneurysms. Ann Vasc Surg 1998; 12:41–45.

44. Lindholt JS, Heickendorff L, Antonsen S, Fasting H, Henneberg EW. Natural history of abdominal aortic aneurysm with and without coexisting chronic obstructive pulmonary disease. J Vasc Surg 1998; 28:226–233.

45. van Laarhoven CJ, Borstlap AC, van Berge Henegouwen DP, Palmen FM, Verpalen MC, Schoemaker MC. Chronic obstructive pulmonary disease and abdominal aortic aneurysms. Eur J Vasc Surg 1993; 7:386–390.

46. Crawford ES, Crawford JL, Safi HJ, Coselli JS, Hess KR, Brooks B, Norton HJ, Glaeser DH. Thoracoabdominal aortic aneurysms: preoperative and intraoperative factors determining immediate and long term results of operations in 605 patients. J Vasc Surg 1986; 3:389–404.

47. Satta J, Immonen K, Reinila A, Pokela R, Juvonen T. Outcome of elective infrarenal abdominal aortic aneurysm repair—an analysis of 174 consecutive patients. An Chir Gynaecol 1996; 85:231–235.

48. Hertzer NR, Mascha EJ, Karafa MT, O'Hara PJ, Krajewski LP, Beven EG. Open infrarenal abdominal aortic aneurysm repair: the Cleveland Clinic experience from 1989 to 1998. J Vasc Surg 2002; 35:1145–1154.

49. Axelrod DA, Henke PK, Wakefield TW, Stanley JC, Jacobs LA, Graham LM, Greenfield LJ, Upchurch GR Jr. Impact of chronic obstructive pulmonary disease on elective and emergency abdominal aortic aneurysm repair. J Vasc Surg 2001; 33:72–76.

50. Eskandari MK, Rhee RY, Steed DL, Webster MW, Muluk SC, Trachtenberg JD, Hoffman RM, Makaroun MS. Oxygen-dependent chronic obstructive pulmonary disease does not prohibit aortic aneurysm repair. Am J Surg 1999; 178:125–128.

51. Arko FR, Newman C, Fogarty TJ. Endovascular stent-grafts for the repair of infrarenal abdominal aortic aneurysms: a brief review. J Intervent Cardiol 2001; 14:475–481.

52. Hinchliffe RJ, Hopkinson BR. Endovascular repair of abdominal aortic aneurysm: current status. J R Coll Surg Edinb 2002; 47:523–527.

53. Arboix A, Morcillo C, Garcia-Eroles L, Oliveres M, Massons J, Targa C. Different vascular risk factor profiles in ischemic stroke subtypes: a study from the Sagrat Cor Hospital of Barcelona Stroke Registry. Acta Neurol Scand 2000; 102:264–270.

54. Limburg M, Wijdicks EF, Li H. Ischemic stroke after surgical procedures: clinical features, neuroimaging, and risk factors. Neurology 1998; 50:895–890.

55. Heit J. Venous thromboembolism epidemiology: implications for prevention and management. Semin Thromb Hemost 2002; 28(Suppl 2):3–14.

56. Lesser BA, Leeper KV Jr, Stein PD, Saltzman HA, Chen J, Thompson BT, Hales CA, Popovich J Jr, Greenspan RH, Weg JG. The diagnosis of acute pulmonary

embolism in patients with chronic obstructive pulmonary disease. Chest 1992; 102:17–22.

57. Hartmann IJ, Hagen PJ, Melissant CF, Postmus PE, Prins MH. Diagnosing acute pulmonary embolism: effect of chronic obstructive pulmonary disease on the performance of D-dimer testing, ventilation/perfusion scintigraphy, spiral computed tomographic angiography, and conventional angiography. ANTE-LOPE Study Group. Advances in new technologies evaluating the localization of pulmonary embolism. Am J Respir Crit Care Med 2000; 162:2232–2237.

58. Amundsen T, Torheim G, Kvistad KA, Waage A, Bjermer L, Nordlid KK, Johnsen H, Asberg A, Haraldseth O. Perfusion abnormalities in pulmonary embolism studied with perfusion MRI and ventilation-perfusion scintigraphy: an intra-modality and inter-modality agreement study. J Magn Reson Imaging 2002; 15:386–394.

59. Carson JL, Terrin ML, Duff A, Kelley MA. Pulmonary embolism and mortality in patients with COPD. Chest 1996; 110:1212–1219.

60. Poulsen SH, Noer I, Moller JE, Knudsen TE, Frandsen JL. Clinical outcome of patients with suspected pulmonary embolism. A follow-up study of 588 consecutive patients. J Intern Med 2001; 250:137–143.

61. Pineda LA, Hathwar VS, Grant BJ. Clinical suspicion of fatal pulmonary embolism. Chest 2001; 120:791–795.

62. Filipecki S, Kober J, Kaminski D, Tomkowski W. Pulmonary thromboembolism. Monaldi Arch Chest Dis 1997; 52:492–493.

63. Sontag SJ. Gastroesophageal reflux disease and asthma. J Clin Gastroenterol 2000; 30:S9–S30.

64. Field SK, Underwood M, Brant R, Cowie RL. Prevalence of gastroesophageal reflux symptoms in asthma. Chest 1996; 109:316–322.

65. Sontag SJ, Schnell TG, Miller TQ, Khandelwal S, O'Connell S, Chejfec G, Greenlee H, Scidel UJ, Brand L. Prevalence of oesophagitis in asthmatics. 1992; Gut 33:872–876.

66. Harding, SM, Richter, JE. The role of gastroesophageal reflux in chronic cough and asthma. Chest 1997; 111:158–163.

67. Boyle JT, Tuchman DN, Altschuler, SM, Nixon TE, Pack AI, Cohen S. Mechanisms for the association of gastroesophageal reflux and bronchospasm. Am Rev Respir Dis 1985; 131:S916–S920.

68. Boeree MJ, Peters FT, Postma DS, Kleibeuker JH. No effects of high-dose omeprazole in patients with severe airway hyperresponsiveness and symptomatic gastro-oesophageal reflux. Eur Respir J 1998; 11:1070–1074.

69. El-Serag HC, Sonnenberg A. Comorbid occurrence of laryngeal or pulmonary disease with esophagitis in United States military veterans. Gastroenterology 1997; 113:755–760.

70. Orr WC, Shamma-Othman Z, Allen M, Robinson MG. Esophageal function and gastroesophageal reflux during sleep and waking in patients with chronic obstructive pulmonary disease. Chest 1992; 101:1521–1525.

71. Mokhlesi B, Morris AL, Huang C-F, Curcio AJ, Barrett TA, Kamp DW. Increased prevalence of gastrophageal reflux symptoms in patients with COPD. Chest 2001; 119:1043–1048.

72. Mokhlesi B, Logemann JA, Rademaker AW, Stangl CA, Corbridge TC. Oropharyngeal deglutition in stable COPD. Chest 2002; 121:361–369.

73. Stein M, Williams AJ, Grossman F, Weinberg AS, Zuckerbraun L. Cricopharyngeal dysfunction in chronic obstructive pulmonary disease. Chest 1990; 97:347–352.
74. Raiha IJ, Ivaska K, Sourander LD. Pulmonary function in gastro-oesophageal reflux disease of elderly people. Age Ageing 1992; 21:368–373.
75. Moallem S, Gross A, Gluck M, Kaplan S, Sanoudos GM, Ray JF III, Clauss RH. Pulmonary complications of gastroesophageal reflux. N Y State J Med 1973; 73:279–283.
76. Pearson JE, Wilson RS. Diffuse pulmonary fibrosis and hiatus hernia. Thorax 1971; 26:300–305.
77. Mays EE, Dubois JJ, Hamilton GB. Pulmonary fibrosis associated with tracheobronchial aspiration. A study of the frequency of hiatal hernia and gastroesophageal reflux in interstitial pulmonary fibrosis of obscure etiology. Chest 1976; 69:512–515.
78. Tobin RW, Pope CE II, Pellegrini CA, Emond MJ, Sillery J, Raghu G. Increased prevalence of gastroesophageal reflux in patients with idiopathic pulmonary fibrosis. Am J Respir Crit Care Med 1998; 158:1804–1808.
79. Ing AJ. Interstitial lung disease and gastroesophageal reflex. Am J Med 2001; 111(suppl 8A):41S–44S.
80. Mannino DM, Homa DM, Akinbami LJ, Ford ES, Redd SC. Chronic obstructive pulmonary disease surveillance, 1971–2000. MMWR 2002; 51:1–18.
81. National Center for Health Statistics. Deaths: Final Data for 1999. Hyattsville, MD: US Department of Health and Human Services, CDC, 2001. (National Vital Statistics Report; vol 49, no. 8) Website: *http://www.cdc.gov/hchs/releases/01facts/99mortality.htm*
82. Coebergh JW, Janssen-Heijnen ML, Post PN, Razenberg PP. Serious comorbidity among unselected cancer patients newly diagnosed in the southeastern part of The Netherlands in 1993–1996. J Clin Epidemiol 1999; 52:1131–1136.
83. Yancik R, Havlik RJ, Wesley MN, Ries L, Long S, Rossi WK, Edwards BK. Cancer and comorbidity in older patients: a descriptive profile. Ann Epidemiol 1996; 6:399–412.
84. van Spronsen DJ, Janssen-Heijnen ML, Breed WP, Coebergh JW. Prevalence of co-morbidity and its relationship to treatment among unselected patients with Hodgkin's disease and non-Hodgkin's lymphoma, 1993–1996. Ann Hematol 1999; 78:315–319.
85. Lopez-Encuentra A, Bronchogenic Carcinoma Co-operative Group. Comorbidity in operable lung cancer: a multicenter descriptive study on 2992 patients. Lung Cancer 2002; 35:263–265.
86. Janssen-Heijnen ML, Schipper RM, Razenberg PP, Crommelin MA, Coebergh JW. Prevalence of co-morbidity in lung cancer patients and its relationship with treatment: a population-based study. Lung Cancer 1998; 21:105–113.
87. Spain DM. The association of terminal bronchiolar carcinoma with chronic interstitial inflammation and fibrosis of the lungs. Am Rev Tuberc 1957; 76:559–567.
88. Turner-Warwick M, Lebowitz M, Burrows B, Johnson A. Cryptogenic fibrosing alveolitis and lung cancer. Thorax 1980; 35:496–499.
89. Nagai A, Chiyotani A, Nakadate T, Konno K. Lung cancer in patients with idiopathic pulmonary fibrosis. Tohoku J Exp Med 1992; 167; 167:231–237.

90. Kawai T, Yakumaru K, Suzuki M, Kageyama K. Diffuse interstitial pulmonary fibrosis and lung cancer. Acta Pathol Jpn 1987; 37:11–19.

91. Hubbard R, Venn A, Lewis S, Britton J. Lung cancer and cryptogenic fibrosing alveolitis: a population-based cohort study. Am J Respir Crit Care Med 2000; 161:5–8.

92. Wells C, Mannino DM. Pulmonary fibrosis and lung cancer in the United States: analysis of multiple cause of death:mortality data. 1979 through 1991. South Med J 1996; 89:505–510.

93. Bouros D, Hatzakis K, Labrakis H, Zeibecoglou K. Association of malignancy with diseases causing interstitial pulmonary changes. Chest 2002; 121:1278–1289.

94. Ma Y, Seneviratne CK, Koss M. Idiopathic pulmonary fibrosis and malignancy. Curr Opin Pulm Med 2001; 7:278–282.

95. Incalzi RA, Gemma A, Marra C, Muzzolon R, Capparella O, Carbonin P. Chronic obstructive pulmonary disease. An original model of cognitive decline. Am Rev Respir Dis 1993; 148:418–424.

96. Incalzi RA, Gemma A, Marra C, Capparella O, Fuso L, Carbonin P. Verbal memory impairment in COPD: its mechanisms and clinical relevance. Chest 1997; 112:1506–1513.

97. Stuss DT, Peterkin I, Guzman DA, Guzman C, Troyer AK. Chronic obstructive pulmonary disease: effects of hypoxia on neurological and neuropsychological measures. J Clin Exp Neuropsychol 1997; 19:515–524.

98. Kozora E, Filley CM, Julian LJ, Cullum CM. Cognitive functioning in patients with chronic obstructive pulmonary disease and mild hypoxemia compared with patients with mild Alzheimer disease and normal controls. Neuropsychiatry Neuropsychol Behav Neurol 1999; 12:178–183.

99. Grasso ME, Weller WE, Shaffer TJ, Diette GB, Anderson GF. Capitation, managed care, and chronic obstructive pulmonary disease. Am J Respir Crit Care Med 1998; 158:133–138.

100. Strassels SA, Smith DH, Sullivan SD, Majajan PS. The costs of treating COPD in the United States. Chest 2001; 119:344–352.

101. Mapel DW, Hurley JS, Frost FJ, Petersen HV, Picchi MA, Coultas DB. Health care utilization in chronic obstructive pulmonary disease. A case-control study in a health maintenance organization. Arch Intern Med 2000; 160:2653–2658.

16

Osteoporosis, Metabolic Bone Disease, and Endocrine Abnormalities

ROBERT M. ARIS, SUE A. BROWN, and DAVID A. ONTJES

University of North Carolina at Chapel Hill
Chapel Hill, North Carolina, U.S.A.

I. Overview

Osteoporosis results in 1.5 million $\times$ 10^6 fractures annually in United States alone (1). Half of all women and one-eighth of men $\geqslant 50$ years old will experience fractures at some time in their lives. Unfortunately, only 20% are diagnosed with osteoporosis and, worse yet, only 5% are adequately treated. Osteoporosis results in 322,000 hospitalizations accounting for 3.5 $\times$ 10^6 bed days and 750,000 office visits annually, leading to 20 $\times$ 10^6 restricted activity days and 60,000 nursing home (NH) admissions. Hip fractures increase mortality two- to fivefold. One-fourth of patients who suffer from a hip fracture die in the first year. When questioned, 80% of women preferred death to hip fracture resulting in nursing home placement, indicating the important psychological impact of osteoporosis in our aging society. The annual medical costs for osteoporosis care in the United States, United Kingdom, and France are $14 billion, £614 million, and 4 billion Fr, respectively. In comparison, the annual United States medical costs for COPD are $13.6 billion and the costs to manage all lung diseases in the United States are $84 billion.

The renewed interest in osteoporosis in the pulmonary community is due to (1) an increased awareness of implications, (2) the impact of lung transplantation, (3) improved and disseminated technology for measuring bone mineral density (BMD) by dual-energy x-ray absorptiometry (DXA), and (4) safe and effective medications (in particular bisphosphonates).

Osteoporosis is defined as a low overall bone mass together with a disruption of normal bone architecture, leading to an increased susceptibility to fractures after minimal trauma. The normal three-dimensional structure of trabecular bone is altered. Osteoporotic bone has fewer connecting bony spicules or "struts," which are thinner than normal. Thus, both the radiological density and mechanical strength of osteoporotic bone are diminished (2,3). Histologically, there is an equivalent decrease in both bone mineral (composed of calcium and phosphorus), and bone matrix (composed of collagen and other bone proteins).

Other metabolic bone diseases that can cause structural weakness of bone include osteomalacia and osteitis fibrosis. Osteomalacia occurs when bone mineral fails to be deposited in normally formed bone matrix. Histologically, osteomalacia is characterized by an increased amount of noncalcified matrix. Rickets in children is the equivalent of osteomalacia in adults. Osteitis fibrosa is due to high circulating levels of parathyroid hormone (PTH). Both primary and secondary (e.g., renal insufficiency) hyperparathyroidism cause increased bone resorption. The histological appearance shows increased numbers of osteoclasts, or bone-resorbing cells.

Bone is a dynamic tissue in which new mineral is constantly being laid down while previously mineralized sections are being resorbed. The cells governing this process are osteoblasts and osteoclasts. Osteoblasts are bone-forming cells derived from connective tissue stem cells. Mature osteoblasts synthesize collagen and other bone matrix proteins such as osteocalcin and a specific isoform of alkaline phosphatase, which are believed to play roles in bone formation and the mineralization process. Osteoclasts, derived from stem cells in the bone marrow resembling macrophages, are the most important cells involved in bone resorption. These cells contain lysosomes that release enzymes to degrade bone matrix proteins.

The World Health Organization defines osteoporosis in terms of bone mineral density measurements (4). Osteoporosis is present when the measured BMD is more than 2.5 standard deviations, or ~25%, below the mean for a normal young individual (when peak bone mass is achieved). Osteopenia refers to a lesser degree of bone loss, in which the measured BMD is between 1.0 and 2.5 standard deviations below normal peak bone mass, or a loss of 10 to 25%.

II. Osteoporosis: Etiology and Pathogenesis

A variety of inherited and acquired factors can lead to osteopenia or osteoporosis. Osteoporosis results when there is too much bone resorption, too little bone formation, or a combination of both. The most common cause of increased bone resorption is estrogen deficiency associated with menopause in healthy women (Fig. 1). Accelerated bone loss continues for ~10 years after

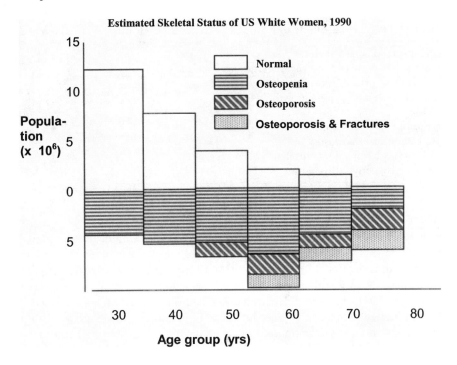

Figure 1 The number of women in the United States suffering from osteopenia and osteoporosis is strongly age-related. Comparable estimates in men are not available, but men are less affected. (Adapted from Ref. 5.)

menopause, then the rate of decline subsides to near the rate associated with normal aging.

Estrogen replacement in the postmenopausal period reduces the rate of resorption and stabilizes bone mass. Men with hypogonadism have accelerated bone loss similar to that of postmenopausal women. Genetic factors play a major role in determining both the peak bone mass and the rate of bone loss in older individuals. In population-based studies, natural variations (polymorphisms) in genes for the vitamin D receptor, the estrogen receptor, and for type 1 collagen matrix protein appear to affect bone mass. Other conditions that cause increased bone resorption include hyperparathyroidism, hyperthyroidism, malabsorptive syndromes, and multiple myeloma. Corticosteroid therapy is by far the most common cause of secondary osteoporosis in western society (see Table 1) (6,7).

Corticosteroids are a significant cause of bone loss. One-third to one-half of patients treated with 0.1 mg/kg of prednisone for 1 year develop vertebral fractures and will lose, on average, 10% of their bone mineral density (BMD). Since trabecular bone is most affected, fractures tend to occur in the spine, ribs, and pelvis, but cortical bone is not resistant to the adverse effects of

Table 1 Detrimental Effects of Corticosteroids on Bone Health

Suppression of bone formation
↓Conversion of precursor cells to mature osteoblast
↓Synthesis of osteoid (bone matrix) by osteoblasts
Local suppression of bone growth factors

Increased bone breakdown
↑Activation of osteoclasts
↓GI calcium absorption and renal tubular resorption
Secondary hyperparathyroidism

corticosteroids. Corticosteroid-induced bone loss is nonlinear and may be partially reversible. Irrespective of underlying disease, the greatest loss in BMD occurs within the first 12 months of corticosteroid therapy; thereafter, the rate of decline slows yet still exceeds the rate expected from normal aging. The rate of loss of BMD immediately after corticosteroid initiation may be two- to fivefold higher than the rate seen during chronic maintenance therapy. Laan et al. demonstrated that rheumatoid arthritis patients treated with 10 mg/day of prednisone (or placebo) for 20 weeks lost 7% of their spine BMD but were able to recover over the next 24 weeks to values close to baseline, reflecting no significant change compared to patients treated with placebo (8). Results such as these suggest that bone is a dynamic tissue that has a compensatory process to remodel after corticosteroid cessation, but the compensation may be incomplete if the duration of therapy is too long or other complicating factors (e.g., postmenopausal status, other) are present.

III. Osteoporosis: Presentation

As bone is lost, there are typically no symptoms until fractures occur, usually with minimal trauma. Compression fractures of the vertebrae are most common, followed by fractures of the proximal femur and the distal radius (Colles' fracture) (Fig. 2) (9).

As a result of vertebral compression with anterior wedging, patients will lose height and develop a kyphosis deformity of the spine. Patients who have experienced vertebral compression fractures may have chronic back pain. Proximal femoral (hip) fractures are the most disabling, often leading to immobilization and a loss of independent living in elderly men and women. Since the entire skeleton is fragile, fractures are more likely to occur at other sites as well, including the pelvis, ribs, and long bones. Once a fracture occurs, the risk for another fracture is two- to fivefold higher than in the general population.

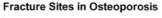

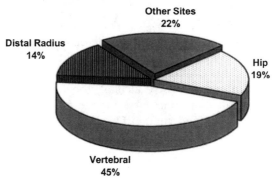

Figure 2 Fracture site distribution in patients with osteoporosis.

IV. Osteoporosis: Diagnostic Approach

Plain chest rays, especially lateral ones, can show several types of abnormalities that suggest osteoporosis or another metabolic bone disease. The most common finding is nonspecific osteopenia or reduced radiographic density. In more advanced disease, deformities, fractures, and kyphosis may occur. In early disease, standard x-rays are normal. At least 30% of total bone mass must be lost before abnormalities in density are detectable by plain radiographs, making this technique very insensitive to early bone loss. However, since chest x-rays are routinely available to lung specialists, they are an easy screen for advanced bone disease.

Quantitative measurement of BMD is the primary means of diagnosing osteoporosis, using World Health Organization standards. The most widely used method for measuring bone mass today is dual-energy x-ray absorptiometry (DXA). The main clinical utility of quantitative BMD measurement is documenting the presence of osteopenia or osteoporosis and predicting the risk of fracture. In general, a decline of one standard deviation below young normal BMD (i.e., T score < -1) doubles the fracture risk. The risk doubles again for each standard deviation decline thereafter (e.g., a T score of -3 equates to a fracture risk that is eightfold higher).

Routine laboratory evaluation is usually limited. Serum creatinine, calcium, phosphorus, alkaline phosphatase and TSH, as well as a complete blood count should be obtained in most patients. Patients with elevated serum calcium should have a measurement of serum PTH. Those at clinical risk for vitamin D deficiency, such as home-bound or institutionalized individuals, should have a measurement of 25-hydroxyvitamin D.

V. Osteoporosis: Management and Therapy

A. Prevention

Osteoporosis is more easily prevented than cured. The health habits of individuals in early and middle life play a role in their risk of osteoporosis in later life. Adequate dietary intake of calcium and vitamin D; active physical exercise; and avoidance of excessive alcohol, tobacco, and drugs known to cause osteopenia are all useful measures for the prevention of osteoporosis. The recommended calcium and vitamin D intake is 1000 to 1200 mg/day and 400 IU, respectively for most adults (10).

B. Drug Therapy

The objectives of therapy in osteoporosis include prevention of further excessive bone loss, promotion of bone formation, prevention of fractures, reduction or elimination of pain, and restoration of physical function. The National Osteoporosis Foundation recommends using antiosteoporotic therapy when either (1) T score < -2 or (2) T score < -1.5 when other risk factors are present, including corticosteroid use, smoking, weight < 127 lb, or history of fracture below the age of 50. All of the agents listed below have been shown to improve BMD, and several have been shown to reduce the incidence of fractures in clinical trials. All of them are considered to be "antiresorptive" agents, acting to reduce rates of bone resorption rather than to stimulate bone formation. Estrogens are commonly used to relieve menopausal symptoms and preserve BMD in postmenopausal women, whether osteoporosis is present or not. The other antiosteoporosis drugs are generally indicated for use in patients having either documented osteoporotic fractures or bone densities at least 2 standard deviations below peak bone mass.

Estrogen replacement in postmenopausal women prevents the excessive bone loss due to estrogen deficiency. Estrogens (providing a minimum or 50 μg of estradiol or equivalent) should be given together with a progestin in women who have an intact uterus to avoid the increased risk of endometrial cancer. Orally administered estrogens have a beneficial effect on the serum lipid profile but adversely affect the risk of venous blood clots in susceptible individuals. Despite decades of use, estrogen replacement remains controversial due to effects on the cardiovascular system.

Selective estrogen receptor modulators (SERMs) are synthetic analogs of estrogen that have some of the biological effects of natural estrogen, but they lack other effects. Drugs in this class include raloxifene, a drug approved for the treatment of osteoporosis (11). Raloxifene acts as an estrogen agonist with respect to bone metabolism. It increases BMD when given to postmenopausal women. Raloxifene is a good choice as an antiosteoporosis drug in women at high risk of breast or uterine cancer, since it does not stimulate the endometrium or breast tissue.

Bisphosphonates are a family of compounds that resemble pyrophosphate and are incorporated into the mineral structure of bone (12). There, they inhibit bone resorption and promote increased bone mass. Clinical trials of several bisphosphonates—including etidronate, alendronate, and risedronate—indicate that BMD is increased in postmenopausal osteoporosis, idiopathic male osteoporosis, and corticosteroid-induced osteoporosis after 2 or more years of treatment. Further trials with alendronate and risedronate provide strong evidence that these drugs can reduce fracture risk by 40 to 60% at various skeletal sites, including the spine and hip. Alendronate and risedronate are the only bisphosphonates currently approved in the United States for treatment of osteoporosis, but other drugs of this class are likely to be approved in the near future.

Calcitonin is a peptide hormone produced by the thyroid gland. The administration of synthetic human or salmon calcitonin in patients with osteoporosis causes a reduction in bone resorption and a modest increase in BMD (13). Clinical trials have found that intranasal calcitonin therapy reduces the occurrence of vertebral fractures in postmenopausal women. However, with the advent of bisphosphonates, calcitonin use has declined.

VI. Osteoporosis in Chronic Obstructive Pulmonary Disease

Among pulmonary disorders, chronic obstructive pulmonary disease (COPD) is most commonly linked to osteoporosis. Systemic corticosteroids decrease bone mineral density, particularly in ribs and vertebrae, where trabecular bone predominates. While corticosteroid therapy for COPD is thought by many to be the most important factor causing osteoporosis in this patient group, a variety of other factors may be important in causing or accelerating bone loss among COPD patients. Lifestyle factors—including reduced dietary calcium intake, reduced physical activity secondary to respiratory limitation, and cigarette and alcohol consumption with their known deleterious effects on bone health—may all contribute to bone demineralization in COPD independent of corticosteroid therapy (14). In addition, as mentioned above, hypoxemia may result in alterations in hypothalamic-pituitary-gonadal axis, resulting in reduced sex hormone levels leading to diminished bone formation (15). More recently, inflammatory cytokines, including TNF-β, IL-6, and IL-1, which emanate from the lung during acute and chronic inflammation, have been implicated in accelerating bone resorption and reducing bone formation at the cellular level contributing to a low BMD (16).

The prevalence and severity of osteoporosis and fractures in patients with COPD has not been determined. On the most severe end of the spectrum, reports from three lung transplantation centers have indicated that COPD patients referred for transplant evaluation almost universally suffer from osteoporosis or osteopenia (17–19). More recently, Iqbal et al. reported that

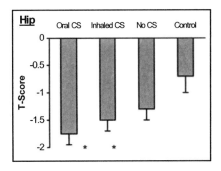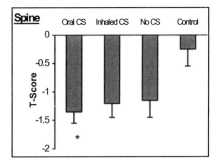

Figure 3 Hip and spine T scores from COPD patients demonstrating that bone mass is lower across all categories of COPD but is the worst for the oral corticosteroid (CS)-treated patients. $*p < 0.05$ versus controls. (From Ref. 20.)

bone mineral density was lower in patients with mild to moderate COPD as well (20). In this study, a large series of chronic lung disease (predominantly COPD) patients from the Atlanta VA Medical Center were screened for osteoporosis by DXA and categorized as to corticosteroid usage. In patients taking oral corticosteroids, the FEV_1 averaged 50.6%, whereas the groups who were taking inhaled corticosteroids and those who had never been treated with corticosteroids had average FEV_1 values of 59 and 69%, respectively (Fig. 3). As expected, those using oral corticosteroids for COPD had lower hip and spine T and Z scores, values that were significantly different from those in an age-matched control population. Interestingly, the inhaled corticosteroid-treated patients and the non-corticosteroid–treated COPD patients also had lower hip and spine T scores than the control population. T scores for the oral steroid-taking COPD patients were slightly lower than in those who took inhaled corticosteroids only, which were, in turn, slightly lower than in those who took no corticosteroids, but these differences among the various COPD groups were not statistically significant. Osteoporosis was ninefold more prevalent in the oral steroid–treated COPD patients and fourfold more prevalent in the non-steroid–treated COPD patients in comparison to controls. The authors concluded that COPD itself was a risk factor for osteoporosis in addition to the well-accepted risk that is attendant on corticosteroid use. These data may extend to patients with chronic bronchitis in addition to those with emphysema. Preat et al. found reduced bone density in chronic bronchitic patients, including those who had never received oral corticosteroids (21).

The consequences of osteoporosis, mainly fractures and kyphosis, have been sparingly studied in COPD patients. McEvoy et al. using a conventional vertebral fracture definition (20% decrease in the anterior vertebral height in comparison to the posterior height), reported that COPD patients suffer considerably more vertebral fractures than an age-matched control population (22) (Fig. 4). The study enrolled 312 men, $\geqslant 50$ years of age, with a smoking

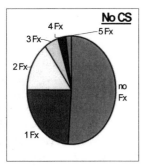 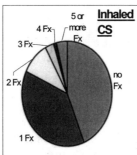 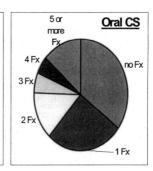

Figure 4 Patients who never received corticosteroids (CS), those who had received inhaled CS, and those receiving oral CS had vertebral fracture (Fx) prevalence rates of 49, 57, and 63%, respectively. (Adapted from Ref. 22.)

history and a spirometric diagnosis of COPD. Subjects were assigned to one of three groups: 117 subjects had never used corticosteroids, 70 had used only inhaled corticosteroids, and 125 had taken an oral corticosteroid for at least 2 weeks during their lives. Subjects with a history of oral corticosteroid use were further grouped into 52 subjects whose lifetime duration of oral corticosteroid use was greater than 6 months and 73 subjects whose lifetime duration less than 6 months.

Subjects who used oral prednisone were nearly two times more likely to have $\geqslant 1$ vertebral fractures than those who never used corticosteroids (odds ratio $= 1.8$; 95% confidence interval: 1.08, 3.07). This observed effect was primarily attributable to subjects whose lifetime use of oral corticosteroids was greater than 6 months (31.2 g of prednisone as a cumulative lifetime dose), in whom there was a threefold increased risk for at least one vertebral fracture (OR $= 2.99$; 1.38, 6.49). The oral corticosteroid–treated COPD patients had a significantly higher prevalence of vertebral fractures than those who had never received oral corticosteroids; but, in addition, these patients were much more likely to have multiple and severe vertebral fractures. Therefore, in this study, the continuous users of corticosteroids were at the greatest risk for vertebral fractures, but those who had not used corticosteroids also had higher fracture rates than controls.

A study of the rates of long bone fractures in COPD has yet to appear in the literature. However, Leech et al. determined a relationship between deterioration in lung function due to kyphosis and the severity of osteoporosis in women (23). They estimated that a 10% decease in vital capacity results from worsening of the kyphosis angle that resulted from each thoracic vertebral fracture. Therefore, in addition to reducing height and causing acute and chronic pain, vertebral compression fractures compromise lung function. Several studies have also demonstrated that vertebral fractures are more common in cigarette smokers. However, neither of these studies was controlled for the presence or absence of COPD.

The effect of inhaled corticosteroids on BMD in patients with COPD has been less well studied than the effect in asthmatics. Nonetheless, a greater effect may be seen in patients with COPD than those with asthma and in postmenopausal than in premenopausal women. The EUROSCOP researchers included an evaluation of osteoporotic vertebral fractures and BMD determination in a subgroup of patients (102 subjects in the budesonide group and 92 in the placebo group) in their randomized, placebo-controlled trial of the effects of inhaled budesonide in persons with mild COPD (24). There was no significant change over time in BMD except for an increase in the density of the femoral trochanter in the active treatment group. New vertebral fractures were rare and occurred in fewer than 5% of the subjects.

A large recent multicenter study evaluating the efficacy of inhaled triamcinolone in treating COPD has shed the first convincing light on the fact that inhaled corticosteroids contribute to a decline in bone density in patients ($n = 559$) who are chronically treated (25). Although the triamcinolone therapy (1200 µg) improved respiratory symptoms and decreased the use of health care services for COPD patients, it did result in statistically significant declines in lumbar spine and femoral neck bone mineral density (-0.35 versus $+0.98\%$, $p = 0.007$; and -2.0 versus -0.22%, $p < 0.001$ respectively). Interestingly, the change in bone mineral density in this 3-year study was not seen at the end of the 1-year therapy period; it was detected only at the end of the third year. Therefore the authors concluded that prolonged monitoring of patients on chronic inhaled corticosteroids might be necessary to assess the impact on bone density. At present, it cannot be determined, based upon the available literature, whether a longer duration of usage or a high dose of inhaled corticosteroid confers an increased risk for osteoporotic fractures.

Therapy for corticosteroid-induced osteoporosis in COPD patients has recently been reviewed (26) and follows the guidelines promulgated by the American College of Rheumatology and the American Association of Clinical Endocrinology (7,27). In large, randomized clinical trials, alendronate, risedronate, etidronate, calcitonin, and hormone replacement therapy (HRT) have all been shown to be effective in improving BMD in corticosteroid-treated patients, but the therapeutic responses are usually less than in patients not taking corticosteroids.

Long-term oral corticosteroids usage, irrespective of underlying disease, also suppresses the hypothalamic-pituitary-adrenal (HPA) axis, but the magnitude of the effect and its persistence following discontinuation of therapy are less certain (28). Schlaghecke et al. found no association between the plasma cortisol response and the dose or duration of corticosteroid therapy, suggesting that both long and short-term therapy suppresses adrenal responsivity (29). However, as accepted in clinical practice, short-term therapy is unlikely to precipitate a clinically evident hypoadrenal crisis, largely because brief steroid therapy does not fundamentally affect long-term adrenal reserve and function (30). Deaths caused by adrenal insufficiency in corticosteroid-dependent patients are rare despite the enormous number of patients receiving such therapy (31). Only a few cases of adrenal insufficiency after withdrawal of inhaled corticosteroid therapy have been reported in adults (32). Of the trials evaluating inhaled corticosteroid use in COPD patients, only Paggiaro et al. found significantly lower cortisol levels in the fluticasone propionate group versus the placebo group ($p = 0.024$), but the clinical significance of this finding was not apparent (33). Some degree of HPA suppression undoubtedly occurs with long-term corticosteroid (oral > inhaled) therapy in COPD, but serious clinical adverse outcomes are rare, probably because clinicians taper corticosteroids slowly rather than stopping them abruptly.

VII. Osteoporosis in Asthma

Inhaled corticosteroids may affect bone mineral metabolism, but results of clinical studies, mostly conducted in asthmatics, are inconsistent (34,35). Most of these studies have been comparisons between asthmatics (children and adults) and normal volunteers. In general, no significant effect on HPA function was found from relatively low doses of inhaled corticosteroids (400–800 mg/day beclomethasone) (34,35). In a metanalysis of systemic adverse effects of inhaled corticosteroids used in asthmatic children and adults, however, Lipworth found significant adrenal suppression with doses above 1.5 mg/day (0.75 mg/day for fluticasone propionate) (34). This finding supports the evidence reported by Brown et al., who found that of 78 adult asthmatics taking 1.5 mg or more inhaled corticosteroid daily, 20.5% showed some biochemical evidence of HPA suppression (36). Risk factors associated with this suppression were previous requirement for long-term systemic corticosteroids and a longer duration of high-dose inhaled therapy. Inhaled corticosteroids probably affect bone mineral metabolism and BMD at doses >1 mg/day.

Convincing evidence that inhaled corticosteroids also lower BMD in patients with asthma has come from a recent study by Wong and colleagues (37). A total of 196 adults with asthma, ages 20 to 40, were studied in a cross-sectional fashion, and higher cumulative doses of inhaled corticosteroids were associated with a decrease in BMD at the lumbar spine and femur. Adjustments for sex, age, and potential confounding factors including asthma severity (i.e., physical activity, FEV_1, and hospital admissions) and past oral and parental corticosteroids use did not weaken the associations. In order to help the readership understand the meaning of these findings, the authors expressed their findings in a real-world example. The bone side effects, on average, mean that the patient who is taking 2000 µg/day of an inhaled corticosteroid for 7 years (i.e., 5 g total dose) will have a lumbar spine bone density that is, on average, 1 standard deviation lower than another patient who has taken a low dose (i.e., 200 µg/day) of inhaled corticosteroids for 1 year. The authors indicated that since millions of Europeans and Americans are taking inhaled corticosteroids at a dose of 800 μg or higher, a small risk in the overall fracture rate would have a substantial public health impact. An additional important finding in this study was that cortical (femoral) bone was affected as much as trabecular (spinal) bone, suggesting that patients taking high doses of corticosteroids for long periods of time may also suffer from increased rates of long bone fractures. While the group of women taking corticosteroids was relatively well matched with those who were not taking corticosteroids, there was a significantly lower level of physical activity scores in the group taking high-dose inhaled coricosteroids, and this may have affected one of the main outcome measures, femoral BMD. Nonetheless, the information is important to pulmonologists because they care for many patients on chronic medium- to high-dose corticosteroids. The authors of this study concluded that patients (both men and women) receiving 1200 μg/day of inhaled corticosteroids over a two-decade period would have a significant reduction in BMD at the femur, at least doubling their fracture risks. Whether all inhaled corticosteroid therapies would produce a similar effect on BMD is unknown. Furthermore, whether oral calcium supplementation or mouth rinsing after corticosteroid use would result in an amelioration of the expected BMD decline are areas for further study.

VIII. Osteoporosis in Cystic Fibrosis

The nature of the underlying bone disease in CF is not known, but osteomalacia is uncommon (38,39). Patients with CF are at increased risk for low BMD due to multiple factors. Delayed puberty, reduced physical activity, decreased sunlight exposure (and thus deceased vitamin D production), decreased sex hormone levels due to chronic illness, chronic malnutrition and low BMI, the use of corticosteroids to relieve airway inflammation, and pancreatic exocrine insufficiency leading to reduced absorption of calcium and vitamin D, resulting in altered calcium homeostasis, may all play a role in reducing BMD in CF patients (40–43). Furthermore, increased levels of inflammatory cytokines (e.g., TNF-α, IL-1, and IL-6), which have been detected in the serum and lungs of patients with CF, may accelerate bone resorption through osteoclastogenesis and osteoclast activation and inhibit bone formation (44). Both accelerated bone resorption and decreased bone formation have been widely reported (45–47).

The prevalence of osteoporosis in the CF population is difficult to define precisely. However, a large number of studies have shown a consistent pattern of low BMD in both CF children and adults. Many CF children suffer inadequate bone growth and fail to reach peak bone mass, a factor that contributes to low BMD as adults. Prior to the redefinition of osteoporosis by the World Health Organization (WHO) (which addresses adults, not children), the cut point for diagnosing osteoporosis was a Z score below 2, and the prevalence of osteoporosis in small groups of CF patients was 19 to 77%, with adults generally experiencing more advanced bone disease than children (47–52). Using the WHO's definition of osteoporosis, the prevalence of osteoporosis in adult CF patients with advanced lung disease was in the range of 23 to 57% (53–55), but osteopenia was almost universal in the patients who failed to meet the definition of osteoporosis. Most recently, large surveys of clinically stable adult CF patients from the United States, United Kingdom, Italy, and Denmark have reported the prevalence of osteoporosis to be 20 to 34% (using a Z score of < -2.0) and 10% (using the WHO definition), respectively, and the prevalence of osteopenia was 31 to 51% (56–61).

A low 25 (OH)D (25 hydroxyvitamin D) levels can occur in CF patients due to malabsorption (62), reduced sunlight exposure (63) or, possibly, accelerated 25(OH)D catabolism (61). Vitamin D deficiency is clearly a factor in some cases of osteomalacia and osteopenia. Serum 25(OH)D levels are the best clinical indicator of the adequacy of the vitamin D supply/production. Hahn et al. were the first to demonstrate a correlation between low 25(OH)D levels and BMD in CF (64). Subsequently, at least 17 studies (nicely reviewed in Ref. 42) have found low 25(OH)D levels and 3 have reported elevated PTH levels in CF. Hanley et al. demonstrated the low efficacy of 800 IU/day of vitamin D (the recommended supplementation in adults) in normalizing 25(OH)D levels in CF patients (65). Although bone disease in CF patients is a complex process and may well involve multiple mechanisms, the above results indicate that vitamin D–dependent processes are very likely to contribute to low BMD in CF.

The main sequelae of osteoporosis in CF are fractures and kyphosis. The prevalence of fragility fractures in some selected populations of adult CF patients may be as high as 10 to 20% (49,53,66). Significantly higher rates of fracture have been reported for nontransplanted CF adults (53). Kyphosis and back pain are also very common in CF. Erkkila et al. (67) first reported an increased prevalence of kyphosis in CF patients, a finding subsequently supported by others (53,68,69). The increased kyphosis angles were due in part to a high prevalence of vertebral compression fractures (70,71).

As a general rule, children and adults with CF should be screened for bone disease by DXA, and if BMD is normal (Z score 0 ± 1 in children and T score 0 ± 1 in adults), rescreening every 2 to 5 years may help determine the rate of bone growth/loss. Z scores are used most often to define bone disease in children, whereas T scores are used most often to define bone disease in adults. Treatment of established bone disease in CF has not been well studied. Encouraging weight-bearing exercise, exposure to sunlight, maintaining a good nutritional status, and the proactive management of pulmonary infection are reasonable measures to maintain or increase BMD. Supplementation of calcium and vitamin D is probably a useful intervention based on clinical studies in non-CF patients with low BMD. ADEK vitamins alone probably are not sufficient if vitamin D deficiency exists in adults, but predicting the optimum vitamin D supplement is not easy due to the variability in vitamin D absorption. Target 25(OH)D levels should be >18 to 20 ng/mL and preferably

> 30 ng/mL. If osteoporosis is present and/or fractures due to minor trauma or kyphosis occur, a more aggressive stance toward therapy should be taken. Preliminary data suggest that intravenous pamidronate is very useful to remineralize bone in CF patients with osteopenia or osteoporosis both before (72) and after lung transplantation (73), but bone pain and fever may occur in non-corticosteroid-taking patients. Oral bisphosphonates or calcitonin may be useful based on anecdotal reports in CF and well-controlled trials in non-CF patients.

IX. Osteoporosis in Sarcoidosis

Osteoporosis and low BMD have frequently been reported in sarcoidosis and may precede the use of corticosteroids, suggesting that the underlying disease places patients at risk (74). Prevalence data are not available. Extrarenal synthesis of calcitriol [1,25(OH)$_2$D$_3$] is central to the pathogenesis of abnormal calcium homeostasis, leading to accelerated bone loss, but alterations in parathyroid hormone (PTH) activity and the expression of PTH-related peptide have also been demonstrated (75–78). Therapeutic efforts to slow bone loss in corticosteroid-treated patients with sarcoidosis have been successful with both calcitonin and alendronate (79,80). The greatest success has been with the initiation of antiresorptive therapy simultaneous with corticosteroid induction.

X. Osteoporosis in Lymphangioleiomyomatosis

Taveira-DaSilva et al. recently studied 104 with lymphangioleiomyomatosis (LAM) patients by DXA and found that 25 (22%) had osteoporosis 38 (36.5%) had osteopenia, and 41 (39.4%) had normal BMD (81). The mean lateral lumbar spine T score for the 104 patients was −1.48. After 21 months, 36 patients receiving progesterone, lumbar spine T scores increased significantly (−1.8 ± 0.22 to −1.2 ± 0.19). In 20 patients treated with bisphosphonates, the increase in lumbar spine T scores from −2.75 ± 0.2 to −1.71 ± 0.22 was significant. In 13 patients who were taking both progesterone and bisphosphonates, the lumbar spine T scores improved significantly, from −2.49 ± 0.26 to −1.44 ± 0.23. Abnormal BMD is frequent in patients with LAM and, despite antiestrogen therapy, BMD scores can actually improve, possibly due to the concurrent treatment with bisphosphonates, calcium, vitamin D, or increased exercise tolerance from improvements in lung disease.

XI. Endocrine Abnormalities

The endocrine problems associated with specific pulmonary disease are presented below. Of course, endocrine problems can arise anew or precede the diagnosis of pulmonary disease without any causal link to the underlying lung disease.

A. Thyroid Disease: Overview

Outside of diabetes, hypothyroidism is the most common endocrine problem that may affect patients with advanced lung disease and is much more prevalent in women ($\sim 2\%$ in some age groups) than in men (prevalence: 0.1%) (82–84). Primary hypothyroidism is the most common cause of thyroid failure, and results in low serum thyroid hormone with elevated TSH levels. There are two major causes of primary hypothyroidism: autoimmune (Hashimoto's disease) thyroiditis (loss of functional thyroid tissue) and interference of thyroid hormone production from ablation therapy (surgical or radioiodine) for hyperthyroidism (85). Secondary hypothyroidism (low TSH or inappropriately normal TSH with low thyroid hormone levels) is usually the result of hypothalamic or pituitary dysfunction, due to either tumors, trauma, surgery, or irradiation. TSH deficiency occurs when the anterior pituitary is unable to secrete adequate amounts of TSH to regulate thyroid hormone production, whereas hypothalamic defects lead to TRH deficiency.

Hypothyroidism can be accurately diagnosed with thyroid function tests. However, these tests can be abnormal in sick but apparently euthyroid patients ("euthyroid sick syndrome") (84,86). These changes are not believed to indicate abnormal thyroid function (because TSH levels are usually normal, thyroid tests return to normal after the underlying illness resolves, and treatment with thyroid replacement has no clinical benefit), but their biological importance is not understood and may represent an adaptive stress response. The existence of these syndromes emphasizes the importance of exercising clinical judgment in the final diagnosis. Table 2 shows the four major patterns of abnormalities in patients with thyroid disease.

B. Thyroid Disease: Diagnostic Approach

Diagnosing the distinct cause of hypothyroidism is usually not necessary, since most cases are iatrogenic or autoimmune thyroiditis. Antithyroid antibodies, thyroid scans, and uptake measurements are rarely necessary since they usually do not change the management of the hypothyroidism. If secondary hypothyroidism is suspected, it is important to assess the adequacy of other pituitary hormones and to obtain magnetic resonance imaging (MRI) of the pituitary/hypothalamus, since replacement of pituitary hormones as well as T_4 may be required. Hyperthyroidism results most commonly from Graves' disease and toxic multinodular goiter, the latter a disease largely of older patients. Hyperthyroidism may lower resting P_{CO_2} levels and increase the drive to breathe (87). A specific diagnosis may assist management; therefore endocrinology consultation may be helpful.

Table 2 The Four Major Patterns of Abnormality in Thyroid Disease

Clinical entity	Thyroid function tests	Presentation
Hypothyroidism (1°)	$\downarrow T_4$, $\uparrow$ TSH	Fatigue, weight gain, dry skin, myxedema, anemia
Hypothyroidism (2°)	$\downarrow T_4$, $\downarrow$ or NL TSH	Same as above
"Euthyroid sick syndrome"[a]	$\downarrow T_4$, NL TSH, NL or $\uparrow T_3$ resin uptake	Clinically euthyroid
Hyperthyroidism	$\uparrow T_4$, $\downarrow$ TSH	Tachycardia, fever, nervousness

[a] Patients on high-dose glucocorticoids or dopamine may have low TSH levels in the face of hypothyroidism because these medications block TSH secretion from the pituitary.

C. Thyroid Disease: Management and Therapy

Hypothyroidism

Levothyroxine is the drug of choice; it is started at 100 to 125 µg/day (~ 1.6 µg/kg/day) and varies depending on age (88). In elderly patients or those with cardiac disease, therapy should be started with smaller doses (25–50 µg/day) and increased gradually to avoid precipitating myocardial ischemia or heart failure. The half-life of levothyroxine is ~ 7 days, so that most symptoms resolve gradually within several days to weeks of initiating therapy. Parenteral levothyroxine is indicated for myxedema coma or severe life-threatening hypothyroidism, which is rare and most often occurs after an intervening illness. Glucocorticoids should also be given in suspected cases, since adrenal insufficiency can commonly coexist with severe hypothyroidism. Subclinical hypothyroidism (an elevated TSH with normal T_4 levels) is common, occurring in $\sim 7.5\%$ of women and $\sim 3\%$ of men. Treatment is controversial and usually not indicated. However, low doses of thyroid hormone can be given to normalize thyroid function tests so as to assess clinical course. The maintenance dose for primary hypothyroidism is adjusted to normalize the TSH level. Because of T_4's long half-life and the delayed fall of chronically elevated TSH levels, dose adjustments should be made no more often than every 5 to 6 weeks. In patients with secondary hypothyroidism, TSH is not regulated normally and cannot be used to adjust the dose. T_4 or free T_4 levels should be maintained within the normal range.

Hyperthyroidism

The main goal in the treatment of hypethyroidism is to suppress synthesis of thyroid hormones with long-term antithyroidal therapy [propylthiouracil (PTU) 100–150 mg every 6–8 hr] or to perform thyroid ablation with radioiodine or surgical intervention (88). Generally speaking, younger patients are treated with long-term antithyroidal therapy or, if noncompliant, subtotal thyroidectomy. Older patients are usually managed with radioactive iodine (^{131}I). If severe thyrotoxicosis (severe hyperthyroidism or thyroid storm) is present, short-term therapy with inorganic iodide more rapidly suppresses hormone release than PTU. In addition, beta-adrenergic antagonists (e.g., propranolol 40–120 mg/day) and glucocorticoids (dexamethasone 2 mg every 6 hr) should be added to control the symptoms and manifestations of excess thyroid hormone. With any of the above therapies, hypothryroidism may result; therefore the patient should be monitored closely.

D. Endocrine Abnormalities Specific for the Underlying Lung Disease

Sarcoidosis

Endocrine abnormalities in sarcoidosis are common. The most widely recognized clinical endocrine abnormality is hypercalcemia, which occurs in approximately 10% (range 2–64%) of patients (89–92). Hypercalciuria is approximately threefold more frequent than hypercalcemia. Both of these abnormalities result from increased activity of 1-α-hydroxlase, a P450-linked mixed function oxidase enzyme capable of synthesizing biologically active $1,25(OH)_2D_3$ from $25(OH)D_3$. This increased enzyme activity probably emanates from extrarenal sites, based on clinical observations that hypercalcemia is observed in anephric patients with sarcoidosis and subsequently by observations that activated macrophages and lymphocytes from areas of granulomatous inflammation are capable of direct synthesis of $1,25\text{-}(OH)_2D_3$. Unlike the normal production of $1,25\text{-}(OH)_2D_3$ in the kidney, the production of this molecule at the site of sarcoidal inflammation is not responsive to negative feedback control. Serum calcium levels rise, since $1,25\text{-}(OH)_2D_3$ results in increased gastrointestinal absorption of calcium and increased osteoclastic activity in bone. Hypercalcemia and hypercalciuria can result in nephrocalcinosis and nephrolithiasis, although these complications are relatively uncommon. Fortunately, treatment of hypercalcemia in sarcoidosis is effective. Guidelines for instituting therapy based on a particular serum or urine calcium level have not been published. Therefore patients with symptomatic hypercalcemia or hypercalciuria deserve therapy, and patients with serum calcium levels >12 mg/L also deserve intervention. Prednisone at doses of 0.5 to 1 mg/kg body weight is highly effective at reducing serum and calcium levels quickly (93). Ketoconazole may be useful in patients who do not require prednisone for lung or systemic disease (94). Nontherapeutic intervention may achieve success if dietary calcium and vitamin D intake are reduced. Likewise, patients who have a high exposure to ultraviolet (UV) light (via sunlight or other) may experience reductions in calcium levels if exposure can be reduced. UV exposure accelerates the production of cholecalciferol from cholesterol precursors in the skin. Rarely is the level of serum calcium so elevated that forced diuresis or intravenous bisphosphonates are necessary.

Osteoporosis and osteopenia are common in patients with sarcoidosis. These conditions may antedate corticosteroid intervention, suggesting that an underlying diathesis for reduced bone mass may be related specifically to sarcoidosis. In addition, as with other lung diseases, corticosteroid therapy exacerbates this problem. Screening and management of osteoporosis have been reviewed above.

Neurosarcoidosis may also cause endocrine abnormalities in addition to neurological ones (95–98). Neurosarcoidosis appears in <10% of all patients with sarcoidosis. While early reports indicated that a partial or complete destruction of the pituitary by sarcoidal granulomatous was causal, more recent studies have indicated that the main cause of hypopituitarism in sarcoidosis is hypothalamic destruction by granulomatous inflammation. In fact, the hypothalamus is the most frequently involved of all the endocrine glands in sarcoidosis (97). Polyuria and polydipsia are the most frequently symptoms in patients with involvement of the pituitary or hypothalamus. While early studies initially attributed these symptoms to diabetes insipidus from vasopressin deficiency, Stuart et al. demonstrated that the main cause of these symptoms is primary polydipsia and disordered control of thirst (96). Other mechanisms for this disorder include diabetes insipidus and vasopression deficiency caused by loss of neurosecretory neurons of the neurohypophysis, destruction of the osmoreceptor, or downward resetting of the osmostat. In addition, the symptoms of polyuria and polydipsia can result from unrelated problems, including hypercalcemia, hypercalciuria, and nephrogenic diabetes insipidus.

Involvement of the HPA axis in sarcoidosis may result in clinically apparent diseases, including hypothyroidism, hypogonadism, hypoadrenalism, and impaired growth. Multiple deficiencies (panhypopituitarism) often coexist. Normal pituitary hormone responsitivity to hypothalamic releasing factors suggests that the primary disorder in sarcoidosis is hypothalamic dysfunction. Deficient secretion of growth hormone and gonadotropins are more common than deficiencies of thyrotropin and adrenocorticotropin. Nonetheless, primary pituitary failure may be seen in addition to hypothalamic dysfunction. While hypoglycemia may be seen in close to one-third of patients with sarcoidosis, clinical evidence of galactorrhea is very uncommon (approximately 1%). Fatal hypoglycemia and dwarfism may result from neurosarcoidosis. In addition, somnolence, insomnia, variations in body temperature, progressive obesity, and personality changes also result from hypothalamic disease.

The next most commonly affected endocrine organ in sarcoidosis is the thyroid gland (99–105). Autopsy studies reveal that approximately 4% of patients with sarcoidosis have granulomatous inflammation of the thyroid gland. In addition, a number of case reports indicate an association between sarcoidosis and thyroiditis, but the case and effect relationship has not been established. Papadopoulos et al. and Nakamra et al. have both found an increased incidence of thyroid autoantibodies in patients with sarcoidosis (100,101). Both of these groups found thyroid autoantibodies in approximately one-third of surveyed patients. It has been suggested that the exaggerated T-helper cell function characteristic of sarcoidosis may facilitate autoantibody production by providing trophic factors for B-cell function. Hashimoto's thyroiditis and Graves' disease have been described in patients with sarcoidosis. Thyroid function test (TSH and T_4 levels, and T_3 resin uptake) are useful screening studies to evaluate thyroid function in patients with sarcoidosis. Additional studies of pituitary function are warranted in the case of primary hypothyroidism.

Adrenal gland involvement in sarcoidosis is rare (105). Granulomatous inflammation of the adrenal gland has resulted in acute addisonian crisis resulting from severe mineralocorticoid deficiency in a patient with sarcoidosis being treated with prednisone. Mineralocorticoid replacement resulted in a dramatic improvement in this patient. Sarcoidosis may also affect the pancreas resulting in diabetes mellitus (106). However, both diabetes mellitus and clinical pancreatitis are no more common in patients with sarcoidosis than the general population. Even more rarely, sarcoidosis may involve both male and female reproductive systems (107,108). The most common sites of involvement include the epididymis, testes, and uterus. Although rare, epididymitis, scrotal masses, oligospermia, infertility, amenorrhea, and menorrhagia have all been described. By and large, all of these abnormalities result from direct granulomatous inflammation of the affected organs.

XII. Langerhans Cell Histiocytosis (Eosinophilic Granuloma)

Langerhans cell histiocytosis (LCH) is a multisystemic disease due to a proliferation of abnormal dendritic histocytes, leading to both pulmonary disease and endocrine abnormalities. Infiltration of the hypothalamopituitary axis (HPA) has been reported in 5 to 50% of autopsy patients with LCH (109). Diabetes insipidus is the most common endocrine abnormality, reported in 15 to 50% of patients. Anterior pituitary dysfunction is well recognized as well in approximately 5 to 20% in LCH patients. In the most comprehensive study to date of multisystem LCH (144 pediatric patients), Nanduri and colleagues found that about one-third of their patients had diabetes insipidus (110). This was an isolated condition in 60% of the cases and was accompanied by other endocrine abnormalities in the other 40%. After diabetes insipidus, growth hormone deficiency is the second most common abnormality in patients with LCH. Growth hormone insufficiency was seen in 15% of patients, 7 of whom had other anterior pituitary deficiencies (gonadotrophic hormones, TSH, the combination, and panhypopituitarism). Posterior pituitary gland involvement is responsible for diabetes insipidus, whereas direct hypothalamic inflammation more commonly results in growth hormone insufficiency. Both diabetes insipidus and growth hormone insufficiency typically are diagnosed within 5 to 10 years of the diagnosis of LCH.

Endocrine abnormalities in adults with LCH have been less well studied. A recent article by Kaltsas et al. found that diabetes insipidus was present in all cases ($n = 12$) of adults with LCH and presented between 1 and 20 years after the original diagnosis (111). Kaltsas et al. found that growth hormone FSH-LH and TSH/ACTH deficiencies were present in 8, 7, and 5 patients, respectively, in their series. Five patients also developed panhypopituitarism. Prolactin levels were elevated in 2 of the 15 adults who were studied. A total of 7 patients with anterior pituitary dysfunction also developed symptoms of other neuroendocrine hormone dysfunction, including 5 with morbid obesity (BMI $\geqslant$ 35), 5 with short-term memory deficits, 4 with sleeping disorders, 2 with disorders of thermoregulation, and 1 with adipsia. All patients had abnormal radiological examinations of the hypothalamus and/or pituitary gland. MRI scanning demonstrated the absence of the bright spot of the posterior pituitary on the T1-weighted images.

Nonendocrinological hypothalamic involvement (including appetite, thirst, and sleep disturbances) can be assessed by the patient history and can be more carefully evaluated with formal neuropsychological-psychometeric evaluation, including general intellectual functioning, memory, attention, and concentration tests and the Halstead-Reitan battery. In addition, a complete endocrinological evaluation is in order, including baseline evaluation of the HPA axis and early morning plasma and urine osmolality measurements. Five patients received radiation therapy to the HPA with partial or complete radiological response, but no form of intervention, including corticosteroids and immunosuppressants, improved any established hormonal deficiency or symptoms of neuroendocrine hormone dysfunction. Growth hormone replacement therapy using the recommended doses of 15 to $20 \, \mathrm{IU/m^2/week}$ divided into daily doses is helpful to achieve greater stature. Diabetes insipidus, whether in children or adults, can be treated with a standard approach.

XIII. Wegener's Granulomatosis

Wegener's granulomatosis is very rarely associated with endocrine abnormalities. There are ~ 20 case reports indicating that Wegener's granulomatosis–associated vasculitis can affect the anterior pituitary gland, resulting in diabetes insipidus and anterior hypopituitarism (112–116). Thyroid abnormalities, including Hashimoto's thyroiditis and thyroid carcinoma, have rarely been reported in Wegener's granulomatosis patients (117). Single case reports also associate adrenal infarction and insulin-dependent diabetes mellitus with Wegener's granulomatosis (118). In all, endocrine complications in Wegener's granulomatosis are quite rare.

XIV. Bronchiolitis Obliterans Organizing Pneumonia

A recent report by Watanabe et al. suggests an association between bronchiolitis obliterans organizing pneumonia (BOOP) and thyroid disease (119). Their manuscript indicates that the thyroid disease present involved the full spectrum, ranging from hypothyroidism to subacute thyroiditis to hyperthyroidism, and that in two of the four cases, the activity of the thyroid disease was similar to that of the underlying BOOP.

XV. Pulmonary Hypertension

A moderate number of reports have linked pulmonary hypertension (PH) and thyroid disease (120–124). The associations between hyperthyroidism and pulmonary hypertension were first described in the early 1980s; subsequently, clinicians have reported improvements in pulmonary hypertension after treatment for hyperthyroidism. The mechanism of disease in these patients may well be related more to high cardiac output and/or sympathetic pulmonary vasoconstriction than to a fundamental remodeling of the pulmonary vasculature. Pulmonary hypertension has been associated with an increased prevalence of autoantibodies. Many patients with both pulmonary hypertension and hyperthyroidism have clinical evidence of an underlying connective tissue disease. Animal model studies have shown that hyperthyroidism affects the tissue levels of endothelin-1, a potent vasoconstrictor peptide, that may contribute to the pathogenesis or consequences of PH. While a mutation within the bone morphogenetic protein type II receptor gene has been identified in both familiar and sporadic cases of primary PH, the presence of thyroid disease may be a modifying factor for the clinical expression of PH. For these reasons, patients with PH should be screened for thyroid disease, both hypo- and hyperthyroidism, especially if abrupt changes in clinical status—such as weight loss, worsening tachycardia, or right heart failure—develop or if a new pericardial infusion occurs.

XVI. Hypogonadism

Hypogonadism is not uncommon in patients with chronic advanced lung disease. Specific incidence and prevalence data are not available. Nonetheless, dozens of reports have confirmed the presence of hypogonadism in the context of a variety of advanced lung diseases, including COPD, IPF, and sarcoidosis (125–129). Secondary hypogonadism (i.e., reduced hypothalamic pituitary function) is the predominant mechanism for low sex hormone levels in patients with severe lung disease. Semple et al. first reported low testosterone levels and clinical symptoms of sexual dysfunction (decreased libido, erectile dysfunction) due to hypoxemia in patients with moderate to severe COPD in 1980 (125). These results have been confirmed and reproduced by others. Further investigation by Semple and colleagues have demonstrated that patients with moderate to severe COPD and resting hypoxemia suffer from reduced levels of luteinizing hormone (LH) and follicle stimulating hormone (FSH) (15). Administration of gonadotropin-releasing hormone intravenously resulted in a normal pituitary response to LH secretion, but the FSH response was subnormal. Similar studies have found a correlation between testosterone levels and P_{O_2} in COPD patients. Treatment of hypoxemia has been shown to lead to increases in serum testosterone levels in patients with low testosterone levels at baseline. For this reason, COPD patients with hypogonadism may have intermittent hypogonadism, and treatment of an exacerbation of underlying lung disease may result in improvements in hypoxemia, which may ultimately lead to improvements in pituitary-hypothalamic function and serum testosterone levels and a reduction in the symptoms of hypogonadism. Should treatments for underlying COPD in its acute and chronic setting fail to improve gonadotropin secretion and testosterone levels, testosterone replacement may improve the clinical symptoms of hypogonadism.

References

1. Osteoporosis prevention, diagnosis, and therapy. NIH Consenus Statement. 2000; 29;17(1):1–45.
2. Shoback D, Marcus R, Bikle D, Strewler G. Mineral metabolism and metabolic bone disease. In: Greenspan FS, Gardner DG, eds. Basic and Clinical Endocrinology, 6th ed. Los Altos, CA: Lange Medical Books, 2001:273–333.
3. Raisz LG, Kream BE, Lorenzo JA. Metabolic bone disease. In: Wilson JD, Foster DW, Kronenberg HM, Larsen PR, eds. Williams Textbook of Endocrinology, 9th ed. Philadelphia: Saunders, 1998:1211–1240.
4. Kanis JA, Melton LJ, Christiansen C, Johnston CC, Khaltaev N. The diagnosis of osteoporosis. J Bone Min Res 1994; 9:1137–1141.
5. Melton LJ. How many women have osteoporosis now? J Bone Min Res 1995; 10:175–177.
6. Canalis E. Clinical review 83: mechanisms of glucocorticoid action in bone: implications to glucocorticoid-induced osteoporosis. J Clin Endocrinol Metab 1996; 81(10):3441–3447.
7. Recommendations for the prevention and treatment of glucocorticoid-induced osteoporosis. American College of Rheumatology Task Force on Osteoporosis Guidelines. Arthritis Rheum 1996; 39(11):1791–1801.
8. Laan RF, van Riel PL, van de Putte LB, van Erning LJ, van't Hof MA, Lemmens JA. Low-dose prednisone induces rapid reversible axial bone loss in patients with rheumatoid arthritis. A randomized, controlled study. Ann Intern Med 1993; 119(10):963–968.
9. Shoback D, Marcus R, Bikle D, Strewler G. Mineral metabolism and metabolic bone disease. In: Greenspan FS, Gardner DG, eds. Basic and Clinical Endocrinology, 6th ed. Lange Medical Books, 2001:273–333.
10. Rodan GA, Martin JA. Therapeutic approaches to bone diseases. Science 2000; 289:1508–1514.

11. Fontana A, Delmas PD. Clinical use of selective estrogen receptor modulators. Curr Opin Rheumatol 2001; 13(4):333–339.
12. Hochberg M. Preventing fractures in postmenopausal women with osteoporosis: a review of recent controlled trials of antiresorptive agents. Drugs Aging 2000; 17:317–330.
13. Silverman SL. Calcitonin. Rheum Dis Clin North Am. 2001; 27(1):187–196.
14. Smith BJ, Phillips PJ, Heller RF. Asthma and chronic obstructive airway diseases are associated with osteoporosis and fractures: a literature review. Respirology 1999; 4(2):101–109.
15. Semple PD, Beastall GH, Watson WS, Hume R. Hypothalamic-pituitary dysfunction in respiratory hypoxia. Thorax 1981; 36(8):605–609.
16. Manolagas SC, Jilka RL. Bone marrow, cytokines, and bone remodeling. N Engl J Med 1995; 332:305–311.
17. Aris RM, Neuringer IP, Egan TM, Weiner M, Ontjes D. Severe osteoporosis before and after lung transplantation. Chest 1996; 109:1176–1183.
18. Shane E, Silverberg SJ, Donovan D, Papadopoulos A, Staron RB, Addesso V, Jorgesen B, McGregor C, Schulman L. Osteoporosis in lung transplantation candidates with end-stage pulmonary disease. Am J Med 1996; 101(3):262–269.
19. Spira A, Gutierrez C, Chaparro C, Hutcheon MA, Chan CK. Osteoporosis and lung transplantation: a prospective study. Chest 2000; 117(2):476–481.
20. Iqbal F, Michaelson J, Thaler L, Rubin J, Roman J, Nanes MS. Declining bone mass in men with chronic pulmonary disease: contribution of glucocorticoid treatment, body mass index, and gonadal function. Chest 1999; 116(6):1616–1624.
21. Praet JP, Peretz A, Rozenberg S, Famaey JP, Bourdoux P. Risk of osteoporosis in men with chronic bronchitis. Osteoporos Int 1992; 2(5):257–261.
22. McEvoy CE, Ensrud KE, Bender E, Genant HK, Yu W, Griffith JM, Niewoehner DE. Association between corticosteroid use and vertebral fractures in older men with chronic obstructive pulmonary disease. Am J Respir Crit Care Med 1998; 157(3 pt 1):704–709.
23. Leech JA, Dulberg C, Kellie S, Pattee L, Gay J. Relationship of lung function to severity of osteoporosis in women. Am Rev Respir Dis 1990; 141(1):68–71.
24. Pauwels RA, Lofdahl CG, Laitinen LA, et al. Long-term treatment with inhaled budesonide in persons with mild chronic obstructive pulmonary disease who continue smoking. N Engl J Med 1999; 340:1948–1953.
25. Effect of inhaled triamcinolone on the decline in pulmonary function in chronic obstructive pulmonary disease. N Engl J Med 2000; 343(26):1902–1909.
26. Goldstein MF, Fallon JJ, Harning R. Chronic glucocorticoid therapy-induced osteoporosis in patients with obstructive lung disease. Chest 1999; 116:1733–1749.
27. Hodgson SF, Johnsoton CC, Jr. AACE clinical practice guidelines for the prevention and treatment of postmenopausal osteoporosis. Endocr Pract 1996; 2:155–171.
28. Miyamoto T, Yosida T, Osawa N, et al. Adrenal response and side reactions after long-term corticosteroid therapy in bronchial asthma. Ann Allergy 1972; 30:587–594.
29. Schlaghecke R, Kornely E, Santen R, et al. The effect of long-term glucocorticoid therapy on pituitary-adrenal responses to exogenous corticotropin-releasing hormone. N Engl J Med 1992; 326:226–230.
30. Axelrod L. Glucocorticoid therapy. Medicine 1976; 55:39–65.

31. Lieberman P, Patterson R, Kunske R. Complications of long-term steroid therapy for asthma. J Allergy Clin Immunol 1972; 49:329–336.
32. Wong J, Black P. Acute adrenal insufficiency associated with high-dose inhaled steroids. Br Med J 1992; 304:1415.
33. Paggiaro PL, Dahle R, Bakran I, et al. Multicentre randomised placebo-controlled trial of inhaled fluticasone propionate in patients with chronic obstructive pulmonary disease. Lancet 1998; 351:773–780.
34. Lipworth BJ. Systemic adverse effects of inhaled corticosteroid therapy. A systematic review and meta-analysis. Arch Intern Med 1999; 159:941–955.
35. Ninan T, Reid I, Carter P, et al. Effects of high doses of inhaled corticosteroids on adrenal function in children with severe persistent asthma. Thorax 1993; 48(6):599–602.
36. Brown P, Blundell G, Greening A, et al. Hypothalamopituitary-adrenal axis suppression in asthmatics inhaling high-dose corticosteroids. Respir Med 1991; 85:501–510.
37. Wong CA, Walsh LJ, Smith CJ, Wisniewski AF, Lewis SA, Hubbard R, Cawte S, Green DJ, Pringle M, Tattersfield AE. Inhaled corticosteroid use and bone-mineral density in patients with asthma. Lancet 2000; 355(9213):1399–1403.
38. Haworth CS, Webb AK, Egan JJ, Selby PL, Hasleton PS, Bishop PW, Freemont TJ. Bone histomorphometry in adult patients with cystic fibrosis. Chest 2000; 118(2):434–439.
39. Elkin SE, Verdi S, Bord S, Garrahan NJ, Hodson ME, Compston JE. Histomorphometric analysis of bone biopsies from the iliac crest of adults with cystic fibrosis. Am J Respir Crit Care Med 2002; 166:1470–1474.
40. Robbins MK, Ontjes DA. Endocrine and renal problems in cystic fibrosis. In: Yankaskas JR, Knowles MR, eds. Cystic Fibrosis in Adults. Philadelphia: Lippincott-Raven, 1999:383–418.
41. Haworth CS, Selby PL, Webb AK, Adams JE. Osteoporosis in adults with cystic fibrosis. J R Soc Med 1998; 91(suppl 34):14–18.
42. Ott SM, Aitken ML. Osteoporosis in patients with cystic fibrosis. Clin Chest Med 1998; 19(3):555–567.
43. Aris RM, Lester G, Dingman S, Ontjes DA. Altered calcium homeostasis in adults with cystic fibrosis. Osteoporos Int 1999; 10(2):102–108.
44. Aris RM, Stephens A, Ontjes DA, Blackwood AD, Lark RK, Hensler M, Lester GE. Adverse alterations in bone metabolism due to lung infection in cystic fibrosis. Am J Respir Crit Care Med 2000; 162(5):1674–1678.
45. DeSchepper J, Smitz J, et al. Low serum bone gamma-carboxyglutamic acid protein concentrations in patients with CF: correlation with hormonal parameters and bone mineral density. Horm Res 1993; 39:197–201.
46. Baroncelli G, De Luca F, Magazzu G, Arrigo T, Sferlazzas C, Catena C, et al. Bone demineralization in CF: evidence of imbalance between bone formation and degradation. Pediatr Res 1997; 41:397–403.
47. Grey AB, Ames, R, et al. BMD and body composition in adult patients with CF. Thorax 1993; 48:589–594.
48. Gibbens DT, Gilsanz V, Boechat MI. Osteoporosis in cystic fibrosis. J Pediatr 1988; 113:295–300.
49. Bachrach LK, Loutit C, Moss R, Marcus R. Osteopenia in adults with CF. Am J Med 1994; 96:27–32.

50. Henderson RC, Madsen CD. Bone density in children and adolescents with CF. J Pediatr 1996; 128:28–34.
51. Mischler EH, Chesney PJ, Chesney RW, Mazess RB. Demineralization in CF. Am J Dis Child 1979; 133:632–635.
52. Aris RM, Neuringer I, Weiner, Egan TM, Ontjes DA. Severe osteoporosis before and after lung transplantation. Chest 1996; 109:1176–1183.
53. Aris RM, Renner J, Lester G, Riggs D, Winder A, Ontjes DA. Increased fractures and severe kyphosis: sequelae of living into adulthood with cystic fibrosis. Ann Intern Med 1998; 128:186–193.
54. Shane E, Silverberg SJ, Donovan D, Papadopoulos A, Staron RB, Addesso V, McGregor C, Schulman L. Osteoporosis in lung transplantation candidates with end-stage pulmonary disease. Am J Med 1996; 101:262–269.
55. Donovan DS, Papadopoulos A, Staron RB, Addesso V, Schulman L, et al. Bone mass and vitamin D deficiency in adults with advanced cystic fibrosis lung disease. Am J Respir Crit Care Med 1998; 157:1892–1899.
56. Haworth CS, Selby PL, Webb AK, Dodd ME, Musson H, McL Niven R, Economou G, Horrocks A, Freemont AJ, Mawer EB, Adams JE. Low bone mineral density in adults with cystic fibrosis. Thorax. 1999; 54(11):961–967.
57. Merkel PA, Herlyn K, Lapey A, Pizzo AS, et al. Osteoporosis in adults with cystic fibrosis. Pediatr Pulmonol 1999; 19(suppl):A456.
58. Melzi M, Bianchi ML, Enfissi L, Columbo C, et al. Factors influencing bone demineralization in CF patients. Pediatr Pulmonol 1999; 17(suppl):A530.
59. Elkin SL, Fairney A, Burnett S, Compson JE, et al. Osteoporosis in adults with CF: a cross-sectional study. Pediatr Pulmonol 1999; 19(suppl):A470.
60. Conway SP, Morton AM, Oldroyd B, Truscott JG, White H, Smith AH, Haigh I. Osteoporosis and osteopenia in adults and adolescents with cystic fibrosis: prevalence and associated factors. Thorax 2000; 55(9):798–804.
61. Laursen EM, Molgaard C, Michaelsen KF, Koch C, Muller J. Bone mineral status in 134 patients with cystic fibrosis. Arch Dis Child 1999; 81(3):235–240.
62. Lark RK, Lester GE, Ontjes DA, Blackwood AD, Hollis BW, Hensler MM, Aris RM. Diminished and erratic absorption of ergocalciferol in adult cystic fibrosis patients. Am J Clin Nutr 2001; 73(3):602–606.
63. Reiter EO, et al. Vitamin D metabolites in adolescents & young adults with CF: effects of sun and season. J Pediatr 1985; 106:21–26.
64. Hahn TJ, Squires AE, Halstead LR, Strominger DB. Reduced serum 25-hydroxyvitamin D concentration and disordered mineral metabolism in patients with cystic fibrosis. J Pediatr 1979; 94:38–43.
65. Hanly JG, et al. Hypovitaminosis D and response to supplementation in older patients with CF. Q J Med 1985; 56:377–385.
66. Henderson RC, Specter BB. Kyphosis and fractures in children and young adults with cystic fibrosis. J Pediatr 1994; 125(2):208–212.
67. Erkkila J, Warwick W, Bradford D. Spine deformities and cystic fibrosis. Clin Orthop 1978; 131:146–149.
68. Denton JR, Tietjen R, Gaerlan PF. Thoracic kyphosis in cystic fibrosis. Clin Orthop 1979; 155:71–74.
69. Logvinoff M, Fon G, Taussig LM, Pitt MJ. Kyphosis and pulmonary function CF. Clin Pediatr 1984; 23:389–392.

70. Salamoni F, Roulet M, Gudinchet F, Filet M, Thiebaud D, Burckhardt P. Bone mineral content in cystic fibrosis patients: correlation with fat-free mass. Arch Dis Child 1996; 74:314–318.

71. Rose J, Gamble J, Schultz A, et al. Back pain and spinal deformity in CF. Am J Dis Child 1987; 141:1313–1316.

72. Haworth CS, Selby PL, Adams JE, Mawer EB, Horrocks AW, Webb AK. Effect of intravenous pamidronate on bone mineral density in adults with cystic fibrosis. Thorax 2001; 56(4):314–316.

73. Aris RM, Lester GE, Renner JB, Winders AW, Blackwood AD, Lark RK, Ontjes DA. Efficacy of pamidronate for osteoporosis in cystic fibrosis patients following lung transplantation. Am J Respir Crit Care Med 2000; 162:941–946.

74. Montemurro L, Fraioli P, Rizzato G. Bone loss in untreated long-standing sarcoidosis. Sarcoidosis 1991; 8(1):29–34.

75. Zehnder D, Bland R, Williams MC, McNinch RW, Howie AJ, Stewart PM, Hewison M. Extrarenal expression of 25-hydroxyvitamin d(3)-1 alpha-hydroxylase. J Clin Endocrinol Metab 2001; 86(2):888–894.

76. Rizzato G. Clinical impact of bone and calcium metabolism changes in sarcoidosis. Thorax 1998; 53(5):425–429.

77. Hamada K, Nagai S, Tsutsumi T, Izumi T. Ionized calcium and 1,25-dihydroxyvitamin D concentration in serum of patients with sarcoidosis. Eur Respir J 1998; 11(5):1015–1020.

78. Zeimer HJ, Greenaway TM, Slavin J, Hards DK, Zhou H, Doery JC, Hunter AN, Duffield A, Martin TJ, Grill V. Parathyroid-hormone-related protein in sarcoidosis. Am J Pathol 1998; 152(1):17–21.

79. Montemurro L, Schiraldi G, Fraioli P, Tosi G, Riboldi A, Rizzato G. Prevention of corticosteroid-induced osteoporosis with salmon calcitonin in sarcoid patients. Calcif Tissue Int 1991; 49(2):71–76.

80. Gonnelli S, Rottoli P, Cepollaro C, Pondrelli C, Cappiello V, Vagliasindi M, Gennari C. Prevention of corticosteroid-induced osteoporosis with alendronate in sarcoid patients. Calcif Tissue Int 1997; 61(5):382–385.

81. Taveira-DaSilva AM, Hedin CJ, Chen CC, Moss J. Bone mineral density studies in 104 patients with lymphangioleiomyomatosis (LAM). Am J Respir Crit Care Med 2001; 163:A560.

82. Lindsay RS, Toft AD. Hypothyroidism. Lancet 1997; 349:413–417.

83. Semple PD, Hume R, Beastall GH, Watson WS. Thyroid function and endocrine abnormalities in elderly patients with severe chronic obstructive lung disease. Thorax 1988; 43(11):945–946.

84. Gow SM, Seth J, Beckett GJ, Douglas G. Thyroid function and endocrine abnormalities in elderly patients with severe chronic obstructive lung disease. Thorax 1987; 42(7):520–525.

85. Toft AD. Drug Therapy: thyroxine therapy. N Engl J Med 1994; 331:174–180.

86. Vasa FR, Molitch ME. Endocrine problems in the chronically critically ill patient. Clin Chest Med 2001; 22(1):193–208.

87. Pino-Garcia JM, Garcia-Rio F, Diez JJ, Gomez-Mendieta MA, Racionero MA, Diaz-Lobato S, Villamor J. Regulation of breathing in hyperthyroidism: relationship to hormonal and metabolic changes. Eur Respir J 1998; 12(2):400–407.

88. Singer PA, Cooper DS, Levy EG, et al. Treatment guidelines for patients with hyperthyroidism and hypothyroidism. JAMA 1995; 273:808–812.

89. Young C, Burrows R, Katz J, Beynon H. Hypercalcaemia in sarcoidosis. Lancet 1999; 353(9150):374.

90. Sharma OP. Vitamin D, calcium, and sarcoidosis. Chest 1996; 109(2):535–539.

91. Sharma OP. Hypercalcemia in granulomatous disorders: a clinical review. Curr Opin Pulm Med 2000; 6(5):442–447.

92. Conron M, Young C, Beynon HL. Calcium metabolism in sarcoidosis and its clinical implications. Rheumatology (Oxf) 2000; 39(7):707–713.

93. Sinha RN, Fraser WD, Casson IF. Long-term management of hypercalcaemia in chronically active sarcoidosis. J R Soc Med 1997; 90(3):156–157.

94. Conron M, Beynon HL. Ketoconazole for the treatment of refractory hypercalcemic sarcoidosis. Sarcoidosis Vasc Diffuse Lung Dis 2000; 17(3):277–280.

95. Stuart CA, Neelon FA, Lebovitz HE. Hypothalamic insufficiency: the cause of hypopituitarism in sarcoidosis. Ann Intern Med 1978; 88(5):589–594.

96. Winnacker JL, Becker KL, Katz S. Endocrine aspects of sarcoidosis. N Engl J Med 1968; 278(9):483–492.

97. Bell NH. Endocrine complications of sarcoidosis. Endocrinol Metab Clin North Am 1991; 20(3):645–654.

98. Guoth MS, Kim J, de Lotbiniere AC, Brines ML. Neurosarcoidosis presenting as hypopituitarism and a cystic pituitary mass. Am J Med Sci 1998; 315(3):220–224.

99. Ilias I, Panoutsopoulos G, Batsakis C, Nikolakakou D, Filippou N, Christakopoulou I. Thyroid function and autoimmunity in sarcoidosis: a case-control study. Croat Med J 1998; 39(4):404–406.

100. Nakamura H, Genma R, Mikami T, Kitahara A, Natsume H, Andoh S, Nagasawa S, Nishiyama K, Chida K, Sato A, Yoshimi T. High incidence of positive autoantibodies against thyroid peroxidase and thyroglobulin in patients with sarcoidosis. Clin Endocrinol (Oxf) 1997; 46(4):467–472.

101. Papadopoulos KI, Hornblad Y, Liljebladh H, Hallengren B. High frequency of endocrine autoimmunity in patients with sarcoidosis. Eur J Endocrinol 1996; 134(3):331–336.

102. Coplu L, Caglar M, Kisacik G, Soylemezoglu F, Altay Sahin A. Sarcoidosis with thyroid involvement. Sarcoidosis Vasc Diffuse Lung Dis 1997; 14(1):86–87.

103. Vailati A, Marena C, Aristia L, Sozze E, Barosi G, Inglese V, Luisetti M, Bossolo PA. Sarcoidosis of the thyroid: report of a case and a review of the literature. Sarcoidosis 1993; 10(1):66–68.

104. van Assendelft AH, Kahlos T. Sarcoidosis of the thyroid gland. Sarcoidosis. 1985; 2(2):154–156.

105. Karlish AJ, MacGregor GA. Sarcoidosis, thyroiditis, and Addison's disease. Lancet 1970; 2(7668):330–333.

106. Cronin CC, Dinneen SF, Mitchell TH, Shanahan FL. Sarcoidosis, the pancreas, and diabetes mellitus. Am J Gastroenterol 1995; 90(11):2068.

107. Haas GP, Badalament R, Wonnell DM, Miles BJ. Testicular sarcoidosis: case report and review of the literature. J Urol 1986; 135(6):1254–1256.

108. White A, Flaris N, Elmer D, Lui R, Fanburg BL. Coexistence of mucinous cystadenoma of the ovary and ovarian sarcoidosis. Am J Obstet Gynecol 1990; 162(5):1284–1285.

109. Howarth DM, Gilchrist GS, Mullan BP, Wiseman GA, Edmonson JH, Schomberg PJ. Langerhans cell histiocytosis: diagnosis, natural history, management, and outcome. Cancer 1999; 85(10):2278–2290.

110. Nanduri VR, Bareille P, Pritchard J, Stanhope R. Growth and endocrine disorders in multisystem Langerhans cell histiocytosis. Clin Endocrinol (Oxf) 2000; 53(4):509–515.

111. Kaltsas GA, Powles TB, Evanson J, Plowman PN, Drinkwater JE, Jenkins PJ, Monson JP, Besser GM, Grossman AB. Hypothalamo-pituitary abnormalities in adult patients with Langerhans cell histiocytosis: clinical, endocrinological, and radiological features and response to treatment. J Clin Endocrinol Metab 2000; 85(4):1370–1376.

112. Rosete A, Cabral AR, Kraus A, Alarcon-Segovia D. Diabetes insipidus secondary to Wegener's granulomatosis: report and review of the literature. J Rheumatol 1991; 18(5):761–765.

113. Hajj-Ali RA, Uthman IW, Salti IA, Zaatari GS, Haddad MC, Nasr FW. Wegener's granulomatosis and diabetes insipidus. Rheumatology (Oxf) 1999; 38(7):684–685.

114. Nishono H, Rubino FA, DeRemee RA, et al: Neurological involvement in Wegener's granulomatosis: an analysis of 324 consecutive patients at the Mayo Clinic. Ann Neurol 1993; 33:4.

115. Garovic VD, Clarke BL, Chilson TS, Specks U. Diabetes insipidus and anterior pituitary insufficiency as presenting features of Wegener's granulomatosis. Am J Kidney Dis. 2001; 37(1):E5.

116. de Groot K, Schmidt DK, Arlt AC, Gross WL, Reinhold-Keller E. Standardized neurologic evaluations of 128 patients with Wegener granulomatosis. Arch Neurol 2001; 58(8):1215–1221.

117. Masor JJ, Gal AA, LiVolsi VA. Case report: Hashimoto's thyroiditis associated with Wegener's granulomatosis. Am J Med Sci 1994; 308(2):112–114.

118. Sugimoto A, Sugimoto S, Tanaka M, Kuribayashi T, Takemura J, Matsukura S, Sugiyama S. Wegener's granulomatosis (WG) and insulin dependent diabetes mellitus (IDDM). Jpn J Med 1989; 28(3):374–378.

119. Watanabe K, Senju S, Maeda F, Yshida M. Four cases of bronchiolitis obliterans organizing pneumonia associated with thyroid disease. Respiration 2000; 67(5):572–576.

120. Ferris A, Jacobs T, Widlitz A, Barst RJ, Morse JH. Pulmonary arterial hypertension and thyroid disease. Chest 2001; 119(6):1980–1981.

121. Kashyap AS, Kashyap S. Thyroid disease and primary pulmonary hypertension. JAMA 2001; 285(22):2853–2854.

122. Arroliga AC, Dweik RA, Rafanan AL. Primary pulmonary hypertension and thyroid disease. Chest 2000; 118(4):1224–1225.

123. Curnock AL, Dweik RA, Higgins BH, Saadi HF, Arroliga AC. High prevalence of hypothyroidism in patients with primary pulmonary hypertension. Am J Med Sci 1999; 318(5):289–292.

124. Thurnheer R, Jenni R, Russi EW, Greminger P, Speich R. Hyperthyroidism and pulmonary hypertension. J Intern Med 1997; 242(2):185–188.

125. Semple PD, Beastall GH, Watson WS, Hume R. Serum testosterone depression associated with hypoxia in respiratory failure. Clin Sci (Lond) 1980; 58(1):105–106.

126. Semple PD, Brown TM, Beastall GH, Semple CG. Sexual dysfunction and erectile impotence in chronic obstructive pulmonary disease. Chest 1983; 83(3):587–588.

127. Semple PD, Beastall GH, Brown TM, Stirling KW, Mills RJ, Watson WS. Sex hormone suppression and sexual impotence in hypoxic pulmonary fibrosis. Thorax 1984; 39(1):46–51.

128. Kamischke A, Kemper DE, Castel MA, Luthke M, Rolf C, Behre HM, Magnussen H, Nieschlag E. Testosterone levels in men with chronic obstructive pulmonary disease with or without glucocorticoid therapy. Eur Respir J 1998; 11(1):41–45.

129. Gosney JR. Atrophy of Leydig cells in the testes of men with long-standing chronic bronchitis and emphysema. Thorax 1987; 42(8):615–619.

17

Cachexia in Chronic Obstructive Pulmonary Disease

EVA C. CREUTZBERG, ANNEMIE M. W. J. SCHOLS,
and EMIEL F. M. WOUTERS

University Hospital Maastricht
Maastricht, The Netherlands

I. Introduction

Weight loss has been recognized as an important phenomenon in the clinical course of patients with COPD. It was a long-held misconception that nutritional depletion was an inevitable and adaptive mechanism to an increased metabolism and that during malnutrition the respiratory muscles were spared. It is now known that body weight loss adversely affects physical performance and health status as well as survival. In this chapter, the prevalence, underlying factors and consequences of cachexia in COPD are discussed.

II. Prevalence of Cachexia in COPD

The weight loss in COPD relates predominantly to the body cell mass (BCM) in contrast to fat mass (FM). BCM is the actively metabolizing and contracting tissue (organ and muscle tissues). Muscle mass can be measured indirectly by assessment of fat-free mass (FFM). In patients with moderate to severe COPD who are in a clinically stable condition, depletion of fat-free mass is present in 20% of the outpatients (1) and in 35% in those eligible for pulmonary rehabilitation (2). Recent data in a large group of patients with stable COPD

($n = 389$) confirm the frequent occurrence of FFM depletion; the prevalence amounted up to 26% in mild to severe COPD (3).

It is therefore evident that the prevalence of FFM depletion is not dependent of the extent of airflow obstruction. In contrast, in patients with emphysema measured with high-resolution computed tomography, weight loss and nutritional depletion are more frequently observed than in chronic bronchitis. This wasting difference concerns mainly the FM; FFM wasting is present in both COPD subtypes (4). No clear information is available on the prevalence of nutritional depletion in acute COPD (patients suffering from respiratory failure), but reports suggest values up to 70%.

III. Underlying Factors of Cachexia in COPD

By definition, weight loss occurs when overall energy expenditure exceeds energy intake. However, the fact that in a substantial proportion of patients with COPD loss of FFM occurs despite relative preservation of fat mass (1) suggest the presence of an imbalance between protein synthesis and protein breakdown. Both mechanisms are discussed below.

A. Energy Balance

Energy Expenditure

Total daily energy expenditure (TDEE) can be divided into three components: (1) resting energy expenditure (REE), which comprises sleeping metabolic rate and the energy expenditure for arousal; (2) diet-induced thermogenesis; and (3) physical activity-induced thermogenesis.

Resting Energy Expenditure

Since the REE accounts for the major component of TDEE in sedentary subjects and can be relatively easily measured, several studies have measured REE in COPD. The most common approach to predict REE for an individual in clinical practice is to apply the Harris and Benedict (HB) equations, which are based on sex, age, height, and body mass (5). Different studies have investigated hypermetabolism in stable patients with COPD on the basis of the HB equations, most studies revealing an increased REE compared to the HB equations or to a control group (6–9) and some not (10,11). The disadvantage of all these studies, however, is that they describe hypermetabolism in relatively small groups of patients (6–19 patients).

Little is known about the prevalence of hypermetabolism at rest in COPD. We investigated, in a large group of patients ($n = 172$), the prevalence of hypermetabolism in COPD. The prevalence of hypermetabolism based on the HB equations (REE > 110% of predicted) amounted up to 54%. However, we also predicted REE adjusted for the influence of FFM using the linear regression equations of REE on FFM generated in 92 healthy elderly subjects, as earlier described by Schols et al (12). The predicted REE adjusted for FFM was obtained by using the FFM of each individual patient in the linear regression equation of REE on FFM generated in the healthy control group. This yielded a prevalence of hypermetabolism at rest of 26%. The difference in prevalence of hypermetabolism between the two methods could be ascribed to the fact that the HB equations do not take body composition into account, while FFM is the most important determinant of REE. Considering FFM is furthermore important in COPD since body compositional changes occur after weight loss; depletion of FFM despite a normal body mass has been described in patients with COPD (1). In the same study, FFM was identified as the most important predictor (65%) of REE in healthy subjects. In the patient group, FFM explained the variation in REE for 51%. Therefore other factors besides the FFM—like work of breathing, medication and systemic inflammation— may explain intersubject variability in REE in patients with COPD.

The suggested increase in oxygen cost of breathing (OCB) is assumed to be one of the main explanations for the elevated REE seen in patients with COPD contributing to weight loss. Several studies have investigated the OCB in patients with COPD and all found a higher OCB in patients compared to healthy controls (8,10,13–16). However, the artifact of these studies is that OCB was measured by augmenting the ventilation or ventilatory effort and not in rest. O'Donnell postulated that increasing the ventilation demands much more energy in patients with COPD than it does in healthy subjects because patients may suffer from dynamic hyperinflation (17). Dynamic hyperinflation will therefore substantially compromise patients with COPD during exercise by elevating the OCB. However, the fact that patients with COPD do not show an elevated ventilation in rest makes it improbable that the OCB is of great impact on REE (17). This is further emphasized by the results of several studies in which the efficiency of breathing in rest was measured by imposing resistance. No difference in breathing efficiency in rest was seen between patients with COPD and healthy subjects (18,19). Another possible explanation for the elevated REE seen in patients with COPD may be a thermogenetic effect of bronchodilating agents such as theophyllines and beta$_2$ sympathicomimetics, which are given in general as an essential part of the pharmacological maintenance treatment approach in patients with COPD. In recent studies both drugs showed an elevating effect on REE in younger healthy subjects (20,21). In a previous study we also found a significant increase in REE of 11% after nebulization of 5 mg of the beta$_2$-sympathicomimetic drug salbutamol in younger subjects. However, the increase in REE in patients with COPD was only 4% and did not differ from an age-matched control group (6%) (22), in line with the rise in REE of 5% found in a comparable study in patients with COPD (23). Together, these slight effects of salbutamol on REE cannot fully explain the elevated REE in patients with COPD.

Another contributing factor to hypermetabolism may be related to systemic inflammation. The polypeptide cytokine tumor necrosis factor alpha (TNF-α) is a proinflammatory mediator produced by different cell types. TNF-α inhibits lipoprotein lipase activity and is pyrogenic. It also triggers the release of other cytokines, which themselves mediate an increase in energy expenditure, as well as mobilization of amino acids and muscle protein catabolism. Using different markers, several studies provided clear evidence for involvement of TNF-α–related systemic inflammation in the pathogenesis of tissue depletion. In an earlier study of our group, elevated levels of the acute phase reactant proteins C-reactive protein (CRP) and LPS-binding protein were reported in hyper- versus normometabolic patients (24). The study of Nguyen et al. showed that resting energy expenditure expressed as percentage of the HB equations was correlated with plasma TNF-α concentration, but not with the degree of airway obstruction, lung hyperinflation, or oxygen cost of breathing (25).

These results were in agreement with the suggested relationship between weight loss and the presence of a systemic inflammatory response. In patients with COPD who had involuntary lost weight, increased serum concentrations of the inflammatory mediator TNF-α were found (26). Furthermore, the LPS-induced production of TNF-α by monocytes was higher in weight-losing versus weight-stable patients (27). Comparison of a group hypermetabolic patients with and without an acute-phase response respectively, revealed a significantly lower FFM in the former group despite a comparable body mass index (BMI; body weight/height^2) between the groups (24). The latter finding suggests that systemic inflammation may not only cause hypermetabolism, but also induce a catabolic response. In a subsequent study such relationship was indeed demonstrated between the acute phase protein LPS-binding protein, REE and decreased plasma amino acid levels as global marker of altered protein metabolism (28). Further studies are indicated to characterize the alterations in substrate metabolism in relation to hypermetabolism and to assess the contribution of decreased anabolic and increased catabolic mediators.

Total Daily Energy Expenditure

Despite measuring TDEE is methodological difficult and expensive, recent studies focused attention on the activity related energy expenditure in patients with COPD. Using the doubly labeled water ($^2H_2O^{18}$) technique to measure TDEE it was demonstrated that patients with COPD had a significantly higher TDEE than healthy subjects (29). Remarkably, the nonresting component of total daily energy expenditure was significantly higher in the patients with COPD than in the healthy subjects, resulting in a ratio between TDEE and REE of 1.7 in patients with COPD and 1.4 in health volunteers. Otherwise, when TDEE was measured in patients with COPD and healthy persons in a respiration chamber, no differences in TDEE were found between patients with COPD and healthy (30), possibly by limitations of activities in the respiration chamber. In line with an increased activity related energy expenditure is the observed decreased mechanical efficiency of leg exercise in patients with COPD (31). Part of the increased oxygen consumption during exercise can be related to an inefficient ventilation in case of increased ventilatory demand especially under conditions of dynamic hyperinflation. Furthermore an inefficient (anaerobic) muscle metabolism may contribute to an increased total daily energy metabolism. Several studies indeed showed a severely impaired oxidative phosphorylation during exercise in COPD, accompanied by an increased and highly anaerobic metabolism involving both the energy release from high energy phosphate compounds as well as an enhanced glycolysis.

The fact that no difference in TDEE between hypermetabolic and normometabolic COPD patients was found and that REE adjusted for FFM did not correlate significantly with total daily energy expenditure (32) indicates that different mechanisms may underlie metabolic alterations in sub-groups of COPD patients.

Energy Intake

Hypermetabolism can explain why some COPD patients lose weight despite an apparent normal or even high dietary intake (33). Nevertheless, it has been shown that dietary intake in weight-losing patients is lower than in weight-stable patients, both in absolute terms as well as in relation to measured REE (34). This is quite remarkable because the normal adaptation to an increase in energy requirements in healthy men is an increase in dietary intake. Furthermore, during an acute exacerbation of COPD, a substantial decrease in appetite and dietary intake was reported, associated with increased subjective sensations of dyspnea and fatigue (35).

The reasons for a relatively low dietary intake in COPD are not completely understood. It has been suggested that patients with COPD eat suboptimally because chewing and swallowing change breathing pattern and decrease arterial oxygen saturation. No changes in arterial oxygen saturation were observed in normoxemic COPD patients during a meal (36). In hypoxemic patients however a rapid decrease in Sa_{O_2} was monitored which slowly recovered after completion of the meal (36). The decrease in Sa_{O_2} was associated with an increased dyspnea sensation. The severity of the drop was significantly different between two meals, but it could not be determined from the study whether this related to the macronutrient composition of the meal (less desaturation after a carbohydrate-rich meal) or meal temperature (more desaturation after a warm meal). Gastric emptying time of a meal may also affect dietary intake since gastric filling in these patients may reduce the functional residual capacity and lead to an increase in dyspnea (37).

Besides these effects on the pulmonary system, systemic factors may also affect dietary intake. Very intriguing is the role of leptin in energy homeostasis. This adipocyte-derived hormone represents the afferent hormonal signal to the brain in a feedback mechanism regulating fat mass. Previous experimental and clinical research indicates the involvement of leptin in energy balance and body weight homeostasis. It regulates the energy balance in a feedback mechanism in which the hypothalamus is involved (38). In animals, administration of leptin results in a reduction in food intake (39) as well as in an increase in energy expenditure (40). In addition, leptin has a regulating role in lipid metabolism and glucose homeostasis and increases thermogenesis.

Few data have been reported on leptin metabolism in COPD. Circulating leptin correlates well with BMI and fat percentage as expected, but significantly lower values were observed compared to healthy subjects (41). In stable disease, plasma leptin corrected for fat mass was inversely correlated with dietary intake (Fig. 1) as well as with the degree of weight change after 8 weeks of nutritional supplementation in depleted patients with COPD (42). During an acute disease exacerbation, systemic leptin concentrations were high and the normal feedback regulation of leptin by FM seemed to be disrupted. On day 7 of the acute exacerbation, plasma leptin concentrations were inversely correlated with dietary intake adjusted for REE (43). In both stable and acute disease, plasma leptin was associated with the systemic inflammatory response. In patients with emphysema as well as in patients suffering from acute exacerbation of COPD, leptin was found to be positively correlated with soluble TNF receptor 55, independently of the amount of FM (42,43). Experimental animal studies have provided evidence for a link between pro-inflammatory cytokines and leptin. Treatment of fasted hamsters with the cytokines TNF-α and interleukin-1 (IL-1) increased leptin messenger RNA (mRNA) in adipose tissue and the circulating concentrations of leptin. Circulating leptin was in turn correlated with a decrease in food intake (44). The hypothesis that cytokine induction of leptin may play a significant role in the anorexia and cachexia of inflammatory diseases was further illustrated by

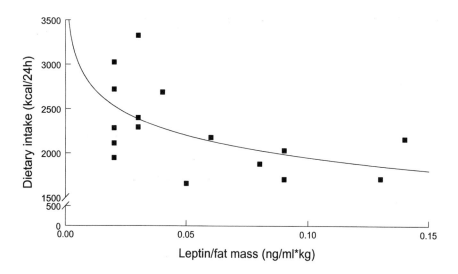

Figure 1 Inverse association between dietary intake and plasma leptin concentration divided by fat mass in depleted patients with COPD ($r = -0.50$, $p = 0.047$). (From Ref. 42.)

Sarraf et al. This group showed that administration of the proinflammatory cytokines TNF-α and IL-1 produced a prompt and dose-dependent increase in serum leptin and leptin mRNA expression in the adipose tissue of mice. In contrast, IL-4 and IL-10, cytokines not known to induce anorexia, did not affect leptin gene expression or serum leptin concentrations (45). Data in humans confirm this influence of systemic inflammation on leptin. In patients with solid tumors, infusion of TNF-α resulted in a transient increase in serum leptin concentration (46). Administration of recombinant human IL-1α to cancer patients also increased leptin concentration dose-dependently, accompanied by a decrease in appetite in the majority of the patients (47). The role of systemic inflammation was confirmed by the data of Creutzberg et al, demonstrating a significant relationship between baseline dietary intake and soluble intercellular adhesion molecule-1 (48).

B. Protein Balance

Besides an overall energy imbalance, there are also indications for disturbances in the protein balance in a subgroup of patients with COPD. Since selective wasting of FFM despite relative preservation of FM is reported (4), a disturbed protein balance can also be present without accompaniment of overall body weight loss. At first, the daily protein intake is reported to be decreased compared to the recommended allowances, especially during the first days of an acute exacerbation of COPD (49). Second, as one mechanism of muscle wasting, a decreased protein synthesis was seen in underweight patients with emphysema (50). Third, recently it was found that whole-body protein synthesis and protein breakdown were enhanced in patients with COPD compared to healthy controls, indicating an elevated protein turnover (51). Since the study group of the latter study comprised weight-stable patients, the enhanced protein turnover did not affect muscle mass yet. However, during unstable disease periods, for instance in patients suffering from an acute exacerbation of COPD, the enhanced protein turnover might eventually lead to FFM wasting.

An enhanced systemic inflammatory response is described as one of the possible causes of a selectively disturbed protein balance. In patients with an elevated REE and an increased C-reactive protein, FFM was decreased together with elevated concentrations of the inflammatory mediators LPS-binding protein (LBP), IL-8 and soluble TNF receptors 55 and 75 compared with those with normal CRP concentrations (24). In addition, an inverse correlation coefficient between elevated plasma LBP concentrations and the total sum of plasma amino acids was reported (28).

Furthermore, decreased levels of anabolic hormones might aggravate the failure of generating an anabolic response needed for muscle anabolism. Indeed low levels of testosterone are reported in COPD, which were even more pronounced in patients on oral glucocorticosteroid (GC) therapy (52). Long-term, low-dose systemic glucocorticosteroids are prescribed as maintenance anti-inflammatory medication in a substantial number of patients. Chronic use of oral glucocorticosteroids further contributes to weakness of both the respiratory and peripheral muscles in patients with COPD (53).

Besides overall loss of muscle mass, intrinsic muscle abnormalities are reported in COPD. Concerning the respiratory muscles, there is evidence that the diaphragm of patients with severe COPD has undergone adaptations resulting in relative resistance to fatigue. The physiological alterations were accompanied by increases in fiber type I proportions and in slow isoforms of myofibrillar proteins (54). In contrast, in the peripheral muscles, a decrease in the proportion of type I fibers corresponding with a relative increase in type II fibers was seen, indicating a shift in function from endurance towards more strength (55,56). These morphological alterations can be accompanied by disturbances in peripheral muscle oxidative enzyme capacity. Patients with COPD exhibiting chronic respiratory failure showed increased activity of the mitochondrial enzyme cytochrome oxidase in skeletal muscle compared with healthy control subjects (57). In addition, elevated concentrations of inosine monophosphate, which is thought to reflect an imbalance between resynthesis and utilization of adenosine triphosphate, were found in the peripheral muscle tissue of stable patients with COPD (58).

In addition, the COPD population comprises merely elderly subjects. Aging per se is already accompanied by a decline in the size of muscle fibers and thereby in muscle function, which is an important determinant of physical performance (59). Furthermore, many patients with COPD reduce their level of exercise dramatically in response to exertional dyspnea. The resulting sedentary lifestyle leads to muscle deconditioning and ultimately to inactivity and disability (60).

IV. Consequences of Cachexia in COPD

It was a long-held misconception that nutritional depletion was an inevitable and adaptive mechanism to increased metabolism and that during malnutrition the respiratory muscles were spared. It is now known that cachexia in COPD is associated with decreased physical capacity, impaired health status, and even increased mortality risk.

A. Muscle Function and Exercise Performance

Dyspnea and exercise intolerance are the most prominent symptoms of patients with COPD. Besides the extent of airflow obstruction and loss of alveolar structure, respiratory and peripheral skeletal muscle weakness are important determinants of these symptoms (61,62). Recent studies have shown that peripheral skeletal muscle dysfunction is predominantly determined by skeletal muscle mass in COPD (63). Besides effects on peripheral muscle strength (64), several studies have also shown that FFM is a significant determinant of exercise capacity and exercise response (65). These findings suggest that the functional consequences of nutritional abnormalities not only relate to muscle wasting per se but also to intrinsic alterations in muscle morphology and metabolism. Significant differences have been observed between patients with COPD and healthy subjects in the activity of enzymes involved in key oxidative and glycolytic pathways (66) and in energy-rich phosphates (58), but the influence of nutritional depletion on these alterations is yet unknown.

B. Health Status

Nutritional depletion in COPD is furthermore associated with a reduced health status. Patients suffering from lean mass depletion exhibited significantly greater impairment in symptom, activity, impact and total score of the St. George's Respiratory Questionnaire. The effects of tissue depletion on health status appeared however to be mediated through increased levels of dyspnea (67). In contrast, Mostert et al. revealed that the relation between tissue depletion and health status was independently of dyspnea, but instead mediated by a decreased exercise performance (68).

C. Acute Disease Exacerbations

Weight loss negatively affects in addition the prevalence and outcome of acute disease exacerbations of COPD. The risk of being hospitalized for an acute exacerbation was increased in patients with a low BMI (69). A low BMI and weight loss were reported as an unfavorable index of outcome during an exacerbation of COPD—i.e., predicting the need for mechanical ventilation (70). Furthermore, the survival time following a disease exacerbation was found to be independently related to the BMI (71).

D. Mortality

Nutritional depletion is furthermore characterized as an independent prognostic factor in patients with COPD. Retrospectively, in a group of 400 patients with COPD, the Cox proportional hazards model was used to quantify the relationship between the variables age, sex, spirometry, arterial blood gases, BMI, smoking, and subsequent overall mortality. The study revealed that low BMI, age and low Pa_{O_2} were significant independent predictors of increased mortality. After stratification of the group into BMI quintiles a threshold value of $25 \, kg/m^2$ was identified below which the mortality risk was clearly increased (72). The disadvantage of this study was however, that it was performed in a highly selective study group, namely in patients eligible for pulmonary rehabilitation. A subsequent study by Landbo et al. prospectively examined whether BMI was an independent predictor of mortality in subjects with COPD from the Copenhagen City Heart Study. In total, 1218 men and 914 women aged 21 to 89 years with airway obstruction defined as an FEV_1/FVC ratio of less than 0.7 were included in the analyses. Spirometric values, BMI, smoking habits, and respiratory symptoms were assessed at the time of study enrollment, and mortality from COPD and from all causes during 17 years of follow-up was analyzed with multivariate Cox regression models. After adjustment for age, ventilatory function, and smoking habits, low BMI was predictive of a poor prognosis (i.e., higher mortality), with relative risks (RRs) in underweight subjects as compared with that in subjects of normal weight of 1.64 [95% confidence interval (CI): 1.20–2.23] in men and 1.42 (95% CI: 1.07–1.89) in women. However, the association between BMI and survival differed significantly with stage of COPD. In mild and moderate COPD there was a non-significant U-shaped relationship, with the lowest risk occurring in normal weight or overweight subjects, whereas in severe COPD, mortality continued to decrease with increasing BMI (test for trend: $p < 0.001$). Similar results were found for COPD-related deaths, with the strongest associations found in severe COPD [RR for low versus high BMI: 7.11 (95% CI: 2.97–17.05)] (73).

V. Treatment of Cachexia in COPD

A. Nutritional Repletion Therapy

Because of the deleterious effects of body weight loss and muscle wasting on morbidity and mortality in COPD, it is important to take the implementation of appropriate therapies under investigation. Several attempts have been made to reverse weight loss and muscle wasting by instituting oral nutritional repletion therapy. The outcome of these interventions were however not unambiguously positive. Significant improvements in respiratory and peripheral skeletal muscle function but also in exercise capacity and health-related quality of life were observed in one inpatient study (74) and one out-patient study (75) after 3 months oral supplementation by about 1000 kcal daily. In other outpatients studies however, despite a similar nutritional supplementation regimen, the average weight gain was less than 1.5 kg in 8 weeks (76,77). The ability of an aggressive nutritional support strategy to provide a sufficient energy supply was studied in patients with severe COPD and weight loss not responding to oral supplementation. Over a prolonged interval of 4 months, nocturnal enteral nutrition support via percutaneous endoscopic gatrostomy tube was provided. The treated group had nightly enteral feeding adjusted to maintain a total daily caloric intake greater than two times measured resting metabolic rate for sustained weight gain. Despite the magnitude of the intervention, a mean weight gain of only 3.3% (0.2 kg/week) was seen in the treated group. The majority of increase in body weight was fat mass and no significant improvement of physiological function was observed (78).

In addition, a recent metanalysis of nine randomized, controlled trials of caloric supplementation given for more than 2 weeks also failed to reveal any significant improvements in anthropometric measures, lung function, or functional exercise capacity among stable patients with COPD (79). Some remarks must, however, be made as to the conclusions of this metanalysis. At first, intervention studies with a duration of 2 or more weeks were included. It is likely that 2 weeks of nutritional supplementation is probably too short a time to achieve substantially changes in body composition and physiological function. Second, most of the nutritional intervention trials were not combined with exercise training. It can be expected that nutritional supplementation without an anabolic stimulus will only result in an expansion of FM. Physiological function will likewise not improve on nutrition alone, since FFM is an important determinant of functional performance. Third, in several studies, the offered nutritional supplementation therapy consisted of an inadequate energy intake relative to the energy requirements needed for body weight gain. In addition, it can be deduced from the above-described evidence on protein balance disturbances in COPD that nutritional supplementation must consist of enough dietary protein.

The importance of incorporating an anabolic stimulus into the nutritional supplementation therapy was emphasized by the study of Schols et al. A daily nutritional supplement of 420 kcal given as an integrated part of a comprehensive pulmonary rehabilitation program resulted in significant gain in body weight as well as in FFM, and inspiratory muscle function also improved (80). Our group reevaluated this nutritional support strategy as integrated part of a pulmonary rehabilitation program on various outcome measures in 64 depleted COPD patients (age 64 years (range 39–77), BMI [20.2 (15.5–24.3 kg/ m^2)], FFMI [15.3 (12.7–18.7) kg/m^2]. Nutritional therapy consisted of the normal diet combined with two to three liquid supplements in order to reach a weight gain of 5% or more after 8 weeks. Actual supplement intake varied between 250 and 875 kcal, with a mean value of 672 kcal. Mean increase in body weight amounted to 4%, equally divided between fat mass and fat-free mass. A comparable percentage increase in measures of respiratory and peripheral skeletal muscle strength was found, while maximal and submaximal exercise performance increased between 10 to 20%. This more pronounced improvement could be related to alterations in muscle oxidative capacity, since the maximal lactic acid value divided by peak work rate significantly decreased ($p < 0.001$) after treatment.

Overall, therefore, the key message is that one should first optimize the treatment designs of nutritional supplementation before stating that the interventions do not sort effect. In other words, the possibility exists that the described nutritional interventions themselves were not of sufficient magnitude to sort an effect; the failure of intervention instead of the failure to intervene might have been responsible for the nonresponse found in several nutritional intervention trials.

B. Nonresponse to Nutritional Repletion Therapy

Even in nutritional supplementation studies with an optimal treatment design, as described above, a substantial number of patients fail to respond to nutritional supplementation therapy in terms of body weight gain. Figure 2

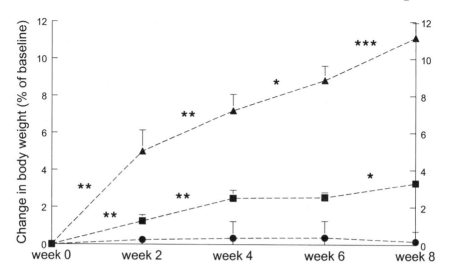

Figure 2 Body weight course per 2 weeks expressed as percentage of baseline body weight in depleted patients with COPD during 8 weeks of nutritional supplementation therapy combined with pulmonary rehabilitation. Circles: weight gain <2%; squares: 2% ≤ weight gain <5%; triangles: weight gain ≥5%. Data are given as mean ±SEM. (From Ref. 48.)

shows the body weight course in depleted patients with COPD nonresponding, moderately responding, and well responding patients to 8 weeks of nutritional supplementation combined with pulmonary rehabilitation (48). Little information is available yet on the underlying causes of nonresponse to nutritional therapy. Nonresponse may be due to factors such as noncompliance to the therapy, an inadequate energy intake relative to energy requirements or the inability of the patient to ingest the extra calories. In addition, nonresponse might be explained by underlying disease-specific problems leading to an inadequate metabolic handling. Indeed, our group previously revealed that patients not responding to optimized nutritional supplementation therapy in terms of weight gain were characterized by, besides a higher age and relative anorexia, an elevated systemic inflammatory response (48). The clinical relevance of nonresponse to nutritional therapy was emphasized by the survival analysis of Schols et al., in which weight gain was identified as a significant independent predictor of the survival rate in patients with COPD (72).

C. Practical Implementation of Nutritional Repletion Therapy

In order to provide optimal response to nutritional repletion therapy, in this section some practical recommendations for the implementation of nutritional therapy in clinical practice are given. Simple screening can be based on measurement of the BMI and the weight course. Based on the BMI, patients are divided into underweight $(BMI < 21 \, kg/m^2$, normal weight $(21 < BMI < 25 \, kg/m^2)$ and overweight patients $(25 < BMI < 30 \, kg/m^2)$. Commonly used criteria for weight loss are >10% in the past 6 months or >5% in the past month. However one should note that every involuntary weight loss that cannot be attributed to daily fluctuations should be taken into consideration. Nutritional supplementation should initially consist of adaptations of the patients' dietary habits (food choice, meal pattern etc). Nutritional support should be given as energy dense supplements spread over the day to avoid loss of appetite and adverse metabolic and ventilatory efforts resulting from a high caloric load.

It was long believed that due to their ventilatory limitation, patients with respiratory disease should consume a fat-rich diet to decrease carbon dioxide load, but scientific evidence is scarce and not convincing. Our group previously observed that transcutaneous oxygen desaturation and dyspnea were more pronounced after a moderate fat compared with a carbohydrate-rich meal in patients with COPD (36). More recent reports show that patients experience less dyspnea after a liquid carbohydrate-rich supplement compared to an equicaloric fat-rich supplement (81). This may not be surprising since gastric emptying time is significantly higher after an equicaloric fat-rich compared to a carbohydrate-rich supplement (37). Furthermore, it was found that the reduced dietary intake of patients with COPD during the acute phase of an exacerbation was characterized by a restricted fat intake (49). Based on data in other chronic wasting conditions, daily protein intake should be at least 1.5 mg/kg body weight to allow optimal protein synthesis (82).

When feasible, patients should participate in an exercise program in order to stimulate an anabolic response rather than fat storage. In view of the adverse effects of inactivity and the pulmonary limitations on exercise capacity, most exercise programs consist predominantly of endurance training. However, since nutritional depletion affects muscle strength at least as much as endurance, a combination of endurance and strength training may be particularly effective in cachectic patients with COPD. For the severely depleted patients unable to perform exercise training, even simple strength maneuvers combined with training in activities of daily living (ADL) and energy conservation techniques may be effective. Exercise not only improves the effectiveness of nutritional therapy but also stimulates appetite. If weight gain and functional improvement occur, therapy is continued or changed into a maintenance regimen. If the desired response is not noted, it may be necessary to identify compliance issues. If compliance is not the problem, more calories may be needed in the form of supplements or by (nocturnal) enteral feeding. Nevertheless, one should recognize that even then some patients might not reach the intended effect due to underlying (metabolic) mechanisms of weight loss described above (83).

Little is known about the effects of nutritional therapy during acute exacerbations of COPD (AECOPD). The main focus during acute exacerbations of COPD should be stabilization of catabolism as well as stabilization of the presumably negative energy and protein balances. Saudny-Unterberger et al. have investigated the effects of 2 weeks of nutritional therapy during acute exacerbation of COPD. A significant improvement of forced vital capacity was found in the treatment group. However, no improvements were found in body composition or nitrogen balance. This could be due to the short intervention period. In addition, a negative correlation was found between nitrogen balance and methylprednisolone intake, suggesting a catabolic effect of glucocorticosteroids. Therefore another explanation for the absence of body compositional improvement could be inadequate protein supplementation that does not meet the increased requirements due to the inflammatory catabolic process (84). This is why Vermeeren et al. suggest that during AECOPD, no additional nutritional therapy is indicated as long as patients adequately respond within a few days to the medical therapy in terms of appetite and energy balance. It is, however, indicated to increase protein intake (1.5 g/kg/day) during the recovery phase of hospitalization in order to optimize conditions for protein synthesis. From a caloric point of view, nutritional support should be targeted to meet 1.3× (estimated or measured) REE to avoid overfeeding in the unstable period.

C. Anabolic Management in the Treatment of Cachexia in COPD

Because in some the patients with COPD tissue depletion was not simply solved by restoring the impaired energy intake relatively to energy expenditure, anabolic endocrinological therapeutic options are worth to take into account for the treatment of wasting in COPD. A second argument for this might be the fact that low circulating anabolic hormones are reported in a part of the patients with COPD (52).

Only few controlled studies on anabolic steroid supplementation are performed in COPD. Previously we investigated the effects of nandrolone decanoate combined with nutritional supplementation versus nutrition alone or placebo as integrated part of an 8-week pulmonary rehabilitation program. In the depleted patients, both treatment regimens resulted in improvements in body weight, FFM and maximal inspiratory mouth pressure (PI_{max}). However, the rises in FFM and PI_{max} differed significantly from the control group only in the group treated with nandrolone decanoate (80). Besides this short-term study, others have evaluated the effects of oral stanozolol treatment during 6 months in depleted male patients with COPD with a low PI_{max}. The treatment was combined with inspiratory muscle training and cycling. Body weight, lean body mass, as well as arm muscle and thigh circumference increased. However, the changes in PI_{max}, the 6-min walking distance and maximal exercise capacity were not different from those of the control group (85).

These previous studies with anabolic steroids have predominantly evaluated their efficacy in the treatment of weight loss. However, imposing anabolic stimuli might be indicated for the improvement of muscle mass in

COPD, irrespectively of weight loss. Furthermore, the effects on physical performance and health status are to be defined.

An additional indication for anabolic steroid treatment in COPD might be stimulation of the erythropoiesis, as suggested by the increases in hematological parameters after nandrolone decanoate. Anabolic steroids are known for their effects on erythropoiesis, predominantly by enhancing the activity of erythropoietin. In the past, anabolic steroids were indeed used for the treatment of anemia in chronic renal failure (86,87). Although erythropoietin is reported to be increased in a part of the patients with COPD (88), an (extra) rise in erythropoietin might be beneficial for the improvement of oxygen delivery.

Other anabolic hormones to be evaluated for the treatment of wasting in COPD are growth hormone and insulin-like growth factors (IGFs). The main rationale for supplementation of these hormones in acute and chronic disease is to improve the nitrogen balance. Aging per se already leads to a decrease in growth hormone and IGF concentrations. Studies in healthy elderly subjects have indicated positive effects of growth hormone therapy on muscle strength and immune function. Although it is not known yet if growth hormone, IGFs, and/or IGF-binding proteins are reduced in patients with COPD, to date two studies on growth hormone supplementation are published. An uncontrolled study suggested positive effects on body weight, nitrogen balance, and inspiratory muscle function (89). However, 3 weeks of growth hormone administration in underweight patients with COPD in a placebo-controlled design increased lean body mass but did not improve muscle strength or exercise tolerance relatively to pulmonary rehabilitation alone (90). Further studies are needed to make a conclusive statement on growth hormone supplementation in COPD.

D. Anticatabolic Management in the Treatment of Cachexia in COPD

From several studies, evidence arose that the systemic inflammatory response is prominently involved in the decreased dietary intake in stable and acute COPD. Plasma leptin as well as plasma-soluble intercellular adhesion molecule-I were inversely associated with dietary intake in depleted, emphysematous patients with COPD (42,48). During an acute exacerbation of COPD, dietary intake was severely depressed. At day 7 of hospitalization, dietary intake relative to REE was inversely correlated with plasma soluble TNF receptor 55 and with plasma leptin (43). Besides evidence for the involvement of the systemic inflammatory response in the energy intake in stable and acute COPD, it was found that systemic inflammation was also associated with nonresponse to nutritional supplementation therapy. Elevated circulating concentrations of soluble TNF receptor 55 and of leptin were found to be independently associated with nonresponse to nutritional supplementation therapy (42,48).

From other work, it has become clear that, besides a local upregulation of inflammatory processes in the lungs (91), an elevated systemic inflammatory response is present in patients with COPD. This was based on elevated concentrations of acute-phase proteins, TNF-α receptors and soluble adhesion molecules in peripheral blood (24,92). In addition, there is clear evidence for a relationship between weight loss and tissue depletion on the one hand and systemic inflammatory parameters on the other (24,26,27). The proposed cytokine involvement in pulmonary cachexia needs an appropriate approach to combat this significant comorbidity in COPD.

The present anti-inflammatory therapeutic strategy in COPD concerns mainly the local inflammatory processes. Inhaled glucocorticosteroids are often prescribed as maintenance anti-inflammatory medication, despite insufficient evidence regarding their efficacy on local inflammation at this time (93). Sometimes prescription of inhaled glucocorticosteroids is accompanied by orally administered glucocorticosteroids. However, it was suggested that the local inflammatory processes were resistant to the anti-inflammatory properties of systemically administered glucocorticosteroids (93). In contrast, long-term treatment with oral glucocorticosteroids can further contribute to weakness and wasting of both the respiratory and the peripheral muscles in patients with severe COPD (53).

For these reasons, other, nonsteroidal anti-inflammatory modulation options, either nutritional or pharmacological, might be indicated for (a subgroup of) patients with COPD. Increasing attention is being paid to the supposed positive effects of omega-3 polyunsaturated fatty acids, as in fish oil, on the inflammatory processes. The possible mechanisms involve suppression of excessive endothelial activity and thereby decreased production of pro-inflammatory mediators like prostaglandins and leukotrienes. After ingestion, omega-3 fatty acids will be preferentially incorporated in the cell membrane and inhibit the metabolizing of arachidonic acid to prostaglandin E2 by cyclooxygenase. Instead, less inflammatory prostaglandins are produced. In line, lipooxygenase converts omega-3 fatty acids to leukotriene B5, which has only a fraction of the chemotactic activity of the leukotriene B4 normally synthesized from arachidonic acid (94). In healthy subjects, dietary supplementation with the omega-3 fatty acid gamma-linolenic acid resulted indeed in increased fractions of this omega-3 polyunsaturated acid in neutrophil phospholipids. This change in phospholipid composition within inflammatory cells such as the neutrophil might attenuate the biosynthesis of arachidonic acid, thereby representing a mechanism by which dietary polyunsaturated fatty acids exert their action (95).

Encouraging effects of omega-3 fatty acid supplementation with respect to improved immune function, decreased systemic inflammatory response and body weight are observed in patients suffering from cancer cachexia (96–98). Studies on supplementation of omega-3 fatty acids in chronic disease, like inflammatory bowel disease, indicate a potential effectiveness on systemic inflammatory response (for instance, decreases in neutrophil leukotriene B4 production) and disease activity (99). Whether omega-3 fatty acid supplementation in COPD will exert positive effects on systemic inflammatory processes and, second, clinical outcome is still to be unraveled. In addition to nutritional anti-inflammatory treatment options, the possibilities with regard to anti-inflammatory modulation by means of pharmacological intervention in COPD are growing (100). However, further research is needed in order to judge the usefulness of these anti-inflammatory mediators in patients with COPD in clinical practice.

In summary, for the subgroup of patients not responding to oral nutritional therapy and characterized by an increased systemic inflammatory response, nutritional or pharmacological anti-inflammatory modulation is worth considering in addition to optimized nutritional supplementation therapy. Furthermore, investigating the consequences of an elevated systemic inflammatory response on muscle fibers per se may open new and more direct approaches to novel anti-inflammatory treatment strategies in patients with COPD.

References

1. Engelen MPKJ, Schols AMWJ, Baken WC, Wesseling GJ, Wouters EFM. Nutritional depletion in relation to respiratory and peripheral skeletal muscle function in out-patients with COPD. Eur Respir J 1994; 7:1793–1797.
2. Schols AMWJ, Soeters PB, Dingemans AM, Mostert R, Frantzen PJ, Wouters EFM. Prevalence and characteristics of nutritional depletion in patients with stable COPD eligible for pulmonary rehabilitation. Am Rev Respir Dis 1993; 147:1151–1156.
3. Smeenk FWJM, Creutzberg EC, Fokkens B, Jagt PH, Wouters EFM on behalf of the COSMIC study group. COPD and Seretide: a multi-center intervention and characterisation (COSMIC) study: prevalence of nutritional depletion in patients with COPD stratified by disease stage. Am J Respir Crit Care Med 2001; 163:A502.
4. Engelen M, Schols A, Lamers RJS, Wouters EFM. Different patterns of chronic tissue wasting among patients with chronic obstructive pulmonary disease. Clin Nutr 1999; 18:275–280.
5. Harris JA, Benedict EG. A Biometric Study of Basal Metabolism. Washington, DC: Carnegie Institute of Washington, 1919.
6. Hugli O, Frascarolo P, Schutz Y, Jequier E, Leuenberger P, Fitting JW. Diet-induced thermogenesis in chronic obstructive pulmonary disease. Am Rev Respir Dis 1993; 148:1479–1483.
7. Fitting JW, Frascarolo P, Jequier E, Leuenberger P. Energy expenditure and rib cage-abdominal motion in chronic obstructive pulmonary disease. Eur Respir J 1989; 2:840–845.
8. Donahoe M, Rogers RM, Wilson DO, Pennock BE. Oxygen consumption of the respiratory muscles in normal and in malnourished patients with chronic obstructive pulmonary disease. Am Rev Respir Dis 1989; 140:385–391.
9. Green JH, Muers MF. The thermic effect of food in underweight patients with emphysematous chronic obstructive pulmonary disease. Eur Respir J 1991; 4:813–819.

10. Sridhar MK, Carter R, Lean ME, Banham SW. Resting energy expenditure and nutritional state of patients with increased oxygen cost of breathing due to emphysema, scoliosis and thoracoplasty. Thorax 1994; 49:781–785.

11. Ryan CF, Road JD, Buckley PA, Ross C, Whittaker JS. Energy balance in stable malnourished patients with chronic obstructive pulmonary disease. Chest 1993; 103:1038–1044.

12. Schols AMWJ, Fredrix EW, Soeters PB, Westerterp KR, Wouters EFM. Resting energy expenditure in patients with chronic obstructive pulmonary disease. Am J Clin Nutr 1991; 54:983–987.

13. Cherniack RM. The oxygen consumption and efficiency of the respiratory muscles in health and emphysema. J Clin Invest 1958; 38:494–499.

14. Shindoh C, Hida W, Kikuchi Y, et al. Oxygen consumption of respiratory muscles in patients with COPD. Chest 1994; 105:790–797.

15. McGregor M, Becklake MR. The relationship of oxygen cost of breathing to respiratory mechanical work and respiratory force. J Clin Invest 1961; 40:971–980.

16. Mannix ET, Manfredi F, Palange P, Dowdeswell IR, Farber MO. Oxygen may lower the O_2 cost of ventilation in chronic obstructive lung disease. Chest 1992; 101:910–915.

17. O. Donnell D, Webb KA. Exertional breathlessness in patients with chronic airflow limitation. The role of lung hyperinflation. Am Rev Respir Dis 1993; 148:1351–1357.

18. Fritts HW, Filler J, Fishman AP, Cournand A. The efficiency of ventilation during voluntary hyperpnea: studies in normal subjects and in dyspneic patients with either chronic pulmonary emphysema or obesity. J Clin Invest 1959; 38:1339–1348.

19. Gosselink RA, Wagenaar RC, Rijswijk H, Sargeant AJ, Decramer ML. Diaphragmatic breathing reduces efficiency of breathing in patients with chronic obstructive pulmonary disease. Am J Respir Crit Care Med 1995; 151:1136–1142.

20. Dash A, Agrawal A, Venkat N, Moxham J, Ponte J. Effect of oral theophylline on resting energy expenditure in normal volunteers. Thorax 1994; 49:1116–1120.

21. Amoroso P, Wilson SR, Moxham J, Ponte J. Acute effects of inhaled salbutamol on the metabolic rate of normal subjects. Thorax 1993; 48:882–885.

22. Creutzberg EC, Schols AMWJ, Bothmer-Quaedvlieg FCM, Wesseling G, Wouters EFM. Acute effects of nebulized salbutamol on resting energy expenditure in patients with chronic obstructive pulmonary disease and in healthy subjects. Respiration 1998; 65 (5):375–380.

23. Burdet L, de Muralt B, Schutz Y, Fitting JW. Thermogenic effect of bronchodilators in patients with chronic obstructive pulmonary disease. Thorax 1997; 52:130–135.

24. Schols AMWJ, Buurman WA, Staal van den Brekel AJ, Dentener MA, Wouters EFM. Evidence for a relation between metabolic derangements and increased levels of inflammatory mediators in a subgroup of patients with chronic obstructive pulmonary disease. Thorax 1996; 51:819–824.

25. Nguyen LT, Bedu M, Caillaud D, et al. Increased resting energy expenditure is related to plasma TNF-alpha concentration in stable COPD patients (see comments). Clin Nutr 1999; 18:269–274.

26. Di Francia M, Barbier D, Mege JL, Orehek J. Tumor necrosis factor-alpha levels and weight loss in chronic obstructive pulmonary disease. Am J Respir Crit Care Med 1994; 150:1453–1455.
27. De Godoy I, Donahoe M, Calhoun WJ, Mancino J, Rogers RM. Elevated TNF-alpha production by peripheral blood monocytes of weight-losing COPD patients. Am J Respir Crit Care Med 1996; 153:633–637.
28. Pouw EM, Schols AMWJ, Deutz NE, Wouters EFM. Plasma and muscle amino acid levels in relation to resting energy expenditure and inflammation in stable chronic obstructive pulmonary disease. Am J Respir Crit Care Med 1998; 158:797–801.
29. Baarends EM, Schols AMWJ, Pannemans DL, Westerterp KR, Wouters EFM. Total free living energy expenditure in patients with severe chronic obstructive pulmonary disease. Am J Respir Crit Care Med 1997; 155:549–554.
30. Hugli O, Schutz Y, Fitting JW. The daily energy expenditure in stable chronic obstructive pulmonary disease. Am J Respir Crit Care Med 1996; 153:294–300.
31. Baarends EM, Schols AMWJ, Akkermans MA, Wouters EFM. Decreased mechanical efficiency in clinically stable patients with COPD. Thorax 1997; 52 (11):981–986.
32. Baarends EM, Schols AMWJ, Westerterp KR, Wouters EFM. Total daily energy expenditure relative to resting energy expenditure in clinically stable patients with COPD. Thorax 1997; 52 (9):780–785.
33. Hunter AM, Carey MA, Larsh HW. The nutritional status of patients with chronic obstructive pulmonary disease. Am Rev Respir Dis 1981; 124:376–381.
34. Schols AMWJ, Soeters PB, Mostert R, Saris WH, Wouters EFM. Energy balance in chronic obstructive pulmonary disease. Am Rev Respir Dis 1991; 143:1248–1252.
35. Vermeeren MAP, Schols AMWJ, Quaedvlieg FCM, Wouters EFM. The influence of an acute disease exacerbation on the metabolic profile of patients with chronic obstructive pulmonary disease. Clin Nutr 1994; 13 (suppl 1):38–39.
36. Schols AMWJ, Mostert R, Cobben N, Soeters P, Wouters EFM. Transcutaneous oxygen saturation and carbon dioxide tension during meals in patients with chronic obstructive pulmonary disease. Chest 1991; 100:1287–1292.
37. Akrabawi SS, Mobarhan S, Stoltz RR, Ferguson PW. Gastric emptying, pulmonary function, gas exchange, and respiratory quotient after feeding a moderate versus high fat enteral formula meal in chronic obstructive pulmonary disease patients. Nutrition 1996; 12:260–265.
38. Campfield LA, Smith FJ, Burn P. The OB protein (leptin) pathway—a link between adipose tissue mass and central neural networks. Horm Metab Res 1996; 28:619–632.
39. Seeley RJ, van Dijk G, Campfield LA, et al. Intraventricular leptin reduces food intake and body weight of lean rats but not obese Zucker rats. Horm Metab Res 1996; 28:664–668.
40. Hwa JJ, Ghibaudi L, Compton D, Fawzi AB, Strader CD. Intracerebroventricular injection of leptin increases thermogenesis and mobilizes fat metabolism in ob/ob mice. Horm Metab Res 1996; 28:659–663.
41. Takabatake N, Nakamura H, Abe S, et al. Circulating leptin in patients with chronic obstructive pulmonary disease. Am J Respir Crit Care Med 1999; 159 (4):1215–1219.

42. Schols A, Creutzberg EC, Buurman WA, Campfield LA, Saris WHM, Wouters EFM. Plasma leptin is related to proinflammatory status and dietary intake in patients with chronic obstructive pulmonary disease. Am J Respir Crit Care Med 1999; 160:1220–1226.

43. Creutzberg EC, Wouters EF, Vanderhoven-Augustin IM, Dentener MA, Schols AM. Disturbances in leptin metabolism are related to energy imbalance during acute exacerbations of chronic obstructive pulmonary disease. Am J Respir Crit Care Med 2000; 162:1239–1245.

44. Grunfeld C, Zhao C, Fuller J, et al. Endotoxin and cytokines induce expression of leptin, the ob gene product, in hamsters. J Clin Invest 1996; 97:2152–2157.

45. Sarraf P, Frederich RC, Turner EM, et al. Multiple cytokines and acute inflammation raise mouse leptin levels: potential role in inflammatory anorexia. J Exp Med 1997; 185:171–175.

46. Zumbach MS, Boehme MW, Wahl P, Stremmel W, Ziegler R, Nawroth PP. Tumor necrosis factor increases serum leptin levels in humans. J Clin Endocrinol Metab 1997; 82:4080–4082.

47. Janik JE, Curti BD, Considine RV, et al. Interleukin 1 alpha increases serum leptin concentrations in humans. J Clin Endocrinol Metab 1997; 82:3084–3086.

48. Creutzberg EC, Schols AM, Weling-Scheepers CA, Buurman WA, Wouters EF. Characterization of nonresponse to high caloric oral nutritional therapy in depleted patients with chronic obstructive pulmonary disease. Am J Respir Crit Care Med 2000; 161:745–752.

49. Vermeeren MAP, Schols AMWJ, Wouters EFM. Effects of an acute exacerbation on nutritional and metabolic profile of patients with COPD. Eur Respir J 1997; 10 (10):2264–2269.

50. Morrison WL, Gibson JN, Scrimgeour C, Rennie MJ. Muscle wasting in emphysema. Clin Sci 1988; 75:415–420.

51. Engelen MP, Deutz NE, Wouters EF, Schols AM. Enhanced levels of whole-body protein turnover in patients with chronic obstructive pulmonary disease. Am J Respir Crit Care Med 2000; 162:1488–1492.

52. Kamischke A, Kemper DE, Castel MA, et al. Testosterone levels in men with chronic obstructive pulmonary disease with or without glucocorticoid therapy. Eur Respir J 1998; 11:41–45.

53. Decramer M, Lacquet LM, Fagard R, Rogiers P. Corticosteroids contribute to muscle weakness in chronic airflow obstruction (see comments). Am J Respir Crit Care Med 1994; 150:11–16.

54. Levine S, Kaiser L, Leferovich J, Tikunov B. Cellular adaptations in the diaphragm in chronic obstructive pulmonary disease. N Engl J Med 1997; 337:1799–1806.

55. Whittom F, Jobin J, Simard PM, et al. Histochemical and morphological characteristics of the vastus lateralis muscle in patients with chronic obstructive pulmonary disease. Med Sci Sports Exerc 1998; 30 (10):1467–1474.

56. Satta A, Migliori GB, Spanevello A, et al. Fibre types in skeletal muscles of chronic obstructive pulmonary disease patients related to respiratory function and exercise tolerance. Eur Respir J 1997; 10:2853–2860.

57. Sauleda J, Garcia-Palmer FJ, Gonzalez G, Palou A, Agust AG. The activity of cytochrome oxidase is increased in circulating lymphocytes of patients with chronic obstructive pulmonary disease, asthma, and chronic arthritis. Am J Respir Crit Care Med 2000; 161:32–35.

58. Pouw EM, Schols AMWJ, vanderVusse GJ, Wouters EFM. Elevated inosine monophosphate levels in resting muscle of patients with stable chronic obstructive pulmonary disease. Am J Respir Crit Care Med 1998; 157 (2):453–457.

59. Klitgaard H, Mantoni M, Schiaffino S, et al. Function, morphology and protein expression of ageing skeletal muscle: a cross-sectional study of elderly men with different training backgrounds. Acta Physiol Scand 1990; 140:41–54.

60. Casaburi R. Anabolic therapies in chronic obstructive pulmonary disease. Monaldi Arch Chest Dis 1998; 53:454–459.

61. Hamilton AL, Killian KJ, Summers E, Jones NL. Muscle strength, symptom intensity, and exercise capacity in patients with cardiorespiratory disorders. Am J Respir Crit Care Med 1995; 152:2021–2031.

62. Gosselink R, Troosters T, Decramer M. Peripheral muscle weakness contributes to exercise limitation in COPD. Am J Respir Crit Care Med 1996; 153:976–980.

63. Bernard S, LeBlanc P, Whittom F, et al. Peripheral muscle weakness in patients with chronic obstructive pulmonary disease. Am J Respir Crit Care Med 1998; 158:629–634.

64. Engelen MP, Schols AM, Does JD, Wouters EF. Skeletal muscle weakness is associated with wasting of extremity fat-free mass but not with airflow obstruction in patients with chronic obstructive pulmonary disease. Am J Clin Nutr 2000; 71:733–738.

65. Palange P, Forte S, Onorati P, et al. Effect of reduced body weight on muscle aerobic capacity in patients with COPD. Chest 1998; 114:12–18.

66. Gosker HR, Wouters EF, van Der Vusse GJ, Schols AM. Skeletal muscle dysfunction in chronic obstructive pulmonary disease and chronic heart failure: underlying mechanisms and therapy perspectives. Am J Clin Nutr 2000; 71:1033–1047.

67. Shoup R, Dalsky G, Warner S, et al. Body composition and health-related quality of life in patients with obstructive airways disease. Eur Respir J 1997; 10:1575–1580.

68. Mostert R, Goris A, Weling-Scheepers CAPM, Wouters EFM, Schols AMWJ. Tissue depletion and health related quality of life in patients with chronic obstructive pulmonary disease. Respir Med 2000; 94:859–867.

69. Kessler R, Faller M, Fourgaut G, Mennecier B, Weitzenblum E. Predictive factors of hospitalization for acute exacerbation in a series of 64 patients with chronic obstructive pulmonary disease. Am J Respir Crit Care Med 1999; 159 (1):158–164.

70. Vitacca M, Clini E, Porta R, Foglio K, Ambrosino N. Acute exacerbations in patients with COPD: predictors of need for mechanical ventilation. Eur Respir J 1996; 9:1487–1493.

71. Connors AF Jr, Dawson NV, Thomas C, et al. Outcomes following acute exacerbation of severe chronic obstructive lung disease. The SUPPORT investigators (Study to Understand Prognoses and Preferences for Outcomes and Risks of Treatments). Am J Respir Crit Care Med 1996; 154:959–967.

72. Schols AMWJ, Slangen J, Volovics L, Wouters EFM. Weight loss is a reversible factor in the prognosis of chronic obstructive pulmonary disease. Am J Respir Crit Care Med 1998; 157 (6):1791–1797.

73. Landbo C, Prescott E, Lange P, Vestbo J, Almdal TP. Prognostic value of nutritional status in chronic obstructive pulmonary disease. Am J Respir Crit Care Med 1999; 160:1856–1861.

74. Rogers RM, Donahoe M, Costantino J. Physiologic effects of oral supplemental feeding in malnourished patients with chronic obstructive pulmonary disease. A randomized control study. Am Rev Respir Dis 1992; 146:1511–1517.

75. Efthimiou J, Fleming J, Gomes C, Spiro SG. The effect of supplementary oral nutrition in poorly nourished patients with chronic obstructive pulmonary disease. Am Rev Respir Dis 1988; 137:1075–1082.

76. Otte KE, Ahlburg P, F DA, Stellfeld M. Nutritional repletion in malnourished patients with emphysema. J Parenter Enteral Nutr 1989; 13:152–156.

77. Knowles JB, Fairbarn MS, Wiggs BJ, Chan Yan C, Pardy RL. Dietary supplementation and respiratory muscle performance in patients with COPD. Chest 1988; 93:977–983.

78. Donahoe M., Mancino J., Constantino J, et al. The effect of an aggressive nutritional support regimen on body composition in patients with severe COPD and weight loss (abstr). Am J Respir Crit Care Med 1994; 149:A313.

79. Ferreira IM, Brooks D, Lacasse Y, Goldstein RS. Nutritional support for individuals with COPD: a meta-analysis. Chest 2000; 117:672–678.

80. Schols AMWJ, Soeters PB, Mostert R, Pluymers RJ, Wouters EFM. Physiologic effects of nutritional support and anabolic steroids in patients with chronic obstructive pulmonary disease. A placebo-controlled randomized trial. Am J Respir Crit Care Med 1995; 152:1268–1274.

81. Vermeeren MA, Wouters EF, Nelissen LH, van Lier AA, Hofman Z, Schols AM. Acute effects of different nutritional supplements on symptoms and functional capacity in patients with chronic obstructive pulmonary disease. Am J Clin Nutr 2001; 73:295–301.

82. Sauerwein HP, Romijn JA. More consideration to dietary protein in the nutrition of chronically ill adults with tendency to weight loss. Ned Tijdschr Geneeskd 1999; 143:886–889.

83. Schols AM, Wouters EF. Nutritional abnormalities and supplementation in chronic obstructive pulmonary disease. Clin Chest Med 2000; 21:753–762.

84. Saudnyunterberger H, Martin JG, Graydonald K. Impact of nutritional support on functional status during an acute exacerbation of chronic obstructive pulmonary disease. Am J Respir Crit Care Med 1997; 156 (3):794–799.

85. Ferreira IM, Verreschi IT, Nery LE, et al. The influence of 6 months of oral anabolic steroids on body mass and respiratory muscles in undernourished COPD patients. Chest 1998; 114:19–28.

86. Ballal SH, Domoto DT, Polack DC, Marciulonis P, Martin KJ. Androgens potentiate the effects of erythropoietin in the treatment of anemia of end-stage renal disease (see comments). Am J Kidney Dis 1991; 17:29–33.

87. Berns JS, Rudnick MR, Cohen RM. A controlled trial of recombinant human erythropoietin and nandrolone decanoate in the treatment of anemia in patients on chronic hemodialysis. Clin Nephrol 1992; 37:264–267.

88. Casale R, Pasqualetti P. Diurnal rhythm of serum erythropoietin circulating levels in chronic obstructive pulmonary disease. Panminerva Med 1997; 39:183–185.

89. Pape GS, Friedman M, Underwood LE, Clemmons DR. The effect of growth hormone on weight gain and pulmonary function in patients with chronic obstructive lung disease. Chest 1991; 99:1495–500.

90. Burdet L, de Muralt B, Schutz Y, Pichard C, Fitting JW. Administration of growth hormone to underweight patients with chronic obstructive pulmonary disease. A prospective, randomized, controlled study. Am J Respir Crit Care Med 1997; 156:1800–1806.

91. Keatings VM, Collins PD, Scott DM, Barnes PJ. Differences in interleukin-8 and tumor necrosis factor-alpha in induced sputum from patients with chronic obstructive pulmonary disease or asthma. Am J Respir Crit Care Med 1996; 153:530–534.

92. Riise GC, Larsson S, Lofdahl CG, Andersson BA. Circulating cell adhesion molecules in bronchial lavage and serum in COPD patients with chronic bronchitis. Eur Respir J 1994; 7:1673–1677.

93. Keatings VM, Jatakanon A, Worsdell YM, Barnes PJ. Effects of inhaled and oral glucocorticoids on inflammatory indices in asthma and COPD. Am J Respir Crit Care Med 1997; 155:542–548.

94. Furst P, Kuhn KS. Fish oil emulsions: what benefits can they bring? Clin Nutr 2000; 19:7–14.

95. Johnson MM, Swan DD, Surette ME, et al. Dietary supplementation with gamma-linolenic acid alters fatty acid content and eicosanoid production in healthy humans. J Nutr 1997; 127:1435–1444.

96. Falconer JS, Fearon KC, Ross JA, Carter DC. Polyunsaturated fatty acids in the treatment of weight-losing patients with pancreatic cancer. World Rev Nutr Diet 1994; 76:74–76.

97. Wigmore SJ, Ross JA, Falconer JS, et al. The effect of polyunsaturated fatty acids on the progress of cachexia in patients with pancreatic cancer. Nutrition 1996; 12:S27–S30.

98. Wigmore SJ, Fearon KC, Maingay JP, Ross JA. Down-regulation of the acute-phase response in patients with pancreatic cancer cachexia receiving oral eicosapentaenoic acid is mediated via suppression of interleukin-6. Clin Sci Colch 1997; 92:215–221.

99. Belluzzi A, Boschi S, Brignola C, Munarini A, Cariani G, Miglio F. Polyunsaturated fatty acids and inflammatory bowel disease. Am J Clin Nutr 2000; 71:339S–3425.

100. Barnes PJ. Novel approaches and targets for treatment of chronic obstructive pulmonary disease. Am J Respir Crit Care Med 1999; 160:S72–S79.

18

Anxiety, Depression, and Coping Skills

SUSAN E. ABBEY

University of Toronto
and University Health Network
Toronto, Ontario, Canada

I. Introduction

Difficulty coping, anxiety, and depression are common problems in individuals with advanced lung disease, as would be expected given the negative impact of advanced lung diseases on multiple life domains and the ever-present threat of respiratory decompensation and death (1). These diseases are typically characterized by a prolonged course of illness with increasing incapacity and the need for a variety of medical interventions, including medications and home oxygen. The challenges are different and may be even greater for those with the precipitous onset of a disease that then rapidly advances. The course of disease is often unpredictable and, in advanced stages, individuals may rapidly and unexpectedly decompensate and die. Ongoing hypoxemia may lead to compromised cognitive functioning. Sleep problems are common. Participation in valued activities, including social and occupational functioning, is typically markedly impaired. The ability to travel freely is impeded. Oxygen supplementation, while often helpful medically, may be distressing to some patients because it is a visible sign of their illness and is therefore, either subjectively or objectively, stigmatizing. All of these factors contribute to markedly impaired quality of life and increased emotional distress (2).

Difficulties in coping, anxiety, and depression may represent transient symptoms that respond to enhanced coping skills or, if of greater duration or intensity, may constitute clinically significant disorders that warrant treatment with pharmacotherapy or psychotherapy. While anxiety and depression may arise from a variety of etiological factors, they clearly have a negative impact on quality of life and often worsen functional status. Wells et al. (3) demonstrated that major depression was associated with a comparable or greater negative impact on quality of life than eight major medical conditions that also affect quality of life negatively. Similarly, Ormel et al. (4) found that depressive symptoms contributed more than chronic medical illness to a sense of impaired well-being, negative health perception, and functional disability in a large cohort of middle-aged and elderly. A study of elderly male veterans with chronic obstructive pulmonary disease (COPD) found that anxiety and depression contributed to the overall variance in functional status over and above the objective medical burden and COPD severity (5). Anxiety has been described as "one of the most important factors determining quality of life in COPD" (6). As well as being distressing to patients and their families, psychiatric comorbid conditions increase health care costs in individuals with chronic medical conditions (7). Yet anxiety and depression continue to be underdiagnosed and undertreated in patients with advanced lung disease (2,5). A recent English study comparing palliative care and quality of life in severe, end-stage COPD with those in lung cancer found that while the COPD group had significantly greater impairments in quality of life and emotional well-being, they received less intervention (2). This chapter reviews new approaches to enhancing coping strategies and treating syndromal level anxiety and depression, offering new hope of reduced suffering to patients and their families.

II. Enhancing Coping Strategies in Distressed Patients

There are a wide variety of interventions that may enhance coping in patients with advanced nonmalignant lung disease who are emotionally distressed or are functionally compromised more than would be expected based upon their objective physiological parameters and disease burden. These approaches may also be helpful in individuals with anxiety or depressive disorders once the disorder is in remission. The major categories of interventions are shown in Table 1. While most of the discussion below focuses on the patient, it is important to remember that caregiver family and friends are also likely to face periods of emotional distress and may benefit from these approaches.

Education and having adequate information is essential to most patients, yet the majority of patients with advanced COPD report unmet information needs (2). While patients want information about their disease, Gore et al. (2) found that "patients' information needs were diverse and sometimes ambiguous and contradictory" and that there was particular reluctance to

Table 1 Interventions to Enhance Coping in Patients with Advanced Nonmalignant Lung Disease

Education
Self-monitoring of symptoms
Exercise
Improving sleep
Cognitive approaches
Physiological calming techniques
Encouraging the expression and processing of emotion
Increasing social support
Building pleasure into every day
Detoxifying death

obtain details about the progression of their disease. The information needs and preferences regarding information delivery have been poorly studied in advanced nonmalignant lung disease patients. Common areas of education that are helpful to COPD patients include exercise, relaxation, and breathing retraining (8,9). Education is often part of multimodal interventions. For example, the importance of an exercise program in addition to education was emphasized by Emery et al. (9) who found increased psychosocial distress and lowered quality of life in those who received education and stress management about their disease without participating in an exercise program as well. Other important areas to consider include the optimal use of medications and in particular puffers, which are often used in a suboptimal way. As disease progresses, education and reinforcement of earlier education about energy conservation techniques assumes heightened importance. Education about cognitive and behavioral strategies for coping with the anxiety and depression associated with advanced lung disease is helpful (10). Patients and families benefit from information about community resources that offer both instrumental and emotional support, including home care, respite care, support groups, and advocacy groups. Education about advanced care directives and end-of-life issues leads to greater use of such directives and improved communication between doctor and patient (11).

Self-monitoring of symptoms refers to a process whereby patients and/or their families monitor symptoms and precipitants to disease exacerbation as well as response to interventions so that they can tailor therapy between medical visits based on prior directives from their health care practitioners (12). Practitioners can provide patients with charts to record symptoms or oxygen saturations and various treatment parameters (e.g., medication dosing, use of "as needed" medications, use of other such treatment modalities, and oxygen flow rates) and review these at scheduled visits. Where possible, suggestions are then made for treatment modifications that the patient or family may institute based on the symptoms and then monitor the effectiveness of the treatment modification. Self-monitoring of symptoms provides a sense of empowerment and greater confidence to patients and families and better information for health care practitioners to base subsequent interventions upon.

Exercise, including stretching for flexibility, strengthening and aerobic activities, is helpful in enhancing adjustment to illness from a variety of perspectives including physiological benefits, improved sense of well-being, improved sleep, and decreased depression and anxiety (13–15). With very advanced, nonmalignant lung disease, the capacity for exercise significantly decreases but is often still a suitable target for intervention. Pulmonary rehabilitation plays an important role earlier in the disease course and may be valuable as disease advances, although at some point the goals must be more limited. The importance of maintaining whatever activity one can must be emphasized to retard further physical deconditioning and the sense of hopelessness and helplessness that accompany it. Many patients who can do nothing else still benefit from very gentle stretching of small muscle groups (e.g., neck rolls) or low demand strengthening exercises.

Improving sleep may be a complex task (1) but typically benefits people through multiple mechanisms. Appropriate sleep hygiene (e.g., regular times to go to sleep and wake up, getting up if one is unable to sleep, limiting time in bed to sleep and lovemaking, limiting naps, decreasing caffeine, etc.) brings significant benefits to many patients. Treatment of sleep apnea and other sleep disorders is important. If all else fails, the judicious use of a medication with sedating properties may help (1).

Cognitive approaches focus on helping the patient to identify unhelpful thoughts that contribute to emotional distress, limit their functional status or may precipitate physiological symptoms of anxiety. This approach encourages patients to identify and evaluate the thoughts they have about their disease and its impact upon their life. Cognitive approaches are derived from cognitive therapy which was initially developed to treat major depression (16) and has been used to facilitate coping with chronic medical illness (17). This approach posits that thoughts about symptoms or lifestyle limitations produce emotional and physiological responses that interfere with successful adaptation to the difficulties that the disease poses for individuals and their families. Cognitive approaches lead to improved coping with medical illness by developing skills in reducing dysfunctional attitudes and beliefs that are limiting, unhelpful, maladaptive, or irrational. A case example follows.

> Naomi is a 64-year-old widow with six children who is now in the advanced stages of COPD. Premorbidly, she was an extremely bright, multitalented, highly active woman who was at the top of her highly competitive profession, was highly involved with her children, her husband's demanding career and both of their parents, did an enormous amount of volunteer work, and had a diverse range of interests, both physical and intellectual. She was referred for psychiatric assessment because she was emotionally distressed and was isolating herself in her home due to her shame at wearing nasal prongs and carrying an oxygen tank. She was able to identify the automatic thought that came every time she thought

of going out of the house, "I can't go out like this because I'm not looking my best." As she explored this, she recognized another belief "Looking one's best in public is everything. You have to do your best or things won't work out." This was a long-standing belief that had always spurred her to carefully groom herself before being seen in public and present only her best work to the world. She credited this belief for her success in multiple life domains. With support, she was able to challenge the usefulness of it at this point in her life given that it barred her from so many activities. She came to see it as limiting and unhelpful. She developed a more balanced thought, "I may not like wearing these nasal prongs and toting the oxygen along but it is keeping me alive and that is important to me and the people who love me."

Other cognitive approaches include using distraction, self-reassuring talk, rationalization, and problem solving. Assistance with problem solving may be very helpful for people who are not able to clearly delineate their problems or generate a range of possible solutions. Cognitive approaches are less helpful in individuals with significant cognitive compromise as the result of decreased cerebral oxygenation, as they have difficulty with concentration, attention, and memory.

Physiological calming techniques are valuable in that they calm both the body and the mind. A wide range of techniques exists. Progressive muscle relaxation involves alternately tensing and then releasing muscles throughout the body and the process releases both bodily and emotional tension (18). It has been demonstrated to reduce dyspnea, anxiety, and airway obstruction in a small sample of COPD patients (19). Autogenic training produces a sense of relaxation through suggestion and deep breathing which reduces autonomic arousal (20). The "relaxation response" described by Benson (21,22) is a concentrative form of meditation that uses concentrating or focusing the mind on a single stimulus (e.g., a word, counting the breath) to calm the body and the mind. Mindfulness meditation changes an individual's relationship with their symptoms by anchoring nonjudgmental awareness of the breath in the present moment and then extending this awareness to incorporate whatever comes into the field of awareness (e.g., physical sensations, emotions, thoughts) (23). As noted above, these approaches are more difficult to use in patients with cognitive compromise secondary to hypoxemia.

Encouraging the expression and processing of emotion is helpful for many patients. This may be accomplished through a range of outlets depending upon a patient's level of distress and the acceptance of this distress by family and friends. Many patients find it helpful to describe their concerns and share their feelings with appropriate family and friends, although others describe a reluctance to do so, given the fear that they will overburden their loved ones at a time that they are already burdening them with instrumental care needs. Some patients may prefer to participate in individual or group support or counseling provided by health care professionals. A wide variety of therapeutic approaches exist and have value for different patient groups (1). While groups led by professionals or trained peers are increasingly common in other disease states, the burdens of advanced lung disease typically preclude this. When such a group is available, patients typically value the support and comfort they receive in the group setting from others struggling with advanced disease. If patients enjoy writing or keeping journals, they should be encouraged to use their writing as a means of processing their experience. Recent research has suggested that writing about stressful life events may improve disease outcome in asthma and rheumatoid arthritis (24); while the data are preliminary and limited to these two diseases, it is consistent with a wider literature documenting the benefits of writing in the processing of emotion (25). Encouraging religious involvement may be helpful for those with experience with faith-based religion, while cultivating a broader sense of spirituality may be helpful to others. Clinically based pastoral care may be helpful to those with religious or spiritual interests and of particular value when patients are distressed about the meaning of their disease, particularly if they see it as a punishment from or abandonment by God.

Increasing social support is helpful on multiple levels. It increases the network of individuals who may be of practical, instrumental support as well as those who may be of emotional support. Many patients with advanced disease withdraw from social interactions because of stigma, fears that they are burdening friends, and reluctance to make social plans for fear that they may not be able to fulfill them when the time comes. It is helpful for health care professionals to provide support around issues of stigma and fears of being a burden and to encourage patients and their families to make flexible plans for social contact rather than not making plans at all. It is also useful to encourage patients to use and value alternative forms of social contact (e.g., telephone, e-mail). Participation in support groups is valuable to many patients, although getting them involved initially may be a challenge if they perceive such participation as stigmatizing or feel that they are being labeled as mentally ill. Normalizing the value of these groups in a diverse range of diseases is helpful. These groups are most effective with a leader who has experience in support and psychotherapeutic issues with the medically ill (26).

Building pleasure into every day acts as a buffer against the many losses and stresses that patients with advanced lung disease and their families face. Health care professionals can suggest that, where possible, people modify formerly pleasurable activities to meet current physical limitations or try to find substitutive interests that can serve some of the functions of their preillness interests. For example, an avid fly fisherman raged against the loss of physical capacity associated with his advanced lung disease. Eventually, after much struggle with family, friends, and health care professionals, he came to enjoy the sedentary pleasures of making fishing lures and watching TV shows about sport fishing—options that he had initially disparaged. Conceiving of such options is often very challenging and requires considerable creativity. Health care professionals may be helpful in encouraging people in this area and in discouraging their devaluation of substitutive activities. Encouraging the patient and his or her support network to find small pleasures in daily life may initially be difficult, but over time people often find that their ability to do so is one of the positive legacies of the disease.

Detoxifying death is a major contribution to decreasing the suffering our patients and their families experience. It is important to sort out for ourselves our own level of comfort in dealing with death and to identify resources for our patients to deal with those aspects of death and dying with which we are not personally comfortable. Responding to covert and overt indications that the patient wishes to discuss end-of-life issues often offers great comfort. Patients commonly describe a profound sense of isolation around these issues, as their families and friends may not want to face the reality of their ultimate demise, yet they have a need to talk about these issues. It is important to discuss availability of palliative care/symptom management teams before they are needed and to address misconceptions about them. There is evidence of underutilization of holistic palliative care approaches in end-stage lung disease (2). It is useful to elicit patients' fears around the dying process and offer them information and appropriate reassurance about our ability to alleviate, if not entirely control, distressing terminal symptoms. Such discussions typically are very reassuring to patients. The management of dyspnea in the end-of-life care for patients with advanced lung disease has recently been reviewed (27).

III. Anxiety and Anxiety Disorders

A. Dignostic Issues

Anxiety is one of the most common emotional symptoms experienced by individuals with advanced lung disease, yet it has received little systematic study. There is some evidence that individuals with advanced lung disease who have comorbid anxiety disorders, particularly panic, are more likely than those without an anxiety disorder to be fearful of bodily sensations and to make catastrophic attributions about them (28). Physiological states such as hypercapnia and medications used in the treatment of advanced lung disease may produce anxiety. Dyspnea has a complex relationship with anxiety and may be the cause or result of it (29).

Brief periods of anxiety are common in this patient group and can be distinguished from pathological or syndromal anxiety in terms of interference with day-to-day functioning (29). When anxiety is of sufficiently severity to interfere with social or occupational functioning, it is likely associated with a syndromal level anxiety disorder as classified by the American Psychiatric Association's *Diagnostic and Statistical Manual of Mental Disorders, Fourth Edition* (DSM-IV) (see Table 2) (30).

Diagnosis may be confounded by symptoms that overlap between respiratory diagnoses and anxiety disorders (e.g., dyspnea, palpitations, chest pain). In some individuals there is a reinforcing relationship between anxiety and the dyspnea associated with respiratory distress. The two interact—anxiety increases dyspnea and increased dyspnea secondary to medical causes provides

Table 2 DSM-IV^{TR} Anxiety Disorders
Common in End-Stage Lung Disease

Panic disorder
Generalized anxiety disorder
Adjustment disorder with anxious mood
Posttraumatic stress disorder

Source: Ref. 30.

a stimulus on which further anxiety may be elaborated. A variety of models
have been proposed to explain the relationship between anxiety, panic, and
dyspnea in patients with lung disease: they include a hyperventilation model, a
false suffocation alarm model, and a cognitive model (31).

A diagnosis of anxiety disorder may result from a focused history by a
health care professional or be detected through screening instruments such as
the PRIME-MD (32), which includes both a patient self-report component and
a professionally administered component following up on the patient's self-
report. The potential role of caffeine, alcohol, and recreational drug
withdrawal in the symptom picture must be considered. Smoking cessation,
nicotine withdrawal, and guilt and anxiety about ongoing smoking are all
associated with increased anxiety in advanced lung disease (29). Bronchodilators, corticosteroids, and other medications may contribute to feelings of
anxiety, as may other medical issues such as hypercapnia, endocrine and
metabolic disturbances, and cardiovascular conditions (33).

Panic Attacks and Panic Disorder

Panic attacks are characterized by four of the eight symptoms shown in Table
3a. Subsyndromal panic attacks have been described, including attacks with a
respiratory focus (34). Nocturnal panic attacks occur in a subset of patients
(29). Panic disorder (see Table 3b) is the most common of the syndromal
anxiety disorders in patients with respiratory disorders (28,31). Rates have
ranged from 2 to 96% in COPD patients, with rates of 10 to 38% being
reported most commonly (31).

Panic anxiety is often a component of the dyspnea experienced by
individuals with respiratory illness, and the relationship between the two has
recently been reviewed from both theoretical and clinical perspectives (31). It is
essential to rule out other respiratory conditions that may potentially present
with panic, such as pneumothorax, pulmonary hypertension, vocal cord or
laryngeal dysfunction, pulmonary embolus, sleep apnea, pulmonary edema,
and pneumonia (31). It is extremely important to help patients, where possible,
to clearly discriminate between the characteristics of the panic attacks they are
experiencing and similar symptoms of shortness of breath, tachycardia, or
other physical symptoms that are related to a medical event that should be

Table 3a Diagnostic Criteria for Panic Attack

Panic attacks are characterized by the sudden and rapid onset of a distinct period of intense fear or discomfort accompanied by some combination of physical and/or psychological symptoms. A minimum of four symptoms which begin abruptly and rapidly reach a peak within 10 min are required for the diagnosis. The symptoms include:
- Feeling dizzy, unsteady, light-headed, or faint
- Sensations of smothering or shortness of breath
- Palpitations, pounding heart, or accelerated heart rate
- Chest pain or discomfort
- Choking sensation
- Nausea or abdominal distress
- Shaking or trembling
- Paresthesias
- Sweating
- Chills or hot flushes
- Derealization (feelings of unreality) or depersonalization (being detached from oneself)
- Fear of losing control or going crazy
- Fear of dying

Source: Ref. 30.

Table 3b Diagnostic Criteria for Panic Disorder

Panic disorder is diagnosed when an individual has recurrent unexpected panic attacks that are not attributable to another medical or psychiatric diagnosis or substance use. At least one of the panic attacks has been followed by 1 month (or more) of:
- Ongoing worry or enduring anxiety about having another attack
- Worry about the perceived implications of the attack (e.g., fearing a catastrophic illness such as multiple sclerosis or a heart attack, worry about having a nervous breakdown)
- Making a significant change in behavior because of the attacks (e.g., not going shopping if an attack occurred in a shopping mall and the individual sees it as a causative or contributory factor)

Source: Ref. 30.

evaluated. In an acute situation where such a distinction is not clear, it is best to first treat or rule out acute respiratory decompensation or a comorbid medical event.

Generalized Anxiety Disorder

Generalized anxiety disorder (GAD) has recently received increased attention as more effective treatments have become available. By definition (Table 4), it is characterized by more than 6 months of excessive worry about a number of

Table 4 Diagnostic Criteria for Generalized Anxiety Disorder

The hallmark of generalized anxiety disorder (GAD) is excessive or unrealistic anxiety or worry about a number of issues. The individual finds the anxiety difficult to control and experiences it on most days for at least 6 months. The generalized anxiety is not attributable to another psychiatric diagnosis, a substance, or a medical condition.

The anxiety and worry are associated with a minimum of three symptoms, some of which have been present for more days than not for at least 6 months:
- Feelings of being on edge, restless or "keyed up"
- Muscle tension
- Irritability
- Easy fatigability
- Problems with concentration or the mind going blank
- Sleep disturbance (difficulty falling asleep, fragmented sleep, difficulty staying asleep, or restless and nonrefreshing sleep)

Source: Ref. 30.

issues (30). Discerning what constitutes "excessive" worry in patients with advanced disease who have many reasons to be worried can be clinically challenging and controversial.

Adjustment Disorder with Anxious Mood

This diagnosis is used to describe psychological distress, in the form of anxious mood, that occurs in response to an identifiable stressor or stressors and is associated with emotional distress in excess of what would be expected given the nature of the stressor or a clinically significant impairment in social, occupational, or recreational functioning (30). Adjustment disorder occurs most commonly at times of change in illness trajectory (e.g., initial diagnosis, beginning to use supplemental oxygen, moving from a rehabilitative to a palliative focus for care). By definition, the disturbance does not meet criteria for another specific disorder.

Posttraumatic Stress Disorder

Posttraumatic stress disorder may develop in response to distressing, life-threatening events that arise as part of the patient's medical course (e.g., sudden respiratory collapse) or occur during the course of medical care (e.g., cardiac arrest during diagnostic bronchoscopy) (Table 5). It may also have antedated the illness and arisen from other traumatic life events (e.g., childhood sexual abuse, rape, witnessing life-threatening events) but be reactivated or increased in intensity by the medical state. There is increasing recent interest in the pharmacotherapy and psychotherapy of posttraumatic stress disorder (35,36).

Table 5   Diagnostic Criteria for Posttraumatic Stress Disorder

Posttraumatic stress disorder (PTSD) is diagnosed when an individual experiences symptoms of more than 1 month duration with significant impairment or distress and these symptoms follow on exposure to a traumatic event. The traumatic event must be one in which there is actual or threatened death or serious injury, or a threat to the physical integrity of self or others. Response to the event includes intense fear, helplessness, or horror. PTSD also requires persistent symptoms of:

- Re-experiencing the trauma
- Avoiding stimuli associated with the trauma or a general numbing of responsiveness
- Increased arousal

Source: Ref. 30.

B. Management

Management of anxiety symptoms and disorders is more complex in advanced lung disease than in milder forms of respiratory disorder or in patients who are medically well. This is because of the overlap in symptoms between the two diagnoses and the limitations that the medical status may pose for some forms of pharmacotherapy and psychotherapy. Management may be directed at the traditional goals of treatment in panic patients without respiratory disease, such as symptom relief, the prevention of secondary complications such as depression and agoraphobia, and improvement in quality of life. In patients with advanced lung disease, additional goals more specific to these individuals may include greater emphasis on coping with breathlessness and decreasing disability as well as improving functional status (31). Management of anxiety symptoms and disorders includes both pharmacological and nonpharmacological interventions. Respirologists and primary care physicians, depending on their experience and orientation, may be quite comfortable with providing front-line treatment and refer only more complicated or treatment-resistant cases. Alternatively, they may feel more comfortable referring early. In either case, it is helpful to make referrals to mental health professionals who are experienced in treating patients with advanced lung disease.

The management of the anxious patient must always include a careful review for depressive symptomatology, as there is a significant comorbidity between the two diagnoses and some treatments (e.g., antidepressants) are effective for both diagnoses while others (e.g., benzodiazepines) are not.

Nonpharmacological Interventions

Nonpharmacological interventions have been described for all of the major anxiety disorders. Anxiety symptoms that do not meet criteria for subsyndromal or syndromal status may respond to a variety of approaches, including a variety of relaxation techniques and cognitive approaches discussed earlier in this chapter.

Cognitive-behavioral therapies are the mainstay of the nonpharmacological treatment of anxiety disorders (1). They include a wide range of therapeutic approaches that all share the goal of decreasing the frequency and severity of symptoms and increasing the individual's capacity to cope with symptoms. The basic model underlying these therapeutic approaches is shown in Figure 1.

Cognitive-behavioral approaches may be targeted at any of the components of the model. Purely cognitive approaches address the patient's initial fearful cognitions by helping him or her to identify the thoughts that fuel the anxiety, such as "This is it—I'm dying," or "It is impossible for me to cope with this feeling of breathlessness" (Table 6). The patient is then taught how to look at the evidence for and against this thought and attempt to come up with a more balanced cognition, as shown in Table 6. In looking for evidence

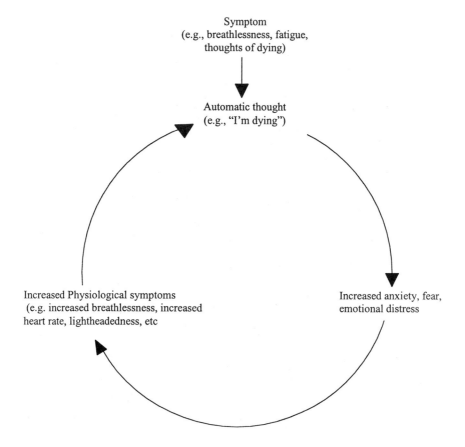

Figure 1 A cognitive model of panic attacks.

Table 6 Thought Record for Panic Attacks

Situation	Mood	Automatic thought(s)	Evidence for thought(s)	Evidence against thought(s)	Alternative balanced thought
Sudden increased shortness of breath	Fear Dread Worry Sense of doom	"I'm dying." "I can't cope with this."	"I feel like I'm going to die." "The sensation of smothering is terrifying." "My COPD is advancing."	"I have had this symptom before and I haven't died." "My doctor says that this type of shortness of breath is panic and it won't kill me." "I can use anxiety reduction strategies to help cope."	"This is a really unpleasant sensation but I can get through this." "I know this panic attack will only last 20 to 30 minutes." "I'll try and use relaxation breathing and talking myself down to help get through this episode."

against their catastrophic thoughts, patients can ask themselves whether past experience contradicts their thoughts in any way, what people who love them would say about their thoughts, what they would tell someone they loved who had these thoughts, whether they feel differently at other times, and what has helped in the past to deal with these thoughts (37). Patients are then encouraged to remind themselves of their more balanced thoughts when they next experience symptoms. Over a period of time, which varies considerably between patients, physical symptoms are no longer met with catastrophic thoughts or the catastrophic thoughts can be quickly dismissed when they arise.

In more behaviorally based interventions, the focus is on providing physiological calming to counteract the increased physical symptomatology that arises from the emotional distress occurring secondary to the distressing automatic thought. A wide variety of approaches exist and are discussed earlier in this chapter. It is important to remember that these techniques may be associated with increased symptoms in a substantial minority of patients, particularly those with panic disorder or generalized anxiety disorder (33).

Pharmacological Interventions

A variety of agents have documented efficacy and effectiveness in the treatment of anxiety disorders although there has been remarkably little systematic study in patients with respiratory disorders. The most commonly used agents are the selective serotonin reuptake inhibitors (SSRIs) and benzodiazepines in those individuals who can tolerate them physiologically. Other antidepressants, such as venlafaxine and the older tricyclic antidepressants, have antianxiety effects in some diagnoses. This patient group requires lower starting doses, slower dosage escalation, and more careful monitoring for drug interactions or problematic side effects. The choice of drug also depends upon the diagnosis— panic disorder responds to clonazepam and alprazolam, the SSRIs, venlafaxine, clomipramine, impiramine, and desipramine (38); generalized anxiety disorder responds to benzodiazepines, buspirone, and antidepressants (venlafaxine, paroxetine, imipramine) (39); adjustment disorder is usually treated nonpharmacologically or with benzodiazepines; and there is preliminary evidence for the use SSRIs in posttraumatic stress disorder (36). The use of these medications in the pulmonary population has recently been reviewed (40).

The SSRIs have become first-line treatments for panic disorder in those without medical illness because of their efficacy, tolerability, and ease of use (31). The most commonly used SSRIs in the medically ill are paroxetine, citalopram, and sertraline because of their shorter half-life compared to fluoxetine (although this may be an advantage in those for whom compliance is problematic) and their improved side-effect profile and less frequent drug interactions compared to fluvoxamine. There has been interest in the effect of serotonin on respiratory drive (31). A case series suggests that SSRIs may have an antidyspneic effect even in the absence of anxiety or mood disorders (41).

SSRIs are also effective in generalized anxiety (39). And there is increasing evidence of their value in posttraumatic stress disorder. Each of the SSRIs has a slightly different cytochrome P450 profile, making it important to check for drug interactions with the patient's other medications, although the chance of drug interactions is much lower with this group of medications than with most of the older tricyclics and monoamine oxidase inhibitors. Recent interest has focused on the role of the selective noradrenergic sertononergic reuptake inhibitor (SNRI) venlafaxine. Both SSRIs and SNRIs have the potential, in the first 7 to 14 days of use, to increase anxiety, including both generalized anxiety and the frequency and severity of panic attacks in panic disorder. For this reason they are typically started at a very low dose and titrated upward slowly. Patients should be advised of this possibility in order to foster compliance and prevent their discontinuing the medication if they do experience this effect. If they are physiologically able to tolerate benzodiazepines, these may be used in this first week or two to prevent an increase in panic symptoms or to treat them should they occur. The major disadvantage of SSRIs and SNRIs is that they do not produce a complete blockade of the anxiety for at least 4 to 8 weeks and patients may notice no improvement at all in the first 2 to 4 weeks. Some tricyclic antidepressants are effective in panic disorder (desipramine is the best tolerated) (38), generalized anxiety disorder (39), and posttraumatic stress disorder (40) but are now most often used as third- or fourth-line treatments because of their anticholinergic side effects, increased likelihood of drug interactions, and lethality in overdose.

Benzodiazepines are also an acceptable first-line treatment for panic disorder, if not medically contraindicated, although they are much less commonly used now that the SSRIs and SNRIs are available. If the patient is able to tolerate them physiologically, they offer more rapid symptom relief but are associated with withdrawal symptoms after long-term use in a significant percentage of patients. The major area of concern is respiratory suppression in individuals with carbon dioxide retention. Benzodiazepine use in this context requires very cautious dosing and close follow-up and is best reserved for the very distressed patient who needs urgent symptom control. When carbon dioxide retention is a problem, there is the option of using buspirone for generalized anxiety, although it is ineffective in panic disorder and takes 3 to 6 weeks to work, or low-dose neuroleptics that do not alter respiratory drive (33). If these agents are not successful and the patient's suffering is impairing his or her quality of life or if anxiety is compromising the patient's respiratory function, benzodiazepines may be cautiously tried, beginning with the lowest possible dose (via cutting the smallest tablet into quarters or halves) and monitoring closely. In older patients, there are concerns about falls secondary to psychomotor impairment with benzodiazepines. Some individuals may also show other signs of central nervous system toxicity, including dizziness, ataxia, weakness, vertigo, confusion, and dysarthria.

Dosing information for drugs used in the treatment of anxiety is shown in Table 7.

Table 7 Drugs Used in the Treatment of Anxiety Disorder

Antidepressants

	Starting dose	Dosing increments	Usual effective dose	Maximum dose[b]
Paroxetine (Paxil)	5–10 mg[a]	10 mg	40–60 mg	60 mg
Sertraline (Zoloft)	25 mg	25 mg	50–200 mg	200 mg
Citalopram (Celexa)	10 mg	10 mg	20–30 mg	50 mg
Venlafaxine (Effexor) XR	18.75 mg– 37.5 mg	37.5 mg	75–150 mg	225–375 mg[c]

Benzodiazepines (if not physiologically contraindicated)

	Starting dose[a]	Dosing increments	Usual effective dose	Maximum dose[b]
Clonazepam (Rivotril, Klonopin)[b]	0.25–0.5 mg	0.25–0.5 mg	0.5–2 mg bid	10 mg
Alprazolam (Xanax)[b]	0.125–0.25 mg	0.25–0.5 mg	0.5–2 mg tid	10 mg
Lorazepam (Ativan)[b]	0.5–1.0 mg	0.5–1.0 mg	1–3 mg tid	10 mg

[a]In the somatically preoccupied patient or patient with severe medical illness.
[b]If physiologically tolerated.
[c]Varies depending on governmental regulatory information.
Source: Ref. 42.

IV. Depression and Depressive Disorders

Sadness, demoralization, and a sense of loss are common responses to advanced nonmalignant lung disease. In addition to transient low mood that may accompany changes in the illness trajectory or periods of heightened frustration or disappointment, many patients suffer from an unrecognized and untreated major depressive episode. The diagnostic criteria for major depression are shown in Table 8. Of note, the assessment of depression in advanced lung disease is complicated by the overlap between symptoms of depression and symptoms of advanced lung disease such as fatigue, cognitive impairment, weight loss, and sleep disturbance (2). Medical-, substance-, and drug-induced causes of depression must also be considered. Mental health professionals familiar with advanced lung disease usually do the best assessments regarding depression.

Rates of major depression in COPD are reported to be as high as 40% (19) or more and yet depression is underdiagnosed and undertreated in this group. There are multiple barriers to the effective diagnosis and management of depression in the medically ill, including stigma, the belief that depression is

Table 8 Diagnostic Criteria for Criteria for Major Depressive Episode

Major depressive episode requires a change from previous functioning with a minimum of five symptoms occurring over most of the day during the same 2-week time period.
- The change from previous functioning is clinically significant and is associated with impairment in daily functioning (e.g., social roles, occupational).
- Symptoms are not counted toward a diagnosis of depression if they directly result from a medical condition, medication, or substance abuse.

Depressed mood **or** loss of ability to experience pleasure or interest must be among the five minimum symptoms.
- Depressed mood that is either subjective or objective
- Significantly decreased capacity to experience pleasure or markedly diminished interest in all, or almost all, activities
- Changes in sleep—insomnia or hypersomnia
- Changes in appetite (increased or decreased) or loss of weight
- Decreased energy or heightened fatigue
- Impaired concentration, decreased ability to think, indecisiveness
- Objective changes in psychomotor status—retardation or agitation
- Significantly lowered self-esteem, feelings of worthlessness, excessive or inappropriate guilt
- Recurrent thoughts of death, wish for a hastened death, suicidal ideation (passive or active) or suicidal behavior

Source: Ref. 30.

normative, health professional time limitations, lack of privacy in most clinic and inpatient settings, and inadequate training of primary care and respiratory medicine specialists in psychiatry. As with anxiety disorders, it is important to consider potential medical etiologies for depression (e.g., thyroid disorders, neurological disorders) and the etiological role of medications and psychoactive substances including corticosteroids and opiates (43).

A. Management

Effective management is multifactorial and may include a combination of approaches as required, including education, support, exercise and pulmonary rehabilitation, empirically validated manualized psychotherapies, antidepressant medication, and electroconvulsive therapy. Decisions as to which treatment or treatments to employ and in what order are based upon the severity of the depression, patient preferences, effective past treatments if applicable, and the availability of resouces. Psychiatric inpatient or day hospitalization may be required by individuals with active suicidal ideation or severe nonpsychotic or psychotic depression.

Psychotherapy

The most commonly used empirically validated psychotherapies in depressed patients with comorbid medical illness are cognitive therapy and interpersonal therapy. Both of these treatments are typically delivered in 12 to 16 individual sessions and may be followed by monthly sessions for a period of time if required to maintain the gains the patient has made. Patients typically continue to show improvements in their mood even without monthly follow-up sessions as benefits accrue over time and as they practice what they have learned in the therapy.

Cognitive therapy for depression is directed towards unhelpful negative thoughts about the self, one's experiences, and the future (16). There is evidence that cognitive therapy is as effective as antidepressant treatment in mildly to moderately depressed medically well populations (44), although it has not been extensively evaluated in medically ill samples. Patients are taught to identify their moods, as this can be surprisingly problematic for a subset of patients who have difficulty in labeling and discriminating their moods. Worksheets may be used initially to record details of low mood and to link moods with situations. Patients are then taught to identify the automatic thought (s) associated with the depressed mood and situation and to record these on worksheets. Finally, they learn to weigh the evidence for and against their automatic thoughts and ultimately attempt to generate more balanced, helpful thoughts. For example, a 64-year-old man who was previously very physically active and enjoyed roughhousing with his grandchildren becomes overwhelmed with sadness whenever he sees his grandchildren and is unable to play with them physically. He identifies the automatic thought "I might as well be dead." This thought could be reworked over time through the process of looking at the evidence for and against the following thought: "It is a struggle to deal with my lung problems but my family love me and would rather have me alive than dead. Even though my pleasures are more limited than before, and I wish I could do more, there are sources of happiness and joy open to me to enjoy, like telling the kids about my earlier adventures and watching adventure videos with them."

Interpersonal therapy (IPT) for depression is based on the importance of disturbances in interpersonal relationships in either the genesis or maintenance of depression (45). Interpersonal relationships and our social worlds are important factors for most of us in the regulation of our mood state. Common disturbances in interpersonal relationships include (1) death of a loved one; (2) transitions secondary to ill health and the changes in social roles and functioning associated with it or secondary to retirement, financial limitations, moves, etc; (3) interpersonal conflict; and (4) deficits in interpersonal skills that leave the individual socially isolated. A therapeutic focus is identified in one of these areas and the therapist then works with the patient to increase meaningful social contact. IPT has been found to be as effective as antidepressant therapy in medically healthy individuals with mild to moderate depression, and its use is being extended to medically ill samples (46).

Pharmacotherapy

There are an increasing number of pharmacotherapy options available for the treatment of depression in the medically ill. Choice of agent depends largely upon (1) side-effect profile, either taking advantage of side effects such as sedation in the insomniac patient or avoiding problematic side effects, and (2) potential for interaction with other medications that the individual is taking. Clinical wisdom advises to "start low, go slow," but it also emphasizes the importance of slowly working up to an effective dose. While the newer medications are much less likely to interact with other drugs, it is important to check for drug interactions before prescribing, given that most patients with advanced nonmalignant lung disease are on a variety of medications. As these newer drugs are used more extensively, case reports of drug interactions are growing; it is therefore essential to check any proposed antidepressant against a current drug interaction database. Worsening of pulmonary function is very uncommon and has typically been associated with drying of secretions, with greater difficulty clearing airways with the much more anticholinergic, older medications. The most common antidepressant agents used in the medically ill are shown in Table 9.

The SSRIs are typically first-line drugs in the treatment of the depressed medically ill patients. They have a range of side effects, but these occur in a minority of patients and usually last for a maximum of 2 weeks. Common side effects include gastrointestinal disturbance (e.g., anorexia, nausea, diarrhea, constipation) and central nervous system cognitive and neurological effects (e.g., insomnia, sedation, lethargy, agitation, sedation, fatigue, headache, etc.) (42). A variety of forms of sexual dysfunction occur in a significant minority of patients on SSRIs and SNRIs. These effects may not resolve in the first few weeks, in which case a decision must be made about the importance to the patient and or partner of the sexual dysfunction and whether to treat it. Treatment approaches include adding a wide range of agents depending upon the type of sexual dysfunction (42) or changing antidepressants.

Bupropion is another popular choice in the medically ill, although it may be too "activating" for anxious patients, and there are concerns about lowering the seizure threshold at higher doses in high-risk patients or with abrupt dosage increases (42). Venlafaxine is a commonly used drug, but concerns about hypertension and the need to monitor blood pressure (42) typically make it a second-line choice. Mirtazepine is a new drug with increasing use. It can be quite sedating, which can be an advantage in the patient with insomnia. It is associated with concerns about weight gain, primarily in the first 4 weeks of treatment, in up to 16% of patients (42). Psychostimulants are an important option in the medically ill population, although they are underutilized and do not have a strong evidence base in large-scale, randomized, placebo-controlled studies.

Table 9 Drugs Commonly Used in the Treatment of Major Depression in the Medically Ill

SSRI (Selective Serotonin Reuptake Inhibitors)

	Starting dose[a]	Dosing increments	Usual effective dose	Maximum dose
Paroxetine (Paxil)	10 mg	10 mg	20 mg	50 mg
Sertraline (Zoloft)	25 mg	25 mg	50–100 mg	200 mg
Citalopram (Celexa)	10 mg	10 mg	20 mg	50 mg

SNRI (Selective Serotonin Norephinephrine Reuptake Inhibitor)

	Starting dose[a]	Dosing increments	Usual effective dose	Maximum dose
Venlafaxine (Effexor) XR	37.5 mg	37.5 mg	75–150 mg	225–375 mg[3]

NDRI (Norepinephrine Dopamine Reuptake Inhibitor)

	Starting dose[a]	Dosing increments	Usual effective dose	Maximum dose[c]
Bupropion (Wellbutrin)[b]	100–150 mg	100–150 mg	300 mg	300–400 mg

NaSSA (Noradrenergic/Specific Serontonergic Antidepressant)

	Starting dose[a]	Dosing increments	Usual effective dose	Maximum dose[c]
Mirtazapine (Remeron)	15–30 mg q hs	15–30 mg	30–45 mg	45 mg

Psychostimulants

	Starting dose[a]	Dosing increments	Usual effective dose	Maximum dose
Methylphenidate (Ritalin)	2.5–5 mg q am, q noon	2.5–5 mg q am, q noon	5–20 mg (total daily dose)	60 mg (total daily dose)
Detroamphetamine (Dexedrine)	2.5–5 mg q am	2.5–5 mg q am	5–30 mg q am	40–60 mg (total daily dose)

[a]In the somatically preoccupied patient or patient with severe medical illness.
[b]Also marketed as Zyban for smoking reduction.
[c]Varies depending on governmental regulatory information.
Source: Ref. 42.

There is a strong anecdotal and case series literature that supports their use (47). Side effects such as tachycardia and dyspnea were documented in less than 3% of a group of heterogeneous medically ill patients in retrospective record review (48). The principal advantage of these drugs lie the rapid remission of depressive symptoms over several days.

V. Conclusions

There is increasing evidence of the importance of emotional distress, and in particular anxiety and depression, in compromising the quality of life and functional status of individuals with advanced nonmalignant lung disease. A better understanding of the range of strategies that enhance coping and advances in psychiatric therapeutics, in the areas of both psychotherapy and pharmacotherapy, offer the potential of decreasing suffering and enhancing daily life for our patients who struggle with their advanced disease. While we await large-scale trials and a stronger evidence base for our treatment, we need to use the modalities currently available to optimize our patients' quality of life. We need to increase the profile of advanced nonmalignant lung disease and of interventions designed to reduce distress and improve quality of life in order to ensure adequate, comprehensive care for our patients and their families.

References

1. Abbey SE, Littlefield C, Bright J. Assisting the patient and family to cope with advanced disease: the psychosocial aspects of end-stage disease. Semin Respir Crit Care Med 1996: 17:534–542.
2. Gore JM, Brophy CJ, Greenstone MA. How well do we care for patients with end stage chronic obstructive pulmonary disease (COPD)? A comparison of palliative care and quality of life in COPD and lung cancer. Thorax 2000; 55:1000–1006.
3. Wells KB, Hays RD, Burnam MA, Rogers W, Greenfield S, Ware JE Jr. Detection of depressive disorder for patients receiving prepaid or fee-for-service care. Results from the Medical Outcomes Study. JAMA 1989; 262:3298–3302.
4. Ormel J, Kempen GI, Deeg DJ, Brilman EI, van Sonderen E, Relyveld J. Functioning, well-being, and health perception in late middle-aged and older people: comparing the effects of depressive symptoms and chronic medical conditions. J Am Geriatr Soc 1998; 46:39–48.
5. Kim HFS, Kunik ME, Molinari VA, Hillman SL, Lalani S, Orengo CA, Petersen NJ, Nahas Z, Goodnight-White S. Functional impairment in COPD patients: the impact of anxiety and depression. Psychosomatics 2000; 41:465–471.
6. Eiser N, West C, Evans S, Jeffers A, Quirk F. Effects of psychotherapy in moderately severe COPD: a pilot study. Eur Respir J 1997; 10 (7):1581–1584.
7. Unutzer J, Patrick DL, Simon G, Grembowski D, Walker E, Rutter C, Katon W. Depressive symptoms and the cost of health services in HMO patient aged 65 years and older. A 4-year prospective study. JAMA 1997; 277:1618–1623.
8. Make B. Collaborative self-management strategies for patients with respiratory disease. Respiratory Care 1994; 39:566–583.
9. Emery CF, Schein RL, Hauck ET, MacIntyre NR. Psychological and cognitive outcomes of a randomized trial of exercise among patients with chronic obstructive pulmonary disease. Health Psychol 1998; 17:232–240.
10. Kunik ME, Braun U, Stanley MA, Wristers K, Molinari V, Stoebner D, Orengo CA. One session cognitive behavioural therapy for elderly patients with chronic obstructive pulmonary disease. Psychol Med 2001; 31 (4):717–723.

11. Heffner JE, Fahy B, Hilling L, Barbieri C. Outcomes of advance directive education of pulmonary rehabilitation patients. Am J Respir Crit Care Med 1997; 155:1055–1059.

12. Clark NM, Becker MH, Janz NK, Lorig KR, Rakowski W, Anderson L. Self-management of chronic disease by older adults. J Aging Health 1991; 3:3–27.

13. Stewart AL, Hays RD, Wells KB, Rogers WH, Spritzer KL, Greenfield S. Long-term functioning and well-being outcomes associated with physical activity and exercise in patients with chronic conditions in the Medical Outcomes Study. J Clin Epidemiol 1994; 47 (7):719–730.

14. Vuori I. Does physical activity enhance health? Patient Educ Counsel 1998; 33 (suppl 1):S95–S103.

15. Durstine JL, Painter P, Franklin BA, Morgan D, Pitetti KH, Roberts SO. Physical activity for the chronically ill and disabled. Sports Med 2000; 30:207–219.

16. Beck AT, Rush AJ, Shaw BR, Emery G. Cognitive Therapy of Depression. New York: Guilford Press, 1979.

17. Devins GM, Binik YM. Facilitating coping with chronic physical illness. In: Zeidner M, Endler NS, eds. Handbook of Coping: Theory, Research, Applications. Toronto: Wiley, 1995:640–696.

18. Bernstein DA, Carlson CR. Progressive relaxation: abbreviated methods. In: Lehrer PM, Woolfolk RL, eds. Principles and Practice of Stress Management. New York: Guilford Publications, 1993:53–58.

19. Gift AG, McCrone SH. Depression in patients with COPD. Heart Lung 1993; 22:289–297.

20. Linden W. The autogenic training method of JH Schultz. In: Lehrer PM, Woolfolk RL, eds. Principles and Practice of Stress Management. New York: Guilford Press, 1993:205–230.

21. Benson H, Klipper MZ. The Relaxation Response. New York: Avon Books, 1976.

22. Benson H, Proctor W. Beyond the Relaxation Response. New York: Berkley, 1985.

23. Kabat-Zinn J. Full Catastrophe Living: Using the Wisdom of Your Body and Mind to Face Stress, Pain and Illness. New York: Delacorte Press, 1990.

24. Smyth JM, Stone AA, Hurewitz A, Kaell A. Effects of writing about stressful experiences on symptom reduction in patients with asthma or rheumatoid arthritis. JAMA 1999; 281:1304–1309.

25. Smyth JM. Written emotional expression: effect sizes, outcome types, and moderating variables. J Consult Clin Psychol 1998; 56:174–184.

26. Spira JL. Understanding and developing psychotherapy groups for medically ill patients. In: Spira JL (ed). Group Therapy for Medically Ill Patients. New York: Guilford Press, 1997.

27. Luce JM, Lance JA. Management of dyspnea in patients with far-advanced lung disease. JAMA 2001; 285:1331–1337.

28. Zaubler TS, Katon W. Panic disorder and medical comorbidity: A review of the medical and psychiatric literature. Bull Menninger Clin 1996; 60 (2, suppl A):A12–A38.

29. Wingate BJ, Hansen-Flaschen J. Anxiety and depression in advanced lung disease. Adv Lung Dis 1997; 18:495–505.

30. American Psychiatric Association: Diagnostic and Statistical Manual of Mental Disorders, 4th ed, text Rev. Washington DC: American Psychiatric Association, 2000.

31. Smoller JW, Pollack MH, Otto MW, Rosenbaum JF, Kradin RL. Panic anxiety, dyspnea, and respiratory disease: theoretical and clinical considerations. Am J Respir Crit Care Med 1996; 154:6–17.
32. Spitzer RL, Williams JBS, Kroenke K, Linzer M, deGruy FV III, Hahn SR, Brody D, Jonhson JG. Utility of a new procedure for diagnosing mental disorders in primary care: the PRIME-MD 1000 study. JAMA 1994; 272:1749–1756.
33. Goldberg RJ, Posner DA. Anxiety in the medically ill. In: Stoudemire A, Fogel BS, Greenberg DB, eds. Psychiatric Care of the Medical Patient. New York: Oxford University Press, 2000:165–180.
34. Rosenbaum J. Limited-symptom panic attacks. Psychosomatics 1987; 28 (8):407–408, 411–412.
35. Yehuda R. Post-traumatic stress disorder. N Engl J Med 2002; 346 (2):108–114.
36. Stein DJ, Zungu-Dirwayi N, van der Linden GJH, Seedat S. Pharmacotherapy of posttraumatic stress disorder. (Cochrane Review) In: The Cochrane Library, Issue 4, 2002, Oxford: Update Software.
37. Greenberger D, Padesky CA. Mind Over Mood: A Cognitive Therapy Treatment Manual for Clients. New York: Guilford Press, 1995.
38. Sheehan DV. Current concepts in the treatment of panic disorder. J Clin Psychiatry 1999; 60 (suppl 18):16–21.
39. Davidson JRT. Pharmacotherapy of generalized anxiety disorder to achieve remission. J Clin Psychiatry 2001; 62 (suppl 11):46–50.
40. Smoller JW. Simon NM. Pollack MH. Kradin R. Stern T. Anxiety in patients with pulmonary disease. Semin Clin Neuropsychiatry 1999; 4 (2):84–97.
41. Smoller JW, Pollack MH, Systrom D, Kradin RL. Sertraline effects on dyspnea in patients with obstructive airways disease. Psychosomatics 1998; 39:24–29.
42. Bezchlibnyk-Butler KZ, Jeffries JJ, eds. Clinical Handbook of Psychotropic Drugs, 11th rev ed. Toronto: Hogrefe & Huber, 2001.
43. Rouchell AM, Pounds R, Tierney JG. Depression. In: Wise MG, Rundell JR, eds. Textbook of Consultation–Liaison Psychiatry. Washington, DC: American Psychiatric Publishing, 2002:307–338.
44. Gloaguen V, Cottraux J, Cucherat M, Blackburn IM. A meta-analysis of the effects of cognitive therapy in depressed patients. J Affect Disord 1998; 49 (1):59–72.
45. Klerman GL, Weissman MM, Rounsaville BJ, Chevron ES. Interpersonal Psychotherapy of Depression. New York: Basic Books, 1984.
46. Markowitz JC, ed. Interpersonal Psychotherapy. Washington, DC: American Psychiatric Press, 1998.
47. Masand PS, Tesar GE. Use of stimulants in the medically ill. Psychiatr Clin North Am 1996; 19 (3):515–547.
48. Masand P, Pickett P, Murray GB. Psychostimulants for secondary depression in medical illness. Psychosomatics 1991; 32 (2):203–208.

19

Measurement of Health Status in Advanced Respiratory Disease

DONALD A. MAHLER

Dartmouth Medical School
Lebanon, New Hampshire, U.S.A.

PAUL W. JONES

St. George's Hospital Medical School
London, England

I. What Is Health-Related Quality of Life? What Is Health Status?

The traditional approach in caring for patients with chronic respiratory disease has been to focus on lung function tests, oxygen saturation, and/or chest radiographs to establish a diagnosis and to assess the response to treatment. However, patients seek medical attention because of symptoms that impair their ability to perform daily activities and/or work. *Functional status* is a general term that refers to the ability of an individual to function in physical, social, and emotional roles.

Two related concepts, health-related quality of life (HRQOL) and health status, are overlapping constructs that describe separate but related patient-assessed health outcomes. HRQOL has been used as a measure of a health outcome for a considerable time. A practical definition of HRQOL is (1):

> Quantification of the impact of disease on daily life and well-being in a formal and standardized manner.

This definition emphasizes the importance of using standardized questionnaires for measurement purposes. However, individuals are not uniform, and it therefore would be difficult to quantify HRQOL in a standard way. Accordingly, the term *HRQOL* is probably best reserved for consideration of *individual patients*.

Nonetheless, it is possible to provide accurate and reliable measurement of the effect of health on the patient's daily life and well-being in a *specific population of patients* to which an individual belongs. One definition of health status is (2):

> The effect of a person's health on the ability to perform and enjoy the activities of daily living.

The approach to measure health status includes various items or questions that are appropriate and applicable to all subjects with a disease. As such, health status instruments explore areas of impaired health common to all patients with a specific condition, and the corresponding scores can be used in the same way as any other standardized measurement, such as pulmonary function tests (1). It is important to recognize that scores from such instruments can determine the health of a population of patients very well, but they will have less precision when used to measure the health of an individual.

Over the past decade interest in health status has increased substantially because (1) health status has been recognized as a unique construct that is distinct from other measures such as blood test results, radiographs, etc; (2) physicians, health care organizations, insurance companies, and the pharmaceutical industry have acknowledged that patients are more concerned about symptoms and their ability to perform activities of daily living rather than physiological outcomes; and (3) the goals of therapy have expanded to include relief of symptoms and improvement in health status. Health status measures are being used as primary endpoints in randomized clinical trials involving patients with advanced respiratory disease (1–3).

II. Measurement Criteria

The two major reasons to measure health status are (4) (1) to discriminate (i.e., differentiate) between individuals or groups with better or worse health status and (2) to evaluate changes as a result of an intervention.

All health status instruments must meet certain measurement criteria (4). *Validity* refers to the actual measurement of what the instrument proposes to evaluate. *Reliable* instruments should demonstrate that the same results are obtained in different settings and with different observers. Repeatability is a specific form of reliability which tests whether health status scores are similar at two different time periods in stable patients. *Responsiveness* represents the ability of the instrument to detect change since it is important to demonstrate an improvement in health status (even if it is small) with a specific intervention.

Thus, a discriminative instrument must be valid and reliable, while an evaluative instrument should, at a minimum, be valid and responsive. Ideally, health status instruments should have both discriminative and evaluative properties, and also be reliable and responsive. Evidence for validation should be obtained in a number of different settings and studies. Furthermore, the responsiveness of an evaluative instrument should not be compromised or limited by *ceiling* (patients with the best score may have substantial improvement) and *floor* (patients with the worst score may deteriorate further) effects.

Another important consideration for a health status instrument is the determination of a minimal important or meaningful change (5,6). A threshold for a clinically significant response or difference between treatment groups can be established by comparing changes in the scores from the instrument with changes in a global estimate of the benefits of therapy (6).

III. Types of Health Status Questionnaires

The simplest way to measure a person's health is to ask the individual a global question such as, "How is your health?" The response could be quantified using a category scale with four or five grades. Generally, such a broad approach may underestimate the real impact that an advanced respiratory disease has on the person's perceived health, especially at the milder end of the disease spectrum (7). In order to estimate an individual patient's health status, both generic and disease-specific questionnaires have been developed (Fig. 1). Ideally, the instruments should combine the features of being comprehensive as well as being brief, so as to enhance applications in clinical research and possibly in clinical practice.

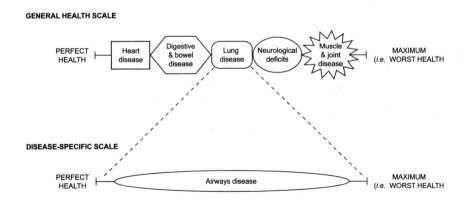

Figure 1   Schema of a general health scale and a scale that is disease-specific for a respiratory illness such as airways disease. (From Ref. 21.)

A.   General Health Questionnaires

The general questionnaires were the first to measure health status in those with respiratory disease. They were designed to measure disturbances in health irrespective of the specific disease. Five major generic instruments have been used to quantify health status in patients with respiratory disease (Table 1).

The Sickness Impact Profile (SIP) was published in 1981 as one of the first general health instruments (8). It incorporates 136 items with 12 components and takes about 20 to 30 min to complete. There are global scores for physical and psychosocial aspects, whereas one total score is transformed into a range of 0 to 100. The SIP was used in the Nocturnal Oxygen Therapy Trial (9) but appears to be insensitive to changes in patients with mild to moderate lung impairment (10). Overall, the SIP has limited applicability because of the time required for a patient to complete the instrument and its relative unresponsiveness.

In 1984 the Quality of Well-Being (QWB) scale (11) was developed as an outcome measure in chronic obstructive pulmonary disease (COPD). It contains 50 items with three components: mobility, physical activity, and social activity. Approximately 10 to 15 min is required for the instrument to be completed via an interview. The overall utility score ranges from 0 (dead) to 1 (optimal health). The advantage of the QWB is that it can be used in cost-effectiveness analysis. However, in a long-term study evaluating the efficacy of pulmonary rehabilitation the QWB failed to show any significant change with rehabilitation even though there were improvements in exercise endurance time and reductions in perceived breathlessness and leg fatigue during exercise (12). Whether the QWB scale can demonstrate responsiveness with an expected improvement associated with another type of treatment remains to be determined.

The Nottingham Health Profile (NHP) (13) includes 38 items covering six dimensions: energy, pain, emotional reaction, sleep, social isolation, and physical mobility. It is self-administered and takes 5 to 10 min to complete. Although scores on the NHP were significantly correlated with the severity of airway obstruction based on the FEV_1 using the American Thoracic Society staging system for COPD, the magnitude of correlation was smaller than observed for a disease-specific health status instrument (14).

In 1990 the EuroQol group developed a five-question instrument (EQ-5D) as a simple and brief method for individuals to rate health status using a visual analog scale "thermometer" for five dimensions (mobility, self-care, usual activities, pain/discomfort, and anxiety/depression) (15). Although this instrument has been translated into numerous different languages, it has not been widely applied up to the present time.

The Medical Outcomes Study Short-Form 36-item (SF-36) questionnaire (16) was published in 1992 as an expansion of a previously developed 20-item questionnaire. The SF-36 covers eight dimensions of health: physical functioning, role limitation due to physical problems, social functioning, role

Table 1 Generic Instruments Used to Measure Health Status in Patients with Chronic Respiratory Disease

Instrument/year	Number of items	Number of components	Scores	Time to complete (min)
Sickness Impact Profile (1981)	136	12	1 total score 2 global scores (physical and psychosocial)	20–30 Self-administered
Quality of Well-Being (1984)	50	3	1 overall utility score	10–15 Interview
Nottingham Health Profile (1985)	38	6	1 total score 1 score for each component	5–10 Self-administered
EuroQol-5D (1990)	5	5	Profile or a single summary score	2–3 Self-administered
Medical Outcome Study 36-item Questionnaire (1992)	36	8	2 global scores (physical and mental) 1 score for each component	5–10 Self-administered

limitation due to emotional state, general health, vitality, mental health, and bodily pain. Each dimension is scored separately and transformed to a scale of 0 to 100. Two global scores are obtained for a physical component summary and a mental component summary. This instrument can be completed by the individual patient in 5 to 10 min. The SF-36 has been validated in patients with asthma (17) and with COPD (18). In an observational study of 76 patients with symptomatic COPD, the physical functioning score on the Medical Outcomes Study 20-item questionnaire was the only health component to show a significant decline over a 2-year period (19). A more recent study in patients with COPD has shown a significant worsening in most of the component scores of the SF-36 over a 3-year period (20).

B. Disease-Specific Questionnaires

Disease-specific instruments were developed to consider the various components or constructs that affect directly the respiratory system (1–3,21). Thus, these types of instruments are likely to be more sensitive (responsive) to small changes observed with therapy. The various disease-specific instruments include components considered important or influence the specific respiratory condition. They vary considerably in the number of items and the number of components that reflect health status. All of these questionnaires have a total score, and most have scores for each of the individual components. The majority of these instruments were developed to be self-administered, although the Asthma Quality of Life Questionnaire by Juniper and colleagues (22) and the Chronic Respiratory Disease Questionnaire developed for patients with COPD by Guyatt and colleagues (23), were intended to be scored, at least in part, by an interviewer based on activities that were selected by the individual patient. Although baseline and treatment scores for these instruments are unique for each individual, this feature limits comparisons of scores obtained with these two instruments between groups of patients who have the same disease but were evaluated in different studies.

Asthma

The major questionnaires used to measure health status in patients with asthma are listed in Table 2. All of these instruments were developed and subsequently published in the 1990s. Recently, Juniper (24) reviewed information about the various quality-of-life measures available for use in patients with asthma.

The Living with Asthma Questionnaire (25) includes 68 items that cover 11 domains (social/leisure, sport, holidays, sleep, work, colds, morbidity, effects on others, medication use, sex, and dysphoric states and attitudes). Impairments due to asthma symptoms are not part of the questionnaire. The patient's responses for each item are graded on a three-point scale. This grading system suggests that the questionnaire may have acceptable

Table 2 Selected Disease-Specific Instruments Used to Measure Health Status in Patients with Asthma

Instrument/year	Number of items	Number of components	Scores	Time to complete (min)
Living with asthma Questionnaire (1991)	68	11	1 total score 1 score for each component	15–20 Self-administered or interview
Asthma QOL Questionnaire (1992)	20	4	1 total score 1 score for each component	5 Self-administered
Life activities Questionnaire (1992)	71			
St. George's Respiratory Questionnaire (1992)	76	3	1 total score 1 score for each component	10 Self-administered
Asthma QOL (1993)	32	4	1 total score 1 score for each component	10 (first time) 5 (subsequent) Interview (for 5 activities) and self-administered for other 27 items

discriminative properties, but the small number of grades may limit its responsiveness.

In 1992 Marks and colleagues (26) presented an Asthma Quality of Life Questionnaire which contains 20 items and four domains (breathlessness and physical restrictions, mood disturbance, social disruption, and concerns for health). Patients rate each item on a five-point scale which takes about 5 min to complete. This instrument has been shown to have both discriminative and evaluative properties (27).

Creer and coworkers (28) published the Life Activities Questionnaire for Adult Asthma in 1992. The instrument has 70 items that cover seven domains (physical activities, work activities, outdoor activities, emotions and emotional behavior, home care, eating and drinking activities, and miscellaneous). A five-point scale is used for each item. As described, the questionnaire focuses primarily on activity limitations, but it does not consider asthma symptoms and other health concerns.

Jones et al. (29) developed the St. George's Respiratory Questionnaire containing 76 items to be used in patients with both asthma and COPD. The three domains included in the instrument are symptoms, activities, and impacts. Although this instrument has been evaluated in patients with asthma (30), its main application has been to examine various interventions in those with COPD. Further description of this instrument is given in the following section on COPD.

In 1993 Juniper and colleagues (22) published a 32-item instrument also called the Asthma Quality of Life Questionnaire. Item selection was based on their importance to patients from a pool of 150 possible topics that affect the lives of those with asthma. The four domains considered were symptoms, emotions, exposure to environmental stimuli, and activity limitation. Each item is graded on a seven-point scale. A unique feature of the questionnaire is that the individual patient identifies five activities that are done regularly and impact the patient's daily activities. At each visit the individual is asked to rate limitations experienced in these activities. Although this feature allows an "individualized" approach to measuring quality of life, it also prevents direct comparisons with other patients or groups, because the five activities are different. The grading of the five activities selected by the patient requires an interviewer, whereas the remaining 27 items are self-administered. Responsiveness of the questionnaire has been demonstrated, and the minimal clinical important difference is a change of 0.5 units for each domain as well as for the total score (22,31,32).

Over the past few years additional instruments have been developed in an attempt to improve the measurement attributes of the above questionnaires. However, these newer instruments have not been included in this review because only limited information is currently available about their performances. For example, a short and simple instrument called the Airways Questionnaire 20 (includes 20 items) has been described for use in patients with asthma and COPD (33). Although this instrument has discriminative properties similar to those of the Asthma Quality of Life Questionnaire and the St. George's Respiratory Questionnaire, it has not yet been tested for responsiveness (33). Furthermore, various authors have modified existing questionnaires used to measure health status in patients with asthma (34–38). These modifications have generally been made to enhance the measurement properties (particularly responsiveness) of the instruments, and/or to reduce the number of questions or items so that the time required for the subject to complete the questionnaire would be shorter. Further testing will be required to establish whether these newer and/or modified questionnaires provide substantial benefits over the more established instruments, as listed in Table 2.

Chronic Obstructive Pulmonary Disease

The Chronic Respiratory Disease Questionnaire was designed by Guyatt and colleagues (23) as an evaluative instrument to quantify changes in health. It consists of four components: dyspnea (five items), fatigue (four items), mastery (four items), and emotion (seven items). Each item is graded by the patient on a seven-point Likert scale. For dyspnea, the subject is asked to describe the five most common activities that caused dyspnea over the past 2 weeks by recall and then by reading a list of 26 different activities. An interviewer is required to assist the patient in making these selections and asking the individual to select a grade. By design, this instrument is specific for an individual patient with chronic lung disease. However, for this reason, results from one study cannot be compared with results of another investigation.

As already described, the St. George's Respiratory Questionnaire (29) was developed for patients with obstructive airway disease, but its primary application since being published in 1992 has been in patients with COPD. The three components include symptoms (distress attributable to cough, wheeze, and acute exacerbations), activity (disturbance of physical activity and mobility caused by dyspnea), and impacts (psychosocial effects of the disease). It was designed for supervised self-administration but has also been validated for use by telephone administration (39). The method of scoring is different than that of other instruments, as each item has its own empirically derived weight independent of age, gender, disease severity and duration (40), and largely independent of country (41).

In 1994, Quirk and Jones (42) described both a 20-item and a separate 30-item Airways Questionnaire as simple and brief instruments for measuring health status in patients with asthma and with COPD. In 1999 Hajiro and coworkers (43) reported that the questionnaire with yes or no responses provided discriminative and responsiveness properties in outpatients with COPD living in Japan. The major advantages of the 20-item Airways Questionnaire are the 2 min necessary for the patients to complete it and the modest correlations observed with this instrument and both the Chronic

Respiratory Disease Questionnaire and the St. George's Respiratory Questionnaire. The authors commented that a high ceiling effect and the limited data available in patients with COPD who speak English were possible disadvantages of the instrument.

Tu and colleagues (44) developed and validated a computer-scannable, self-administered questionnaire to monitor health-related quality of life in patients with COPD. The Seattle Obstructive Lung Disease Questionnaire consists of 29 items measuring four dimensions: physical function, emotional function, coping skill, and treatment satisfaction. In developing the instrument, the authors used the Chronic Respiratory Disease Questionnaire as a model. One of the main purposes of the questionnaire was to survey large numbers of patients on a regular basis using computerized operations for data entry and scoring. Although there are scores for each dimension, the authors report that no overall score can be generated.

Interstitial Lung Disease

Consideration and measurement of health status of patients with interstitial lung disease have been far less extensive compared than in those with asthma and COPD. Presently, the general health instruments have been used primarily to measure health status in this population (45–49). For example, Martinez et al. (45) and Change et al. (46) described the use of the SF-36 questionnaire in patients with idiopathic pulmonary fibrosis and with sarcoidosis. Based on focus groups and individual interviews, De Vries and colleagues (47) reported that hobbies/leisure activities, mobility, transport, social relationships, working capacity, energy, and doing things more slowly were important aspects of quality of life identified by patients with idiopathic pulmonary fibrosis. Subsequently, De Vries et al. (48) have suggested that the World Health Organization Quality of Life 100-item questionnaire (49) was be more useful in idiopathic pulmonary fibrosis than the disease-specific instruments. Moreover, these investigators found that physical health and level of independence were impaired in 41 patients with idiopathic pulmonary fibrosis as measured on the World Health Organization instrument compared with 41 healthy persons matched for age and gender (48).

Although developed for patients with asthma and COPD, the St. George's Respiratory Questionnaire has been reported to be valid in 50 patients with various types of interstitial lung disease (46).

Bronchiectasis

Wilson et al. (50) reported that the St. George's Respiratory Questionnaire appeared to have good validity in patients with bronchiectasis. Furthermore, the scores on this questionnaire were worse in patients colonized with *Pseudomonas* compared to those who were not colonized with this organism (51).

Cystic Fibrosis

In adult patients with cystic fibrosis, Orenstein et al. (52,53) have described the use of the Quality of Well-Being scale, whereas Busschbach et al. (54) reported on the EuroQol and the Nottingham Health Profile to measure health status.

IV. Minimal Important Difference

There has been increasing interest in identifying clinically relevant changes in evaluative instruments used to measure health status (2–5). Why? Although an experienced clinician may be comfortable interpreting the measured change in one or more parameters of lung function, the meaning of a specific change in a score for a health status instrument is not intuitively obvious. Therefore various methods have been used to examine the interpretability of the changes in health status scores. the complex issues around the establishment of these thresholds have recently been reviewed (55). Jaeschke et al. (56) have defined the minimal important difference as:

> The smallest difference in score in the domain of interest which patients perceive as beneficial and would mandate, in the absence of troublesome side effects and excessive cost, a change in the patient's management.

One of the most common methods used to interpret health status data is an "anchor approach," whereby the changes in the scores on the instrument are compared, or anchored, to global ratings by the patient and/or the physician (57). Thus, to determine the minimal important difference, the change in a health status score is judged to be that which corresponds to the smallest important change perceived by the patient and/or the physician (5,6,57). For example, small, medium, and large effects correspond to changes of approximately 0.5, 1.0, and > 1.0 per question for instruments that use a seven-point scale (56), such as the Asthma Quality of Life Questionnaire (22) and the Chronic Respiratory Disease Questionnaire (23)

Another approach to determining the minimal important difference is to use standard statistical methods to calculate relevant intraindividual change over time as identified by the standard error of measurement. Such studies are ongoing to define a minimal important difference in certain health status instruments based on statistical methodology.

A. Published Data

The following information represents published data on calculated values for the minimal important differences of selected instruments listed in Tables 1 to 3.

General Health Questionnaire

Although statements in the literature have suggested that differences of three to five points for the domains of the SF-36 questionnaire may be clinically

Table 3 Selected Disease-Specific Instruments Used to Measure Health Status in Patients with Chronic Obstructive Pulmonary Disease

Instrument/year	Number of items	Number of components	Scores	Time to complete (min)
Chronic Respiratory Disease Questionnaire (1987)	20	4	1 total score 1 score for each component	20 (first time) 10–15 (subsequent) Interview
St. George's Respiratory Questionnaire (1992)	76	3	1 total score 1 score for each component	10 Supervised, self-administered
Airways Questionnaire 20 (1994)	20	1	1 total score	2 Self-administered
Seattle Obstructive Lung Disease Questionnaire (1997)	29	4	1 score for each component No total score	5–10 Supervised, self-administered

meaningful, a formal determination of the minimal important difference has not been established for this instrument.

Asthma

Juniper et al. (22) and Rowe and Oxman (31) reported that a change in the score of 0.5 is the minimal important difference both for the overall score and for each of the individual domains for the Asthma Quality of Life Questionnaire. Furthermore, responses of 1.0 and 2.0 represent moderate and large changes, respectively (22,31).

Jones and colleagues (58) found that a change of four points for the total score on the St. George's Respiratory Questionnaire represents the minimal important difference.

Chronic Obstructive Pulmonary Disease

In an initial report, Guyatt et al. (59) indicated that "a change in score of 4 or more represents a clinically important difference in physical function" domain of the Chronic Respiratory Disease Questionnaire. Further analyses have revealed that a change of 0.5 *per question* is the minimal important difference for this instrument (6,56). As the Chronic Respiratory Disease Questionnaire consists of 20 questions or items, a change in the total score of 10 is therefore considered to be the minimal important difference.

A change of at least four points is the minimal important difference for patients with COPD using the St. George's Respiratory Questionnaire, which is the same as described above for patients with asthma (58).

Tu et al. (44) reported that a change of approximately five points on the Seattle Obstructive Lung Disease Questionnaire represented the minimal important difference.

V. Clinical Applications

Selected studies that have used health status measures to evaluate various treatments in patients with asthma and in patients with COPD are summarized below. It is clear from these studies that statistical analyses of the changes in standard physiological outcomes and the changes in health status scores demonstrate only modest correlations among the variables. These results confirm that measurement of health status provides unique information that has become necessary for a comprehensive assessment of treatment effect in patients with advanced respiratory disease.

A. Asthma

Bronchodilator Therapy

At least five randomized controlled trials have evaluated the effects of inhaled beta-agonist therapy on health status in patient with asthma (32,60–63).

Juniper et al. (32) compared salmeterol (50 µg twice daily), albuterol (200 µg four times a day), and placebo in a crossover trial with each medication taken for 4 weeks. The subjects included 140 adults with mild to moderate asthma. Overall and individual domain scores on the Asthma Quality of Life Questionnaire were better (statistically and clinically important) for salmeterol compared with placebo and with albuterol (Fig. 2). Furthermore, changes in the overall score on the Asthma Quality of Life Questionnaire were significantly correlated with changes in morning peak flow ($r = 0.58$) and daytime symptoms ($r = 54$).

Rutten-van Molken and colleagues (60) compared two disease-specific instruments and two generic instruments in evaluating the effects of salmeterol (50 µg twice daily) versus albuterol (400 µg twice daily) on health status in 120 patients with moderate asthma. As expected, the long-acting salmeterol led to significant improvements over albuterol in all clinical outcomes. However, the disease-specific Asthma Quality of Life Questionnaire and the generic patient rating scale showed significantly greater improvement with salmeterol than with albuterol, whereas the Living with Asthma Questionnaire and the Sickness Impact Profile showed only a favorable trend for salmeterol.

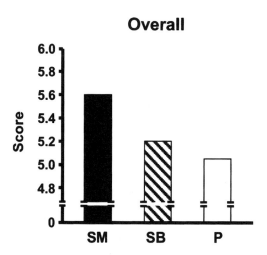

Figure 2 Overall scores at the end of the treatment period (4 weeks) on the Asthma Quality of Life Questionnaire with salmeterol (SM), salbutamol (SB), and placebo (P) in 140 adults with mild to moderate asthma. Salmeterol was more effective than placebo (mean difference = 0.55; $p < 0.0001$) and salbutamol (mean difference + 0.40; $p < 0.0001$). (From Ref. 24.)

Furthermore, only the Asthma Quality of Life Questionnaire correlated with the patient's overall assessment of efficacy ($r = 0.64$); the other three instruments failed to show any significant correlation. The authors concluded that of the two disease-specific instruments, the Asthma Quality of Life Questionnaire was more valid and more responsive to detect clinically important changes with salmeterol.

van der Molen et al. (61) investigated the benefits of formoterol (24 µg twice daily) or placebo for 6 months in 110 patients with moderate asthma (daily inhaled corticosteroids and beta$_2$-agonist use of five or more inhalations per week). Although formoterol improved the total score of the Living with Asthma Questionnaire (mean change, -0.05, $p = 0.048$), there were no significant differences observed in the scores on the Asthma Quality of Life Questionnaire or with two generic health status instruments (Short Form 36-item questionnaire and the General Well-Being Scale). The authors concluded that improvement in health status reported after 6 months with formoterol was very small and was observed with only one questionnaire.

Lockey et al. (62) compared the efficacy of salmeterol versus placebo in patients with asthma who experienced significant nocturnal symptoms and continued theophylline and/or inhaled corticosteroids. The mean change from baseline for the overall and individual domain scores on the Asthma Quality of Life Questionnaire were significantly greater with salmeterol than with placebo at 12 weeks.

Juniper et al. (63) evaluated the role of formoterol (24 µg twice daily) or placebo in 470 patients with asthma randomized to receive either 200 µg or 800 µg of budesonide for 1 year. Improvements in the scores for the Asthma Quality of Life Questionnaire were greatest in the group who received both formoterol and the higher dose of budesonide.

Anti-inflammatory Therapy

Jones and colleagues (30) used both the St. George's Respiratory Questionnaire and the Sickness Impact Profile to examine the efficacy of nedocromil sodium compared with placebo in 719 total patients with asthma who were also receiving either inhaled corticosteroids or inhaled and/or oral bronchodilators. After 48 weeks of treatment, the score for the impacts domain on the St. George's Respiratory Questionnaire was significantly greater than with placebo. In general, both patients and physicians judged that nedocromil was more effective than placebo.

In a 13-week placebo-controlled trial the efficacy of zafirlukast (20 mg twice daily), a leukotriene receptor antagonist, was evaluated in adults and adolescents with moderate asthma (64). Zafirlukast was significantly more effective in improving asthma symptoms and scores on the Asthma Quality of Life Questionnaire.

In a 12-week trial, 347 adults with moderate asthma were treated with hydrofluoroalkane-134a (HFA) beclomethasone dipropionate (400 µg per day), chlorofluorocarbon (CFC) beclomethasone (800 µg per day), or HFA placebo following withdrawal of 7 to 12 days of prednisone therapy (65). As expected, there was a deterioration in the Asthma Quality of Life Questionnaire score in the placebo group, whereas there was stability in these scores with both the HFA beclomethasone and CFC beclomethasone therapy.

These collective randomized, controlled trials demonstrated that long-acting inhaled beta-agonist bronchodilators and anti-inflammatory agents improve health status compared with placebo in patients with symptomatic asthma. Furthermore, these studies demonstrated that the different medications enhanced health status scores that generally exceeded the threshold values considered to be the minimal important difference.

B. Chronic Obstructive Pulmonary Disease

Pulmonary Rehabilitation

Various randomized controlled trials have demonstrated improvements in health status after pulmonary rehabilitation in patients with COPD (66–73), and this has been confirmed in a metanalysis (74). These studies incorporated inpatient (66,67), outpatient (68–71), and home-based (67,72,73) pulmonary rehabilitation and used either the Chronic Respiratory Disease Questionnaire or the St. George's Respiratory Questionnaire to measure health status. Overall, the improvements occurred in all four components of the Chronic Respiratory Disease Questionnaire with the greatest changes observed for dyspnea and the least changes for emotional function. The mean values for improvement exceeded the threshold for the minimal important difference in these studies. In the investigation by Guell et al. (71) improvements in scores on the Chronic Respiratory Disease Questionnaire were evident at the third month and continued with somewhat diminished magnitude in the second year of follow-up.

In the studies by Wedzicha and colleagues (69) and by Finnerty et al. (70) there were improvements with pulmonary rehabilitation in the St. George's Respiratory Questionnaire that reached the threshold for both clinical and statistical significance. A recent study demonstrated that the improved scores on the Chronic Respiratory Disease Questionnaire and on the St. George's Respiratory Questionnaire after rehabilitation exceeded the thresholds for the clinically important differences, while the clinical benefits on the St. George's Respiratory Questionnaire were maintained for 1 year (75).

In contrast, two controlled studies examining pulmonary rehabilitation did not show any benefit in health status using generic instruments such as the Quality of Well-Being (11) and the Short SF-36 questionnaire (69). However, an improvement in the SF-36 physical function score has been reported following pulmonary rehabilitation (75).

Rivera and colleagues (76) have shown that inspiratory muscle training at a training load of 60 to 70% of maximal sustained inspiratory pressure for 30 min daily, 6 days a week for 6 months led to significant and clinically meaningful improvements in health status measured on the Chronic Respiratory Disease Questionnaire compared with a control group who trained at zero load.

These overall findings demonstrate the advantage of the disease-specific instruments for measuring health status in evaluating the response to various pulmonary rehabilitaiton programs.

Bronchodilator Medications

Guyatt et al. (59) were the first investigators to show the benefits of bronchodilator therapy on health status in patients with COPD. They reported that patients treated with albuterol or theophylline for 2-week periods improved not only lung function and exercise capacity but also health status using the Chronic Respiratory Disease Questionnaire. The combination of both medications provided additional improvement.

Van Schayck et al. (77) reported that there were no significant differences in the Nottingham Health Profile between albuterol (400 µg per day) and ipratropium bromide (160 µg per day) over a 2-year period in 93 patients with mild COPD. The authors commented that a disease-specific health status instrument might have been more sensitive to detect a difference.

In 1997 Jones and colleagues (78) showed that salmeterol at a dose of 50 µg twice a day led to significant and clinically important improvements on the St. George's Respiratory Questionnaire, whereas the 100-µg dose given twice daily was no different than the placebo group. The authors proposed that the higher dose of salmeterol contributed to side effects such as central nervous system stimulation as evident by results of the SF-36 questionnaire. Of note, the pattern of changes in the SF-36 questionnaire was similar to that seen with the St. George's Respiratory Questionnaire (Fig. 3).

In two separate investigations using identical study designs the efficacy of salmeterol (50 µg twice a day) and ipratropium bromide (36 µg four times a day) were compared with placebo (two puffs four times a day) in patients with symptomatic COPD (79,80). The benefits of these bronchodilators on health status were inconsistent. After 12 weeks of therapy, the mean overall score for the Chronic Respiratory Disease Questionnaire was significantly higher for salmeterol (7.1 ± 1.4) and for ipratropium bromide (6.8 ± 1.2) compared with placebo (2.1 ± 1.3) in the study by Mahler et al. (79); however, there were no significant improvements in health status with either bronchodilator compared to placebo in the study by Rennard et al. (80).

ZuWallack and colleagues (81) examined the combination of salmeterol and theophylline compared with either agent alone in 943 patients with COPD. Although combination therapy provided significant improvements in pulmonary function and decreases in dyspnea scores, there were no significant differences in the overall Chronic Respiratory Disease Questionnaire scores at week 12 among the three treatment groups. However, a significantly higher percentage of patients in the combination group (52–54%) experienced a

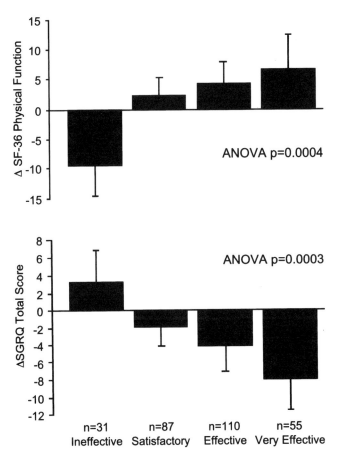

Figure 3 Relationship between the patients' global estimate of treatment efficacy and the St. George's Respiratory Questionnaire (SGRQ) total score and the Short Form-36 (SF-36) physical functioning score in 283 patients with COPD. Data from all three treatment groups are included. (From Ref. 78.)

clinically important difference (≥ 10 points) compared with salmeterol alone (36–45%) or theophylline alone (31–42%) at weeks 4 and 12.

Cook and colleagues (82) compared regular use of albuterol (two puffs four times a day) versus "as needed" use in 53 patients with COPD. All patients received ipratropium bromide and inhaled corticosteroids as routine therapy. Despite greater beta-agonist therapy with regular prescription, there were no differences in any outcomes between the two groups. In particular, there were no differences in any of the four domains on the Chronic Respiratory Disease Questionnaire.

Dahl et al. (83) examined the effectiveness of 12 or 24 μg of formoterol twice daily with ipratropium bromide (40 μg four times a day) and with placebo in a total of 780 patients with COPD over 12 weeks. Both doses of formoterol resulted in significant improvements in health status on the St. George's Respiratory Questionnaire, although only the 12-μg dose (-5.1 in total score) exceeded the threshold for the minimal important difference (-4).

Casaburi et al. (84) reported that tiotropium, a once-daily inhaled anticholinergic bronchodilator, produced a significant improvement in health status as measured on the St. George's Respiratory Questionnaire compared to placebo over one year. Similar improvements were observed with tiotropium in physical health domains (physical function, role function, and general health) on the SF-36 questionnaire.

These numerous studies demonstrate the clinical benefits of different bronchodilator medications and pulmonary rehabilitation in improving health status in patients with COPD.

Inhaled Corticosteroids

Spencer et al. (20) reported that inhaled fluticasone (500 μg twice daily) slowed the decline in health status by 39% as measured by the St. George's Respiratory Questionnaire compared with placebo over a 3-year period in a total of 751 patients with moderate to severe COPD.

VI. Summary

The measurement of health status has become an important outcome variable in evaluating the response to treatment in patients with advanced respiratory disease. The majority of questionnaires used to quantify health status have been developed within the past decade. Thus, the use of these instruments in randomized controlled trials has just started to become standard for examining efficacy and effectiveness of a specific intervention. Furthermore, the current literature reveals that these questionnaires have been used predominantly in patients with asthma and with COPD. This is really no surprise, as these airway diseases represent the two most common chronic respiratory illnesses in the world today.

What is the future of measuring health status? We believe that there will be increasing interest in this outcome measure by federal and state health care agencies, health care organizations, insurance companies, regulatory agencies, and pharmaceutical companies. This anticipated greater application represents the simple recognition that symptoms, such as breathlessness and cough, of chronic respiratory disease and their impact on an individual's ability to perform and enjoy the activities of daily living are clearly as important as the "hard data" of chest radiographs, computed tomography (CT) scans, and physiological tests considered essential in caring for our patients. Moreover, we expect that health status will become a routine measure in trials examining treatment effects in other advanced respiratory disorders including interstitial lung disease, cystic fibrosis, pulmonary vascular disease, diseases involving the respiratory muscles, etc.

What instruments should be used to measure health status? That is a difficult question to answer. Certainly, there are ongoing efforts directed toward the development of new instruments as well as modification of existing questionnaires in an attempt to improve the measurement qualities. We anticipate that such interest will continue in the future. Whether agreement will be reached on which one or two instruments are the "best" and therefore preferred remains to be determined. It is possible and even likely that certain questionnaires will perform better and be preferred in certain diseases. For example, the Asthma Quality of Life Questionnaire (22) has been used in many studies of patients with asthma, while the Chronic Respiratory Disease Questionnaire (23) and the St. George's Respiratory Questionnaire (29) have been the major instruments used to measure health status in trials of patients with COPD. It is clear from the results of published studies that the disease-specific instruments are more responsive to demonstrate both statistically significant and clinically meaningful changes with various medications and with exercise training. Furthermore, the generic instruments provide information on the overall burden of the disease on other health problems such as everyday functioning and emotional well-being (85,86). Thus, a generic instrument may indicate an unfavorable side effect of a medication that might not be detected with a disease-specific instrument. It may therefore be reasonable to use both a disease-specific and a generic questionnaire to quantify health status in clinical trials.

References

1. Jones PW, Quirk FH, Bayerstock CM. Why quality of life should be used in the treatment of patients with respiratory disease. Monaldi Arch Chest Dis 1994; 49:79–82.
2. Curtis JR, Martin DP, Martin TR. Patient-assessed health outcomes in chronic lung disease. Am J Respir Crit Care Med 1997; 156:1032–1039.
3. Mahler DA. How should health-related quality of life be assessed in patients with COPD? Chest 2000; 117:54S–57S.
4. Guyatt GH, Feeny DH, Patrick DL. Measuring health-related quality of life. Ann Intern Med 1993; 118:622–629.
5. Juniper EF, Guyatt GH, Willan A, Griffith LE. Determining a minimal important change in a disease-specific quality-of-life questionnaire. J Clin Epidemiol 1994; 47:81–87.
6. Redelmeier DA, Guyatt GH, Goldstein RS. Assessing the minimal important difference in symptoms: a comparison of two techniques. J Clin Epidemiol 1996; 49:1215–1219.

7. Barely EA, Jones PW. A comparison of global questions versus health status questionnaires as measures of the severity and impact of asthma. Eur Respir J 1999; 14:591–596.
8. Bergner M, Bobbitt RA, Carter WB, Gilson BS. The sickness impack profile: development and final revision of a health status measure. Med Care 1981; 19:787–805.
9. McSweeney JA, Grant I, Heaton RK, Adams RK, Timms RM. Life quality of patients with chronic obstructive pulmonary disease. Arch Intern Med 1982; 142:473–478.
10. Carone M, Jones PW. Health status "quality of life." In: Donner CF, Decramer M, eds. Pulmonary Rehabilitation: European Respiratory Monograph. Sheffield, UK: European Respiratory Society Journals, 2000:22–35.
11. Kaplan RM, Atkins CJ, Timms R. Validity of a quality of well-being scale as an outcome measure in chronic obstructive pulmonary disease. J Chronic Dis 1984; 37:85–95.
12. Ries AL, Kaplan RM, Limberg TM, Prewitt LM. Effects of pulmonary rehabilitation on physiologic and psychosocial outcomes in patients with chronic obstructive pulmonary disease. Ann Intern Med 1995; 122:823–832.
13. Hunt SM, McEwen J, McKenna SP. Measuring Health Status. Kent, UK: Croom Helm, 1986.
14. Ferrer M, Alonso J, Morera, Marrades RM, Khalaf A, Aguar MC, Plaza V, PrietoL, Anto JM. Chronic obstructive pulmonary disease stage and health-related quality of life. Ann Intern Med 1997; 127:1072–1079.
15. The EuroQol Group. EuroQol—a new facility for the measurement of health-related quality of life. Health Policy 1990; 16:199–208.
16. Ware JE Jr, Sherbourne CD. The MOS short-form health survey (SF-36). 1. Conceptual framework and item selection. Med Care 1992; 30:473–483.
17. Bousquet J, Knani J, Dhivert H, Richard A, Chicoye A, Ware JE Jr, Michel FB. Quality of life in asthma: internal consistency and validity of the SF-36 questionnaire. Am J Respir Crit Care Med 1994; 149:371–375.
18. Mahler DA, Mackowiak JI. Evaluation of the short-form 36-item questionnaire to measure health-related quality of life in patients with COPD. Chest 1995; 107:1585–1589.
19. Mahler DA, Tomlinson D, Olmstead EM, Tosteson ANA, O"Connor GT. Changes in dyspnea, health status, and lung function in chronic airway disease. Am J Respir Crit Care Med 1995; 151:61–65.
20. Spencer S, Calverley PMA, Burge PS, Jones PW, ISOLDE study group. Health status deterioration in patients with chronic obstructive pulmonary disease. Am J Respir Crit Care Med 2001; 163:122–128.
21. Jones PW. Quality of the measurement for patients with diseases of the airways. Thorax 1991; 46:676–682.
22. Juniper EF, Guyatt GH, Ferrie PJ, Griffith LE. Measuring quality of life in asthma. Am Rev Respir Dis 1993; 147:832–838.
23. Guyatt GH, Berman LB, Townsend M, Pugsley SO, Chambers L. A measure of quality of life for clinical trials in chronic lung disease. Thorax 1987; 42:773–778.
24. Juniper EF. Quality-of-life measures. In: Kotses H, Harver A, eds. Lung Biology in Health and Disease Series: Vol 113. Self-Management of Asthma. New York: Marcel Dekker, 1998:91–116.

25. Hyland ME, Finnis S, Irvine SH. A scale for assessing quality of life in adult asthma suffers. J Psychosom Res 1991; 35:99–110.
26. Marks GB, Dunn SM, Woolcock AJ. A scale for the measurement of quality of life in adults with asthma. J Clin Epidemiol 1992; 45:461–472.
27. Marks GB, Dunn SM, Woolcock AJ. An evaluation of an asthma quality of life questionnaire as a measure of change in adults with asthma. J Clin Epidemiol 1993; 46:1103–1111.
28. Creer TL, Wigal JK, Kotses H, McConnaughy K, Winder JA. A life activities questionnaire for adult asthma. J Asthma 1992; 29:393–399.
29. Jones PW, Quirk FH, Baveystock CM, Littlejohns P. A self-complete measure of health status for chronic airflow limitation: the St. George's Respiratory Questionnaire. Am Rev Respir Dis 1992; 145:1321–1327.
30. Jones PW and the nedocromil sodium quality of life study group. Quality of life, symptoms and pulmonary function in asthma: long-term treatment with nedocromil sodium examined in a controlled multicentre trial. Eur Respir J 1994; 7:55–62.
31. Rowe BH, Oxman AD. Performance of an asthma quality of life questionnaire in an outpatient setting. Am Rev Respir Dis 1993; 148:675–681.
32. Juniper EF, Johnston PR, Borkhoff CM, Guyatt GH, Boulet LP, Haukioja A. Quality of life in asthma clinical trials: comparison of salmeterol and salbutamol. Am J Respir Crit Care Med 1995; 151:66–70.
33. Barely EA, Quirk FH, Jones PW. Asthma health status measurement in clinical practice: validation of a new short and simple instrument. Respir Med 1998; 92:1207–1214.
34. Juniper EF, Buist AS, Cox FM, Ferrie PJ, King DR. Validation of a standardized version of the Asthma Quality of Life questionnaire. Chest 1999; 115:1265–1279.
35. Juniper EF, Guyatt GH, Cox FM, Ferrie PJ, King DR. Development and validation of the mini asthma quality of life questionnaire. Eur Respir J 1999; 14:32–38.
36. Gupchup GV, Wolfgang AP, Thomas J III. Reliability and validity of the asthma quality of life questionnaire—Marks in a sample of adult asthmatic patients in the United States. Clin Ther 1997; 19:1116–1125.
37. Katz PP, Eisner MD, Henke J, Shiboski S, Yelin EH, Blanc PD. The Marks asthma quality of life questionnaire: further validation and examination of responsiveness to change. J Clin Epidemiol 1999; 52:667–675.
38. Bayliss MS, Espindle DM, Buchner D, Blaiss MS, Ware JE. A new tool for monitoring asthma outcomes: the ITG asthma short form. Qual Life Res 2000; 9:451–466.
39. Anie KA, Jones PW, Hilton SR, Anderson HR. A computer-assisted telephone interview technique for assessment of asthma morbidity and drug use in adult asthma. J Clin Epdemiol 1996; 49:653–656.
40. Quirk FH, Jones PW. Patients' perception of distress due to symptoms and effects of asthma on daily living and an investigation of possible influential factors. Clin Sci 1990; 79:17–22.
41. Quirk FH, Baveystock CM, Wilson RC, Jones PW. Influence of demographic and disease-related factors on the degree of distress associated with symptoms and restrictions on daily living due to asthma in six countries. Eur Respir J 1991; 4:167–171.

42. Quirk FH, Jones PW. Repeatability of two new short airways questionnaires. Thorax 1994; 49:1075P.

43. Hajiro T, Nishimura K, Jones PW, Tsukino M, Ikeda A, Koyama H, Izumi T. A novel, short, and simple questionnaire to measure health-related quality of life in patients with chronic obstructive pulmonary disease. Am J Respir Crit Care Med 1999; 159:1874–1878.

44. Tu SP, McDonell MB, Spertus JA, Steele BG, Fihn SD. A new self-administered questionnaire to monitor health-related quality of life in patients with COPD. Chest 1997; 112:614–622.

45. Martinez TY, Pereira CAC, dos Santos ML, Ciconelli RM, Guimaraes SM, Martinez JAB. Evaluation of the short-form 36-item questionnaire to measure health-related quality of life in patients with idiopathic pulmonary fibrosis. Chest 2000; 117:1627–1632.

46. Chang JA, Curtis JR, Patrick DL, Raghu G. Assessment of health-related quality of life in patients with interstitial lung disease. Chest 1999; 116:1175–1182.

47. De Vries J, Seebregts A, Drent M. Assessing health status and quality of life in idiopathic pulmonary fibrosis. Which measure should be used? Respir Med 2000; 94:273–278.

48. De Vries J, Kessels BLJ, Drent M. Quality of life of idiopathic pulmonary fibrosis patients. Eur Respir J 2001; 17:954–961.

49. WHOQOL group. The World Health Organization quality of life assessment (WHOQOL): position paper from the World Health Organization. Soc Sc Med 1995; 41:1403–1409.

50. Wilson CB, Jones PW, O'Leary CJ, Cole PJ, Wilson R. Validation of the St. George's Respiratory Questionnaire in bronchiectasis. Am J Respir Crit Care Med 1997; 156:536–541.

51. Wilson CB, Jones PW, O'Leary CJ, Hansell DM, Cole PJ, Wilson R. Effect of sputum bacteriology on the quality of life of patients with bronchiectasis. Eur Respir J 1997; 10:1754–1760.

52. Orenstein DM, Pattishall EN, Nixon PA, Ross EA, Kaplan RM. Quality of well-being before and after antibiotic treatment of pulmonary exacerbation in patients with cystic fibrosis. Chest 1990; 98:1081–1084.

53. Orenstein DM, Kaplan RM. Measuring the quality of well-being in cystic fibrosis and lung transplantation. Chest 1991; 100:1016–1018.

54. Busschbach JJV, Horikx PE, van den JMM, de la Riviere AB, de Charro FT. Measuring the quality of life before and after bilateral lung transplantation in patients with cystic fibrosis. Chest 1991; 105:911–917.

55. Jones PW. Interpreting thresholds for a clinically significant change in health status in asthma and COPD. Eur Respir J 2002; 19:398–404.

56. Jaeschke R, Singer J, Guyatt GH. Measurement of health status. Ascertaining the minimal clinically important difference. Control Clin Trials 1989; 10:407–415.

57. Lydick E, Epstein RS. Interpretation of quality of life changes. Qual Life Res 1993; 2:221–226.

58. Jones PW, Quirk FH, Baveystock CM. The St. George's Respiratory Questionnaire. Respir Med 1991; 85(suppl B):25–31.

59. Guyatt GH, Townsend M, Pugsley SO, Keller JL, Short HD, Taylor DW, Newhouse MT. Bronchodilators in chronic air-flow limitation: effects on airway function, exercise capacity, and quality of life. Am Rev Respir Dis 1987; 135:1069–1074.

60. Rutten-van Molken MPMH, Custers F, Van Doorslaer EKA, Jansen CCM, Heurman L, Maesen FPV, Smeets JJ, Bommer AM, Raaijmakers JAM. Comparison of performance of four instruments in evaluating the effects of salmeterol on asthma quality of life. Eur Respir J 1995; 8:888–898.

61. van der Molen T, Sears MR, de Graff CS, Postma DS, Maeyboom-de Jong B. Quality of life during formoterol treatment: comparison between asthma-specific and generic questionnaires. Eur Rerspir J 1998; 12:30–34.

62. Lockey RF, DuBuske LM, Friedman B, Petrocella V, Cox F, Rickard K. Nocturnal asthma: effect of salmeterol on quality of life and clinical outcomes. Chest 1999; 115:666–673.

63. Juniper EF, Svensson K, O'Byrne PM, Barnes PJ, Bauer CA, Lofdahl CG, Postma DS, Pauwels RA, Tattersfield AE, Ullman A. Asthma quality of life during 1 year of treatment with budesonide with or without formoterol. Eur Respir J 1999; 14:1038–1043.

64. Nathan RA, Bernstein JA, Bielory L, Bonuccelli CM, Calhoun WJ, Galant SP, Hanby LA, Kemp JP, Kylstra JW, Nayak AS, O'Connor JP, Schwartz HJ, Southern DL, Spector SL, Williams PV. Zafirlukast improves asthma symptoms and quality of life in patients with moderate reversible airflow obstruction. J Allergy Clin Immunol 1998; 102:935–942.

65. Juniper EF, Buist AS. Health-related quality of life in moderate asthma: 400 µg hydrofluoroalkane beclomethasone dipropionate vs 800 µg chlorofluorocarbon beclomethasone dipropionate. Chest 1999; 116:1297–1303.

66. Goldstein RS, Gort EH, Stubbing D, Avendano MA, Guyatt GH. Randomised controlled trial of respiratory rehabilitation. Lancet 1994; 344:1394–1397.

67. Behnke M, Taube C, Kirsten D, Lehnigk B, Jorres A, Magnussen H. Home-based exercise is capable of preserving improvements in severe chronic obstructive pulmonary disease. Respir Med 2000; 94:1184–1191.

68. Bendstrup KE, Ingemann Jensen J, Holm S, Bengtsson B. Out-patient rehabilitation improves activities of daily living, quality of life and exercise tolerance in chronic obstructive pulmonary disease. Eur Respir J 1997; 10:2801–2806.

69. Wedzicha JA, Bestall JC, Garrod R, Garnham R, Paul EA, Jones PW. Randomized controlled trial of pulmonary rehabilitation in severe chronic obstructive pulmonary disease patients, stratified with the MRC dyspnoea scale. Eur Respir J 1998; 12:363–369.

70. Finnerty JP, Keeping I, Bullough I, Jones J. The effectiveness of outpatient pulmonary rehabilitation in chronic lung disease: a randomized controlled trial. Chest 2001; 119:1705–1710.

71. Guell R, Casan P, Belda J, Sangenis M, Morante F, Guyatt GH, Sanchis J. Long-term effects of outpatient rehabilitation of COPD. Chest 2000; 117:976–983.

72. Wijkstra PJ, Altena RV, Kraan J, Otten V, Postma DS, Koeter GH. Quality of life in patients with chronic obstructive pulmonary disease improves after rehabilitation at home. Eur Respir J 1994; 7:269–273.

73. Cambach W, Chadwick-Strayer RVM, Wagenaar RC, van Keimpema AR, Kemper HC. The effects of a community-based pulmonary rehabilitation programme on exercise tolerance and quality of life: a randomized controlled trial. Eur Respir J 1997; 10:104–113.

74. Lacasse Y, Wong E, Guyatt GH, King D, Cook DJ, Goldstein RS. Meta-analysis of respiratory rehabilitation in chronic obstructive pulmonary disease. Lancet 1996; 348:1115–1119.

75. Griffiths TL, Burr ML, Campbell IA, Lewis-Jenkins V, Mullins J, Shiels K, Turner-Lawlor PJ, Payne N, Newcombe RG, Ionescu AA, Tunbridge TJ, Lonescu AA. Results at 1 year of outpatient multisciplinary pulmonary rehabilitation: a randomised controlled trial. Lancet 2000; 355:362–368.

76. Rivera HS, Montemajor Rubio T, Ortega Ruiz F, Cejudo Ramos P, del Castillo Otero D, Elias Hernandez T, Castillo Gomez J. Inspiratory muscle training in patients with COPD: effect on dyspnea, exercise performance, and quality of life. Chest 2001; 120:748–756.

77. van Schayck CP, Rutten-van Molken MPMH, van Doorslaer EKA, Folgering H, van Weel C. Two-year bronchodilator treatment in patients with mild airflow obstruction. Chest 1992; 102:1384–1391.

78. Jones PW, Bosh TK. Quality of life changes in COPD patients treated with salmeterol Am J Respir Crit Care Med 1997; 155:1283–1289.

79. Mahler DA, Donohue JF, Barbee RA, Goldman MD, Gross NJ, Wisniewski ME, Yancey SW, Zakes BA, Rickard KA, Anderson WH. Efficacy of salmeterol xinafoate in the treatment of COPD. Chest 1999; 115:957–965.

80. Rennard SI, Andeerson W, ZuWallack R, Broughton J, Bailey W, Friedman M, Wisniewski M, Rickard K. Use of a long-acting inhaled β_2-adrenergic agonist, salmeterol xinafoate, in patients with chronic obstructive pulmonary disease. Am J Respir Crit Care Med 2001; 163:1087–1092.

81. ZuWallack RL, Mahler DA, Reilly D, Church N, Emmett A, Rickard K, Knobil K. Salmeterol plus theophylline combination therapy in the treatment of COPD. Chest 2001; 119:1661–1670.

82. Cook D, Guyatt G, Wong E, Goldstein R, Bedard M, Austin P, Ramsdale H, Jaeschke R, Sears M. Regular versus as-needed short-acting inhaled beta-agonist therapy for chronic obsttructive pulmonary disease. Am J Respir Crit Care Med 2001; 163:85–90.

83. Dahl R, Greefhorst LAPM, Nowak D, Nonikov V, Byrne AM, Thomson MH, Till D, Della Cioppa G. Inhaled formoterol dry powder versus ipratropium bromide in chronic obstructive pulmonary disease. Am J Respir Crit Care Med 2001; 164:778–784.

84. Casaburi R, Mahler DA, Jones PW, Wanner A, San Pedro G, ZuWallack RL, Menjoge SS, Serby CW, Witek T Jr. A long-term evaluation of once-daily inhaled tiotropium in chronic obstructive pulmonary disease. Eur Respir J. 2002; 19:217–224.

85. Harper R, Brazier JE, Waterhouse JC, Walters SJ, Jones NMB, Howard P. Comparison of outcome measures for patients with chronic obstructive pulmonary disease (COPD) in an outpatient setting. Thorax 1997; 52:879–887.

86. Engstrom CP, Persson LO, Larsson S, Sullivan M. Health-related quality of life in COPD: why both disease-specific and generic measures should be used. Eur Respir J 2001; 18:69–76.

20

Traveling with Supplemental Oxygen for Patients with Chronic Lung Disease

LOUTFI SAMI ABOUSSOUAN

Wayne State University School of
  Medicine
Detroit, Michigan, U.S.A.

JAMES K. STOLLER

Cleveland Clinic Foundation
Cleveland, Ohio, U.S.A.

I. Introduction

As medical advances have improved the quality of life of patients with lung disease, many are now considering travel by air. Also, many patients with advanced lung disease are referred for further evaluation at specialized centers. This may include evaluation for lung transplantation, lung volume reduction surgery, second opinions, etc. This chapter provides a comprehensive review of issues regarding air travel by such individuals. We discuss the fundamental physics of atmospheric pressure at altitude and in aircraft, followed by the physiological consequences of air travel, particularly for the patient with lung disease. We then review the available literature on the risks of in-flight emergencies and deaths and the contribution of hypoxemia and lung disease to those events. The different currently available methods for the prediction of in-flight oxygen levels and the literature on specific oxygen recommendations are reviewed. Finally, we summarize practical recommendations for the air traveler who requires in-flight oxygen and for health care providers advising such individuals.

II. Environmental Oxygen at Altitude and in Aircraft

Atmospheric pressure depends on the mass of atmosphere at a certain altitude and is determined by gravitational influences. Accordingly, there is an exponential decrease in gas density and atmospheric pressure as altitude increases:

$$PB \text{ in mmHg} = 760 \times e^{-\text{altitude in feet}/26,000} \tag{1}$$

$$\text{Gas density (relative to ground level)} = e^{-\text{altitude in feet}/26,000} \tag{2}$$

where 26,000 represent atmospheric scale height, a useful measure of the vertical extent of the atmosphere, and 760 an estimate of ground level atmospheric pressure in millimeters of mercury.

While the fractional concentration of inspired oxygen (F_{IO_2}) remains constant at 0.21 with increasing altitude up to about 70,000 ft (1), the drop in barometric pressure results in a decline in alveolar oxygen pressure (P_{AO_2}) according to the alveolar air equations:

$$P_{AO_2} = P_{IO_2} - P_{ACO_2} \times [F_{IO_2} + (1 - F_{IO_2})/R] \tag{3}$$

$$P_{IO_2} = (P_B - P_{H_2O}) \times F_{IO_2} \tag{4}$$

where P_{IO_2} is the pressure of inspired oxygen in trachea, P_{H_2O} is airway water vapor pressure in the trachea and is determined by temperature (47 mmHg at 37°C, 55 mmHg at 40°C), P_{ACO_2} is the pressure of alveolar carbon dioxide and is usually assumed to be equal to arterial carbon dioxide pressure (P_{aCO_2}), and R is the respiratory exchange ratio. The respiratory exchange ratio depends on the predominant fuel used for cellular metabolism and increases with increasing altitude from 0.85 at ground level up to 1.05 at 22,000 ft but is generally assumed to be constant at 0.8 (3).

For general economy and efficiency of operation, modern aircraft fly at altitudes of up to around 44,000 ft, where PB is < 160 mmHg and P_{IO_2} is about 20 mmHg (4,5). Sudden exposures to these altitudes, as after accidental depressurization, can be associated with nitrogen embolism and severe hypoxemia, with subsequent useful consciousness lasting for fewer than 15 sec (4). Aircraft are therefore pressurized with the maximal cabin pressures that are determined by the structurally allowable maximal differential pressure between the cabin and the outside atmospheric pressure. Maintaining the pressure inside the aircraft cabin (cabin pressure) at the ground level pressure would require stronger and impracticably heavy aircraft structures and would unacceptably reduce fuel economy. Recognizing this, the Federal Aviation Administration currently specifies that cabin altitude should be maintained at < 8000 ft, with short excursions above 10,000 ft allowable—e.g., when necessary to avoid adverse weather. Although most of the altitude tolerance information has been obtained from military studies (4), a National Academy of Sciences report concluded that cabin pressurization to 5000 to 8000 ft is physiologically safe with no need for oxygen supplementation in most individuals (6).

Structural differences cause significant variation in the cabin altitude reached by different aircraft. For instance, at their maximal differential pressure, different airplanes reach a cabin altitude of 8000 ft at different altitudes, ranging from 35,000 ft for the B-737 to 46,200 feet for the B-747 (6). In one study of direct measurements of in-flight cabin altitude in 204 commercial flights, the cabin altitude was found to range from sea level to 8915 feet, with no significant difference between domestic and international flights. With some exceptions, notably the Concorde, which flies higher and maintains lower cabin pressures, more modern aircraft cruise at higher altitudes and at higher cabin pressures, thereby exposing passengers to lower oxygen levels (7).

III. Physiological Consequences of Air Travel

A. Decompression Sickness and Barobariatrauma

Altitude-induced decompression sickness occurs when nitrogen gas normally stored in a dissolved state in tissues and fluids is released under hypobaric conditions with formation of bubbles, following Henry's law. It can manifest with joint pains ("the bends"), mottled skin, or more seriously with "the chokes," which present nearly universally with substernal chest pain and occasionally also with dyspnea and cough comprising the classically described triad (8). Additional symptoms include petechiae in the neck, shoulder, or axilla; pallor; and tachycardia. There is no safe altitude threshold below which decompression sickness cannot occur. However, there is little evidence that it occurs at altitudes below 18,000 ft, with most instances occurring at altitudes above 25,000 ft, making decompression illness an unlikely occurrence within the context of commercial air travel (9). Notable exceptions include individuals who have Scuba-dived fewer than 24 hours earlier (who can develop symptoms of decompression sickness at altitudes as low as 5000 ft) (9), and the markedly obese patient (barobariatrauma) because of the high concentration of nitrogen in adipose tissue (1). Advanced age, exertion at altitude, and alcohol consumption have been cited as other risk factors (10,11).

B. Effects on Pulmonary Function and Ventilatory Response in Chronic Obstructive Pulmonary Disease

Exposure to altitude can exert physiological effects on lung function. For example, in one study of chronic obstructive pulmonary disease (COPD) and healthy subjects, hypobaric hypoxia was associated with a decline in forced vital capacity (FVC) by an average of 0.123 L, which correlated with an increased residual volume (RV). Maximum voluntary ventilation (MVV) decreased by 1.24 L/min in the COPD patients, correlating with a decreased

FVC and increased RV. Resting arterial blood gases were not changed (12). In another study, exposure to a hypoxic gas mixture increased respiratory frequency and minute ventilation (VE), with no significant change in V_{CO_2}, V_{O_2}, and the respiratory exchange ratio $R(V_{CO_2}/V_{O_2})$ (13). This increase in ventilation has been proposed to explain the decreased variability between supine and sitting Pa_{O_2} in altitude compared to sea level in patients with interstitial lung disease and COPD (14). Last, while most studies concerning the effect of air travel have generally included patients with COPD, there may be differences in the response of patients with other type of lung diseases. For instance in one study, patients with restrictive pulmonary disease experienced greater decreases in pulse oximetry saturations and had more serious discomfort than patients with asthma or COPD (15).

C. Effects on Cardiovascular Function in Chronic Obstructive Pulmonary Disease

Studies have examined the effects of altitude exposure on cardiovascular function in patients with COPD. For example, blood pressure and pulsus paradoxus were not significantly changed in subjects with severe COPD (mean FEV_1 31% predicted) exposed to a simulated altitude of 8000 ft in a hypobaric chamber, although subsequent oxygen supplementation decreased systolic and pulse pressures and pulsus paradoxus (16). Cardiac arrhythmias were rare and heart rate was unchanged in that study. These results contrast those of Gong et al. who studied patients with less severe chronic but stable airway obstruction (mean FEV_1 44% predicted), who had increased heart rate upon exposures to progressively hypoxemic gas mixtures (i.e., hypoxic hypoxia) (13). Asymptomatic premature atrial and ventricular beats were noted in 45% of those subjects (13). A potential reason for the discrepancy of those results is that hypoxic exposure is achieved progressively (at a rate of 500 ft/min) during hypobaric exposure and more acutely while breathing hypoxic mixtures.

D. Effects of Smoking on Air Travel

Many airlines voluntarily ban smoking on their flights and official regulations are likewise increasingly restrictive. For instance, the U.S. Department of Transportation has banned smoking on all scheduled passenger flights to and from the United States effective June 4, 2000. Smokers are therefore likely to smoke just before a flight and may have a decreased altitude tolerance (17). In one study of physically fit volunteer smokers and nonsmokers, smokers who smoked before a simulated flight had elevated heart rate, decreased transcutaneous P_{CO_2}, decreased task performance, and higher error rates at altitude compared to nonsmokers (17).

E. Effects of Diet on Hypoxemia During Air Travel

Dietary considerations may compound the effects of hypoxemia during air travel, though much remains to be determined before firm recommendations can be made. For instance, because carbohydrate metabolism elevates the respiratory quotient R to 1, thereby increasing alveolar ventilation and Pa_{O_2} [Eq. (3)], carbohydrate-rich foods and drinks have been advocated for air travelers with borderline hypoxemia (18). However, excessive dietary carbohydrate also increases lipogenesis, CO_2 production, and ventilatory requirements and cannot be recommended uniformly at altitude for patients with advanced lung disease (19). Conversely, alcohol metabolism decreases the respiratory quotient towards 0.67 and may decrease PA_{O_2} and Pa_{O_2} [Eq. (3)] (19). However, moderate consumption of two glasses of wine every evening for 6 weeks was not associated with demonstrable changes in the respiratory quotient (20). There may be other reasons to recommend avoidance of alcohol, such as the risk of compounding the effects of hypoxemia on cognition. Another consideration is the expansion of intestinal gases as cabin pressure decreases, with bloating and discomfort, which in turn may aggravate the postprandial dyspnea and desaturation experienced commonly by travelers with COPD (21). Heavy meals before and during a flight should be avoided.

IV. Risks of Air Travel

The available data on in-flight emergencies are limited by the lack of a systematic or centralized mechanism to collect and report those incidents. The available studies are therefore skewed towards cases collected from a specific airport (22,23) or airline (24) or those in which a death occurred (25) or the emergency kit was used (26,27). Moreover, the method of ascertainment of in-flight incidents differs between studies (Table 1). In general, larger studies that include more serious incidents, such as those lasting for more than 1 hr and those requiring the emergency kit use or the assistance of a telemedicine company, indicate a low frequency of 2.6 to 13 emergencies per million passengers (Table 1). Less serious events are more frequent, with up to 30 events per million passengers (Table 1). The Office of Aviation Medicine recently compiled data from two airlines and two in-flight medical care companies representing a total of nine U.S. carriers and 65% of the domestic U.S. enplanements from 1990 to 1993 (28). These data indicate a doubling in the incidence of in-flight medical emergencies from fewer than 2 emergencies per million enplanements in 1990 to nearly 4 emergencies per million enplanements in 1993, suggesting that the increase in emergencies is not solely due to the increase in number of travelers (Fig. 1). Syncope, neurological, and cardiac episodes were the most frequent, whereas cardiac, neurological, and respiratory conditions accounted for most of the diversions to nearby airports (28). Respiratory conditions including dyspnea, asthma, and COPD account for 6 to 12% of all reported medical events during air travel (22–27,29). Up to

Table 1 Summary of Available Reports of In-flight Medical Emergencies and Deaths

First author	Period covered	Source	Ascertainment method	Number of travelers $\times 10^3$	Deaths/billion passengers (n)	Medical interventions/ million passengers (n)
Cummins (25)	1977–1984	IATA	Reports of deaths by airlines	1,962,600	294 (578)	—
Cummins (22)	Sept. 1986–Aug. 1987	SEA	Emergency calls to the airport	7,230[a]	0 (0)	25.3 (183)
Speizer (23)	Oct. 1985–Mar. 1986	LAX	Complaints by arriving passengers	8,735	800 (7)	29.8 (260)
Cottrell[c] (26)	July 1986–June 1987	United Airlines	Emergency kit use	55,000	50 (3)	13.1 (115)[b] 6.6 (362)
Hordinsky (27)	Aug. 1986–July 1988	FAA	Emergency kit use	900,000[a]	40 (33)	2.6 (2322)

| Skjenna (24) | 1982–1988 | Air Canada | Emergency kit use, medical assistance | 84,565 | 320 (27) | 29.1 (2461)[d] |
| DeJohn (28) | Jan. 1990–Dec. 1993 | FAA | In-flight medical emergencies[f] | 940,000[a] | — | 11.0 (928)[e] 2.6 (2388) |

Key: FAA, Federal Aviation Administration; IATA, International Air Transport Association; LAX, Los Angeles International Airport; SEA, Seattle-Tacoma Airport.

[a] Calculated from data or figures provided in the paper.
[b] Symptoms lasting more than 1 hr.
[c] Reflects data from an FAA mandated monitoring included in the larger Hordinsky report.
[d] All incidents requiring assistance by medical professionals.
[e] Incidents requiring use of the emergency kit.
[f] As reported by participating air carriers and in-flight medical care delivery companies.

Source: Adapted from Ref. 29.

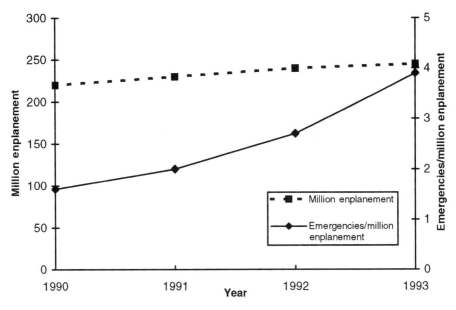

Figure 1 In-flight medical emergency rate per million enplanements, 1990 to 1993. (From Ref. 28.)

18% of patients with COPD who travel by air experience transient symptoms (such as dyspnea, edema, wheezing, cyanosis, chest pain) and 4.5% request oxygen while on board (30). Moreover, COPD is a common diagnosis in individuals seeking posttravel medical attention (31).

There are also 40 to 800 deaths per billion (1×10^9) passengers (Table 1). In the largest survey by the International Air Transport Association (IATA) between 1977 and 1984, there were 577 deaths, representing one death event per 3.2 million passengers (25). In a subsequent 2-year reporting period (1986–1988) on the use of emergency medical equipment mandated by the U.S. Department of Transportation, there were 33 deaths, representing 1 death event per 27 million passengers (32). In both those reports, cardiac events accounted for 48 to 56% of death events (25,32), whereas pulmonary causes accounted for 6% (25). The variability in death rates in the studies outlined in Table 1 may reflect differences between international and domestic travelers and travel circumstances, such as longer flight distance and sicker patients on international flights. For instance, studies originating from international airports or from the IATA member airlines report higher death rates (Table 1). Also, several deaths in the IATA survey were in aeromedical patients, with 6% already being accompanied by medical personnel (25).

Although those incidents are rare, further increases may be expected due to:

1. The increase in number of travelers. Data from the Air Transport Action Group reveal that more than 1600 million passengers were carried by the world's airlines in 1998 and passenger and freight traffic are expected to increase at an average annual rate of around 4 to 5% between 1998 and 2010.
2. An increase in age of the traveling population.
3. A possible increase in altitude exposure as more efficient airplanes fly higher (7).
4. An increase in travel by individuals with medical conditions (24).
5. The Air Carrier Access Act of 1986 and the Americans with Disability Act of 1990, which ensure that disabled individuals are treated without discrimination and encourage their travel.

Hypoxemia may clearly be contributing to a large portion of in-flight cardiac and pulmonary complications. It is reasonable to conclude that many of those complications are potentially preventable if a need for oxygen supplementation is identified before the flight. However, the impact of such early intervention on in-flight emergencies, oxygen requests, and posttravel symptoms and medical complications remains to be determined.

Though presumably unrelated to the hypobaric hypoxic conditions during flight, deep venous thrombosis and pulmonary embolism have attracted increasing attention as complications of air travel, especially in coach class (where the name *economy class syndrome* has been applied). Recent incidence data indicate a mean rate of clinically severe pulmonary embolism up to 4.77 per million passenger arrivals, with the frequency rising as the distance flown exceeds 2500 km (1550 mi) (33).

V. Assessment of In-Flight Oxygenation

Because federal regulations limit the cabin altitude pressure to < 8000 ft, this altitude represents a reasonable "worst case" from which to asses the exposure risk. Different strategies have been proposed to predict Pa_{O_2} during flight and therefore determine the need for oxygen supplementation. These strategies have included actual measurement of oxygenation during air travel (altitude stress test), simulation of exposure to high altitude (hypobaric simulation and hypoxia altitude simulation tests), or, more conveniently, use of prediction equations and associated nomograms.

A. Altitude Stress Test

The altitude stress test involves actual monitoring of oxygen levels during air flight with noninvasive pulse oximetry (34,35) or with blood gas sampling at altitude (36–38). While more accurate than other approaches, these tests are more practically used during aeromedical evacuation of injured or sick patients

(34,35,37) and have limited applicability in the management of patients with lung disease who wish to travel.

B. Hypobaric Chamber

Exposing individuals on the ground to hypobaric hypoxia can closely approximate the physiological effects of air travel. Several studies have evaluated the use of hypobaric chambers (12,39,40). While potentially more accurate, hypobaric chambers are neither widely available nor cost-effective, making the test impractical outside of research studies to validate more readily available tests, or facilities where chambers are used for other clinical purposes (e.g., military sites).

C. Hypoxia Altitude Simulation Test

The hypoxia altitude simulation test (HAST) replicates the inspired partial pressure of oxygen (P_{IO_2}) at altitude by asking the traveler to inhale a hypoxic mixture. At an altitude of 8000 ft, the P_B is around 560 torr [Eq. (1)], corresponding to a P_{IO_2} of 108 torr [Eq. (4)]. Substituting a P_B of 760 torr for ground level, an equivalent P_{IO_2} can be calculated with an F_{IO_2} of 15%. For a lower altitude of 5400 ft, an equivalent F_{IO_2} of 17% can be calculated. Similarly, using an oxygen analyzer calibrated at ground level, Aldrette and Aldrette determined the lowest oxygen concentration during flight at a cabin pressure ranging between 6050 and 8450 ft to correspond to an equivalent oxygen concentration of 15.2% (41). These hypoxemic gases can be premixed or customized and administered via a mouthpiece with a nose clip. An alternative technique is to use a commercially available Venturi device to allow entrainment of room air by a nitrogen gas flow, resulting in a range of hypoxic gas mixtures (42). This latter technique also allows determination of the oxygen supplementation rate required to correct the resultant hypoxemia (42).

HAST has been used to reproduce hypoxemia in patients with a wide range of lung diseases, (42–46) and accurately reflects values obtained during actual air travel (38) and hypobaric exposure (39). An additional advantage is that unlike sea level Pa_{O_2}, HAST correlates well with altitude Pa_{O_2} even when performed up to 4 months before the flight (38,47).

D. Prediction Equations

The simplest method to predict the Pa_{O_2} during air travel is to estimate in-flight Pa_{O_2} by transposing the expected cabin pressure in the alveolar air equation (48). However appealing, this technique does not take into account the variability of ventilatory and cardiac responses to altitude in patients with advanced lung disease, and consequent alterations in ventilation/perfusion relationships that may affect the reliability of a calculated Pa_{O_2}. Other sources of variability include variable cabin pressure, duration of flight, variability in the disease, and nature of the disease.

Table 2 Prediction Equations for In-flight Pa_{O_2}

First Author	Pa_{O_2} at altitude	r^a
Henry (36)	$20.38 - 3.0 \times CA + 0.67 \times Pa_{O_2\ ground}$	0.83
Gong (13)	$22.8 - 2.74 \times CA + 0.68 \times Pa_{O_2\ ground}$	0.94
Dillard (49)[b]	$0.410 \times Pa_{O_2\ ground} + 17.652$	0.59
Dillard (49)[b]	$0.519 \times Pa_{O_2\ ground} + 11.855 \times FEV_1 - 1.760$	0.85
Dillard (49)[b]	$0.453 \times Pa_{O_2\ ground} + 0.386 \times (FEV_1\%\ pred) + 2.440$	0.85
Dillard (50)[c]	$Pa_{O_2\ ground} \times e^{-[0.02002 - (0.00976) \times (FEV_1)] \times (P_{I_{O_2}\ ground} - P_{I_{O_2}\ altitude})}$	0.83
Dillard (50)[c]	$Pa_{O_2\ ground} \times e^{-[0.01731 - (0.00019) \times (FEV_1\%\ pred)] \times (P_{I_{O_2}\ ground} - P_{I_{O_2}\ altitude})}$	—

Key: CA, cabin altitude in thousands of feet; $Pa_{O_2\ ground}$, Pa_{O_2} at ground level in mmHg; FEV_1, forced expiratory volume in the first second in liters; FEV_1 %pred, percent of predicted FEV_1; $P_{I_{O_2}\ ground}$ and $P_{I_{O_2}\ altitude}$, pressure of inspired oxygen at ground and altitude level, respectively.
[a] Pearson correlation coefficient between measured and predicted Pa_{O_2} at altitude.
[b] Predict Pa_{O_2} at an altitude of 8000 ft.
[c] Allows prediction of altitude Pa_{O_2} in individuals whose ground evaluation is performed at elevations above sea level.
Source: Adapted from Ref. 29.

In several studies, a ground-level Pa_{O_2} was found to be a good predictor of altitude Pa_{O_2} when obtained shortly before simulated (13,43,49) or actual air travel (37,38) (Table 2). The timing of the blood draw appears to be important. For instance, one study found no correlation between ground-level Pa_{O_2} and altitude Pa_{O_2} unless the ground-level Pa_{O_2} was drawn within 2 hr of the flight (38). Similarly, in other reports, a ground-level Pa_{O_2} obtained as recently as 3 weeks before the flight could not accurately determine in-flight Pa_{O_2} (37,47).

Studies by Dillard et al. have found that both ground level Pa_{O_2} and FEV_1 are significant predictors of altitude Pa_{O_2} (49,50). More specifically, the addition of FEV_1 to the model improves the prediction of altitude Pa_{O_2} (49). These results were confirmed in a subsequent metanalysis of studies in which both ground-level and simulated Pa_{O_2} values were available (50). The authors speculated that FEV_1 acted as a surrogate of markers that could affect the altitude Pa_{O_2} independently of ground Pa_{O_2} such as ventilatory drive, age, and ventilation/perfusion matching (50). However, in other studies, altitude Pa_{O_2} was not correlated with FEV_1, FVC, or DL_{CO} (13,37).

Prediction equations should be used with caution because they may not generalize to populations that differ from those in which they have been derived. Most of those equations have studied patients with stable COPD, and patients with restrictive disease may have more significant desaturation than patients with obstructive impairment (15). Also, in other studies, the calculated Pa_{O_2} at altitude overestimated the Pa_{O_2} as assessed by a hypoxic inhalation test (51) or by a hypobaric chamber evaluation (44). This underscores the variability of some lung disease and the impact of medications on the predictive accuracy of those equations. Finally, prospective validation of those equations is needed.

VI. Fitness to Fly and Oxygen Supplementation

For most healthy individuals exposed to altitudes of 8000 to 10,000 ft, the drop in arterial oxygen pressure (Pa_{O_2}) to 50 to 60 mmHg with arterial oxygen saturation between 80 and 90% is well tolerated (19). Guidelines for air travel by patients with COPD generally recommend that arterial oxygen pressure be maintained above 50 mmHg (52) or 55 mmHg (53), with oxygen supplementation recommended for anticipated drops below those levels. In one HAST study, sea-level Pa_{O_2} values of 68 and 72 mmHg adequately identified over 90% of patients who developed a Pa_{O_2} of greater than 55 mmHg at 5000 and 8000 ft, respectively (13). Similarly, in a study by Cottrell, a sea-level Pa_{O_2} of > 70 mmHg was required to maintain adequate saturation at 6214 ft (7). Based on these findings, current recommendations are that a preflight Pa_{O_2} of > 70 mmHg is adequate to allow air travel without supplemental oxygen (53). However, these guidelines do not address the effects of ambulating at altitude and are not uniformly accepted. For instance, in altitude chamber tests of COPD subjects with an $FEV_1 < 50\%$ and a sea-level $Pa_{O_2} > 70$ mmHg, 53% could be expected to develop a $Pa_{O_2} < 55$ mmHg at a simulated altitude of 8000 ft (44). Moreover, 86% of those individuals had a $Pa_{O_2} < 55$ mmHg during light ambulation at this altitude (44).

A simple and potentially more accurate assessment of fitness to fly may be the patient's capacity to exercise. In one study, all patients with a maximal oxygen consumption during a graded bicycle test of >12.1 mL/min/kg had a Pa_{O_2} of > 50 mmHg at 8000 ft of simulated altitude (44). Similarly, the ability to walk 50 yards or climb a flight of stairs has been recommended to assess fitness to fly (53–55).

Oxygen supplementation should aim for a minimum Pa_{O_2} of 50 to 55 mmHg during flight (19,55,56). Although direct assessment of the required oxygen flow rate is feasible during HAST (42), it is often empirically set. In patients with COPD and a mean FEV_1 of 31%, oxygen at 4 L/min at 8000 ft of hypobaric simulated altitude augmented the Pa_{O_2} by 34.9 mmHg, an increase that exceeded by nearly 10 mmHg the ground-level Pa_{O_2} (57). Oxygen via a Venturi mask at 24 and 28% did not cause mean Pa_{O_2} to increase above ground-level value (57). For individuals not using oxygen at sea level, empirically giving 2 L/min is therefore usually adequate (52,53,56). For those already receiving oxygen, increasing the flow rates by 1 to 2 L/min has been recommended (55).

A special case warranting further discussion is that of the patient undergoing air medical transport. In this case, the following equation can be used:

$$F_{I_{O_2} \text{altitude}} = F_{I_{O_2} \text{ground}} \times P_{B\text{ground}} / P_{B\text{altitude}} \qquad (5)$$

where $P_{B\text{altitude}}$ is the cabin pressure at altitude which can be easily determined from Eq. (1) or from tables (1).

For patients with higher oxygen requirements, the maximum altitude of equal oxygenation can be estimated by placing the patient on 100% oxygen ($FI_{O_2 altitude} = 1$) and using Eq. (5) to determine $PB_{altitude}$, from which the maximal tolerable cabin altitude can be determined (1).

VII. Practical Considerations

Careful planning is necessary for the individual with lung disease anticipating travel. Such planning is particularly necessary given the lack of standard regulations for the medical use of oxygen in airports and aboard commercial aircraft and the variability in oxygen policies, costs, and services among commercial air carriers (55,58).

A. Interactions with Physicians

A physician can assess fitness to travel and need for in-flight oxygen and can assist in completing the forms required by airlines and in providing names of physicians at destinations and layover sites in case of need. A physician can also provide prescriptions, including emergency medications such as antibiotics or corticosteroids in case of exacerbation. Certification letters specifying the diagnosis, whether the traveler needs oxygen, and, if so, the flow rate and whether it is continuous, may be required. Several copies may be needed depending on the number of segments on the trip. The airlines may require a standard IATA medical information form (MEDIF), usually available from travel agents, airlines, or airline websites for this purpose. This form contains two parts: one to be completed by the passenger or his or her travel agent/ airline sales office and another part to be completed by the passenger's physician if required. The form is confidential and used by the airline's medical department to assess fitness to travel and to accommodate the patient's special needs. For individuals who need frequent medical clearance, a standard IATA Frequent Traveler's Medical Card (FREMEC) can be registered in computer booking systems for physical travel requirements. As an alternative to a personal physician's evaluation, some airlines may refer prospective travelers to a medical evaluation service, which will provide the necessary certifications.

B. Interactions with Air Carriers and Travel Agents

Current U.S. Federal Aviation Administration regulations prohibit travelers from using their own portable oxygen systems on board commercial aircraft. While many airlines provide medical oxygen, the policies on oxygen needs and its costs vary substantially among airlines. The traveler (rather than insurance companies) often assumes the costs of in-flight oxygen (29,58). The prospective traveler requiring on-board oxygen would therefore be well advised to consider these charges when planning travel and selecting airlines and to contact airlines

Table 3   Practical Tips for Planning Travel for the Patient Requiring In-flight Oxygen

Interaction with physician
Determine whether need for in-flight oxygen exists.
Get multiple copies of:
- Letter describing condition
- Liter flow and duration of in-flight oxygen
- Medication prescriptions

Consider emergency supply of antibiotics, corticosteroids.
Ascertain names of physicians en route to and at destination.
Get summary of medical records including ECG tracings.

Interaction with air carrier/travel agent
Questions to ask airlines:
- Does the airline accommodate patients who need oxygen?
- Are there charges for providing oxygen?
- Does the airline provide nasal cannulas or masks?
- What is the liter flow capability of in-flight equipment?
- What is the required documentation?
- Is special assistance available?

Notify of need for oxygen ≥ 48 hr before flight.
Fly nonstop if possible or with direct flight as an alternative.
- Less inconvenient
- Less expensive (especially if oxygen cost is per coupon)

Travel during business hours so vendor personnel are available.
Prearrange motorized cart or wheelchair if layover is scheduled.
Try to be seated near lavatory on plane.
Call airline at least 48 hr before flight to confirm.
Consider using a travel agent specializing in travel for patients with medical needs.

Interaction with oxygen vendor
Favor a company that has or can arrange nationwide coverage.
Arrange for oxygen during layovers (if needed).
Try to learn the type of systems that will be supplied (i.e., to check adapters).

Personal planning for travel day and during travel
Arrives at least 1 1/2 hr early
- Must pay for oxygen on day of travel
- Charge is either per coupon or per canister

Bring your own nasal cannula and extra length of tubing.
Pack medications in carry-on luggage.
Have multiple copies of prescriptions.
Some first aid stations may have oxygen if not otherwise available.
Have cash (to pay for oxygen if needed).
Avoid alcohol and heavy meals.

Source: Adapted from Ref. 29.

early regarding their policies, requirements, and fee structures. As an example of the variation among carriers, the oxygen service fee may depend on the number of flight segments (flight coupons) or on the number of oxygen cylinders used. Also, at least 48 hr of advance notice is required by most airlines for domestic on-flight oxygen, but some carriers require longer advance notice. Some suggestions are (1) arrange travel during business hours to ensure that the personnel from vendor companies are available to deliver oxygen supplies at layover sites or at the final destination, (2) choose nonstop flights if possible or direct flights (where the layover does not necessitate a change of plane) to reduce inconvenience and added cost of oxygen (depending on the fee structure of the airline), (3) prearrange special transportation needs at layover sites or destination, and (4) choose seating near the lavatory.

C. Interactions with the Oxygen Vendor

Oxygen is usually no longer necessary once the plane lands unless the patient is routinely on oxygen at home or if the destination is at an elevated altitude that would necessitate initiation of oxygen. In the latter case, the patient's physician can best make a determination of oxygen need at destination with the same methods as those used for determination of in-flight oxygen need. The airline will provide only on-board oxygen and an oxygen vendor should be contacted in advance to ensure that oxygen is available at layovers or at the destination site. Vendors that can offer such off-site services or those with a nationwide network may be preferable.

D. Personal Planning on Travel Day

The traveler should come early to ensure that all arrangements are in place and to process the oxygen service charge at the ticket counter, as this procedure may require as much as 20 min to complete (19). Medications (in their original container), prescriptions, physician's letters, a summary of medical records, and possibly electrocardiogram (ECG) tracings should be readily available in the carry-on luggage. A nasal cannula, extra length of tubing, different adapters or connectors, and even tape may be needed to ensure that the patient's delivery device interfaces with the aircraft's oxygen source (19). If oxygen is needed at the airport and prearrangements have not been made or are not available, oxygen may be obtained at the airport's First Aid station, though an informal poll suggests that only 35% of these stations can provide oxygen (29). Heavy meals and alcohol should be avoided before and during the trip.

VIII. Future Directions

There is a trend for increased travel by air by patients with lung disease who may be at risk for in-flight complications. For instance, it has been estimated that 19% of individuals with COPD travel by air at least once per year (30). Moreover, many cystic fibrosis patients now survive into adulthood and consider travel by air (59). About 62% of in-flight emergencies (27) and 20% of deaths (25) occur in individuals with a pre-existing condition directly or indirectly related to the event. Yet as many as 73% of individuals with COPD initiate air travel without prior medical consultation (30). Inasmuch as there may be different approaches to such patients in determining or improving fitness to fly, it is important to secure early medical evaluation and/or treatment to optimize travel candidacy. These approaches may include intensified chest physiotherapy in patients with cystic fibrosis (59) or close evaluation of exercise tolerance and oxygen needs of individuals with COPD.

Whether the responsibility for promoting preflight evaluation rests with the patient, physician, or the airlines is unclear, but physicians may need to be more proactive. For instance, in one survey, fewer than 76% of physicians routinely offered advice, and while most of the others offered advice on request, approximately 8% gave no advice (60). A recognized problem is the lack of evidence-based guidelines for recommending in-flight oxygen. The current methods for determining the risk of hypoxemia during flight and the need for oxygen vary widely. Moreover, these methods are not uniformly applied, with few physicians using predictive equations or hypoxic challenge tests (60).

As expected from the lack of uniform regulations for the medical use of oxygen in airports and aboard commercial aircraft, the availability, costs, and ease of implementing in-flight oxygen vary greatly among commercial air carriers (55,58). The American Medical Association Council on Scientific Affairs has recommended a revision of federal regulations to accommodate passengers who require oxygen and to facilitate an uninterrupted source of oxygen from departure to destination (55).

Last, better studies of in-flight medical emergencies and of the quality of the delivered care are needed. Such endeavors will require standardized and industrywide data on the frequency and cost of emergencies and related diversions, and on the outcome including following hospital admissions (28).

IX. Summary

Medical complications attributable to air travel remain rare. However, current trends suggest that there will be further increases in the number of travelers at risk for complications, with pulmonary conditions accounting for about 10% of in-flight emergencies and hypoxemia for a majority. Prearranged on-board oxygen may therefore be useful, though few patients seek medical advice and many physicians do not routinely offer it to prospective passengers. The best available evidence suggests that a ground-level $Pa_{O_2} > 70$ mmHg usually indicates no need for in-flight supplemental oxygen unless the FVC is < 50% of predicted value or activity tolerance is limited (unable to walk 50 yards or climb a flight of stairs). Individuals with ground level $Pa_{O_2} < 70\,mmHg$ and those with poor activity tolerance or $FVC < 50\%$ should be evaluated for oxygen need, ideally by a hypoxia altitude simulation test (HAST) if available. An alternative would be to evaluate stable and adequately treated patients with the use prediction equations that incorporate the FEV_1 and a room air Pa_{O_2} value from a blood gas obtained as close as possible to the actual travel. If the HAST or prediction equations indicate a flight Pa_{O_2} of < 50 to $55\,mmHg$, then $2\,L/min$ O_2 via nasal cannula should be prescribed for the flight. For individuals already on oxygen at ground level, increasing the flow rates by 1 to $2\,L/min$ has been recommended.

Close interactions with the physician, the air carrier, and the oxygen vendor are necessary. Future directions should include promotion of preflight evaluation, better evidence-based guidelines for recommendation of in-flight oxygen for patients with a variety of lung disorders, revision of federal regulations to facilitate an uninterrupted oxygen supply from departure to destination, and better studies of in-flight medical emergencies and of delivered care. Revising the 8000-ft-altitude-equivalent ceiling and structural modifications of aircraft hulls to achieve lower altitude pressures are options that should await objective and strong outcome measures before implementation.

References

1. Blumen IJ, Abernethy MK, Dunne MJ. Flight physiology. Clinical considerations. Crit Care Clin 1992; 8(3):597–618.
2. Martin L. Abbreviating the alveolar gas equation: an argument for simplicity. Respir Care 1986; 31(1):40–44.
3. Sheffield PJ, Heimbach RD. Respiratory physiology. In: DeHart RL, ed. Fundamentals of Aerospace Medicine. Philadelphia: Lea & Febinger, 1985.
4. Mohler SR. Physiologically Tolerable Decompression Profiles for Supersonic Transport Type Certification. AM 70–12. Washington, DC: US Federal Aviation Administration, Office of Aviation Medicine, 1970.
5. Stoller JK. Oxygen and air travel. Respir Care 2000; 45(2):214–221.
6. The Airliner Cabin Environment: Air Quality and Safety. Washington, DC: National Academy Press, 1986.
7. Cottrell JJ. Altitude exposures during aircraft flight. Flying higher. Chest 1988; 93(1):81–84.
8. Rudge FW. Variations in the presentation of altitude-induced chokes. Aviat Space Environ Med 1995; 66(12):1185–1187.
9. Brown JR, Antuñano MJ. Medical Facts for Pilots: Altitude-Induced Decompression Sickness. Publication AM-400-95/2. Oklahoma City, OK: FAA Civil Aeromedical Institute, Aeromedical Education Division, 1995.
10. Rudge FW. Decompression sickness in a private pilot. South Med J 1995; 88(2):227–229.
11. Neubauer JC, Dixon JP, Herndon CM. Fatal pulmonary decompression sickness: case report. Aviat Space Environ Med 1988; 59(12):1181–1184.

12. Dillard TA, Rajagopal KR, Slivka WA, Berg BW, Mehm WJ, Lawless NP. Lung function during moderate hypobaric hypoxia in normal subjects and patients with chronic obstructive pulmonary disease. Aviat Space Environ Med 1998; 69(10):979–985.

13. Gong H Jr, Tashkin DP, Lee EY, Simmons MS. Hypoxia-altitude simulation test. Evaluation of patients with chronic airway obstruction. Am Rev Respir Dis 1984; 130(6):980–986.

14. Knutson SW, Dillard TA, Mehm WJ, Phillips YY. Effect of upright and supine posture on hypoxemia during air transport. Aviat Space Environ Med 1996; 67(1):14–18.

15. Vea H, Aasebo U. Experiences of pulmonary disease on jet planes. Tidsskr Nor Laegeforen 1990; 110(10):1219–1220.

16. Berg BW, Dillard TA, Derderian SS, Rajagopal KR. Hemodynamic effects of altitude exposure and oxygen administration in chronic obstructive pulmonary disease. Am J Med 1993; 94(4):407–412.

17. Nesthus TE, Garner RP, Mills SH, Wise RA. Effects of simulated general aviation altitude hypoxia on smokers and nonsmokers. Final Report DOT/FAA/AM-97/7. Washington, DC: Federal Aviation Administration, Office of Aviation Medicine, 1997.

18. Hansen JE. Diet and flight hypoxemia. Ann Intern Med 1989; 111(10):859–860.

19. Gong H. Air travel and oxygen therapy in cardiopulmonary patients. Chest 1992; 101(4):1104–1113.

20. Cordain L, Bryan ED, Melby CL, Smith MJ. Influence of moderate daily wine consumption on body weight regulation and metabolism in healthy free-living males. J Am Coll Nutr 1997; 16(2):134–139.

21. Wolkove N, Fu LY, Purohit A, Colacone A, Kreisman H. Meal-induced oxygen desaturation and dyspnea in chronic obstructive pulmonary disease. Can Respir J 1998; 5(5):361–365.

22. Cummins RO, Schubach JA. Frequency and types of medical emergencies among commercial air travelers. JAMA 1989; 261(9):1295–1299.

23. Speizer C, Rennie CJ, III, Breton H. Prevalence of in-flight medical emergencies on commercial airlines. Ann Emerg Med 1989; 18(1):26–29.

24. Skjenna OW, Evans JF, Moore MS, Thibeault C, Tucker AG. Helping patients travel by air. Canadian Medical Association Journal 1991; 144(3):287–293.

25. Cummins RO, Chapman PJ, Chamberlain DA, Schubach JA, Litwin PE. In-flight deaths during commercial air travel. How big is the problem? JAMA 1988; 259(13):1983–1988.

26. Cottrell JJ, Callaghan JT, Kohn GM, Hensler EC, Rogers RM. In-flight medical emergencies. One year of experience with the enhanced medical kit. JAMA 1989; 262(12):1653–1656.

27. Hordinsky JR, George MH. Response capability during civil air carrier inflight medical emergencies. Aviat Space Environ Med 1989; 60(12):1211–1214.

28. DeJohn CA, Veronneau S.J.H., Hordinsky JR. Inflight Medical Care: An Update. Final Report DOT/FAA/AM-97/2. Washington, DC: Federal Aviation Administration, Office of Aviation Medicine, 1997.

29. Stoller JK. Travel for the technology-dependent individual. Respir Care 1994; 39(4):347–360.

30. Dillard TA, Beninati WA, Berg BW. Air travel in patients with chronic obstructive pulmonary disease. Arch Intern Med 1991; 151(9):1793–1795.

31. Richards PR. The effects of air travel on passengers with cardiovascular and respiratory diseases. Practitioner 1973; 210(256):232–241.
32. Hordinsky JR, George MH. Utilization of Emergency Kits by Air Carriers. Final Report DOT/FAA/AM-91/2. Washington, DC: Federal Aviation Administration, Office of Aviation Medicine, 1991.
33. Lapostolle F, Surget V, Borron SW, Desmaizières M, Sordelet D, Lapandry C, Cupa M, Adnet F. Severe pulmonary embolism associated with air travel. N Engl J Med 2001; 345(11):779–783.
34. Bendrick GA, Nicolas DK, Krause BA, Castillo CY. Inflight oxygen saturation decrements in aeromedical evacuation patients. Aviat Space Environ Med 1995; 66(1):40–44.
35. Kramer MR, Jakobson DJ, Springer C, Donchin Y. The safety of air transportation of patients with advanced lung disease. Experience with 21 patients requiring lung transplantation or pulmonary thromboendarterectomy. Chest 1995; 108(5):1292–1296.
36. Graham WG, Houston CS. Short-term adaptation to moderate altitude. Patients with chronic obstructive pulmonary disease. JAMA 1978; 240(14):1491–1494.
37. Henry JN, Krenis LJ, Cutting RT. Hypoxemia during aeromedical evacuation. Surg Gynecol Obstet 1973; 136(1):49–53.
38. Schwartz JS, Bencowitz HZ, Moser KM. Air travel hypoxemia with chronic obstructive pulmonary disease. Ann Intern Med 1984; 100(4):473–477.
39. Dillard TA, Moores LK, Bilello KL, Phillips YY. The preflight evaluation. A comparison of the hypoxia inhalation test with hypobaric exposure. Chest 1995; 107(2):352–357.
40. Rose DM, Fleck B, Thews O, Kamin WE. Blood gas-analyses in patients with cystic fibrosis to estimate hypoxemia during exposure to high altitudes in a hypobaric-chamber. Eur J Med Res 2000; 5(1):9–12.
41. Aldrette JA, Aldrette LE. Oxygen concentrations in commercial aircraft flights. South Med J 1983; 76(1):12–14.
42. Vohra KP, Klocke RA. Detection and correction of hypoxemia associated with air travel. Am Rev Respir Dis 1993; 148(5):1215–1219.
43. Chi-Lem G, Perez-Padilla R. Gas exchange at rest during simulated altitude in patients with chronic lung disease. Arch Med Res 1998; 29(1):57–62.
44. Christensen CC, Ryg M, Refvem OK, Skjonsberg OH. Development of severe hypoxaemia in chronic obstructive pulmonary disease patients at 2,438 m (8,000 ft) altitude. Eur Respir J 2000; 15(4):635–639.
45. Cramer D, Ward S, Geddes D. Assessment of oxygen supplementation during air travel. Thorax 1996; 51(2):202–203.
46. Oades PJ, Buchdahl RM, Bush A. Prediction of hypoxaemia at high altitude in children with cystic fibrosis. Br Med J 1994; 308(6920):15–18.
47. Schwartz JS. Hypoxemia during air travel. Ann Intern Med 1990; 112(2):147–148.
48. Apte NM, Karnad DR. Altitude hypoxemia and the arterial-to-alveolar oxygen ratio. Ann Intern Med 1990; 112(7):547–548.
49. Dillard TA, Berg BW, Rajagopal KR, Dooley JW, Mehm WJ. Hypoxemia during air travel in patients with chronic obstructive pulmonary disease. Ann Intern Med 1989; 111(5):362–367.
50. Dillard TA, Rosenberg AP, Berg BW. Hypoxemia during altitude exposure. A meta-analysis of chronic obstructive pulmonary disease. Chest 1993; 103(2):422–425.

51. Lebzelter J, Fink G, Kleinman E, Rosenberg I, Kramer MR. Preflight assessment by hypoxic inhalation test in cardiopulmonary patients. Harefuah 2000; 138(8):635–639, 711.
52. American Thoracic Society. Standards for the diagnosis and care of patients with chronic obstructive pulmonary disease. Am J Respir Crit Care Med 1995; 152(5 pt 2):S77–S121.
53. Aerospace Medical Association, Air Transport Medicine Committee. Medical guidelines for air travel. Aviat Space Environ Med 1996; 67(10 suppl):B1-B16.
54. Harding RM, Mills FJ. Aviation medicine. Problems of altitude I: Hypoxia and hyperventilation. Br Med J (Clin Res Ed) 1983; 286(6375):1408–1410.
55. Lyznicki JM, Williams MA, Deitchman SD, Howe JP. Medical oxygen and air travel. Aviat Space Environ Med 2000; 71(8):827–831.
56. Lien D, Turner M. Recommendations for patients with chronic respiratory disease considering air travel: a statement from the Canadian Thoracic Society. Can Respir J 5(2):95–100.
57. Berg BW, Dillard TA, Rajagopal KR, Mehm WJ. Oxygen supplementation during air travel in patients with chronic obstructive lung disease. Chest 1992; 101(3):638–641.
58. Stoller JK, Hoisington E, Auger G. A comparative analysis of arranging in-flight oxygen aboard commercial air carriers. Chest 1999; 115(4):991–995.
59. Kamin WE, Fleck B, Rose D. Intensified physiotherapy improves fitness to fly in cystic fibrosis patients. Eur J Med Res 2000; 5(9):402–404.
60. Coker RK, Partridge MR. Assessing the risk of hypoxia in flight: the need for more rational guidelines. Eur Respir J 2000; 15(1):128–130.

21

Advanced Lung Disease
End-of-Life Care

JOHN HANSEN-FLASCHEN

University of Pennsylvania School of Medicine
Philadelphia, Pennsylvania, U.S.A.

I. Introduction

Chronic lung disease is the fourth leading cause of death in the United States, accounting primarily for more than 110,000 deaths a year. Most of these deaths are anticipated and occur after prolonged suffering. Most people who die of chronic lung disease pass through the care of one or more physicians who specialize in pulmonary medicine. Yet it is unclear how much pulmonologists contribute to their terminal care. Review of the literature suggests that the contribution may be limited. Until recently, next to no articles could be found in Medline-accessible journals focusing specifically on the terminal and palliative care of patients with advanced lung disease. Two recently published books on death and dying in critical care units begin to close this gap in the medical literature (1,2).

This article outlines an approach to the palliative care of patients who are dying of advanced lung disease. Recent identification of six attributes of a "good death" derived from interviews with terminally ill patients and their caregivers provides a framework for care. Palliation begins with frank disclosure of a poor prognosis based on statistical evidence. Mutual understanding that death may be near sets the stage for medical advanced planning, not only of life support but also of other issues of concern to patient and family. Symptomatic management is paramount and should address dyspnea, cough, pain, insomnia, anxiety, depression, and delirium. Hospice referral should be considered when a terminally ill patient is largely confined to a bedroom and in need of the specialized services offered by hospice. Because sustained dyspnea at rest is distressing to caregivers as well as patients and is difficult to manage, the option of terminal hospitalization for symptom control and hygiene should be kept open, even for those who express a preference to die at home.

II. Attributes of a Good Death

A study published by Steinhauser and colleagues provides a framework for palliative and terminal care of adults who suffer from an irreversible progressive chronic disease (3). To identify attributes of a good death, these authors convened 12 focus groups, each averaging 6 adults, drawn from the university and local communities of Durham, North Carolina. Participants included physicians, nurses, chaplains, social workers, patients, and recently bereaved family members who ranged in age from 26 to 77 years. Focus group meetings were conducted, audiotaped, transcribed, and analyzed using accepted techniques of qualitative research. From this process, six components of a good death were identified (Table 1). Most important was pain and symptom management. Patients and family members expressed a strong desire to avoid needless suffering. Patients also wanted clear, timely decision making and participation in treatment decisions. To prepare for death, they wanted to know what to expect, and they wanted to plan for the events that would likely precede and follow their deaths. Participants conveyed the importance of spirituality and meaningfulness at the end of life as well as the importance of life review and closure of unresolved issues with family and friends. People want to continue contributing to others as long as possible, and they want to be understood by others as unique and whole persons, even as their function declines. Interwoven through all of these components is the importance of uninhibited, two-way communication with family members, close friends, and caregivers.

III. Prognosis

Consideration of palliative care begins with a frank discussion about prognosis (4). For at least 2500 years, the thoughtful provision of an accurate medical prognosis has been one of the most important and difficult services provided by physicians. In the fifth century B.C., Hippocratic physicians distinguished themselves from other competing schools of health care largely by offering their patients a prognosis that was based on an understanding of disease as a natural process. At that time, a physician's reputation was determined largely by his ability to predict the outcome of an illness or injury. Even to this day,

Table 1 Components of a "Good Death"

Recent qualitative research has identified the following six attributes of a good death as commonly perceived by terminally ill patients and their caregivers (3):
1. Pain and symptom management
   People fear dying unattended in distress.
2. Clear decision making
   Patients feel empowered by participating in treatment decisions.
3. Preparation for death
   Many patients want to know what to expect during the course of their illness. They want to plan for the events that precede and follow death.
4. Completion
   Completion includes faith and spiritual experiences and also life review, resolution of conflicts, spending time with family and friends, and saying good-bye.
5. Contributing to others
   Many people want to contribute to the well-being of others, even as they decline and die.
6. Affirmation of the whole person
   Terminally ill patients appreciate empathic caregivers who understand their current condition in the context of their lives, values, and preferences as whole and unique persons.

patients judge physicians to a considerable extent by how well or poorly they address the question of prognosis. Yet remarkably, for many years until the mid 1960s, clinicians in the United States routinely withheld a poor prognosis from their patients to spare them the pain of bad news. Today, full disclosure of diagnosis and prognosis is the standard of practice across North America and western Europe. Nevertheless, obstacles continue to arise that interfere with full disclosure of poor prognosis in chronic or progressive illness.

A. Obstacles to Talking Frankly About Prognosis

The first of these is cultural. Many physicians in eastern Europe, South America, and the Far East continue to withhold or soften disclosure of a fatal prognosis. Some people who come from those locations still expect physicians in western nations to do the same. Thus, physicians are sometimes asked by family members to refrain from revealing knowledge of a terminal condition to a patient.

How should a physician respond to those requests? One approach is to consider the adverse effects of withholding material information about prognosis. Might the withholding of the diagnosis or prognosis undermine the patient's trust in the physician? Will the patient or others be placed unknowingly at risk from certain behaviors that are not appropriate for the diagnosis or prognosis? Will the physician be restrained from answering questions about the purpose of proposed or potential future medical interventions? Will the patient not be able to participate in important decisions about his or her medical care or personal affairs?

Under some circumstances, the answers to these and other related questions may be no. For example, if the physician is asked as a one-time consultant to provide an opinion on a specific issue not directly related to a terminal condition or prognosis or if a hospitalized patient requires urgent attention for severe distress or is cognitively impaired, disclosure of the overall prognosis might not be immediately relevant to the task at hand. In such situations, it may be reasonable for the physician not to volunteer information about prognosis while still reserving the authority to answer questions honestly and completely if asked directly by the patient.

If the withholding of information about diagnosis or prognosis at the request of a family member is likely to compromise a continuing relationship between physician and patient, the physician should ask why he or she is being asked not to provide the information. The discussion that ensues may lead to a mutually acceptable plan. If not, the physician might best serve the patient by declining to enter into an ongoing professional relationship, "I feel so strongly about this that I am probably not the right doctor for your [relative]. If you wish, I will see him this once to answer his questions and yours."

A second obstacle to complete disclosure of prognosis arises commonly in the care of young adults afflicted by chronic, fatal, inherited diseases such as cystic fibrosis and muscular dystrophy. Despite awareness for many years that they are expected to die prematurely, many such people are understandably unable to telescope a full life experience into a substantially shortened time span. Mention of death by a physician rekindles strong emotions of betrayal and anger in young adults, "Why am I to be deprived?" They may grow silent and look away or change or close the subject, "I don't want to talk about that." Family members report afterwards that the patient was unhappy about the conversation. Overcoming this obstacle sometimes requires full exploration of the feelings and beliefs that underlie an expressed reluctance to talk about death—a task that is beyond the ability or time constraints of many physicians in subspecialty medical practice. Barring such an exploration, younger patients should not be drawn reluctantly into advance medical planning. Instead, the physician might respond to initial resistance by saying, "If you want to talk with me about dying and what you would want, let me know, and we'll set up a special time."

A third obstacle to full disclosure of a poor prognosis rests with the patient's expectations and fears. People seek out and reward physicians who offer hope. In turn, physicians tend to promote hope by offering some treatment—no matter how marginally efficacious—and describing that treatment in the most positive possible terms, "With a positive attitude, at least I can offer a little placebo effect." Hope is preserved in this way, at least temporarily, but attention to planning for death is deferred or denied.

A fourth obstacle is particularly germane to advanced lung disease. Physicians do not know how long an individual will live. Relative to lung cancer, the prognosis for many chronic, progressive lung diseases is particularly uncertain (5–7). Chronic obstructive pulmonary disease (COPD), for example, progresses at a slow rate that varies considerably among individuals and within individuals over time. Most patients who suffer from COPD die not from intractable respiratory failure but rather from some unanticipated acute event, such as bronchitis, pneumonia, pulmonary embolism, myocardial infarction, or stroke. For that reason, the 95% confidence interval around the median survival of a group of patients with advanced COPD is particularly broad. Indeed, among 19 indications for referral to hospice, only dementia has a more uncertain prognosis than COPD (5,8). Out of fear of being wrong, physicians may try to avoid the subject of prognosis altogether or give unhelpful answers when asked, such as "I can't possibly predict; now let's talk about your colchicine treatment."

B. Approach to Conveying a Prognosis

Estimation of prognosis begins with identification of a cumulative survival curve for a group of patients who are most comparable to the individual patient (6,7). The expected median survival can be adjusted to a limited extent by additional knowledge about the patient, such as age, current performance status, and rate of progression of disease or intercurrent illness. For example, the median survival for patients with the usual interstitial pneumonitis (UIP) form of idiopathic pulmonary fibrosis (IPF) from the time of surgical lung biopsy is about 3 years (9). If a patient with advanced IPF also has severe three-vessel coronary artery disease and uncontrolled angina, the median survival for a similarly afflicted group of patients is likely to be less than 2 years.

This information should be presented to the patient in a straightforward manner that is not unduly framed to encourage a false impression. For example, "Idiopathic pulmonary fibrosis is a fatal condition, but survival is somewhat unpredictable. About half of patients with your condition live longer than 3 years, and will live 4 to 6 years or even longer. Half live less than 3 years. Some may die within weeks or a few months after diagnosis." Speak slowly and pause afterwards to invite a response. Encourage hope, not by offering therapy of doubtful benefit but by moving beyond prognosis to discussion of measures the patient, family, and physician can take to maximize quality of life and minimize suffering. Then come back to prognosis. Realistic expectations for a terminal illness are so important and so easily misinterpreted that it is useful to test the patient's comprehension later in the conversation or early in a subsequent visit, "I want to be sure that you understand. How would you explain your prognosis to someone else?"

IV. Advance Medical Planning

For more than 20 years, the primary tool in the United States for planning care near the end of life has been the medical advance directive (10,11). These legal documents were introduced in the late 1970s as a way for physicians to obtain protection from litigation and prosecution in the event that someone challenged the decision to withhold or withdraw life support. Reflecting their legal origins, advance directives were often called "living wills" or "durable powers of attorney." Thousands of court cases later, the fear of legal sanction that gave rise to these documents is no longer justified in the United States provided that physicians act in the best interests of their patients with full regard for their expressed or imputed wishes (12). From a current perspective, conventional written directives perform a limited planning function at best (12–15). Standardized, preprinted forms, signed at the kitchen table and filed away in safe deposit boxes, frequently enter late into medical decision making if at all. Except for some patients who fall unexpectedly into permanent unconsciousness, standardized medical directives often serve to validate rather than drive decisions actually made for patients by others.

Given these considerations, experts in end-of-life care are increasingly recommending a primarily medical approach to advance planning for preterminal health care that is directed by the patient's principal physician and constrained but not dictated by legal concerns (12). Unfortunately, many physicians continue to delay or avoid substantive discussions regarding terminal care. In agreement with several previous studies, a recent survey of Canadian pulmonologists revealed that many respondents initiated discussions about mechanical ventilation late in the progression of advanced lung disease if at all (16). This practice is counter to patients expectations. In a survey of pulmonary rehabilitation patients, virtually all of the study participants expressed interest in discussing end-of-life decisions with their physicians (17).

Given the inherent unpredictability of survival for many advanced lung diseases, preparation for dying should be considered when death is anticipated within about a year or when a patient with advanced lung disease is being prepared for a major therapeutic intervention such as lung reduction surgery or lung transplantation. The door to medical advance planning opens with frank disclosure of prognosis. If the patient does not then raise the subject of planning for terminal care, the physician should do so. Physicians can open a discussion of medical advance planning without implying that death is necessarily imminent by stating simply, "It is good to hope for and expect the best, but it is also wise to prepare for the worst." If initial reticence is encountered, the physician might respond with, "I share your hope—we plan to get you through. But bad things happen. I don't think you want to dump all the decision making on your family members if you get suddenly very sick. That won't be good for you or for them."

Medical advance planning is best pursued as a three-way conversation between a patient, the patient's designated medical proxy, and the patient's principal physician. Preferably the discussion should be held in an outpatient setting during a visit scheduled for this purpose. The physician might begin with a brief statement about the purpose of the meeting and the patient's current condition or prognosis. Then the physician should turn to the patient with an open-ended invitation to speak, "I expect that you have been thinking about this meeting. What are your thoughts?" Other helpful, open-ended questions include, "What are your hopes for the future?" and "What are your greatest concerns and fears?" Answers to these broad questions remind physicians that patients with advanced lung disease often have other concerns that may be more important to them than the technical aspects of medical life support or cardiopulmonary resuscitation. The patient's surrogate is given an opportunity to speak next. Finally, the physician raises or clarifies specific medical decisions that should be considered in advance. The characteristics of a good death identified by Steinhauser et al. (Table 1) can serve as a general guide for the discussion.

Depending on the circumstances, four practical issues are often appropriate for shared decision making between patient, family, and physician in meetings devoted to advance planning for terminal care (Table 2). First, is the patient likely to die at home or in an institutional setting? Many who express a desire to die at home considerably underestimate the associated effort and expense and the degree of expertise necessary to ensure their comfort and hygiene (18). Victims of advanced lung disease may be confined to bed on and off or continuously for weeks or months before they die. For some or much of this time, they cannot be left unattended. With rare exceptions, health insurance policies do not provide for prolonged, continuous bedside care at home. Because of work or family commitments or their own health care needs,

Table 2 Issues for Advance Medical Planning

---

1. Discuss the most appropriate location for terminal care: the patient's or a family member's home versus an institutional setting.
2. Identify preferred providers for terminal home or institutional care.
   a. Home care organization
   b. Acute care hospital
   c. Skilled nursing facility
3. Determine patient preferences for initiation and termination of life support.
   a. Should mechanical ventilation be initiated in the event of respiratory failure?
   b. Terminal withdrawal of life support in the event of irreversibly impaired consciousness?
   c. Terminal withdrawal versus institutional care in the event of prolonged dependency on mechanical ventilation?
4. Plan for anticipated "what ifs," such as
   a. "What if I find him unconscious on the kitchen floor?"
   b. "What if she starts coughing up blood again?"

---

many family members are ill equipped to provide this level of home care for longer than a few days. Consequently, the physician should focus this component of medical advance planning on the caregivers. What level of care can they realistically support at home?

Often the appropriate answer is an open one that anticipates possible or probable conversion from to home to institutional care at some time during the progression of the illness. Three-way agreement on this point helps to allay the guilt of family members if a patient who prefers home care ultimately dies in a hospital or a nursing home. This point also sets the stage for a second goal of medical advance planning, which is to identify preferred providers for home or institutional skilled nursing care. By preparing in advance, the patient and family members establish a relationship with one or more selected organizations that are then prepared to provide service on short notice. For a patient who is expected to die, a full-service home care organization that includes an accredited hospice is often most appropriate.

Because patients with advanced lung disease rarely experience sudden cardiac arrest, discussions regarding cardiopulmonary resuscitation with this group of patients should focus primarily on ventilatory support. There are limited choices to consider—these should be laid out in the same manner that a physician describes options for the treatment of lung cancer. A patient with advanced emphysema might, for example, be guided through the following options as a starting point for discussion: (1) home care only; (2) hospitalize if indicated for comfort care, but do not initiate mechanical ventilation or other major life support; (3) initiate appropriate life support, to be continued only so long as the physician and the proxy both believe there is a reasonable chance for recovery to functional independence; and (4) indefinite life support so long as the patient retains the potential for self-awareness, to be continued in a chronic nursing facility if necessary. These options encompass a spectrum in the timing and circumstances of a transition from life-sustaining to palliative care that can be refined by further discussion. If the patient favors a limited trial of life support (third option), the role of the patient, the proxy and the physician in the decision to abandon the trial is clarified. If the patient chooses indefinite ventilatory support (fourth option), the impact of that decision on the patient's financial resources and family should be discussed openly.

If the planning session predates major surgery such as lung transplantation or lung volume reduction surgery, the physician should discuss the special considerations that apply to intraoperative and immediate postoperative care (11). In the perioperative period, the need for cardiopulmonary resuscitation or other life-supporting interventions often has a more favorable prognostic significance than at other times. Indeed, many surgeons and anesthesiologists consider perioperative life support an integral component of the surgical procedure itself. If, as is often recommended, the patient's general preferences are to be suspended at the time of surgery, the transition back to those preferences should be discussed in advance.

Family members who provide home care for terminally ill patients are often concerned about certain "what ifs." "What should I do if I find him unconscious on the kitchen floor?" "What if she starts coughing up blood again?" Not every eventuality can be anticipated and planned. Nevertheless, home caregivers appreciate guidance in advance on how they should respond if an uncontrolled or frightening situation develops suddenly or at an inconvenient hour. Who should be called? Should the patient be transported urgently to an emergency room? How should the patient's preferences be communicated to emergency personnel? This planning is essential to respect the wishes of those patients who want to limit life support, and particularly those who prefer to die at home.

Shortly after completion of initial discussions, the patient ideally or the proxy or physician should write a brief summary of the decisions that were made in the form of a letter or declaration. In addition to defining the role of the proxy and the primary physician in medical decision making should the patient become incapacitated, the document lays out goals of therapy, limitations on treatment that can be identified in advance, and outcomes to be avoided. If circumstances warrant, the document can then be modified in form, with the help of a lawyer, to meet the requirements of applicable state laws. In addition to the patient, both the proxy and the physician might also sign the document, indicating that they will do their best to ensure that the patient's stated wishes are fulfilled. Copies should be filed by all three participants in readily accessible locations. If surgery is planned, a copy should be provided to the surgeon for further discussion during a preoperative meeting.

This approach offers several advantages. Unlike a standardized form completed at home, an advance planning agreement reached by three-way discussion benefits from the guidance and advice of the physician and is tailored to the patient's individual circumstances. Just as importantly, the initial discussion opens lines of communication among the three key decision makers that can be continued for the duration of the patient's life. During the planning discussion, the patient can ensure that both the proxy and the primary physician are in agreement with the plan. The three-way discussion, as documented in the summary statement, serves as a foundation for negotiations between proxy and physician at the time decisions must be made, thereby maintaining focus on the patient's preferences. Also, a written advance directive prepared in this way empowers the principal physician to play an active role in medical decision making if the patient is hospitalized under the care of another physician.

V. Hospice Home Care

Patients with advanced lung disease should be encouraged to consider hospice home care (19–21). The hospice movement developed in the United States primarily as an extension of medical oncology. Even today, many hospices report that most of their patients suffer from incurable cancer (8), even though terminally ill patients with diagnoses other than cancer are also likely to benefit from home care and professional assistance (22,23). Although many hospices welcome patients with other diagnoses, they receive relatively few referrals of patients with advanced lung disease. Indeed, patients with COPD comprised only 3.1% of a representative group of Medicare beneficiaries enrolled in hospice programs in 1990 (22). The reason is unclear but may relate in part to common misperceptions about hospice among physicians who care for patients with advanced lung disease.

Prior to enrollment in a hospice program, Medicare and most other insurers require that the patient sign an agreement indicating understanding and acceptance of the hospice approach to palliative health care. Also, the referring physician and the hospital medical director both must certify that the patient is expected to die within 6 months.

Because of the uncertainties associated with determining such a prognosis, in 1996 an expert committee of the National Hospice Organization issued criteria to help physicians identify patients with nonmalignant terminal illnesses, including advanced lung disease (24). The Health Care Financing Administration (HCFA) codified the guidelines in 1997 into auditable criteria by which Medicare intermediaries are to judge the appropriateness of hospice referral (25). These criteria have been used by the Office of Inspector General in a campaign to reduce fraud and abuse by hospice organizations known as Operation Restore Trust. Specialists in respiratory medicine recognize inconsistencies within the HCFA hospice review policy for pulmonary diseases. The criteria are not evidence based. Prognostic criteria derived from the guidelines failed to distinguish patients enrolled in the SUPPORT study (26) who died within 6 months after hospital discharge from those who did not (8). Indeed, no set of criteria have yet been devised that confidently identify medically stable patients with advanced lung disease who will die within 6 months.

Fortunately, there is no penalty to patients for failing to die within 6 months. Given the uncertainty inherent in prognosis for advanced lung disease, Abrahm and Hansen-Flaschen (20) have proposed three alternative "commonsense" guidelines for referral to hospice that are not based directly on predicted duration of survival (Table 3). These guidelines target patients with advanced, irreversible lung disease who have little or no cardiopulmonary reserve and are likely to benefit from the specialized services offered by hospices.

In the United States, certified home hospices receive a fixed daily payment from Medicare Part A for the comprehensive care of qualifying patients (approximately $110 per day for routine hospice home care and approximately $580 per day for short-term continuous home care). All medical expenses other than physician's fees are covered by the payment, including the cost of medications, supplies, durable medical equipment, and long-term

Table 3 Referral to Hospice: Commonsense Guidelines for Patients with Advanced Lung Disease

1. Despite an adequate trial of therapy, cardiopulmonary reserve has been exhausted by progressive disease such that death can occur at any time.
2. Because of distressing symptoms or a severely limited performance status, the patient can be expected to benefit from the specialized services offered by hospice programs.
3. The patient accepts the fact that death may be near and does not want to suffer needlessly.

Source: Ref. 20.

oxygen. Home assessment, education, and counseling are provided by nurses, social workers, dietary counselors, pastoral counselors, and therapists as appropriate. Telephone consultation and coordination of care is often available 24 hr per day. Home health aides are typically provided for 2 or 3 hr a day. Home nursing care may be available for up to 24 hr a day during a medical crisis. Some hospices provide volunteers for transportation to a doctor's office or to cover family care givers for short trips out of the house. Brief hospitalizations for symptom control and up to several days of inpatient respite care to provide caregivers with personal time may also be covered by the hospice program.

Hospice coverage lapses during longer-term residential care or acute-care hospitalization for reasons other than palliation of the major illness. However, hospice care can be renewed repeatedly provided the patient is recertified each time as terminally ill. Many private insurers provide comparable coverage.

The flexibility of the Medicare hospice benefit serves many terminally ill patients well. Unfortunately, Medicare capitated payments for hospice services work against some patients with advanced lung disease who are dependent on unusually expensive therapies. The high cost of home mechanical ventilation and such drugs as nebulized tobramycin, transplant immunosuppression drugs, dornase alpha, and epoprostenol (prostacyclin) effectively preclude enrollment in hospice, especially for those who already incur the expense of home oxygen. Continuous intravenous prostacyclin infusion is especially problematic in that patients with severe pulmonary hypertension risk sudden death if this drug is discontinued even momentarily. Thus, most Medicare patients with severe pulmonary hypertension must relinquish their hospice benefit for life in order to receive intravenous prostacyclin because few hospice organizations can afford the cost of this treatment in addition to other hospice services.

Terminally ill patients who are unwilling to enroll in a hospice program may obtain some of the same benefits from a visiting nurse agency, although most insurers restrict the quantity and duration of palliative home care services available by this route.

VI. Dying at Home

Although most patients with advanced lung disease express a desire to die at home, relatively few in North America actually do so. Unless a fatal complication supervenes, many spend an extended period of time confined to bed completely dependent on others for sustenance, hygiene, and comfort. Constant attendance and considerable skill are often required. Dyspnea at rest and accompanying anxiety/panic are distressing to onlookers and difficult to manage, even under the best of circumstances. Hospice programs can provide considerable support, including 24-hr-a-day bedside care for a few days. For others, the patient may best be served by terminal hospitalization. Provided that the intent is palliative, these hospital admissions are covered on a per diem rather than capitated basis by the Medicare hospice benefit. Some hospitals have established specialized inpatient units specifically for this purpose (27). To avoid undesired invasive emergency care, this possibility should be planned for in advance whenever possible.

Funeral arrangements are also best planned in advance. Many older Americans appreciate the opportunity to discuss their own preferences for funeral arrangements. In the event that a person dies at home, a mortuary service can be summoned at the time of death. The presence of a physician is not required. The funeral home can arrange for the physician to complete the death certificate at a convenient time afterwards.

Physicians who learn palliative care recognize that death is not a failure but an opportunity to practice a form of professional care that is as old as medicine and as gratifying as any other service we offer.

References

1. Curtis JR, Rubenfeld GD, eds. Managing Death in the ICU: The Transition from Cure to Comfort. Oxford, UK: Oxford University Press, 2000.
2. Seymore JE. Critical Moments—Death and Dying in Intensive Care. New York: Open University Press, 2001.
3. Steinhauser KE, Clipp, EC, McNeilly M, et al. In search of a good death: observations of patients, families, and providers. Ann Intern Med 2000; 132:825–832.
4. Christakis NA. Prophecy and Prognosis in Medical Care. Chicago: University of Chicago Press. 1999.
5. Fox, E, Landrum-McNiff, K, Zhong, Z, et al. Evaluation of prognostic criteria for determining hospice eligibility in patients with advanced lung, heart, or liver disease. JAMA 1999; 282:1638–1645.
6. Herbst LH. Prognosis in advanced pulmonary disease. J Palliat Care 1996; 12:54.
7. Manaker S, Tino G. Natural history and prognosis of advanced lung disease. Clin Chest Med 1997; 18:435–455.

8. Fox E, Landrum-McNiff K, Zhong Z, et al. Evaluation of prognostic criteria for determining hospice eligibility in patients with advanced lung, heart, or liver disease. JAMA 1999; 282:1638–1645.

9. Bjoraker JA. Ryu JH. Edwin MK. Myers JL, et al. Prognostic significance of histopathologic subsets in idiopathic pulmonary fibrosis. Am J Respir Crit Care Med. 1998; 157:199–203.

10. Emanuel LL. Structured advanced planning: is it finally time for physician action and reimbursement? JAMA 1995; 274:510.

11. Cohen C, Cohen P. Do-not-resuscitate orders in the operating room. N Engl J Med 1991; 325:1879.

12. Gillick M. A broader role for advance medical planning. Ann Intern Med 1995; 123:621.

13. Kapp M. State statutes limiting advanced directives: death warrants or life sentences? J Am Geriatrics Soc 1992; 40:722.

14. Danis M, Multran E, Garrett J, et al. A prospective study of the impact of patient preferences on life-sustaining treatment and hospital cost. Crit Care Med 1996; 24:1811.

15. Schneiderman L, Pearlman R, Kaplan R, et al. Relationship of general advanced directive instructions to specific life-sustaining treatment preferences in patients with serious illnesses. Arch Intern Med 1992; 152:2114.

16. Sullivan KE, Hebert PC, Logan J, et al. What do physicians tell patients with end-stage COPD about intubation and mechanical ventilation? Chest 1996; 109:258.

17. Heffner J, Fahy B, Hilling L, Barbieri C. Attitudes regarding advance directives among patients in pulmonary rehabilitation. Am J Respir Crit Care Med 1996; 154:1735.

18. Emanuel EJ, Fairclough DL, Slutsman J, et al. Assistance from family members, friends, paid caregivers, and volunteers in the care of terminally ill patients. 1999; 341:956–63.

19. Byock I. Hospice and palliative care: a parting of ways or a path to the future? J Palliat Med 1998; 1:165–175.

20. Abrahm J, Hansen-Flaschen J. Hospice care for patients with advanced lung disease. Chest 2002; 121:220–229.

21. Rhymes J. Hospice care in America. JAMA 1990; 264:369–372.

22. Christakis NA, Escarce JJ. Survival of Medicare patients after enrollment in hospice programs. N Engl J Med 1996; 335:172–178.

23. von Gunten CF, Twaddle ML. Terminal care for noncancer patients. Clin Geriatr Med 1996; 12:349–358.

24. Stuart B, Alexander C, Arenella C, et al. Medical Guidelines for Determining Prognosis in Selected Non-cancer Diseases. 2nd ed. Arlington, VA: National Hospice Organization, 1996.

25. Medicare Part A Intermediary Hospice Medical Policy Manual. Determining terminal status in non-cancer diagnoses: pulmonary disease, Policy Identifier 98007. Revised, April 9, 1999. Assessable at: http://www.wellmedicare.com/provider/lmrp/meda.htm.

26. SUPPORT Principal Investigators. A controlled trial to improve care for seriously ill hospitalized patients. The study to understand prognoses and preferences for outcomes and risks of treatments (SUPPORT). JAMA 1995; 274:1591.

27. Fainsinger R, Miller M, Bruera E, et al. Symptom control during the last week of life on a palliative care unit. J Palliat Care 1991; 7:5.

AUTHOR INDEX

Italic numbers give the page on which the complete reference is listed.

Z

SUBJECT INDEX

A

Air travel, 711–730
  fitness to fly/oxygen supplementation,
    722–723
  in-flight oxygenation, assessment of,
    719–721
  oxygen pressures, altitude and, 712–713
  physiology, 713–715
  practical considerations, 723–727
  risks of, 715–719
Anxiety/depression, 661–683
  anxiety, 667–676
    adjustment disorder, 670
    generalized anxiety disorder, 669–670
    management, 671–676
      cognitive/behavioral, 671–674
      pharmacological, 674–676
    panic attack/panic disorder, 668–669
    posttraumatic stress disorder, 670–
      671
  coping strategies, 662–667
  depression, 676–681
    diagnosis, 677

[Anxiety/depression]
    management, 677–681
    pharmacotherapy, 679–681
    prevalence, 676
    psychotherapy, 678–679
Autoimmune pulmonary disease, 39–43,
    205 (*see also* individual diseases)
  histopathology, 41–43
  pathological patterns, 43

B

Bronchiectasis, 17–21
  bronchoscopy, 350
  causes of, 18, 342–343
  clinical features, 346–349
    physical examination, 346
    pulmonary function tests, 348
    radiology, 346–347
    symptoms, 346
  congenital, 18
  definition, 17
  diagnosis, 349–350
  diffuse, 343–346